Venous and Lymphatic Diseases

Venous and Lymphatic Diseases

edited by

Nicos Labropoulos
New Jersey Medical School
Newark, New Jersey, U.S.A.

Gerard Stansby
University of Newcastle upon Tyne
Newcastle upon Tyne, U.K.

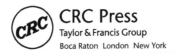

CRC Press
Taylor & Francis Group
Boca Raton London New York

CRC Press is an imprint of the
Taylor & Francis Group, an **informa** business

CRC Press
Taylor & Francis Group
6000 Broken Sound Parkway NW, Suite 300
Boca Raton, FL 33487-2742

First issued in paperback 2019

© 2010 by Taylor & Francis Group, LLC
CRC Press is an imprint of Taylor & Francis Group, an Informa business

No claim to original U.S. Government works

ISBN-13: 978-0-8247-2923-3 (hbk)
ISBN-13: 978-0-367-39085-3 (pbk)

A CIP record for this book is available from the British Library.

Library of Congress Cataloging-in-Publication Data available on application

Visit the Taylor & Francis Web site at
http://www.taylorandfrancis.com

and the CRC Press Web site at
http://www.crcpress.com

Preface

"The best preparation for tomorrow is to do today's work superbly well."
—*William Osler (1849–1919)*

The new millennium is an exciting time to be involved with the care of venous disorders, and there have probably been more key advances in the last 20 years than in the previous 200. Despite this, phlebology remains a relatively under-represented specialty in many countries, and there is sometimes a lack of high-quality data and access to training materials. As a result, sufferers of venous and lymphatic problems are often inadequately investigated or mismanaged. This is a situation that cannot be allowed to continue. Venous and lymphatic diseases are both common and distressing for suffers. They also impose a large financial burden on the health services of most industrialized countries. These alone are reasons why the topic is worthy of study, and patients have the right to be seen by physicians and nurses with a special interest in the management of their condition.

This book, *Venous and Lymphatic Diseases*, is an attempt to draw together a wide range of experts in various aspects of venous disease to cover the full range of conditions encountered in clinical practice. The aim has been to produce chapters that are both definitive and readable, so that they will be of utility to both the expert in the subject and the novice. To aid this, most chapters have a clear "key points" section. In addition, we have deliberately chosen to invite a mixture of North American and European authors to produce a genuinely international, multidisciplinary approach to the subject. The book is subdivided and organized into related sections and includes sections on investigation as well as treatment, including complex venous surgery and radiological therapies. However, it has been the deliberate aim of the editors that this should not simply be a surgical textbook; as a result, there are extensive sections on non-surgical topics, including drug therapy, venous disorders in pregnancy, compression therapy, and conservative therapies in lymphedema. The first three chapters set the scene by reviewing the historical context, the anatomical terminology, and the physiology of the veins and lymphatics.

If the book is useful to those involved in caring for patients with venous or lymphatic disease, then we will have accomplished our aim.

ACKNOWLEDGMENT

The editors express their sincere thanks to the contributors who have given so much of their valuable time to produce their sections. Thanks also go to Geoff Greenwood who initially saw the need for such a book and who was pivotal in taking the idea forward to fruition.

Nicos Labropoulos
Gerard Stansby

Contents

SECTION F: OTHER VENOUS CONDITIONS

Contributors

Yues S. Alimi Service de Chirurgie Vasculaire, Centre Hospitalier Universitaire Nord, Marseille, France

Sachiendra V. Amaragiri Freeman Hospital, University of Newcastle upon Tyne, Newcastle upon Tyne, U.K.

Enrico Ascher Division of Vascular Surgery, Department of Surgery, Maimonides Medical Center, Brooklyn, New York, U.S.A.

Ahmad Bhatti Division of Vascular Surgery, Loyola University Medical Center, Maywood, Illinois, U.S.A.

Paul H. Blair Regional Vascular Surgery Unit, Royal Victoria Hospital, Belfast, Northern Ireland

Marc Borge Interventional Radiology, Department of Radiology, Loyola University Medical Center, Maywood, Illinois, U.S.A.

Alberto Caggiati Department of Anatomy, University "La Sapienza," Rome, Italy

Bruce Campbell Royal Devon and Exeter Hospital, Exeter, U.K.

Joseph A. Caprini Feinberg School of Medicine, Northwestern University, Chicago, Illinois; Evanston Northwestern Healthcare, Evanston, Illinois; and Glenbrook Hospital, Glenview, Illinois, U.S.A.

Keith F. Cutting Vascular Unit, Ealing Hospital, Southall, U.K.

Michael C. Dalsing Indiana University School of Medicine, Indianapolis, Indiana, U.S.A.

Gudmundur Danielsson Department of Vascular Diseases, Lund University, Lund, Sweden

Alun H. Davies West of London Vascular Service, Charing Cross Hospital, London, U.K.

Meryl Davis West of London Vascular Service, Charing Cross Hospital, London, U.K.

Linda de Cossart   Countess of Chester, NHS Foundation Trust, Chester, U.K.

Walter N. Durán   New Jersey Medical School, Newark, New Jersey, U.S.A.

Ronald K. G. Eifell   Department of Vascular and General Surgery, Queen Elizabeth Hospital, Gateshead, U.K.

Bo Eklöf   Department of Vascular Diseases, Lund University, Lund, Sweden

Anna Falanga   Department of Haematology–Oncology, Ospedali Riuniti, Bergamo, Italy

F. G. R. Fowkes   Wolfson Unit for Prevention of Peripheral Vascular Diseases, University of Edinburgh, Edinburgh, U.K.

George Geroulakos   Vascular Unit, Ealing Hospital, Southall, and Department of Vascular Surgery, Imperial College, London, U.K.

Athanasios D. Giannoukas   University of Thessaly Medical School and Division of Vascular Surgery, University Hospital of Larissa, Larissa, Greece

Jonathan Golledge   School of Medicine, James Cook University, Townsville, Queensland, Australia

Hany Hafez   St. Richard's Hospital, Chichester, U.K.

George Hamilton   University Department of Surgery, Royal Free Hospital, UCL and Royal Free Medical School, London, U.K.

Denis W. Harkin   Regional Vascular Surgery Unit, Royal Victoria Hospital, Belfast, Northern Ireland

Olivier Hartung   Service de Chirurgie Vasculaire, Centre Hospitalier Universitaire Nord, Marseille, France

Anil Hingorani   Division of Vascular Surgery, Department of Surgery, Maimonides Medical Center, Brooklyn, New York, U.S.A.

Claude Juhan   Service de Chirurgie Vasculaire, Centre Hospitalier Universitaire Nord, Marseille, France

Stavros K. Kakkos   Vascular Unit, Ealing Hospital, Southall, U.K.

Steven S. Kang   South Miami Heart Center, Miami, Florida, U.S.A.

Patrick Kesteven   Department of Haematology, Freeman Hospital, Newcastle upon Tyne, U.K.

Shankat N. Khan   Northern Vascular Centre, Freeman Hospital, Newcastle upon Tyne, U.K.

Nicos Labropoulos   Vascular Laboratory, Division of Vascular Surgery, New Jersey Medical School, Newark, New Jersey, U.S.A.

Brajesh K. Lal   New Jersey Medical School, Newark, New Jersey, U.S.A.

Tim A. Lees   Department of Vascular Surgery, Freeman Hospital, Newcastle upon Tyne, U.K.

Luis Leon   Division of Vascular Surgery, Loyola University Medical Center, Maywood, Illinois, U.S.A.

Sumaira Macdonald   Northern Vascular Centre and the Department of Radiology, Freeman Hospital, Newcastle upon Tyne, U.K.

Derek Manas   Hepatic Surgery Unit, Freeman Hospital, Newcastle upon Tyne, U.K.

James E. McCaslin   Department of Vascular and General Surgery, Queen Elizabeth Hospital, Gateshead, U.K.

Jonathan Michaels   Department of Vascular Surgery, University of Sheffield, Sheffield, U.K.

Peter Neglén   River Oaks Hospital and University of Mississippi Medical Center, Jackson, Mississippi, U.S.A.

Ian Nichol   Department of Vascular Surgery, The James Cook University Hospital, Middlesbrough, U.K.

Klaus Overbeck   Northern Vascular Centre, Freeman Hospital, Newcastle upon Tyne, U.K.

Frank T. Padberg, Jr.   New Jersey Health Care System–Veterans Affairs Medical Center, East Orange, New Jersey, U.S.A.

Simon Palfreyman   Department of Vascular Surgery, University of Sheffield, Sheffield, U.K.

Peter J. Pappas   New Jersey Medical School, Newark, New Jersey, U.S.A.

Michel Perrin   University of Lyon, Lyon, France

Andrea Piccioli   Department of Medical and Surgical Sciences, University of Padua, Padua, Italy

Paolo Prandoni   Department of Medical and Surgical Sciences, University of Padua, Padua, Italy

Seshadri Raju   River Oaks Hospital and University of Mississippi Medical Center, Jackson, Mississippi, U.S.A.

Jill Robson   Freeman Hospital, Newcastle upon Tyne, U.K.

Frank C. T. Smith   Bristol Royal Infirmary, Bristol, U.K.

Philip D. Coleridge Smith   Royal Free and University College Medical School, London, U.K.

Gerard Stansby   University of Newcastle upon Tyne, Newcastle upon Tyne, U.K.

Sriram Subramonia   Northern Vascular Centre, Freeman Hospital, Newcastle upon Tyne, U.K.

Alok Tiwari   University Department of Surgery, Royal Free Hospital, UCL and Royal Free Medical School, London, U.K.

Fiona J. Tsang   West of London Vascular Service, Charing Cross Hospital, London, U.K.

Dereck W. Wentworth   U.S. Medical Affairs, New York, New York, U.S.A.

Robert W. Zickler   UMDNJ–New Jersey Medical School, Newark, New Jersey and New Jersey Health Care System–Veterans Affairs Medical Center, East Orange, New Jersey, U.S.A.

1
Historical Background

Alberto Caggiati

Department of Anatomy, University "La Sapienza," Rome, Italy

Venous disorders have been recognized since ancient times, although real knowledge came only with an understanding of the anatomy of the venous and lymphatic systems developed over many centuries. This hard-won knowledge still underpins any modern study of venous and lymphatic function in both health and disease.

THE "DISCOVERY" OF THE VENOUS DRAINING SYSTEMS

Meticulous but partial descriptions of the venous system are to be found in the works of Aristotle (384–322 BC), who described the vena cava and the superficial veins of the upper extremities. However, the real beginning of the study of vascular and lymphatic anatomy is due to Herophilus of Chalcedon (300–250 BC), a Greek physician living in Egypt. He practiced in Alexandria, where human dissections were permitted, even performing some in public. Herophilus furnished the first anatomical and functional discrimination between arteries and veins. In addition, he was the first to note and describe lacteals, which he observed in the mesentery of man. Galen of Pergamum (130–200 AD) subsequently described the course of the veins of the whole body and called the smallest vessels *"tricoidé,"* i.e., "hair-like." He confirmed that these small vessels connect arteries and veins throughout the body. He believed that blood originated in the liver and moved back and forth through the body, passing through the heart, where it was mixed with air ("pneuma") by pores in the septum. Galen also introduced the concept of the "spirit" system, consisting of natural spirit or "pneuma" (he thought air was found in the arteries), vital spirit (blood mixed with air found in the arteries), and animal spirit (which he believed to be found in the nervous system). The first complete and systematic description of the whole venous system was finally furnished by André Vesale (1514–1564) in the *De Humanis Corporis Fabrica*, illustrated by the magnificent drawings of Jan Stefan van Kalkan (Fig. 1).

A depiction of venous valves did not appear in the original *Fabrica*. They were first described in the renal, azygos, and external iliac veins by Giovanni Battista Canano (1515–1579) from Ferrara in 1540. They were included in the subsequent editions of the *Fabrica*. Many decades later, Hyeronimus Fabricius of Acquapendente (1533–1619) was

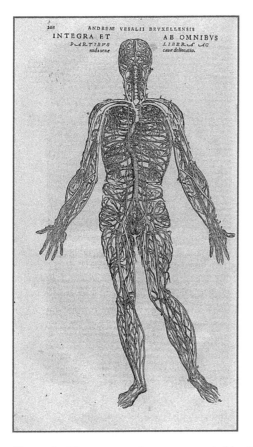

Figure 1   The venous system as represented by Vesale in his *Fabrica*.

the first to furnish a good description of the valves of the veins and of their role (Fig. 2). He was Harvey's teacher at Padua and undoubtedly must have stimulated his interest in the circulation of the blood.

A description of the perforating veins did not appear until two centuries later. In 1803, they were first described by Justus Christian Von Loder (Fig. 3). In 1824, Paul Briquet described the anatomy of the calf venous pump but believed that blood would be pushed by the calf pump from deep to superficial veins via the perforators. The correct hemodynamic role of perforators was finally stated by Aristide August Verneuil, a French surgeon, in 1855.

LYMPHATIC VESSELS

Herophilus (third century BC) mentioned the existence of the lymphatics. Bartolomeus Eustachii (1500–1574), Professor at *La Sapienza* University of Rome, described in 1563 the thoracic duct nearly a century before Pecquet (1651); *"...a whitish canal going from the clavicular area to lower parts...."* Sixty years later (1622) Gaspare Aselli (1581–1626) described the lymphatics. In a posthumous account published in 1627, he stated that lacteals contained milky or creamy fluid. Aselli described also the valves placed along lymphatics, especially at their confluences. His book *De Lactibus Sive Lacteis Venis*

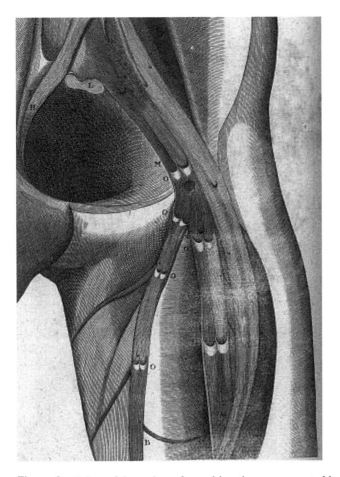

Figure 2 Valves of the sapheno-femoral junction as represented by Fabricius in 1603.

was published just before the *De Motu* of Harvey, who had not appreciated Aselli's discovery and perhaps was not aware of it. Paolo Mascagni (1752–1815) was prosector in anatomy at the University of Siena (Italy). In 1787, Mascagni published a large folio volume entitled *Vasorum lymphaticorum corporis humani historia et iconographia*. This important monograph contained the first systematic and definitive description of the human lymphatic system (Fig. 4). Mascagni has been credited with discovering some 50% of the lymphatic vessels.

THE "DISCOVERY" OF THE CIRCULATION OF THE BLOOD

William Harvey (1578–1657) is correctly credited with the "discovery" of the circulation of the blood. He proved that the heart receives and expels blood during each cycle by observing the action of the heart in small animals and fishes. By compressing the visible veins of the forearm, he simply but persuasively confirmed Fabricius' observation that the venous valves permitted flow in only one direction, toward the heart. But the concept of blood circulation was not new. In fact, Wang Shu So reported in the *Mei Ching* (China, third century AD) that *"the heart regulates all the blood in the body...The blood*

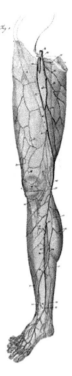

Figure 3 The first drawing in which perforators are reported (Van Loder, 1803).

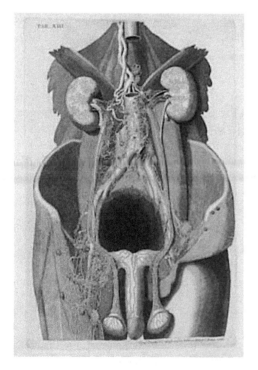

Figure 4 The lymph trunks of the pelvis and of the abdomen as represented by Mascagni (1787).

current flows continuously in a circle and never stops." The Spanish anatomist Ludovicus Vassaeus in 1544 depicted exactly the anatomy of the cardiovascular system and the flow direction in the main vessels. The Spanish theologian Miguel Servede, alias Servetus of Villanueva (1509–1553), described in 1564 the pulmonary circulation: he stated that the blood enters the lungs by the way of the pulmonary artery in greater quantities than necessary for their nutrition, mixes with the *"pneuma"* and returns by way of the pulmonary veins. The discovery of Servetus did not disseminate to contemporary physicians, probably because it was reported in a theological work. Andrea Cesalpino (1519–1603) from Arezzo, was Professor of Medicine at Pisa and at Rome. He first delineated that blood flows into the heart (*"…the blood enters the right ventricle by the vena cava…exit from the heart to open into the lungs…from the left ventricle opens the orifice of the aorta…"*). Furthermore, Cesalpino identified the function of the valves (*"…certain membranes placed at the openings of the vessels prevent the blood from returning…"*) and coined the term "circulation" supposing the existence of *"vasa in capillamenta resoluta."* Finally, Realdo Colombo (c. 1510–1577) from Cremona, successor of Vesalius as the chair of anatomy in Padua, furnished an exact description of the circulatory system, denying the previously suggested existence of porosity in the interventricular septum.

Harvey's theory of blood circulation was completely accepted only in 1661, when the Italian Marcello Malpighi (1628–1694) demonstrated using rudimentary microscopes, the existence and hemodynamic role of the capillaries. Mechanisms of venous return were better defined by: (1) Richard Lower, who emphasized the role of the muscular pump and theorized the *vis a tergo*: *"the return of the venous blood is the result of the impulse given to the arterial blood…,"* (2) Antonio Maria Valsalva, pupil of Malpighi and teacher of Morgagni, who in 1710 described the respiratory forces that enhance venous return to the heart: the *"vis a fronte,"* and (3) Giovanni Lancisi, who in 1728 demonstrated experimentally the spontaneous rhythmical contraction of the larger veins.

SCLEROTHERAPY

Sclerotherapy is based upon the observation reported in 1815 by Joseph Hodgson (1788–1869) who noted that *"thrombosis extinguished varicose veins."* Sclerotherapy developed after the invention of the hypodermic needle in 1845 by Francis Rynd and of the syringe by Pravaz in 1851. However, former attempts of venous cannulation were made by Francesco Folli (1623–1685) who in 1654 accomplished artero-venous blood transfusion by insertion of a silver tube into the artery of the donor and a bone cannula into the vein of the recipient, uniting the two by means of a tube especially made from an animal blood vessel. In 1665, Sigismond Johann Elsholz (1623–1688) used a chicken bone as a needle and the bladder of a pigeon as a syringe to irrigate ulcers by intravenous injection of distilled water or of essences from plants.

Many substances have been used to induce venous obstruction. Here are a few examples: Monteggio and De Leroy d'Etoilles (1840) proposed absolute alcohol for sclerotherapy. Pravaz (1851) used ferric chloride. Benedetto Schiassi from Bologna used a combination of iodine and potassium iodide. Kausche (1917) proposed inverted sugar for sclerotherapy of varicose veins. After having used sodium carbonate for 4 years, Sicard came to prefer sodium salicylate because *"it occluded varicose veins and, at the same time, it mitigated the arthritis that occurred in so many patients with varicose veins."* In 1921, Genevrier, a military surgeon, discovered that injection of quinine solution to treat malarial crisis could cause venous sclerosis. He suggested injecting a concentrated quinine solution in the diseased veins of malarial varicose patients thereby treating both diseases. In 1925, Linser of Dresden reported the use of a 20% solution of ordinary table salt to sclerose varicose veins.

Different techniques of venipuncture and strategies for sclerotherapy developed in the last century. Benedetto Schiassi from Bologna, was the first to perform intraoperative injections. In 1944, Horbach introduced the technique called "air block" to enhance the effects of sclerotherapy. In 1963, Fegan described his methods of sclerosing varicose veins based upon tight post injective compression and in the 1990s Shadek introduced the Duplex evaluation of the effect of sclerosing agents. Duplex monitoring has recently allowed the use sclerosing foam obtained chemically (Juan Cabrera) or by a mechanical procedure (Lorenzo Tessari).

SURGERY

Historically, venous surgery started in the second century BC with Heliodorus. He gave the first description of ligation and torsion of blood vessels to control hemorrhage. The Roman Celsus extirpated varicose veins with a blunt hook and used cauterization with a red hot iron. Oribasius of Pergamum (325–405 BC) was the first of the Byzantine surgeons who dealt with varicose veins. He devoted three chapters of his Book XLV to this subject and recommended: (1) shaving and bathing the leg to be operated, (2) with the leg still warm, the surgeon has to mark varicose veins with the patient standing (they marked them by small incisions!), (3) the use of a special hook, called a *cirsulce,* (4) to extirpate varicose vein of the lower leg firstly, then at the thigh, (5) to remove the veins because, if only ligated, they can form new varices.

"Open surgery" of varicose veins started with Paulus of Aegina (625–690). He recommended isolation of varicose veins at the thigh by a longitudinal incision, and, after bloodletting, to ligate them at both ends. The tied-off portion was excised or allowed to slough off later with the ligatures. Arab surgeons operated on varicose veins by cautery. Guglielmo Saliceti, from Piacenza (Italy), alias Williams of Saliceto (1210–1277), had the great merit of reintroducing the use of the knife into surgery, which had been abolished by the Arabs. Giovanni da Vigo (1460–1525), surgeon to Pope Julius II, ligated the veins *"...intromittendo acum sub vena desuper filium stringendo..."* (by introducing a needle beneath the vein and tightening the thread from above) (1514). In 1545, Ambroise Parè (1510–1590), after initially treating varicose veins by external cauterization (Arab tradition), reintroduced the use of ligature of varicose veins.

Modern venous surgery started with the Swiss surgeon Tommaso Rima (1777–1843), who was the first to propose in 1806, a hemodynamic treatment of varicose veins with ligation of the upper portion of the great saphenous vein, an operation generally credited to Trendelemburg (1896). In 1816, Sir Benjamin Collins Brodie (1783–1862) operated on varicose veins: *"...after the skin over a varix was incised, the varix was divided with a curved bistoury and pressure was applied to prevent haemorrhage....."* Alfred Armand Louis Marie Velpeau (1795–1864) introduced a pin or needle through the skin, which was passed underneath the vein, and at right angles to it. A twisted suture was then applied round the two ends of the pin, so as to compress the vein sufficiently to produce its obliteration. In 1877, Max Schede reported a technique for radical removal of varicosities based upon multiple ligature or venesections and percutaneous ligations. In 1884, Madelung proposed the complete excision of the great saphenous vein through a long incision much like those used today in vein harvest for coronary bypass. In 1906, Delbet proposed to treat varicose veins by re-implantation of the terminal portion of the great saphenous vein just below a healthy femoral valve.

In 1905, W.L. Keller described a rigid intraluminal stripper to extirpate the Great Saphenous Vein. Two years later, Babcock modified the technique of Keller and devised the acorn tip and used a flexible rod. Finally, in 1907 Mayo proposed an extraluminal ring stripper that was modified by Myers and Smith in 1947. In 1956, Robert Muller elaborated a modern technique for ambulatory stab avulsion of varicose veins. In 1963, Jean Van der Stricht described the "saphenectomy by invagination" refining similar techniques proposed in the past. Utilizing Duplex preoperative evaluation of the varicose bed, in 1988 Claude Franceschi proposed a minimally-invasive and conservative treatment of varicose veins designated with the acronym CHIVA ("conservative haemodynamic treatment of incompetent and varicose veins in the ambulatory patient").

Endovascular treatment of the Saphenous vein started in 1964 when Politowski destroyed varicosities by endovenous electrosurgical dessication. In 1972 Watts described the treatment of saphenous varicosities by endovenous diathermy. In 1981 Milleret and Le-Pivert proposed a freezing technique to treat saphenous insufficiency. In 1989, Puglisi and his colleagues of the School of Malan (Milan) firstly reported at the IUP Congress in Strasbourg, the use of endovenous Laser to treat varicose saphenous veins. At the end of the 1990s, radiofrequency probes were introduced into clinical practice to induce endovenous obliteration of the Saphenous veins.

Selective surgery of perforating veins was proposed in 1938 by R.R. Linton, who proposed a medial subfascial approach to treat incompetent perforating veins. In 1953, Cockett and Jones proposed the epifascial ligature of medial ankle perforators. Two years later, Felder recommended that subfascial incision for ligation of perforating veins should be placed in the posterior midline of the calf to avoid placing the lower end of the incision over the ulcer itself or in the compromised skin of the medial leg, the so-called "posterior stocking seam" approach. Bassi suggested avulsion of perforators by use of a hook. Finally, in 1985, Hauer performed the first subfascial endoscopic interruption of perforating veins.

2
Venous and Lymphatic Anatomy

Alberto Caggiati

Department of Anatomy, University "La Sapienza," Rome, Italy

THE ROOTS OF THE DRAINING SYSTEMS: THE MICROVASCULAR BED

The microvascular bed includes the terminal arterioles, the precapillary sphincters, the capillaries and the small venules. The microvascular bed also includes the initial lymphatics, the lymphatic capillaries and artero-venous anastomoses (AVA). The wall of the arterioles contains smooth muscle cells and these are the major site of systemic vascular resistance. The rhythmical contractile activity of the precapillary sphincter causes intermittent flow in the capillaries (vasomotion) and allows a large number of capillaries to remain open or closed for long periods. The walls of the capillaries are made up of flat endothelial cells lying on a basal lamina (BL) and oriented with the vessel's long axis. In some organs, capillaries have pericapillary cells (pericytes) imbedded within the BL, which play a contractile role. Endothelial cells secrete vasoconstrictor, vasodilator, mitotic agents, and their own BL.

Capillaries are drained by venules. Initially, the venular wall is strengthened by pericytes, then by smooth muscle cells, increasing in number and layers. Initial lymphatics are blindly ending tubes, 5–50 μm wide, making up a net of lymphatic capillaries. Their wall is made up of flat endothelial cells, a discontinuous BL and fine anchoring fibrils. The wall permits the capillary to drain water, solutes, cells or cellular remnants from the tissue spaces. Then, the lymph passes into larger and richly valvulated lymphatic vessels with a very thin wall composed of endothelium, basal lamina and collagen, with scattered smooth muscle cells.

The microvascular bed of some tissues (e.g., skin) contains direct connections between arterioles and venules. Such AVA allow blood to bypass the capillary bed. Accordingly, the flow in these shunts does not participate in transfer of gases, nutrients or wastes. The arrangement of these connections may be extremely simple (direct connections) or extremely complex, like in the skin, where AVA play an important role in heat regulation.

THE SUPERFICIAL VENOUS SYSTEM OF THE LOWER LIMB

The capillaries of the subcutaneous tissue are drained by two main venular plexuses. The more superficial is situated in the dermal papillae. The deeper venular plexus is placed

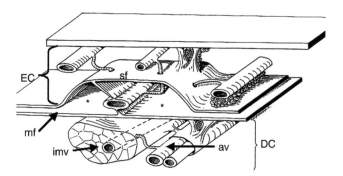

Figure 1 Planar anatomy of the veins of the lower limb. The saphenous compartment (*) is delimited by the saphenous fascia (sf) and the muscular fascia (mf) and hosts only the great saphenous vein. Epifascial veins course in the epifascial compartment (EC). The deep compartment (DC) hosts intramuscular veins (imv) and axial veins (av).

at the boundary between the papillary and the reticular layers of the dermis. These plexuses are drained by a tremendously complicated net of interconnected veins that lie superficially with respect to all the fasciae of the limb: the *epifascial veins* (Fig. 1) These are very thin-walled and run close to the dermis surrounded only by amorphous fat. For these reasons, epifascial veins are more prone to varicose changes (dilatation, elongation, and tortuosity). Epifascial veins are extremely variable in number, size, and path. Nevertheless, there is some order in their variability, because a few of them are quite constant in size, path, and connections. These have been designated in longitudinal and oblique groups (Table 1).

    Longitudinal epifascial veins are parallel to the saphenous veins (SVs) and richly connected with them. For these reasons, they have been designated "accessories" of the relative *saphenae*, and in order to allow their easy identification, they are discriminated on the basis of their topography [for the great SV: anterior,[a] posterior, and superficial accessories (Figs. 2 and 3); for the small SV: superficial accessory]. Besides the accessories of the saphenae, longitudinal epifascial veins also include the lateral venous plexus, whose veins course along the lateral leg and thigh.

    Oblique epifascial veins connect main longitudinal veins, SVs, or their accessories (Fig. 4). In the thigh, oblique veins are called "*circumflex veins*" due to their path. The *anterior thigh circumflex vein* (ATCV) connects the lateral venous plexus with the GSV. The *posterior thigh circumflex vein* (PTCV) originates from the SSV, from the lateral plexus, or from reticular veins of the posterior thigh to drain into the GSV or its posterior accessory. These veins are responsible for reflux transmission between the great and the small SVs.

    Interfascial (saphenous) veins course in an intermediate plane between epifascial and deep veins and are the *great saphenous vein* (GSV), the *small saphenous vein* (SSV), and its *thigh extension* (not mentioned in the CEAP). They course deeply in the subcutaneous tissue, close to the deep fascia (DF). They are covered by a continuous

---

[a] The anterior accessory of the GSV at the upper thigh, courses deeply (just above the muscular fascia, like the GSV) and below a hyperechoic fascia that resembles the GSV covering (Fig. 4). However, the AAGSV can be easily identified because it courses more anteriorly with respect to the GSV with a path corresponding to that of the underlying femoral artery and veins.

Table 1 Nomenclature of the Superficial Veins

Great saphenous vein:
Sapheno-femoral junction
Terminal valve
Pre-terminal valve
External pudendal vein
Superficial circumflexiliac vein
Superficial epigastric vein
Superficial dorsal vein of clitoris or penis
Anterior labial veins
Anterior scrotal veins
Anterior accessory of the great saphenous vein
Posterior accessory of the great saphenous vein
Superficial accessory of the great saphenous vein
Small saphenous vein:
Sapheno-popliteal junction
Terminal valve
Pre-terminal valve
Cranial extension of the small saphenous vein
Superficial accessory small saphenous vein
Anterior thigh circumflex vein
Posterior thigh circumflex vein
Intersaphenous veins
Lateral venous system
Dorsal venous network of the foot
Dorsal venous arch of the foot
Superficial metatarsal veins (dorsal and plantar)
Plantar venous subcutaneous network
Superficial digital veins (dorsal and plantar)
Lateral marginal vein
Medial marginal vein

Source: Modified from Ref. 1.

connective membrane, the *saphenous fascia* (SF). DF and SF fuse at the sides of the SVs, delimiting the *saphenous compartment* (SC) (Fig. 1). The superficial venous arcade of the dorsum of the foot, which connect the saphenous veins (medial marginal vein, dorsal arcuate vein, and lateral marginal vein), show the same topography and fascial

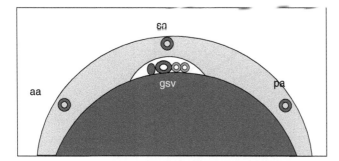

Figure 2 The great saphenous vein (GSV) course with related nerve, artery, and lymphatics within its compartment (white space). Its accessories course in a more superficial plane of the subcutaneous tissue. *Abbreviations*: aa, anterior accessory; sa, superficial accessory; pa, posterior accessory.

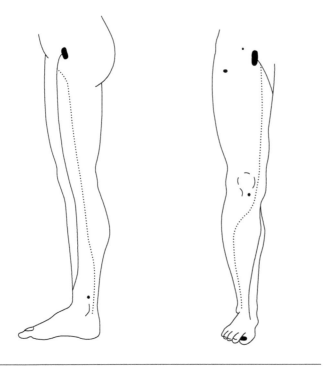

Figure 3   Dotted lines indicate the path of the posterior (*left*) and anterior (*right*) accessories of the great saphenous vein.

relationships. Varicose changes in refluxing SVs are relatively slow to develop and less pronounced than those of nonsaphenous, being visible only by Duplex sonography in many limbs. This is due to the deep position of the SVs, to their thicker wall, and to the *fasciae* of the SC, which oppose their dilatation.

Sapheno-Femoral Junction

The GSV terminates at the groin in the common femoral vein (CFV). In about 70% of limbs, a valve is placed just above its opening (supra-saphenic valve) to protect the lower limb vasculature from the abdomino-pelvic hydrostatic column (Fig. 5). There is also usually a valve at the GSV opening (terminal valve, TV), to prevent reflux from the CFV.

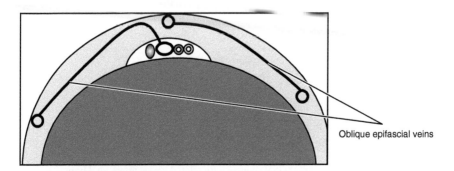

Figure 4   Oblique epifascial veins connect longitudinal epifascial with the great saphenous vein or with deep veins, via perforators.

A few centimeters below the terminal valve is the pre-terminal valve (PTV), which prevents reflux from tributaries of the SFJ into the GSV trunk. The TV is present in 100% of limbs and the PTV in about 70%. SFJ tributaries reach the GSV between the PTV and the TV. All SFJ tributaries may be the source of reflux, especially those connected to pelvic veins (external pudendal vein, genital veins). Full Duplex evaluation of the SFJ should assess PFV, TV, PTV competence and flow patterns in SFJ tributaries.

Classic descriptions of the SFJ tributaries include the following vessels: external pudendal, superficial dorsal vein of clitoris or penis, anterior labial or scrotal veins (from the external genitalia), superficial circumflex iliac vein (from the lateral abdominal and pelvic wall), and the superficial epigastric vein (from the anterior abdominal wall). The accessories of the GSV must also be included in the group of SFJ tributaries. The termination of the SFJ tributaries varies greatly. In fact, they usually end into the GSV, but, less frequently, they can join directly the common femoral vein. Further, saphenous tributaries can join themselves before ending, forming large trunks that can be confused with the GSV (Fig. 6).

In about one-third of limbs with an incompetent GSV, the reflux does not originate from the CFV, but it comes from one of the GSV inguinal tributaries. This occurs more frequently from the external pudendal or from veins draining the external genitalia. In most cases, junctional reflux descend along the GSV. It is not rare to observe a junctional reflux passing from the GSV in one of its inguinal tributaries at the groin or at the upper thigh. This occurs more frequently into the anterior accessory.

SSV Termination and SPJ

The morphology of the SSV termination varies greatly. This is because in the embryo, the SSV extends along the posterior face of the thigh (the so-called "post-axial vein") to end into the inferior gluteal vein. In most limbs, the thigh portion of the embryonic SSV disappears when the deep system develops and the SSV ends in the popliteal vein. In about one-third of limbs, the thigh portion of the SSV persists in part (Fig. 7). It is of particular clinical relevance when the termination of the SSV is into the GSV via the posterior thigh circumflex vein (Giacomini's anastomosis).

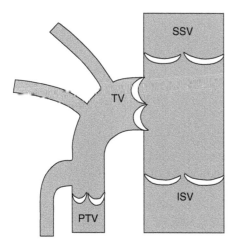

Figure 5 Valves of the sapheno-femoral junctions. *Abbreviations*: SSV, suprasaphenic valve; ISV, infrasaphenic valve; TV, terminal valve; PTV, preterminal valve.

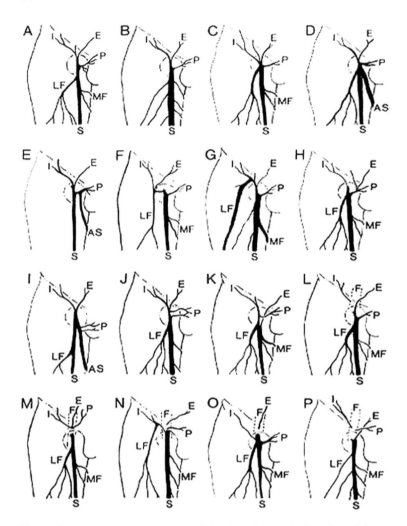

Figure 6 Variability of the veins draining into the terminal portion of the great saphenous vein. *Abbreviations*: I, superficial circumflex iliac vein; E, superficial epigastric vein; P, pudendal vein; LF, lateral superficial femoral vein; MF, medial and superficial femoral vein; AS, accessory saphenous vein; SS, double saphenous vein; S, vena saphena magna; F, femoral vein. *Source*: Modified from Ref. 5.

DEEP VEINS OF THE LOWER LIMB

The term *deep veins* designates indiscriminately all veins that course below the deep (muscular) fascia. In turn, this group of veins is quite heterogeneous from both anatomic and functional points of view (Table 2).

 Intramuscular veins are arranged as a plexus around bundles of myocites. They are particularly developed in the muscles of the foot sole, of the calf, and of the buttock, where they actively contribute to the propulsion of blood (muscle pumps). Isolated thrombosis of muscular sinusoids may simulate muscular disease but are easy to be evidenced by Duplex.

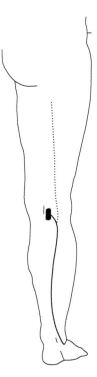

Figure 7 The path of the thigh extension of the small saphenous vein (dotted line).

Axial veins, whose role is to conduct blood toward pelvic collectors, are satellite of the corresponding arteries. They are constantly double at the leg. Anterior tibial, posterior tibial, and peroneal veins join to form the popliteal at different levels of the popliteal fossa. For this reason, in many limbs the popliteal may appear double. The popliteal passes into the femoral vein, which receives the deep femoral vein at the upper thigh to form the common femoral vein. The common femoral vein, after receiving the great saphenous, continues into the external iliac. Duplex investigation of limbs with clinical evidence of DVT must take into account that occlusion may occur in only one branch of a duplicated femoral or popliteal.

In case of thrombosis of the popliteal-femoral axis, the drainage of the limb can be allowed by other veins, which, in normal conditions, are small sized and hemodynamically irrelevant. Main collateral path are:

1. A double femoral vein
2. The deep femoral venous axis. In fact, the popliteal vein is connected with the roots of the deep femoral by anonymous muscular veins, which can enlarge when the femoral vein is occluded
3. The obturator vein, which normally drains only a small portion of the medial thigh to confluence into the internal iliac
4. The sciatic vein, which normally drains only the sciatic nerve and drains into the inferior gluteal veins. It may be connected with the deep and superficial veins of the posterior leg. The sciatic vein can be the source of a reflux responsible for leg varicose veins.
5. Perforating veins (PVs) (Table 3 and Fig. 8).

Table 2 Nomenclature of the Deep Veins

Thigh	Common femoral vein
	Femoral vein
	Deep femoral vein
	Deep femoral communicating veins (accompanying veins of perforating arteries)
	Medial circumflex femoral vein
	Lateral circumflex femoral vein
	Sciatic vein
Knee	Popliteal vein
	Genicular venous plexus
Leg	Sural veins
	Soleal veins
	Gastrocnemius veins
	Medial gastrocnemius veins
	Lateral gastrocnemius veins
	Intergemellar vein
	Anterior tibial veins
	Posterior tibial veins
	Fibular or peroneal veins
Foot	Medial plantar veins
	Lateral plantar veins
	Deep plantar venous arch
	Deep metatarsal veins (plantar and dorsal)
	Deep digital veins (plantar and dorsal)
	Pedal vein

Source: Modified from Ref. 1.

PERFORATING VEINS

PVs are the vessels that connect superficial collectors with subfascial veins. Most of them are valvulated and permit only flow toward the subfascial compartment. Most of them are microscopically sized and hemodynamically irrelevant. PVs have been designated in "direct PVs" (those connecting a superficial vein with an axial deep vein) and "indirect PVs" (those connecting a superficial vein with a intramuscular vein).

More than 100 PVs are in the lower limbs. In fact, one or two veins accompany all the perforating arteries that supply the subcutaneous layer. Theoretically, each of these PVs can dilate and assume clinical relevance in varicose syndromes or in DVT. However, PVs, which more frequently assume clinical relevance, are quite constant and have been grouped and designated according with their topography. CEAP designates only thigh (AP17) and leg (AP18) PVs. PVs may represent the starting point of a reflux or its point of re-entry. In both conditions, they play a pivotal role in the hemodynamics of varicose limbs and need specific treatment for their selective interruption. PVs have been designated on the basis of their topography (Fig. 8).

The Veins of the Pelvis

Pelvic veins are of great clinical importance due to their role in venous thrombo embolism (VTE), pelvic congestive syndromes, and varicose veins of the lower trunk and limbs.

Table 3 Nomenclature of the Perforating Veins (PVs)

Foot perforators	Dorsal foot PV or intercapitular veins	1
	Medial foot PV	2
	Lateral foot PV	3
	Plantar foot PV	4
Ankle perforators	Medial ankle PV	5
	Anterior ankle PV	6
	Lateral ankle PV	7
Leg perforators	Medial leg PV	
	Paratibial PV	8
	Posterior tibial PV (cockett PV)	9
	Anterior leg PV	10
	Lateral leg PV	11
	Posterior leg PV	
	Medial gastrocnemius PV	12
	Lateral gastrocnemius PV	13
	Intergemellar PV	14
	Para-achillean PV	15
Knee perforators	Medial knee PV	16
	Suprapatellar PV	17
	Lateral knee PV	18
	Infrapatellar PV	19
	Popliteal fossa PV	20
	Medial thigh PV	
	PV of the femoral canal	21
	Inguinal PV	22
	Anterior thigh PV	23
	Lateral thigh PV	24
Thigh perforators	Posterior thigh PV	
	Postero-medial	25
	Sciatic PV	26
	Posterolateral	27
	Pudendal PV	28
Gluteal perforators	Superior gluteal PV	29
	Mid gluteal PV	30
	Lower gluteal PV	31

Source: Modified from Ref. 1.

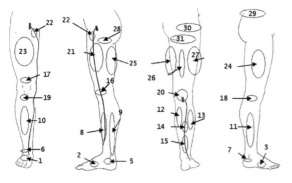

Figure 8 Topography of main groups of perforating veins.

Pelvic venous anatomy is extremely complex, due to the presence of many veins and plexuses, showing variable pathways, size, and connections (Table 4).

The pelvic walls and the pelvic organs are covered by plexuses of tiny avalvulated veins. These plexuses are connected by numerous avalvulated anonymous vessels and drained by larger (mostly avalvulated) veins that (Table 5) open into mayor collectors (poorly valvulated).

Pelvic venous congestive hypertension can be transmitted to the venous system of the lower limb due to many "latent" connections. The more important occur at the level of the:

(1) obturator vein, which connect the hypogastric vein with veins of the upper medial thigh
(2) sciatic vein, which connect with deep and superficial veins of the posterior thigh and leg
(3) gluteal veins, which connect with the sciatic vein or with superficial veins of the posterior thigh
(4) pudendal veins, which connect the hypogastric venous district with superficial veins of the perineum
(5) the veins of the round ligament, which connect uterine plexus with the superficial inguinal veins.

Table 4   Nomenclature of Pelvic Veins

Plexuses and peripheral veins		Draining veins		Main collectors	
1	Pampiniform plexus	2	Ovarian veins	4	Inferior vena cava
5	Sacral venous plexus	3	Testicular veins	10	Common iliac vein
11	External rectal plexus	6	Median sacral vein	14	Inferior mesenteric vein
	Internal rectal plexus	7	Ileolumbar vein	38	Internal iliac vein
12	(Hemorrhoidal)	8	Internal iliac (hypogastric)		(Hypogastric)
20	Deep perineal veins	8	External iliac	43	External iliac vein
21	Superficial perineal veins	13	Superior rectal vein		
22	Deep dorsal veins	15	Middle rectal veins		
	of clitoris	16	Inferior rectal veins		
23	Deep veins of clitoris	17	Superior gluteal veins		
24	Deep dorsal veins	18	Inferior gluteal veins		
	of penis	19	Lateral sacral veins		
25	Deep veins of penis	27	Internal pudendal vein		
26	Urethral bulb veins	28	Obturator veins		
29	Pudendal plexus	35	Vesical veins		
30	Vesical plexus	36	Uterine veins		
31	Prostatic plexus	37	Vaginal veins		
32	Uterine plexus	39	Pubic veins (accessory		
33	Vein of the broad ligament		obturator veins)		
34	Vaginal plexus	40	Sovrapubic veins		
		41	Inferior epigastric vein		
		42	Deep circumflex iliac vein		

Source: Modified from Ref. 2.

Table 5   Designation of Lymphatics

Name	Number	Topography	Provenience of afferents	Destination of efferents
Lateral group	4–6	Medial and posterior aspects of the axillary vein	From the whole arm with the exception of the lymphatics, which course along the cephanlic vein	Part to the central and apical axillary nodes, part to the inferior deep cervical glands
Anterior or pectoral group	4–5	Along the lower border of the pectoralis minor, close the lateral thoracic artery	From the anterior and lateral thoracic walls, and the central and lateral parts of the mamma	To the central and apical group of axillary glands
Posterior or subscapular group	6–7	Lower margin of the posterior wall of the axilla close to the subscapular artery	From the back of the neck and of the posterior thoracic wall	To the apical and central group of axillary glands
Central group	3–4	Adipose tissue near the base of the axilla	From all the preceding groups of axillary glands	To the apical glands
Apical group	6–12	Posterior to the upper portion of the pectoralis minor and above the upper border of this muscle	From all the preceding groups and lymphatics accompanying the cephalic vein	Consitute the subclavian trunk, which joins directly the junction of the internal jugular and subclavian veins

The Venous System of the Upper Limb

The general arrangement of the venous system of the upper limb resembles that of the inferior one, being divided into two sets, *superficial* and *deep*; the two sets are richly anastomosed by perforating vessels. Both groups of veins are valvulated.

The *deep veins* follow the course of the arteries, forming their venæ comitantes. They are generally arranged in pairs situated one on either side of the corresponding artery, connected at intervals by short avalvulated oblique. Paired deep veins accompany the arteries in the hand, forearm and arm, to confluence into the axillary vein, which continues into the subclavian at the outer border of the first rib. This vein passes behind the clavicle and subclavius and in front of the subclavian artery, from which it is separated by the scalenus anterior and the phrenic nerve. The subclavian vein ends at the sterno-clavicular joint, where it joins with the internal jugular to form the brachiocephalic trunk.

Main *superficial veins* originate from a tiny plexus of subdermic veins. The cephalic vein originate from the radial side of the dorsal network of the hand to course along the radial border of the forearm. At the elbow it joins the basilic vein by the median basilic vein, which corresponds to the vein of Giacomini of the inferior limb. Then, the cephalic vein courses in the groove between the brachioradialis and the biceps brachii. In the upper third of the arm, it passes between the pectoralis major and deltoideus. Finally, it pierces the coracoclavicular fascia to end in the axillary vein.

The *basilic vein* begins in the ulnar side of the dorsal venous network and runs up the posterior surface of the ulnar margin of the forearm. At the elbow, it is joined by the vena mediana cubiti. It ascends obliquely in the groove between the biceps brachii and pronator teres and perforates the deep fascia at the middle of the arm, to reach the axillary vein after having sided the brachial artery.

Lymphatic System

The lymph passes from initial lymphatics to lymphatic capillaries, which join to form *lymphatic vessels*. These are richly valvulated and provided with smooth muscle. The segments of lymphatic vessels comprised between two sets of valves are called *lymphangions*. Smooth muscles in the walls of the lymphatic vessels cause the lymphangions to contract sequentially allowing the flow of lymph toward the thoracic region. Valves prevent backward flow.

Lymphatic Vessels of the Lower Extremity

The lymphatic vessels of the lower extremity consist in a superficial and a deep set, like veins. The existence of connections between these two systems by perforating lymphatics has been postulated but never clearly demonstrated.

The main *superficial lymphatic vessels* arise from a plexus of tiny lymphatics that pervade the skin everywhere. They are divisible into two groups: a medial, which follows the course of the GSV, and a lateral, which accompanies the SSV. The vessels of the medial group are larger and more numerous than those of the lateral group They commence on the dorsum of the foot and ascend close to the GSV to end in the subinguinal group of superficial nodes. The vessels of the lateral group arise from the fibular margin of the foot and accompany the SSV to enter the popliteal glands.

The *deep lymphatic vessels* accompany the deep axial veins. They are few in number and smaller in size, if compared with the superficial ones. Leg deep lymphatics enter the popliteal lymph glands. Six or seven small popliteal glands are embedded in the fat contained in the popliteal fossa. One of them is close to the terminal part of the SSV, while the others lie at the sides of the popliteal vessels. Most of popliteal efferents course along the femoral vessels to enter the deep inguinal glands.

Twelve to twenty inguinal glands are in the upper portion of the femoral triangle. A horizontal line at the level of the termination of the GSV divides them into the *superficial inguinal glands*, which are designated in a proximal and a distal group. Proximal glands are located just below the inguinal ligament and receive afferents from the gluteal region and from the abdominal wall (lateral glands) and from the external genitalia and perineum (medial glands). The glands of the distal group are located close to the saphenous ending, and they drain all the superficial lymphatics that course close to the GSV.

One to three *deep subinguinal glands* are on the medial side of the common femoral vein. Usually, the lowest is just below the SFJ, the middle in the femoral canal, and the highest in the femoral ring. They receive the femoral lymphatics and small lymphatics from the external genitalia and superficial inguinal nodes.

The efferentes of the inguinal glands reach the *external iliac glands*, from eight to ten in number, which lie along the external iliac vessels and the *common iliac glands*, four to six in number, located along the common iliac artery and below the bifurcation of the aorta. Common iliac glands also drain the hypogastric collectors, and their efferents pass to the lateral aortic glands.

Most of the vessels originating from the lateral aortic glands converge to form the *right and left lumbar trunks*, which join the cisterna chyli to continue into the thoracic duct. The *thoracic duct* enters the thorax through the aortic hiatus of the diaphragm and ascends between the aorta and azygos vein. It ends in the left subclavian vein, at its angle of junction with the internal jugular vein. Its termination is protected by two semilunar valves, which prevent the passage of venous blood into the duct.

The Lymphatics of the Upper Extremity

Also in the upper extremity, lymphatic vessels are arranged into two sets, superficial and deep. The superficial lymphatic vessels originate in the lymphatic plexus of the palm and on the flexor aspect of the digits. From the dense plexus of the palm, main lymphatics run upward in front of and behind the wrist, and they are collected into radial and ulnar groups, which accompany the cephalic and basilic veins respectively. Most of ulnar (or basilic) lymphatics end in the lateral group of axillary glands. Some of the radial (or cephalic) vessels are collected into a trunk which ascends with the cephalic vein to the deltoideo-pectoral glands, located below the clavicle. The efferents from this group pass either to the subclavicular axillary glands or to the inferior cervical glands.

The deep lymphatic vessels course close to the deep veins and arteries. In the forearm, they consist of four sets, corresponding with the radial, ulnar, volar, and dorsal interosseous arteries. At the elbow, (Fig. 9) they unite to form small collectors that course

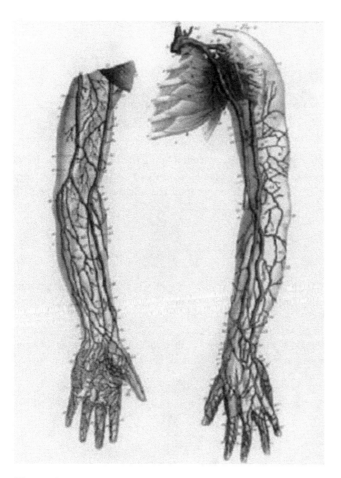

Figure 9 The venous system of the upper limb. *Source*: Modified from Ref. 3.

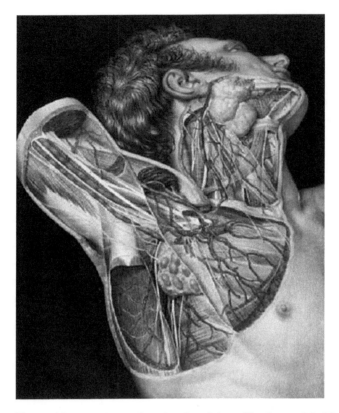

Figure 10 Lymph vessels and nodes of the axilla. *Source*: Modified from Ref. 4.

toward the axilla. A few of them end in glands scattered along the brachial artery. Most of
them pass into the lateral group of the axillary glands. Twenty to thirty nodes are located in
the axilla (Fig. 10). They are designated topographically. Table 5 summarizes their
connections.

REFERENCES

1. Caggiati A, Dorgan JJ, Gloviczki P, Jantet G, Wendell-Simith CP, Partsch H. Nomenclature of
    the veins of the lower limbs: an international interdisciplinary consensus statement. J Vasc Surg
    2002; 36:416–422.
2. Caggiati A. J Vasc Surg, in press.
3. Caggiati A, Bergan JJ, Gloviczki P, Eklof B, Allegia C, Partsch H. Nomenclature of the veins of
    the lower limbs: extensions, refinements, and clinical applications. J Vasc Surg 2005;
    41:719–724.
4. Traité complet de l'anatomie de l'homme Bourgery. Marc Jean 1831–1854.
5. Venous Drainage at the Fossa Ovails. Ronald A. Bergman, PhD Adel K. Afifi, MD, MS Ryosuke
    Miyauchi, MD.

3
Physiology of the Veins and Lymphatics

Philip D. Coleridge Smith
Royal Free and University College Medical School, London, U.K.

INTRODUCTION

The venous and lymphatic systems are very important in the maintenance of the health of all tissues. In the lower limbs these systems are particularly adapted to man's erect posture with modifications for the high venous pressures to which the lower limb tissues would normally be exposed. The Edinburgh Vein Study found that 32% of women and 40% of men had clinical evidence of venous disease in the lower limb (1), making this group of diseases some of the most common vascular disorders.

THE CIRCULATION AND THE VENOUS SYSTEM

The heart is ultimately responsible for all flow in the circulatory system. The pressure produced by contraction of the left ventricle is transmitted through the arterial system, and via the capillary bed to the venous system. This capillary venous filling pressure is known as the *vis a tergo*. This depends on arterial pressure which is dependent on cardiac output and on peripheral resistance. Cardiac output, in turn, is dependent on venous return via the left atrium, the *vis a fronte*. Cardiac output is extremely sensitive to cardiac filling pressure. Stroke volume may change up to 50% in response to a change in venous filling pressure of as little as 1 cm H_2O. Reflex changes in heart rate, cardiac contractility, peripheral vascular resistance and venous capacitance minimise this effect, however, central venous pressure remains pivotal in cardiovascular homeostasis.

At any one time, 70% of the total blood volume lies within the veins. This is made possible by the physical properties of the vein wall. At low transmural pressures, veins collapse, their walls approximating. On filling, the major veins assume an elliptical shape. Passive distension then occurs with little increase in pressure within the walls, allowing a large volume of blood to be accommodated. Only when the cross-section becomes circular does pressure rise appreciably (Fig. 1). A very much larger volume of blood is then required to stretch the vein wall than was required for passive distension. Blood may be rapidly mobilized from these capacitance vessels to improve central venous pressure. This is achieved partly by contraction of smooth muscle within the vein wall, which is mediated by the sympathetic nervous system, and partly by elastic recoil of the vein wall in the face

Vein empty

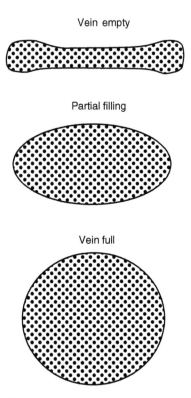

Partial filling

Vein full

Figure 1 One of the main functions of large veins is to act as capacitance vessels and contain about 70% of circulating blood volume.

of reduced flow. Although all veins have similar properties, the splanchnic veins are the main capacitance vessels. Veins of skeletal muscle and skin are more concerned with temperature regulation.

Most of the large veins in the lower extremity lie within the muscular compartments of the leg and are subject to external compression during calf muscle contraction. Using Duplex ultrasound B-mode scanning to observe the large axial veins that are not subject to muscular compression, it was found that they collapsed in a circular rather than elliptical configuration is response to a decrease in venous volume (2). These veins are supported on all sides by connective tissue and/or fat and are subject to equal external pressure vectors at all points on the vein wall. They expand or collapse in response to changes in venous volume through changes in circular diameter rather than change in the shape of the vein resulting from external compression. Once the vein reaches a circular shape, further increases in venous volume require increased intra-luminal pressure to increase the venous circumference and venous volume. Due to the thinness of the vein walls, minimal pressure increases are needed to overcome the inherent stiffness of the adventitial layer. The venous volume is increased by over 250% as a result of an increase in the venous transmural pressure from 0 to 15 mmHg (3).

The veins of the lower limb are influenced by gravity due to man's erect posture. On standing, about 250 mls of venous blood fills the veins of each lower limb resulting in an increase in calf volume of about 2%. This leads to a fall in central venous pressure and, therefore, a transient fall in cardiac output. A new equilibrium between venous return and cardiac output is quickly achieved by reflex mechanisms. Pressure in the veins of the leg is

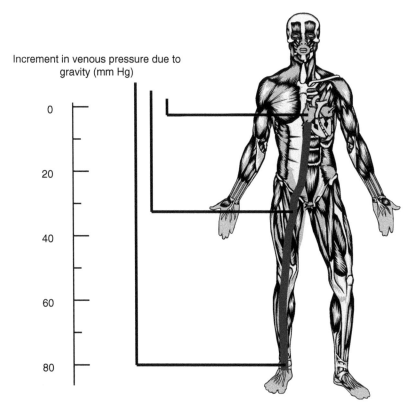

Increment in venous pressure due to gravity (mm Hg)

0

20

40

60

80

Figure 2 The venous pressure in the lower limb on standing are attributable to the hydrostatic effects of a column of blood extending to the right atrium. (*See color insert.*)

now increased as a result of hydrostatic pressure (P_h). This is proportional to the weight of the column of blood extending from the right atrium to the level at which pressure is being measured.

$$P_h = -\rho gh$$

where ρ is the density of blood, g is the gravitational acceleration constant and h is the distance from the heart (Fig. 2).

The same hydrostatic pressure is added to the arteries and as a result the pressure differential across the capillary bed remains the same in supine and standing positions. Flow is therefore maintained but at the price of a high venous pressure. A series of muscle pumps within the lower limb augments the return of venous blood and the action of these lowers venous pressure in the leg considerably. As a result, the pressure differential between arterial and venous limbs of the capillary bed increases, and blood flow increases dramatically.

THE VENOUS VALVES

Valves are present in lower extremity veins and are bicuspid with a fine connective tissue skeleton and are extremely strong even though they are just a thin layer of collagen fibres covered with endothelium (4). The valve cusps are stronger and more elastic than the vein wall. The valve sinus is always wider than the vein above and below the cusps (5). The calf muscle pump in combination with functioning venous valves provides the force necessary to overcome venous compliance and hydrostatic pressure and promotes venous return in the upright position. There are more valves in the distal leg veins and they decrease in numbers proximally. The inferior vena cava and common iliac veins have no valves and 75% of external iliac veins have no valves, but only 25% of common femoral veins are valveless (6). Valves in the internal iliac systems are less frequent, occurring in about 7% of the population (7). It has been suggested that the lack of valves in the iliac and common femoral veins is the starting point for the development of a progressive descending valvular incompetence that causes varicose veins (8), although this hypothesis has largely been rejected in the light of more modern evidence. The valves in the axial veins ensure that blood flows from caudal to cephalad and from superficial to deep in the communicating veins of the calf with the exception of foot communicating veins where venous flow is from the deep veins in the muscles of the sole of the foot to the superficial veins on the dorsum (9,10). The valves close in response to cephalad to caudal blood flow and a reverse flow velocity of at least 30 cm/s appears to be required for venous valve closure (11).

SUPERFICIAL VENOUS SYSTEM

The lower extremity veins can be divided into three types: superficial, deep and perforating veins (Fig. 3). The superficial venous system lies above the investing fascial layer of the leg and thigh and consists of the long and short saphenous veins and their tributaries. These veins are not compressed by muscle contraction. The great saphenous vein (GSV) and small saphenous vein (SSV) are the major superficial veins, although each of these veins has numerous tributaries.

COMMUNICATING OR PERFORATING VEINS ASSOCIATED WITH THE LONG SAPHENOUS VEIN

Numerous communications exist between the superficial and deep veins. Some of these have eponymous names such as the Cockett medial calf perforating veins, Boyd's perforating vein lying just below the knee, and the Hunter perforating vein in the mid-thigh region. The purpose of these veins is to drain blood from the superficial venous system into the deep veins of the lower limb. Some perforating veins contain valves, but many travel an oblique track through the fascia of the limb resulting in a functional valve which prevents outward flow of blood during normal muscle activity.

DEEP VENOUS SYSTEM

The deep veins lie beneath the fascial covering and are subject to compressive forces when the muscles of the limb contract. Most venous return from the lower extremities flows though the deep veins. In the calf the major axial veins are accompanied by pairs of venae comitantes. The veins accompanying the posterior tibial and peroneal veins are especially large (up to 10 mm in diameter in male subjects) and participate in the pumping mechanism that returns blood from the leg. In addition, the medial and lateral heads of gastrocnemius and soleus also contain pairs of veins accompanying the major arteries

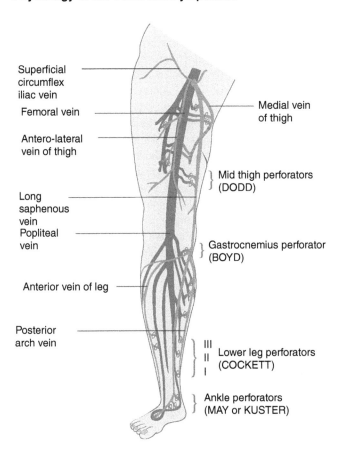

Figure 3 The deep and superficial veins of the lower limb. (*See color insert.*)

to these muscles. These are also often of large diameter and participate in the calf muscle pump. The calf veins empty into the popliteal vein which is often duplicated. Flow from the popliteal vein returns via the femoral vein in the thigh. The muscles of the thigh are drained via the deep femoral vein which joins the femoral vein to form the common femoral vein in the inguinal triangle. This is joined by the GSV and is the major route of venous drainage from the lower limb.

NORMAL VENOUS PHYSIOLOGY OF THE LOWER LIMBS

There are many factors that influence the return of blood from the lower extremities to the heart and the relative importance of each factor varies with body position and activity.

In the Supine Position

When the subject is in the supine position, the respiratory cycle plays an important part in the venous return from the lower extremities. The foot vein pressure in the supine position is approximately 15 mmHg. The right atrial pressure is normally between 0 and 2 mmHg so the venous return to the heart in the supine position is generated by a pressure gradient of 13–15 mmHg. During inspiration, the volume of the veins of the thorax increases and the pressure decreases in response to reduced intrathoracic pressure (12,13). Expiration leads to the opposite effect, with decreased venous volume and increased pressure. The venous response to respiration is reversed in the abdomen, where the pressure increases during inspiration because of the descent of the diaphragm, and decreases during expiration as the diaphragm ascends. Increased abdominal pressure during inspiration decreases pressure gradients between peripheral veins in the lower extremities and the abdomen, thus reducing flow in the peripheral vessels (14). During expiration, when intra-abdominal pressure is reduced, the pressure gradient from the lower limbs to the abdomen is increased and the flow in the peripheral veins rises correspondingly. The respiratory effects are usually associated with clear phasic changes in venous flow in the extremities. These can be detected by various instruments, including many forms of plethysmography and Doppler flow detectors. The respiratory changes in venous velocity may be exaggerated by respiratory manoeuvres, such as the Valsalva manoeuvre, which increases intra-thoracic and abdominal pressures and decreases, abolishes, or even reverses flow in some peripheral veins.

From the Supine to the Upright Position

When the subject moves from the supine position to the upright position, the influence of the respiratory cycle changes and the effect on the venous blood flow patterns has been demonstrated in the common femoral vein using duplex ultrasonography with simultaneously recordings of the cardiac and respiratory cycles using an electro-cardiogram (ECG) monitor and a respiratory monitor (2). The subject was placed in the non weightbearing supine position and on a tilt table and gradually moved until fully upright. At minus 10 degrees head down, the weight of the abdominal viscera presses on the diaphragm and this is sufficient to counteract the descent of the diaphragm during inspiration. In this position, the outward movement of the chest wall generates the negative intra-thoracic pressure that is required for inspiration with little change in the intra-abdominal pressure. The venous blood flow patterns were shown to be primarily dependent upon the cardiac cycle but virtually independent of the respiratory cycle. Blood leaving the legs essentially flows downhill into the passively dilating right atrium until it is stopped by the onset of the cardiac contraction. As the subject becomes more upright, the influence of the cardiac cycle on the venous return rapidly diminishes as the respiratory cycle becomes more important. It has been shown in the study above that with the subject in the non weightbearing and 30 degree head-up position on a tilt table, the respiratory monitor indicated presence of flow in the common femoral vein during expiration and flow ceased with normal inspiratory effort.

In the Fully Upright Position

In the upright position, the column of blood between the level of the manubrium sterni, the point used as the zero reference for the pressure measurement, and the foot exerts a gravitational force known as the hydrostatic pressure. The pressure in the foot vein then becomes 15 mmHg plus the hydrostatic pressure (Fig. 1). In this position, the expiratory promotion of venous flow is not enough to overcome the gravitational hydrostatic forces and promote adequate venous return. The contraction of the calf muscles is required to overcome this gravitational forces and promote venous return.

THE RETURN OF BLOOD TO THE HEART

Blood returning from the lower extremity must flow against the forces of gravity to return to the right atrium. The foot vein pressure in the supine position is about 100 mmHg, so in order for blood to return from the foot, it has to reach this pressure to ensure adequate return. Since the vascular system is a closed series of tubes, the return pressure on the venous side is balanced by an equal hydrostatic arterial pressure supplying the limb. The pumping force of the heart results in the blood leaving the capillary system having a small residual pressure of 15–20 mmHg. This is sufficient to ensure venous return whether in the supine or erect position. In the supine position, the venous return takes place at the expense of a high venous pressure in the extremity. A highly specialised pumping mechanism has been evolved to actively pump venous blood back to the heart from the lower limb. It is thought that the principal participants in the pumping mechanism are the calf veins, gastrocnemius and soleus, within the calf muscles. Failure of this system results in symptoms ranging from varicose veins to severe ulceration of the lower limb.

THE CALF MUSCLE PUMP

It is thought that the principal participants in the pumping mechanism are the veins of the calf within the calf muscles, gastrocnemius and soleus. These contain as much as 250 ml of blood (15). Additional muscle pumps are also recognized in the thigh and foot (9,16). The latter has a much smaller capacity (about 25 ml), but assists in the return of blood from the foot. It may have a "pump priming" effect on the calf muscle pump. The calf pump is often referred to as the peripheral heart. Venous flow is also dependent upon the contractile force of the heart, static filling pressure and gravity. During calf contraction, the pressure within the deep fascia becomes raised to as much as 250 mmHg resulting in all the intra-muscular veins becoming completely compressed (Fig. 4). Blood that was present in these veins is emptied into the outflow tract, the first part of which is the popliteal vein. The large veins within the gastrocnemius and soleus muscles form the main chamber of the pump but the venae comitantes of the posterior tibial and peroneal veins and all other deep veins participate (16). Distal deep venous valves prevent axial reflux and functional or physiological valves in the communicating veins prevent reflux from the deep venous system to the superficial venous system (17). With continuous exercise, the calf blood volume is reduced by 1.5–2.0 ml/100 ml mainly as a result of the compression of the veins in the pump chamber and the average expelled volume is approximately 100–120 ml, that is, about 50% of all the blood within the pump. The pump will normally expel this volume in four or five contractions though one single sustained contraction can expel as much. The popliteal vein is a large bore vein which offers virtually no resistance to outflow. As the gradient of 10–15 mmHg between the small veins and the heart is sufficient to ensure venous blood flow in the supine position, the increase in gradient produced by the calf muscle pump during contraction is more than enough to ensure an adequate rapid venous return to the heart during vigorous erect muscle exercise.

As the calf muscles relax, valves cephalad to the muscle pump close and prevent reflux of blood from more proximally in the axial veins. The pressure within the muscle fascia falls to low levels. The valves in the communicating veins open and allow normal blood flow from the superficial to the deep venous system. In addition, arterial inflow from the lower extremity capillary beds re-primes the calf muscle pump for a subsequent contraction. At the moment when the calf muscles relax, their contained veins are empty, at low pressure and as yet unfilled by arterial inflow. As the veins are collapsed, they are unaffected by hydrostatic pressure. On the other hand, the superficial veins are full and subjected to hydrostatic pressure plus the remnant of cardiac generated pressure, the "vis a tergo." The pressure gradient between the two compartments becomes 100–110 mmHg resulting in blood immediately flowing from the superficial to the deep compartment through the many communicating veins (18). This empties the superficial compartment and reduces its pressure (19). Therefore, the function of the calf muscle pump is vital in ensuring venous return from the lower limbs during exercise and the reduction of the superficial venous pressure, thus removing the damaging effects of the hydrostatic pressure ever present as a result of man's upright posture.

The effectiveness of the calf muscle pump can be investigated by air plethysmography and ambulatory venous pressure measurement technique which measures deep venous pressure directly by placing a needle in a dorsal foot vein and connecting it to a standard pressure transducer and a recording device during rest and exercise.

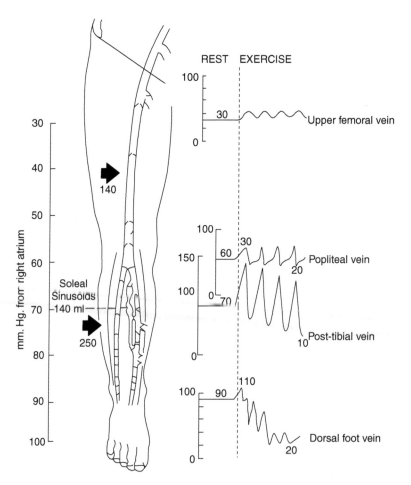

Figure 4   The physiological events during the operation of the calf muscle pump.

LOWER LIMB VENOUS PATHOPHYSIOLOGY

In venous disease some components of the venous system become damaged, and the well-organized physiology described above becomes less efficient. The most commonly affected structure is the venous valve. In varicose veins the valves of the superficial veins spontaneously become incompetent permitting reverse flow in the GSV, SSV and their tributaries. This does not normally cause any problem since the pumping capacity of the muscle pumps can usually compensate for incompetent superficial veins. Should the superficial veins become very dilated then the volume of venous reflux may be considerable resulting in ankle edema, skin changes or even leg ulceration. The valves of the deep veins may also be damaged, most commonly as a consequence of deep vein thrombosis. In some patients spontaneous incompetence of the deep vein valves may occur. Veins may also become temporarily or permanently occluded by venous thrombosis. In the major axial veins this results in considerable disturbance of normal flow with large collateral channels of venous drainage developing. The pressure in the lower limb remains permanently elevated and edema is a common clinical problem in these patients.

VALVULAR REFLUX OR RETROGRADE FLOW

Venous reflux is the flow of blood in the opposite direction from physiological flow. This reflux may be natural, physiological or pathological. The duration of the reflux flow depends on the physiological or pathological state of the valvular apparatus. There have been studies (20) to show that the duration of reflux in the deep venous trunks in normal subjects was less than 0.5 sec in 95% of subjects scanned. Other studies (21,22) have also shown that reflux is significant if the duration of the retrograde flow within the veins exceeds 0.5 sec. Although it is not necessarily correlated to the development of varicose disease, this minimum duration of 0.5 sec does seem to be universally recognised as indicative of pathological reflux (23–25). Kistner proposed a classification of deep vein reflux according to the level of descent of radiological contrast medium, during descending venography (26). He defined four classes in increasing order of severity, with class 1 corresponding to reflux descending to mid-thigh, class 2 corresponding to reflux descending to the knee, class 3 corresponding to reflux descending to the mid-calf and class 4 corresponding to reflux descending to the ankle.

There are several ways of eliciting reflux flow in the lower limb venous system, and the most effective ones include manual compression of the calf by means of a cuff. Compression with the cuff placed on the calf and inflated to 120 mmHg and then rapidly deflated, thus mobilizing the blood from the superficial and deep veins, is the method that is easy to reproduce systematically since automatic cuffs that can inflate and deflate rapidly are available.

The accurate quantification of venous reflux in individual veins has not yet been fully established. Several methods of quantifying venous reflux in individual veins have been described using duplex scanning. These include measurements of valve closure time (27), venous reflux index or the Doppler efficiency index (EId) (28), velocity at peak reflux, and quantitative volume flow measurements by calculating the cross-sectional area of the vessel and the time-averaged velocity.

EDEMA

Starling Forces and How Edema Is Formed

Edema is described as a perceptible expansion of the interstitial fluid volume. While the clinical importance of edema is usually that of its underlying cause, the accumulation of edema fluid and elevation of tissue pressure may directly interfere with various physiological activities.

Most of the fluid that enters the tissue space by ultrafiltration from the arterial end of the capillary bed is absorbed back into the circulation at the venous end of that network (Fig. 5). Ernest Starling, in 1896, described interstitial fluid formation and absorption in terms of the pressure gradients acting across the capillary endothelium, the surface area available for fluid transfer and the permeability of the capillary membrane to protein. The direct and immediate causes of edema are alterations in the Starling forces that lead to an increase in the capillary-absorption ratio and a decrease in lymphatic drainage.

In the capillary circulation the capillary endothelium is slightly permeable to plasma proteins allowing a small amount to enter the interstitial space. In general, there is little protein in extracellular fluid compared to blood and the colloid osmotic pressure due to the plasma proteins (which amounts to about 25 mmHg) favors reabsorption of fluid into the capillaries. At the arterial end of the capillary bed the capillary pressure may be as high as 50 mmHg. This would favor egress of water into the tissues, since this exceeds, the colloid osmotic pressure. Near the venous end of the capillary, when the pressure is 15 mmHg, the osmotic pressure is higher than the capillary pressure and fluid is reabsorbed by the capillary. This situation is summarized by Fig. 5. It must be recognized that this diagram is a considerable simplification of what actually happens in the capillary network but it depicts the net consequences of many complex events.

Edema is observed in a wide variety of diseases in which one or more of the Starling forces are modified by the disease process. In most cases, there is a complex interaction among the factors that control transcapillary fluid exchange and interstitial volume. A simple example of edema is the orthostatic edema that occurs in the dependent parts of the body. In this case, gravity acts to impair venous return resulting in increased capillary filtration rate as a result of increased capillary volume and capillary pressure. The single affected element of the system is the capillary pressure. Any procedure that will facilitate

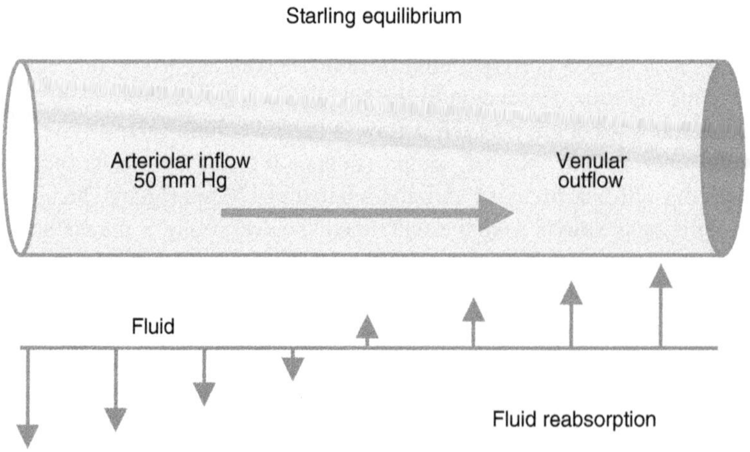

Figure 5   Diagrammatic representation of the Starling equilibrium.

venous return, such as muscle activity or compression stockings, will alleviate the condition. It is clear from this consideration that if capillary pressure was allowed to rise to that of the potential hydrostatic pressure in the veins at the ankle, considerable edema would develop. The need for an efficient pumping system which maintains a low pressure in the superficial veins of the leg becomes obvious.

In lower limb chronic venous insufficiency, edema may occur as a result of increased capillary pressure, secondary to an elevation in venous pressure due to venous obstruction, or increased venous hypertension due to valvular incompetence. Other causes of clinical edema include pregnancy, congestive heart failure, and renal or hepatic insufficiency. Edema may also occur in inflammatory conditions of any type since these tend to increase the amount of protein escaping into the tissues. This reduces the difference in colloid osmotic pressure between the interstitial fluid and the capillaries favoring the development of edema.

Plasma proteins that escape into the interstitial fluid cannot be reabsorbed by the capillaries since there is no active mechanism to achieve this. In order to prevent a steady rise in interstitial protein levels, these must be removed continuously. Failure to do this would result in the development of edema as the osmotic pressure rose in the interstitial fluids. The lymphatic system is responsible for removing plasma proteins from the interstitial fluid. The volumetric flow in these vessels is very small in comparison to the arterial inflow. For example, at rest the flow of blood to the lower limbs is about 1 L per minute whereas the total flow of lymph returning via the thoracic duct is 100 mL per hour. This small volume of fluid contains much protein ($40–60\ \mathrm{gL}^{-1}$) and it is this which is of great importance to the tissues. These proteins would otherwise remain trapped in the interstitial tissues (29).

LYMPHATIC SYSTEM

In most tissues of the body a network of lymphatic "capillaries" is present. These comprise a single layer of endothelial cells that are held together by connective tissue structures. The junctions between lymphatic cells are not tight junctions but formed by overlapping cells. These permit entry of interstitial fluid, including large protein molecules, into the lumen of the lymphatic vessels. It is considered that the junctions between endothelial cells act as flap valves preventing exit of fluid from within the vessels. The pressure within the lymphatics is approximately 1 mmHg, similar to that of the interstitial space. The lymphatic capillary endothelial cell contains myoendothelial fibres which contract rhythmically allowing the vessels to pump lymph proximally toward the larger lymphatic vessels. During pumping the overlapping endothelial cells provide a valve mechanism which prevents lymph from returning to the interstitial space. The connective tissue fibers anchoring the endothelial cells pull the lymphatic capillary open again after contraction, allowing it to refill with interstitial fluid.

The small lymphatic capillaries join to form larger lymphatic vessels. These have an inner endothelial layer and an outer muscle layer conferring contractility on these vessels. The walls of these vessels are impermeable to protein and contract rhythmically actively pumping lymph more proximally. The pressures with the larger lymphatic vessels reach as much as 25 mmHg. The lymphatic vessels are also compressed by adjacent structures such as muscle, arterial pulsation and compression by clothes. Immobilisation of a limb may result in swelling due to loss of this extra impetus to lymphatic propulsion. The lymphatic vessels contain many tiny bicuspid valves which ensure that lymph is pumped in the correct direction.

In the lower limbs the lymphatics are arranged in two distinct layers which run separately. One set lies in the superficial tissues outside the investing fascia of the limb. The other set lies deeply beneath the fascia draining the muscles and other deep structures (30).

At intervals along the lymphatic vessels lymph nodes are present. Lymph flows through the lymph nodes in order to reach more proximal lymphatic vessels. These vary in size between 0.2 mm and 20 mm in length. Collections of lymph nodes are found in the axilla and inguinal region, the neck and in the thorax and abdomen. These structures facilitate interaction of the immune system with the lymph. This is a further function of the lymphatic system and is crucially important in protection of the body against infection and tumors, functions which are provided by the complex components of the immune system.

The lymphatic vessels unite to form large vessels. Those from the lower limb enter the posterior wall of the abdomen after leaving the inguinal lymph nodes and eventually reach the cysterna chyli, a sac-like dilation situated in front of the bodies of the first and second lumbar vertebrae. From here the lymph enters the thoracic duct which also receives lymphatic flow from the left side of the thorax, left arm and left side of the head and neck. The thoracic duct enters the venous system at the junction of the left subclavian vein and left internal jugular vein. The right lymph duct drains lymph from the right side of the thorax, the right side of the head and neck and the right arm. The normal total return of lymph to the venous system is about 2–4 litres per day.

The lymph is similar in electrolyte composition to other extracellular fluids but contains substantial amounts of protein (40–60 gL^{-1}) of which albumin is the main part (23–34 gL^{-1}). The white cell count in peripheral lymph is about 5×10^8 cells per litre of which half are lymphocytes. The lymph entering the thoracic duct contains about 1×10^{10} lymphocytes per litre, emphasising the role of this system in the immune response. The return of lymph from the peripheral tissues maintains the interstitial fluid protein level at about 15 $g L^{-1}$, which is usually sufficiently low to ensure that edema does not arise. This has a low colloid osmotic pressure (about 5 mmHg) ensuring that a substantial gradient exists between the interstitial tissues and capillary lumen favoring reabsorption of water from the tissues.

LYMPHEDEMA

Lymphedema arises when the lymphatic system fails to drain lymphatic fluid and interstitial fluid contains increased amounts of protein. This may arise as a congenital deficiency when lymphatic channels are absent or ineffective. More commonly this is seen as a secondary problem arising following trauma, such as surgery, radiation or infection. The lymphatics may become blocked by parasitic infection such as filariasis or by malignant disease. The distribution of the resulting lymphedema will depend upon the anatomical location of the affected vessels.

REFERENCES

1. Evans CJ, Fowkes FG, Ruckley CV, Lee AJ. Prevalence of varicose veins and chronic venous insufficiency in men and women in the general population: Edinburgh Vein Study. J Epidemiol Community Health 1999; 53:149–153.
2. Moneta GL, Bedford G, Beach K, Strandness DE. Duplex ultrasound assessment of venous diameters, peak velocities, and flow patterns. J Vasc. Surg 1988; 8:286–291.
3. Moreno AH, Katz AI, Gold LD, Reddy RV. Mechanics of distension of dog veins and other thin walled tubular structures. Circ Res 1970; 27:1069–1080.

4. Ackroyd JS, Pattison M, Browse NL. A study of the mechanical properties of fresh and preserved human femoral vein wall and valve cusps. Br J Surg 1985; 72:117.

5. Cotton LT. Varicose veins. Gross anatomy and development. Br J Surg 1961; 48:589.

6. Powell T, Lynn RB. The valves of the external iliac, femoral and upper third of the popliteal vein. Surg Gynec Obstet 1951; 92:453.

7. Basmajian JV. Distribution of valves in femoral, external iliac and common iliac veins and their relationship to varicose veins. Surg. Gynecol. Obstet 1952; 95:537–542.

8. Ludbrook J, Beales G. Femoral venous valves in relation to varicose veins. Lancet 1962; 1:79.

9. Gardner AMN, Fox RH. The venous pump of the human foot. Bristol Med Chir J 1983; 109:112.

10. Pegum JM, Fegan WG. Physiology of venous return from the foot. Cardiovasc Res 1967; 1:249.

11. van Bemmelen PS, Beach K, Bedford G, Strandness DE. The mechanism of venous valve closure. Its relationship to the velocity of reverse flow. Arch Surg 1990; 125:617–619.

12. Moreno AH, Burchell AR, Vanderwonde R, Burke JH. Respiratory regulation of splanchnic and systemic venous return. Am J Physiol 1967; 213:455.

13. Moreno AH, Katz AI, Gold LD. An integrated approach to the study of the venous system with steps toward a detailed model of the dynamics of venous return to the right heart. IEEE Trans Biomed Eng 1969; 16:308.

14. Duomarco JL, Rimini R. Energy and hydraulic gradients along systemic veins. Am J Physiol 1954; 178:215.

15. Ludbrook J, Louchlin J. Regulation of volume in posarteriolar vessels of the lower limb. Am Heart J 1964; 67:493–507.

16. Gardner AMN, Fox RH. The return of blood to the heart: venous pumps in health and disease. London: John Libbey & Co Ltd, 1989.

17. Almen T, Nylander G. Serial phlebography of the normal lower limb during muscular contraction and relaxation. Acta Radiol Scand 1962; 57:264.

18. Bjordal R. Simultaneous pressure and flow recordings in varicose veins of the lower extremity. Acta Chir Scand 1970; 136:309.

19. Pollack AA, Wood EH. Venous pressure in the saphenous vein at the ankle in man during exercise and changes in posture. J Appl Physiol 1949; 1:649.

20. Van Bemmelen PS, Beach K, Bedford G, Strandness DE. The mechanism of venous valve closure. Its relationship to the velocity of reverse flow. Arch Surg 1990; 125:617–619.

21. Neglen P, Raju D. A comparison between descending phlebography and duplex Doppler investigation in the evaluation of reflux in chronic venous insufficiency: A challenge to phlebography as the 'gold standard'. J Vasc Surg 1992; 16:687–693.

22. Neglen P, Raju S. A rational approach to detection of significant reflux with duplex Doppler scanning and air plethysmography. J Vasc Surg 1993; 17:590–595.

23. Sarin S, Scurr JH, Coleridge Smith PD. Mechanism of action of external compression on venous function. Br J Surg 1992; 79:499–502.

24. Moulton S, Bergan JJ, Beeman S, Poppiti R. Gravitational reflux does not correlate with clinical status of venous stasis. Phlebology 1993; 8:2–6.

25. Coleridge Smith PD. How should we investigate patients with venous disease? Phlebology 1993; 8:1.

26. Kistner RL. Transvenous repair of the incompetent femoral vein valve. Chicago: Year Book Medical Publishers, 1978 (Bergan JJ, Yao JST, eds. Venous Problems).

27. Welch HJ, Faliakou EC, McLaughlin RL, Umphrey SE, Belkin M, O'Donnell TF. Comparison of descending phlebography with quantitative photoplethysmography, air plethysmography, and duplex quantitative valve closure time in assessing deep venous reflux. J Vasc Surg 1992; 16:913–920.

28. Beckwith TC, Richardson GD, Sheldon M, Clarke GH. A correlation between blood flow volume and ultrasonic Doppler waveforms in the study of valve efficiency. Phlebology 1993; 8:12–16.

29. Pflug JJ. The lymphatic system and lymphedema. Br J Hospital Medicine 1972;270–363.

30. Pflug JJ, Calnan JS. The normal anatomy of the lymphatic system in the human leg. Br J Surg 1971; 58:925–930.

4

Epidemiology of Venous Disorders

F. G. R. Fowkes
Wolfson Unit for Prevention of Peripheral Vascular Diseases, University of Edinburgh, Edinburgh, U.K.

Venous disorders in the legs are extremely common and can range from minor asymptomatic incompetence of venous valves to severe chronic leg ulceration. In this chapter on epidemiology, the frequency of varicose veins, asymptomatic venous insufficiency, venous skin changes and chronic ulceration in the general population will be described. Epidemiological evidence on risk factors for varicose veins and ulceration will also be discussed.

VARICOSE VEINS: PREVALENCE AND INCIDENCE

The prevalence of varicose veins observed in selected studies (1–20) conducted during the last 40 years is shown in Table 1. The study populations varied widely because they were based in different countries, were often derived from selected groups in the population, used different methods of assessment, and had slightly different age ranges. There was no standard definition of varicose veins. Some authors included varices of all sizes ("all varicosities") while others only included trunk (stem) varices and excluded some of the smallest, e.g., telangiectasia or reticular varices. Given these study differences it is not surprising that the prevalences varied markedly, even in the same country. In Switzerland, for example, the prevalence in females in three surveys (4,5,7) ranged from 29% to 68%.

In order to obtain a reasonable estimate of the prevalence of varicose veins in Western populations, the data from studies based on general population samples in the United States (6), New Zealand (8), Israel (11), Turkey (16), Scotland (17), Finland (18) and Italy (19) are of interest. Although the definitions of disease and methods of measurement were slightly different, Figure 1 shows that the prevalence of varicose veins in females was remarkably consistent with around one-quarter to one-third of women affected.

There is little doubt from the majority of epidemiological studies that a higher prevalence of varicose veins has been observed in females than in males (Table 1). Prevalences derived from earlier surveys in the general population between 1973 and 1981 (6,8,11), suggest that the female:male ratio was approximately 2:1. However, in two studies, one in Switzerland (7) and one in the Rarotongan Cook Islanders (21), no sex

Table 1 Prevalence of Varicose Veins in Adult Males and Females in Selected Epidemiological Surveys

Year	Country	Population	Definition used	n	Female (%)	Male (%)
1966	Wales (1)	Population sample	All varicosities	289	53.1	37.2
1969	Egypt (2)	Cotton mill workers	Excl. tel	467	5.8	–
1969	England (2)	Cotton mill workers	Excl. tel	504	31.1	–
1972	India (South) (3)	Railway sweepers	All varicosities	323	–	25.1
1972	India (North) (3)	Railway sweepers	All varicosities	354	–	6.8
1973	Switzerland (4)	Chemical industry employees	All varicosities	4529	55.0	56.0
1973	Switzerland (5)	Shop and factory employees	Excl. tel	610	29.0	–
1973	United States (6)	Population sample	All varicosities	6389	25.9	12.9
1974	Switzerland (7)	Chemical industry employees	All varicosities	4376	68.0	57.0
1975	New Guinca (9)	Villagers	All varicosities	1457	0.1	5.1
1976	New Zealand (8)	General population	All varicosities	356	37.8	19.6
1977	Tanzania (10)	Outpatients	All varicosities	1000	5.0	6.1
1981	Israel (11)	Population sample	Excl. small varicosities	4888	29.3	10.4
1986	Brazil (12)	Health center patients	Excl. tel. and retics	1755	50.9	37.9
1988	Sicily (13)	Villagers	All varicosities	1122	46.2	19.3
1990	Japan (14)	Patients, hospital staff, elderly residents	All varicosities	541	45.0	–
1991	Czechoslovakia (15)	Shop employees	All varicosities	696	60.5	–
1994	Turkey (16)	General population	All varicosities	850	38.3	34.5
1995	Scotland (17)	General population	Trunk varicosities	1566	32.2	39.7
1995	Finland (18)	General population	Varicose veins	7217	24.6	6.8
1998	Italy (19)	General population	All varicosities	1319	35.2	17.0
2000	United States (20)	University employees	Trunk varicosities	600	33.0	17.3

Abbreviations: Excl, excluding; tel, telangiectasia; retics, reticular veins.

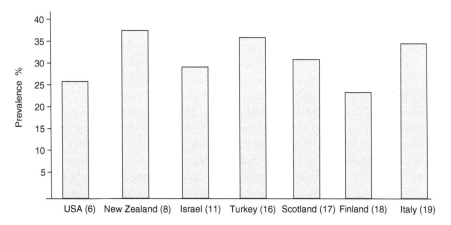

Figure 1   Prevalence of varicose veins in females in general population surveys.

difference was found, but neither of these were large studies based on random samples of the general population. On the other hand, males were found to have a higher prevalence in New Guinea (9), Kenya (22) and Hong Kong (23). It has been suggested that the prevalence rises first in males in developing countries due to their earlier contact with Western culture, although this is purely hypothetical. However, in the Edinburgh Vein Study a slightly higher prevalence was found in men (17), and this was also noted in young adults in the Bochum Study in Germany (24). These are recent studies and there is a possibility that the prevalence of varicose veins may be increasing in men. Also, the higher prevalence in women in some studies may be due partly to recruitment bias because relatively more women concerned about the cosmetic appearance of their varicosities may volunteer to take part.

A common finding in epidemiological studies is that the prevalence of varicose veins increases with age. For example, Table 2 shows that in men in the Edinburgh Vein Study (17) prevalence increased from around 16% in those aged 25–34 years to 61% in those 55–64 years. For women aged 25–34 years, prevalence was 14% rising to 51% in those 55–64 years of age. In the Bochum Study, examination of schoolchildren aged 10–12 years demonstrated the presence of only discrete reticular varices in 10% of the pupils, but four years later this figure had increased to 30%, and a few children had developed stem and branch varices (25).

The prevalences of different categories of varicose veins (trunk, reticular, etc.) in populations are difficult to determine because most studies do not provide such information, and the classification of the categories and their severity varies between

Table 2   Prevalence of Varicose Veins by Age and Sex in Edinburgh Vein Study

Age (years)	% Varicose Veins (n)	
	Men	Women
18–24	20 (11)	5 (4)
25–34	16 (16)	14 (22)
35–44	36 (57)	23 (42)
45–54	42 (76)	42 (95)
55–64	61 (124)	51 (111)

Note: Varicose veins comprise only trunk varices of any grade of severity.
Source: From Ref. 15.

studies. In the Basle Study (Survey II), 5.2% of men and 3.2% of women were considered to have trunk varices, and 51.8% of men and 64.8% of women to have reticular varices and/or telangiectasia (7). On the other hand, in the Basle Study (Survey III), the prevalence of trunk varices in men had risen to 20% and in women to 16% (4). Such differences would however be affected by variation in the age of subjects between the two surveys. By comparison, a survey in Japan on highly selected groups of women found that 10% had trunk varices, 16% had isolated non-trunk varices, 13% had reticular varices and 7% had telangiectasia (14). In the Edinburgh Vein Study both reticular varices and telangiectasia were found in over 80% of subjects although most were relatively mild. Clearly, more information is required on the relative distributions of different categories of varices.

During the early 1970s, several authors produced anecdotal evidence derived from clinical observations in developing countries, suggesting that varicose veins were rare in Africa and other developing countries in comparison to the West (26). Some believed that there was an equal prevalence throughout the world but the occurrence of fewer complications in tropical Africa resulted in the condition presenting very rarely (27). Meaningful comparisons between countries, however, can only be made if studies use the same methods and are based on population surveys. In this regard, a study investigating varicose veins in New Zealand and the South Pacific is of interest because any differences were more likely to be real than to be due to methodological biases (8,21). A marked difference in prevalence was found between the populations; for example, 44% of New Zealand Maori women had varicose veins compared to less than 5% of Atoll islanders. Furthermore, the prevalence among the New Zealand Maoris was similar to that of New Zealand caucasians. More recently in Southern California, no differences were found in the prevalence of trunk varices between Caucasian, Hispanic, Black and Asian Americans (20).

Although there have been many studies examining the prevalence of varicose veins, very little data is available on the incidence, that is, the rate of development of new cases. In the Framingham Study (28) the annual incidence was found to be 1.9% per annum in men and 2.6% in women. Interestingly, the incidence did not increase with age (Fig. 2) so that the observed increase in the prevalence of varicose veins would therefore appear to be a result of the relatively constant development of cases as people grow older. Thus, increasing age per se would not appear to be a risk factor for the development of varicose veins.

ASYMPTOMATIC VENOUS VALVE INCOMPETENCE: PREVALENCE

In recent years, the availability of duplex scanning has permitted vein reflux to be measured non-invasively in epidemiological studies. In the Edinburgh Vein Study, for example, duplex scanning was carried out on a random sample of men and women in the general population aged 18 to 64 years. In individuals who had no evidence on clinical observation of significant venous disease (other than minor telangiectasia or reticular varicosities) around 35% had significant reflux (≥ 0.5 sec) in at least one of eight venous segments measured in each leg (29). Thus venous insufficiency in the legs may occur with no evidence of varicose veins or other clinical manifestation.

Indeed, the Bochum studies in Germany have demonstrated that in the teenage years venous reflux occurs much more commonly than clinical varicosities and that asymptomatic reflux may be a normal precursor of clinical disease (24). For example, among 14–16 years olds examined in Bochum Study II, 12.3% had saphenous reflux but

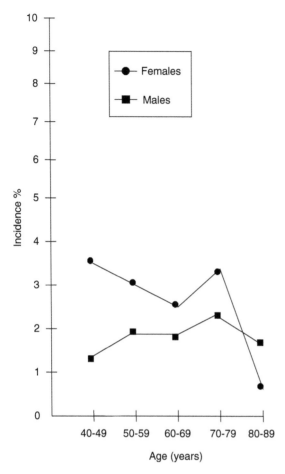

Figure 2 Annual incidence of varicose veins in males and females in the Framingham Study, United States. *Source*: Adapted from Ref. 28.

only 1.7% had trunk varices, 0.8% had tributary varices and 4.1% incompetent perforators. Four years later, nearly 20% had saphenous reflux with only 3.3% having trunk varices.

RISK FACTORS FOR VARICOSE VEINS

Numerous genetic, lifestyle, and physiological characteristics have been put forward as possible risk factors for the development of varicose veins. Many of these factors, such as low fibre diet and lack of exercise, are associated with "westernization" and have been suggested as possible explanations for the apparent geographical variation in the prevalence of varicose veins. However, the evidence linking most of these factors to the development of varicose veins is extremely limited, particularly as there have been very few properly conducted epidemiological studies. Table 3 summarizes the levels of evidence available on possible risk factors for varicose veins.

Obesity

Obesity is commonly believed to be important in predisposing individuals to increased risk of varicose veins. In a large case control study with over 500 subjects in each group (30), obesity, defined as $>20\%$ over ideal weight, was much more common in those with trunk varicosities and telangiectasia than in controls (15% vs. 3%, $p<0.0001$). Similarly, in the Basle Study of chemical workers in which the results were age-adjusted, varicose veins were more common in overweight women. But, in men, only telangiectasia and reticular varicosities, and not trunk varices, were more common in overweight individuals (4).

Population-based studies have also shown a relationship between body mass and varicose veins. In the community survey in West Jerusalem, people with varicose veins had a higher body mass index (kg/m^2) than normal (11). In multivariate analyses including weight and height, weight remained significantly related to the occurrence of varicose veins in women, but not in men. Similarly among caucasian New Zealanders, body mass index was related to severity of varicose veins only in women and independently of parity (8). In the Framingham Study, the incidence of varicose veins over a 16-year follow up period was higher in subjects with a baseline body mass index of over 27 kg/m. On multivariate analysis the difference was maintained in women, but not in men (28). Likewise, in another longitudinal population study in the Netherlands, the incidence of varicose veins in overweight women was higher than in those of normal weight at all ages (31) but no increased risk was found in men.

Thus, the balance of evidence would suggest that a high body mass index is related to the occurrence of varicose veins, but the evidence is much more convincing for women than for men. It is also not clear whether the risk increases above a certain cut-off point or is apparent across the range of body mass index.

Pregnancy

It is a widely held view that in many women, varicose veins appear for the first time during pregnancy. However, pregnancy may merely be an exacerbating factor in those already predisposed, rather than a primary cause (32). Epidemiological studies have sought to determine whether a previous history of pregnancy or the number of pregnancies are related to the occurrence of varicose veins. In the population based study in New Zealand,

Table 3   Risk Factors Implicated in the Etiology of Varicose Veins by Level of Research Evidence

Good evidence
   Female
   Obesity (only in women)
   Number of pregnancies
Limited evidence
   Inherited factors
   Prolonged standing and sitting
   Constipation
Poor evidence
   Low dietary fiber
   Tight undergarments
   Oral contraceptive use
   Hormone replacement therapy
No evidence
   Smoking
   Lack of exercise
   Social class

The level of evidence relates to the demonstration of a positive association between the risk factor and occurrence of varicose veins.

a greater number of pregnancies in women of European origin was associated with an increasing prevalence of varicose veins, and in Maoris with a greater severity of varicose veins (8). The relationships between pregnancy and varicose veins was maintained on adjustment for age, height and weight. In a study in a more selected population in Brazil attending a health centre, a positive correlation was found between prevalence of varicose veins and number of previous pregnancies, independently of age (12).

In the Basle Study (Survey III), age-adjusted rates of varicose veins were higher in multiparous than primiparous women, who in turn had higher rates than nulliparae (4). The Framingham Study is the one longitudinal study to relate the incidence of varicose veins to various risk factors; it was found that the number of pregnancies was associated with incidence, although the association was statistically nonsignificant ($p > 0.05$) (28). The only population-based study which has not found a relationship with number of pregnancies was in Tecumseh, USA (6). In the above studies, associations were age adjusted but not all were adjusted for obesity. Nevertheless, the balance of the evidence at present would indicate that number of pregnancies is a risk factor for the development of varicose veins. The precise relative risks are difficult to determine but results from the Basle and Framingham Studies indicate that women with two or more pregnancies, compared to those with a single pregnancy or no previous pregnancy, have an approximately 20% to 30% increased risk of developing varicose veins (4,28).

It is not clear why pregnancy might increase the risk of developing varicose veins. The common belief that pregnancy leads to varicose veins due to pressure of the pregnant uterus obstructing venous return from the legs has been refuted, because the majority of varices appear during the first three months of pregnancy when the uterus is not large enough to cause mechanical obstruction. A hormonal factor or the additional burden of increased circulating blood volume could be important.

Inherited Factors

Evidence on the role of genetic predisposition in the development of varicose veins is limited and prone to considerable methodological difficulties. In one study investigating the role of heredity in the etiology of varicose veins (33), the risk of varicose veins was higher in those with affected relatives and if the relative was a male. However, such a study relied on the patient's history for the assessment of relatives, and this method has been shown to be highly inaccurate (1). On the other hand Cornu-Thénard et al. clinically examined the parents of 67 cases of varicose veins and 67 spouse controls (34). They found that both the mothers and fathers of cases were more likely than parents of the controls to have varicosities and a history of treatment (Table 4). In a study of several hundred twins in Germany, (35) 76 pairs were found on examination to have varicose veins in at least one twin. Of monozygous pairs, 42% both had primary varicose veins compared to 11% of dizygous pairs (concordant quotient 4:1).

Thus, the few studies on heredity are inconclusive but indicate that genotype could well have an important effect on the risk of acquiring varicose veins. A study on the cadavers of black Africans showed that they have a higher number of valves than Caucasians when comparing the same section of leg vein (36). This suggests that the number of valves is an inherited factor differing between races and may account for the differences in prevalence of varicose veins seen in different parts of the world. Clearly, there is a need for substantial research on the genetics of varicose veins including family studies of modes of inheritance, twin studies, and the investigation of certain genotypes, such as collagen genes which may influence the structure and biochemical composition of the vein wall.

Table 4   Venous Status of Parents of Cases of Varicose Veins and Controls

	% Mothers		% Fathers	
	No. of Cases (n=67)	No. of Controls (n=67)	No. of Cases (n=67)	No. of Controls (n=67)
Varicose veins				
Long saphenous	46.3	26.9	38.8	14.9
Short saphenous	32.8	16.4	23.9	4.5
Nonsaphenous	19.4	10.4	10.4	6.0
Telangiectasia	83.6	73.1	41.8	28.8
Varicose vein treatment				
Surgery	28.4	6.0	19.4	0.0
Sclerotherapy	44.8	19.4	21.9	3.0

Source: From Ref. 34.

Lifestyle Factors

Prolonged standing has often been blamed for the development of varicose veins. Standing at work was shown to be positively associated with varicose veins in the study in Israel (11). However among women in Czechoslovakia, an association with standing was found only for varices of the main trunk veins (15). In the Framingham Study, the two-year incidence of varicose veins was higher with the length of time women spent sitting or standing (28) but no significant difference was found relating posture to varicose veins in a study from Brazil (12). Comparing railway sweepers in north and south India, both groups were engaged in the same job, and therefore posture at work could not account for the observed difference in prevalence (3).

Sitting in a chair has also been implicated. This practice is a Western habit not adopted by primitive communities in which prevalence of varicose veins is apparently low. In New Guinea, varicose veins were common in men who sat "with the legs dangling", but rare in women who sat cross-legged on the ground, suggesting that variation in sitting positions might be the cause of this sex difference (9). Alexander proposed that sitting in a chair increased the hydrostatic pressure exerted on the leg veins, leading to pooling of blood in the legs, venous dilatation and increased tension in the wall itself (23). The effect of chair-sitting during childhood could therefore produce veins of an increased calibre which would be more susceptible to factors such as pregnancy, standing and tight clothes.

Tight undergarments may raise intra-abdominal pressure, and in theory might promote the development of varicose veins. In cotton workers in England and Egypt in the 1960s, the prevalence of varicose veins increased with the tightness and stiffness of the undergarment being worn (2). In Jerusalem, habitual corset-wearing was also a positive risk factor, (11) but in Swiss women the association between corset-wearing and varicose veins was lost on correcting for age (5).

A positive risk factor for the development of varicose veins in a study in Sicily was constipation (13), but this was not important in the study of cotton workers (2). Such results are however of dubious value because of the difficulty of measuring constipation in a valid and reliable way. Among inhabitants of the South Pacific, the prevalence of varicose veins was low in primitive peoples, but high in more westernized cultures where the diet contained more refined carbohydrate and less dietary fiber (21). A typical low fibre Western diet produces small, hard stools which are difficult to pass, leading to regular straining and repeated increases in intra-abdominal pressure. In the Edinburgh Vein Study, straining in men was related to a higher risk of trunk varices (37). Cleave postulated that during constipation, the loaded bowel compresses the iliac vein thus obstructing venous return from the legs, ultimately leading to the development of varicose veins (38). Alternatively, raised intra-abdominal pressure from straining at stool may be transmitted down the veins of the legs, leading to dilation of the veins and non-apposition of the valve cusps, thus rendering the valves incompetent.

Many other factors have been implicated in the development of varicose veins. These include lack of exercise, cigarette smoking, and use of oral contraceptives. However, the evidence linking these and most of the other factors above to the occurrence of varicose veins is tenuous. The relationship between obesity, pregnancy and the occurrence of venous insufficiency is the most convincing but for many factors, the relationship with varicose veins may be related more to confounding by other factors than a direct causal association.

VENOUS SKIN CHANGES: PREVALENCE

The prevalence in the general population of skin changes due to venous insufficiency, such as hyperpigmentation, eczema and edema, have not been well documented. In the population study in Tecumseh, USA (6), 3.7% of women and 3.0% of men had evidence of skin changes. The prevalence increased markedly with age so that, for example, in women, only 1.8% of those aged 30–39 years had skin changes compared to 20.7% of those over 70 years of age. In the Basle Study (II), the prevalence of "pronounced" skin changes (dilatation of subcutaneous veins, hyper- or hypo-pigmentation) was found in 9.6% of women and 8.7% of the men (7). Mild skin changes in the form of a venous flare occurred in 15% of women and 10% of men. These results were, however, based on active chemical industry employees and not on the general population. Nevertheless, the results from both the Basle and Tecumseh studies suggest that there is not such a large female to male preponderance of skin changes as there is for varicose veins.

In surveys of individuals with varicose veins, a considerable proportion have evidence of skin changes. For example, in a survey of varicose vein patients in Brazil (12), edema was the commonest manifestation occurring in nearly 20% of subjects. Hyperpigmentation occurred in 6% and eczema in 1–2%. The community-based study in Tecumseh, USA found that 10% of men and 20% of women with varicose veins had edema (6). In female cotton workers in the 1960s in England, 10% of women with varicose veins had skin changes or ulceration (2), whereas only 2.5% of South India railworkers with varicose veins had such signs (3). In the Basle Study, (Survey II), the prevalence and severity of various grades of skin change was found to relate to the severity of varicose veins (7). Among those with severe varicose veins (marked trunk varices), the prevalence of skin changes or ulceration was 81% and among those with minor varicose veins (reticular veins and/or telangiectasia or "scarcely visible trunk varices") the prevalence was 30%.

VENOUS ULCER: PREVALENCE, INCIDENCE, AND PROGNOSIS

The prevalence of chronic leg ulcers found in several epidemiological surveys (4,6,39–48) in the general population is shown in Table 5. It is important to distinguish between the occurrence of open (active) ulcers in the population and the combination of open and healed ulcers because very different figures will prevail. The prevalences also vary greatly because of the different sampling methods, ages of the populations, and definitions of ulceration. Furthermore, some studies include all chronic ulcers whereas others include

Table 5 Prevalence of Venous Ulcers in Adult Males and Females in Selected Epidemiological Surveys

Year	Location	Survey method	n	Population	Type of ulcer	Prevalence of ulcer	
						Male (%)	Female (%)
1973	Tecumseh, USA (6)	Examination	6389	General, 10 yrs+	Venous, active or healed	0.1	0.3
1978	Basle, Switzerland (4)	Examination	4529	Chemical workers, 25 yrs+	Chronic, active or healed	1.0	1.0
1985	Lothian/Forth Valley, Scotland (41)	Health Service	1 million	General, 20 yrs+	Chronic active		0.15
1986	Ireland (41)	Health Service	92,100	General, 40 yrs+	Chronic active		0.38
1986	Harrow, England (40)	Postal	2,012	General, all ages	Chronic active	1.0	2.1
1991	Perth, Australia (42)	Health Service	238,000	General, 20 yrs+	Chronic active		0.11
1991	Skaraborg, Sweden (43)	Health Service	270,800	General, all ages	Chronic active	0.22	0.39
1992	Malmo, Sweden (44)	Health Service	232,908	General, all ages	Chronic active		0.12
1992	Newcastle, England (45)	Health Service	107,400	General, 45 yrs+	Chronic active		0.19
1993	Gothenburg, Sweden (46)	Postal	5,140	General, 65 yrs+	Chronic active	3.2	1.5
1996	Skovde, Sweden (47)	Postal and examination	2785	Industrial workers, 30–65 yrs	Chronic, active or healed	1.6	
2000	Village, Sweden (48)	Postal and examination	541	General, 70 yrs+	Chronic, active or healed	12.6	

only those believed to be primarily of venous origin. Reviewing the results overall, a very approximate estimate of the prevalence of open venous ulceration in the adult population over 18 years of age in Western countries is about 0.3%. That is, about one in 350 adults are affected at any one time. For every patient with an open ulcer in the population, there would appear to be between two and four individuals with healed ulcers, so that the population prevalence of open and healed ulcers combined could be around 1% (43). These summary figures are, however, very rough estimates.

In many of the epidemiological studies, the prevalence of ulceration is not given separately for males and females. Table 5 shows that in the studies reviewed, three studies found a female predominance of two to three times that in males, (6,41,43) one found no difference, (4) and another a male predominance (46). However, other epidemiological studies have found a female:male ratio ranging from approximately 2:1 to 3.5:1. Thus, overall it would appear that the prevalence of ulcers is around two to three times more common in females than males. Chronic leg ulceration is relatively uncommon below the age of 60 years (40). Above that, the prevalence increases consistently with age in both men and women (39–43) with the female predominance being maintained at all ages.

The prognosis of chronic venous ulcers is often poor. Typically, in patients attending for treatment, only half the ulcers are healed within four months (49). Information on the duration of ulcers existing in the general population at any point in time has been obtained in prevalence surveys in which the duration of ulcers was assessed retrospectively (44,45,50–52). The results of these studies were similar; for example, in the Lothian and Forth Valley Leg Ulcer Study in Scotland, 20% of ulcers had not healed after two years, and 8% had been open for five years. The longest duration was 62 years in an 85 years old woman (51).

In a similar way the duration of the ulcer diathesis, i.e. the length of time in which ulcer patients in a community have experienced ulcers irrespective of whether they were consistently open, has been investigated retrospectively. In the Lothian and Forth Valley Study, 45% had had episodes for more than 10 years and 21% for between five and ten years. The number of episodes of active ulceration has also been recorded in some surveys (50–52). Approximately one-third were shown to have had one episode and at least another third were likely to have had four or more episodes. Although these figures were based on all chronic leg ulcers, and not just venous ulcers, they do reflect the situation for venous ulcers which comprise the majority of all leg ulcers.

Limited data is available on the incidence of development of new chronic ulcers in the general population. In a retrospective survey in England, the annual incidence rate was estimated to be 3.5 per 1000 in those aged over 45 years of age, (15) whereas in the population over 15 years of age in Olmsted County, Minnesota, it was nearly two per 10,000 (53).

RISK FACTORS FOR VENOUS ULCERS

Venous ulcers are at the severe end of the spectrum of venous disease in the legs. It is not surprising therefore that less severe forms of venous disease, such as varicose veins and skin changes are associated with mild chronic venous disease, and increase the risk of the development of varicose ulcers. In the Basle Study, for example, the risk of developing varicose ulcers during an 11 years follow-up period was 0.8% for those with mild varicosities but 20% for those with severe varicose veins (Fig. 3).

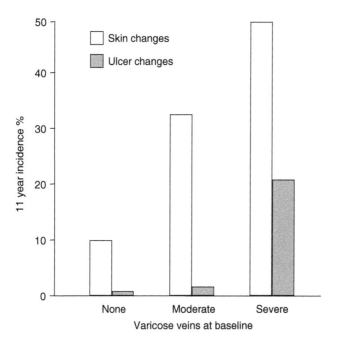

Figure 3 Incidence of skin changes and chronic ulceration during 11 years of follow up by severity of varicose veins at baseline: Basle Study. *Source*: Adapted from Ref. 59.

There is also some evidence that the severity of venous incompetence, as indicated by objective measures such as the ambulatory venous pressure of the foot, may be related to the risk of ulceration. In one study of 220 unselected patients with venous problems (54), no ulceration occurred in limbs with ambulatory venous pressure <30 mmHg. A consistent increase in the prevalence of ulceration occurred with higher ambulatory venous pressure, ranging from 14% in limbs with pressure between 31 and 40 mmHg to 100% in limbs with pressure >90 mmHg. This relationship occurred in both those with superficial venous reflux and those with deep venous reflux with or without occlusion.

Deep vein thrombosis (DVT) is known to be an antecedent risk factor for the skin changes, edema and ulceration associated with venous disease in the legs. Under these circumstances the venous condition is often referred to as the post thrombotic syndrome. Although most studies do not separately identify ulcers or the number of ulcers are too small for meaningful analysis, the results linking DVT and the postthrombotic syndrome (55,56) are probably also meaningful in relation to ulcer alone.

In the population-based study of chronic venous ulcers in Perth, Western Australia, (50) 17% of patients had a history of DVT and a large number had a history of conditions that might predispose to DVT. Although this prevalence seemed relatively high, results were unfortunately not available from a healthy comparison group. On the other hand, in a population based study of 3,600 people in Copenhagen, Denmark, various risk factors were related to the occurrence of objective signs of venous disease (57). Previous thromboembolism (history of DVT or pulmonary embolism) was related to the occurrence of venous disease, independently of age, sex and other possible risk factors. The incidence of ulcers has been shown in follow-up studies of patients having a diagnosis of DVT (55,56) to be around 1% to 2% per annum.

Arterial disease per se in the lower limbs is considered to be a cause of chronic leg ulceration, but the extent to which arterial disease might increase the risk of venous ulceration is less clear. Some studies have reported a relatively high prevalence of arterial disease in leg ulcer patients (40,42) but this may be partly accounted for by the presence of patients with ulcers primarily of arterial origin. Also, no comparisons were made with the occurrence of ulcers in a healthy control group. However, in a case control comparison in Edinburgh, Scotland, arterial disease (angina, intermittent claudication, hypertension, and low ankle brachial pressure index) did not occur more commonly in 331 leg ulcer patients compared to an equal number of age and sex matched population controls (58).

Finally, several other factors may be possible contributory factors to the development of venous ulceration. These include minor trauma, edema (not necessarily related to venous insufficiency), obesity, and co-existing conditions such as arthritis or neuropathies. However, the extent to which these factors are important is not well established.

CONCLUSION

In conclusion, varicose veins are an extremely common disorder in the population in which the risk factors are not well established. Further epidemiological research, including genetic studies, are required to elucidate the aetiology of this condition. Venous ulceration is the most serious complication in which the prognosis is often poor. In order to prevent ulceration, further research is required to establish the risks of this condition, particularly in subjects with varicose veins. The prevalence of venous disorders increases with age so that the changing age structure of the population will result in an increasing burden of these conditions in society.

KEY POINTS

- Varicose veins occur commonly in the general population affecting around one quarter to one-third of adults in western countries. The prevalence in most surveys is higher in females than males.
- Minor varicosities such as reticular varices and telangiectasia are almost the norm and occur in around 80% of adults.
- In individuals with no obvious trunk varices, around one-third have significant valvular reflux in at least one segment of either leg.
- Venous abnormalities, including valvular reflux, may begin in childhood and, although prevalence increases with age, limited evidence suggests that the risk of acquiring venous disease is constant throughout life.
- Number of pregnancies and obesity (only in women) have been shown consistently to be risk factors for varicose veins. Limited evidence suggests that inherited factors, prolonged standing and/or sitting and constipation may be important.
- The frequency of skin changes associated with varicose veins, such as hyper/hypo-pigmentation, eczema and edema, varies greatly between surveys but the prevalence appears to increase with the severity of the varicosities.
- Venous ulcers, which account for about 75% of all chronic ulcers, occurs in 1% of the adult population during their lifetime. The prevalence of open ulceration is about 0.3%.

- Ulceration is more common in women than men and is relatively uncommon below the age of 60 years. The prognosis is poor with only half healed within four months and two thirds having more than one episode of active ulceration.
- Although DVT and raised ambulatory venous pressure increase the risk of ulceration, other risk factors that might lead to an ulcer developing in patients with varicose veins are not well established.

REFERENCES

1. Weddell JM. Varicose veins pilot study, 1966. Brit J Prev Soc Med 1969; 23:179–186.
2. Mekky S, Schilling RSF, Walford J. Varicose veins in women cotton workers. An epidemiological study in England and Egypt. Br Med J 1969; 2:591–595.
3. Malhotra SL. An epidemiological study of varicose veins in Indian railroad workers from the south and north of India, with special reference to the causation and prevention of varicose veins. Int J Epid 1972; 1:117–183.
4. Widmer LK, ed. Peripheral Venous Disorders—Prevalence and Socio-medical Importance. Bern: Hans Grudber, 1978:1–90.
5. Guberan W, Widmer LK, Glaus L, et al. Causative factors of varicose veins: myths and facts. VASA 1973; 2:115–120.
6. Coon WW, Willis PW, Keller JB. Venous thromboembolism and other venous disease in the Tecumseh community health study. Circulation 1973; 48:839–846.
7. da Silva A, Widmer LK, Martin H, Mall TH, Glaus L, Schneider M. Varicose veins and chronic venous insufficiency—prevalence and risk factors in 4376 subjects in the Basle Study II. VASA 1974; 3:118–125.
8. Beaglehole R, Salmond CE, Prior IAM. Varicose veins in New Zealand: prevalence and severity. NZ Med J 1976; 84:396–399.
9. Stanhope JM. Varicose veins in a population of New Guinea. Int J Epid 1975; 4:221–225.
10. Richardson JB, Dixon M. Varicose veins in tropical Africa. Lancet 1977; 1:791–792.
11. Abramson JH, Hopp C, Epstein LM. The epidemiology of varicose veins—a survey of Western Jerusalem. J Epidemiol Comm Health 1981; 35:213–217.
12. Maffei FHA, Magaldi C, Pinho SZ, et al. Varicose veins and chronic venous insufficiency in Brazil: prevalence among 1755 inhabitants of a country town. Int J Epid 1986; 15:210–217.
13. Novo S, Avellone G, Pinto A, et al. Prevalence of primitive varicose veins in a randomised population sample of Western Sicily. Int Angio 1988; 7:176–181.
14. Hirai M, Kenichi N, Nakayama R. Prevalence and risk factors of varicose veins in Japanese women. Angiology 1990; 41:228–232.
15. Stvrtinova V, Kolesar J, Wimmer G. Prevalence of varicose veins of the lower limbs in the women working at a department store. Int Angio 1991; 10:2–5.
16. Komsuoğlu B, Göldeli O, Kulan K, Cetinarsalan B, Komsuoğlu SS. Prevalence and risk factors of varicose veins in an elderly population. Gerontology 1994; 40:25–31.
17. Evans CJ, Fowkes FGR, Ruckley CV, Lee AJ. Prevalence of varicose veins and chronic venous insufficiency in men and women in the general population. J Epidemiol Comm Health 1999; 53:149–153.
18. Sisto T, Reunanen A, Laurikka J, et al. Prevalence and risk factors of varicose veins in lower extremities: Mini-Finland Health Survey. Eur J Surg 1995; 161:405–414.
19. Canonico S, Callo C, Paolisso G, et al. Prevalence of varicose veins in an Italian elderly population. Angiology 1998; 49:129–135.
20. Langer RD, Criqui MH, Denenberg J, Fronek A. The prevalence of venous disease by gender and ethnicity in a balanced sample of four ethnic groups in southern California. Phlebology 2000; 15:99–105.
21. Beaglehole R, Prior IAM, Salmond CE, Davidson F. Varicose veins in the South Pacific. Int J Epid 1975; 4:295–299.

22. Kakande I. Varicose veins in Africans as seen at Kenyatta National Hospital, Nairobi. East Afr Med J 1981; 58:667–676.
23. Alexander CJ. The epidemiology of varicose veins. Med J Aust 1972; 1:215–218.
24. Schultz-Ehrenburg U, Weindorf N, Matthes U, Hirche H. New epidemiological findings with regard to initial stages of varicose veins (Bochum Study I–III). In: Raymond-Martinbeau P, Prescott R, Zummo M, eds. Phlebologie 92. Paris: John Libbey Eurotext, 1992:234–236.
25. Schultz-Ehrenburg U, Weindorf N, Von Uslar D, Hirche H. Prospective epidemiological investigations on early and preclinical stages of varicosis. In: Davy A, Stemmer R, eds. Phlébologie '89. Paris: John Libbey Eurotext Ltd, 1989:163–165.
26. Burkitt DP, Townsend AJ, Patel K, Skaug K. Varicose veins in developing countries. Lancet 1976; ii:202–203.
27. Rivlin S. Varicose veins in tropical Africa. Lancet 1974; i:1054.
28. Brand FN, Dannenberg AL, Abbott RD, et al. The epidemiology of varicose veins: the Framingham Study. Am J Prev Med 1988; 4:96–101.
29. Evans CJ, Allan PL, Lee AJ, Bradbury AW, Ruckley CV, Fowkes FGR. Prevalence of venous reflux in the general population on duplex scanning: The Edinburgh Vein Study. J Vasc Surg 1998; 28:767–776.
30. Sadick NS. Predisposing factors of varicose veins and telangiectatic leg veins. J Dermatol Surg Oncol 1992; 18:883–886.
31. Seidell JC, Bakx KC, Deurenberg P, van den Hoogen HJM, Hautvast JGAJ, Stijnen T. Overweight and chronic illness—a retrospective cohort study, with a follow up of 6–17 years, in men and women of initially 20–50 years of age. J Chron Dis 1986; 39:585–593.
32. Fanfera FJ, Palmer LH, Mawr B. Pregnancy and varicose veins. Arch Surg 1968; 96:33–35.
33. Gundersen J, Hauge M. Hereditary factors in venous insufficiency. Angiology 1969; 20:346–355.
34. Cornu Thenard A, Boivin P, Baud JM, de Vincenzi I, Carpentier PH. Importance of the familial factor in varicose disease. Clinical study of 134 families. J Dermatol Surg Oncol 1994; 20:318–326.
35. Nierman H. Genetik und Varizen. In: Salfeld K, ed. Phlebologie, Lymphologie und Proktologie in Verschiedenen Hebensaltern: Aktuelles aus Diagnostik u Therapie. Stuttgart: FK Schautter Verlag, 1978.
36. Banjo AO. Comparative study of the distribution of venous valves in the lower extremities of black Africans and caucasians: pathogenetic correlates of the prevalence of primary varicose veins in the two races. Anat Rec 1987; 217:407–412.
37. Lee AJ, Evans CJ, Hau CM, Fowkes FGR. Fibre intake, constipation and risk of varicose veins in the general population. Edinburgh Vein Study. J Clin Epidemiol 2001; 54:423–429.
38. Cleave TL. The Saccharine Disease. Bristol, England: John Wright and Sons, Inc, 1974 pp. 44–65.
39. Callam MJ, Ruckley CV, Harper DR, Dale JJ. Chronic ulceration of the leg: extent of the problem and provision of care. Br Med J 1985; 290:1855–1856.
40. Cornwall JV, Doré CJ, Lewis JD. Leg ulcers; epidemiology and aetiology. Br J Surg 1986; 73:693–696.
41. Henry M. Incidence of varicose ulcers in Ireland. Irish Med J 1986; 79:65–67.
42. Baker SR, Stacey MC, Singh G, Hoskin SE, Thompson PJ. Aetiology of chronic leg ulcers. Eur J Vasc Surg 1992; 6:245–251.
43. Nelzen O, Bergquist D, Hallbook T, Lindhagen A. Chronic leg ulcers: an underestimated problem in primary health care among elderly patients. J Epidemiol Comm Health 1991; 45:184–187.
44. Lindholm C, Bjellerup M, Christensen OB, Zederfeldt B. A demographic survey of leg and foot ulcer patients in a defined population. Acta Derm Venereol 1992; 72:227–230.
45. Lees TA, Lambert D. Prevalence of lower limb ulceration in an urban health district. Br J Surg 1992; 79:1032–1034.

46. Andersson E, Hansson C, Swanbeck G. Leg and foot ulcer prevalence and investigation of the peripheral arterial and venous circulation in a randomised elderly population. An epidemiological survey and clinical investigation. Acta Derm Venereol 1993; 73:57–61.

47. Nelzen O, Bergquist D, Framsson I, Lindhagen A. Prevalence and aetiology of leg ulcers in a defined population of industrial workers. Phlebology 1996; 11:50–54.

48. Marklund B, Sulan T, Lindholin C. Prevalence of non-healed and healed chronic leg ulcers in an elderly population. Scand J Primary Health Care 2000; 18:58–60.

49. Skene AI, Smith JM, Doré CJ, Charlett A, Lewis JD. Venous leg ulcers: a prognostic index to predict time to healing. Br Med J 1992; 305:1119–1121.

50. Baker SR, Stacey MC, Jopp-McKay AG, Hoskin SE, Thompson PJ. Epidemiology of chronic venous ulcers. Br J Surg 1991; 78:864–867.

51. Callam MJ, Harper DR, Dale JJ, Ruckley CV. Chronic ulcer of the leg: clinical history. Br Med J 1987; 294:1389–1391.

52. Nelzen O, Bergquist D, Lindhagen A. Venous and non-venous leg ulcers: clinical history and appearance in a population study. Br J Surg 1994; 81:182–187.

53. Heit JA, Rooke TW, Silverstein MD, et al. Trends in the incidence of venous stasis syndrome and venous ulcer: a 25 year population based study. J Vasc Surg 2001; 33:1022–1027.

54. Nicolaides AN, Hussein MK, Szendro G, Christopoulos D, Vasdekis S, Clarke H. The relation of venous ulceration with ambulatory venous pressure measurment. J Vasc Surg 1993; 17:414–419.

55. Strandness DE, Langlois Y, Cramer M, Randlett A, Thiele BL. Long-term sequelae of acute venous thrombosis. JAMA 1983; 250:1289–1292.

56. Mudge M, Leinster SJ, Hughes LE. A prospective 10-year study of the post-thrombotic syndrome in a surgical population. Ann R Coll Surg Engl 1988; 70:249–252.

57. Wille-Jørgensen P, Jørgensen T, Andersen M, Kirchaff M. Post phlebitic syndrome and general surgery: an epidemiological investigation. Angiology 1991; 42:397–403.

58. Fowkes FGR, Callam MJ. Is arterial disease a risk factor for chronic leg ulceration? Phlebology 1994; 9:87–90.

59. Widmer LK. Unpublished observations, 1992.

5

Health Economics and Quality of Life— Impact of Venous Disorders

Meryl Davis, Fiona J. Tsang, and Alun H. Davies
West of London Vascular Service, Charing Cross Hospital, London, U.K.

INTRODUCTION

Health is a difficult entity to evaluate and this particularly holds true for venous disease. There is a lack of precise classification for venous disease and, as a consequence, an underestimate of the impact on the health economy of a nation. Using The International Classification of Disease (ICD-9), venous disease includes categories numbers 454 (varicose veins of the lower extremities), 459 (venous insufficiency and postphlebitic syndrome), and 451 (phlebitis and thrombophlebitis).

HEALTH ECONOMICS

Most medical practitioners will have some involvement in health economics during their career with the aim being to optimize the resources available. This can be described in terms of efficiency (technical, productive, and allocation) or in terms of cost.

Efficiency

1. Technical efficiency—the relationship between the resource available and the health outcome
2. Productive efficiency—the relationship between different patterns of the resource available and health outcome
3. Allocation efficiency—the relationship between the cost and the outcome at a social level

Chronic venous insufficiency and venous leg ulceration are debilitating conditions. In developed countries chronic venous insufficiency affects approximately 5% of the adult population with leg ulcers affecting between 0.2 and 0.5% of the population. Venous disease consumes 1–2% of the health care budgets of European countries. The extent of the disease burden in developing countries is not known. In 1992 it was estimated that

Table 1 The Cost of Venous Diseases of the Legs in the U.K.

Cost	UK £ million
Hospital inpatient	89
Hospital outpatient	n/a
District nursing services	180
General practitioners	8
Prescription medicines	7
Compression hosiery	10
Total	£294 million

Note: Venous diseases includes varicose veins, venous insufficiency, post phlebitic syndrome and phlebitis and thrombophlebitis.

venous disease cost 318–1135 million ECUs per annum (1). Venous ulcers are a chronic and often recurring disease; in the United Kingdom approximately 1,00,000 patients have active leg ulcers. The cost to the National Health Service is approximately £400 million per annum and represents 2.0% of the costs for all conditions (2). Venous diseases absorb approximately 1% of hospital in patient costs in the major EEC countries. Treating venous disease is one of the most time-consuming of district nurses' activities. In 1992 it was estimated that district nurses spend 30–50% of their time dealing with patients with leg ulcers, which translates into a figure of £180 million (3). Table 1 summarizes the overall costs of venous diseases of the legs based on 1989 figures.

The "cost of illness" incorporates the costs of productive capacity lost as a consequence of illness. These are usually described as "indirect" costs in contrast to the "direct" costs of healthcare services. In 1989 the indirect costs of invalidity in the United Kingdom was estimated at £73 million (Table 2).

Leg ulcers are treated by many medical specialities with a majority being treated in the community, therefore a true perspective of the disease is difficult to gain. Approximately 75% of chronic leg ulcers are treated solely in the community, subsequently there is a lack of awareness of the magnitude of the problem as a user of health resources (4).

Chronic leg ulcers are perceived as a disease of the elderly with the peak prevalence being in the seventh and eighth decade and is estimated at between 0.18 and 1.9 per 1000. The costs of leg ulcer treatment are considerable, with an unhealed leg ulcer estimated to be £1067 per year with an annual total cost to the NHS approximately £300 million (3). In 1995 the total direct and indirect costs of treating two hundred patients with venous ulcers over twenty-four weeks were greater than £1,93,000. The costs per healed ulcer was calculated at £1654 (in 1995), however, this only represented 59% of the patients, for the 41% of ulcers which were not healed the cost continued to rise (5). It has been calculated that in 1998 the mean cost per ulcer clinic attendance was £29.90 while the mean cost per home visit was £10.60. The median healing times were 20 and 43 wk for patients in the

Table 2 Indirect Costs in 1989 of Invalidity Attributed to Venous Diseases in the U.K.

	Days of invalidity	As % of invalidity	Cost £ million
All venous diseases	1.8 million	0.4	73
ICD 454	818,000	0.2	33
ICD 459	903,000	0.2	36

Source: From Ref. 1.

clinic and control groups, respectively. These figures again are inaccurate as they fail to take into account the personal costs due to invalidity and time spent receiving treatment (3).

Approximately 15–20% of the adult population have varicose veins with an annual incidence of 2.5% (6). This translates into 60,000 varicose veins operations in the National Health Service and a further 15,000 operations in the private sector (7).

The National Institute for Clinical Excellence (NICE) offers advice on providing the best attainable standards of care. Clinical effectiveness is insufficient for maintaining or introducing a clinical procedure; cost must also enter the decision making process. NICE and its advisory bodies have adopted a ratio up to £15,000/quality adjusted life year (QALY) as a figure at which they would be unlikely to reject a procedure solely on the grounds of cost ineffectiveness. Values achieved in the region of £25,000–£35,000/QALY would need special reasons to be accepted as cost effective (8). In a randomized trial of treatment for symptomatic, uncomplicated varicose veins, surgery was both clinically and cost effective. Surgical treatment produced an estimated incremental benefit of 0.083 quality adjusted life years resulting in an incremental cost effectiveness ratio of £4682 per quality adjusted life year (9).

QUALITY OF LIFE

Quality of life as defined by the World Health Organization is a state of complete physical, mental and social well being, and not merely the absence of disease. However, Price described quality of life as the impact of an illness and its treatment on disability and daily living (10). Quality of life assessment is of value in demonstrating the benefit of interventions of patients and can be used to plan care.

The criteria for an ideal quality of life measure are:

- Equally applicable to any disease process or outcome
- Equally applicable across all levels and degrees of invalidity
- Proven validity with a high level of convergence within patient groups when applied across geographic, linguistic and cultural boundaries (11)

Currently there is no single quality of life tool that fulfils the above criteria; this means that a generic tool has to be adopted, and options include the Nottingham Health Profile (NHP) or the Short Form Survey (SF-36/SF-12). The International Quality of Life Assessment (IQOLA) project was an undertaking to translate and adapt the SF-36 questionnaire and validate it in all major languages thereby making it an international scale of health related quality of life (12).

Studies on the impact of chronic venous disease on quality of life are scarce. Instruments used to measure quality of life are classified into generic and disease-specific instruments. Generic instruments allow comparison across populations of patients with different diseases, whereas disease-specific instruments are sensitive to key dimensions of quality of life that are affected by specific diseases. Therefore combining the two is a preferred strategy when examining quality of life. In a review article twenty-five studies were identified which described the development or use of a quality of life instrument in patients with chronic venous disease. The findings are summarized in Table 3 (13).

Ten disease-specific questionnaires were identified which measured quality of life in specific groups with chronic venous disease and are summarized in Table 4. The use of a

Table 3 Studies on the Quality of Life in Patients with Chronic Venous Disease

Author (year)	Sample size	Method of evaluation	Note
Chronic venous insufficiency			
Franks (1992) (17)	114	QoL questionnaire for patients with venous disease and symptom rating test	
Launois (1996) (18)	2001	CIVIQ	
Augustin (1997) (19)	246	Freiburger questionnaire of quality of life in venous diseases	Patients matched with healthy controls
Klyscz (1998) (20)	142	Tubingen questionnaire for measuring QoL in patients with CVI (TLQ-CVI)	Evaluated in 4 countries
Lamping (1998) (21)	615	VEINES-QOL	
Venous thrombosis			
Beyth (1995) (22)	124	Interview with symptoms and SF-36 items	
Mathias (1999) (23)	111	QoL questionnaire for patients with DVT	
Ziegler (2001) (24)	161	CIVIQ (modified)	All patients had post-thrombotic syndrome
Kahn (2002) (25)	41	SF-26, VEINES QOL	19 with PTS, 22 without PTS
Venous leg ulceration			
Hyland (1986) (26)	50	QoL questionnaire for patients with leg ulcers	
Lindholm (1993) (27)	125	NHP	
Phillips (1994) (28)	73	Interview	
Franks (1994) (29)	185	SRT, adapted version of QoL questionnaire	
Charles (1995) (30)	4	Interview	
Walters (1999) (31)	233	SF-36, EQ, SF-MPQ, FAI	
Smith (2000) (14)	98	SF-36 and the Charing Cross venous ulcer questionnaire	
Franks (2001) (32)	383	NHP	
Varicose venis			
Garratt (1993) (33)	281	SF-36 and QoL questionnaire for patients with varicose veins	542 controls
Kurz (2001) (34)	1054	SF-36, VEINES QoL	259 controls

Abbreviations: CIVIQ, chronic lower limb venous insufficiency; CVI, chronic venous insufficiency; DVT, deep vein thrombosis; EQ, Euro-QoL; FAI, Frenchay Activities Index; NHP, Nottingham Health Profile; PTS, post thrombotic syndrome; QoL, quality of life; SF-36, short form 36; SF-12, short form 12; SF-MPQ, McGill short form pain questionnaire; VAS, visual analogue score; VEINES-QOL, venous insufficiency epidemiologic and economic study questionnaire.

wide range of instruments in the studies indicates a lack of consensus concerning the ideal way to measure quality of life in the field of chronic venous disease. The majority of studies used generic quality of life measures such as the SF-36 which allowed comparison of patients with venous disease with a healthy population.

Table 4 Disease-Specific Quality of Life Instruments

Author (year) (Ref.)	Questionnaire and population studied	Criteria			
		Social	Physical	Psychological	Other
Chronic venous insufficiency					
Franks (1992) (17)	Health questionnaire for venous disease		*	*	
Launois (1996) (18)	CIVIQ (for chronic venous insufficiency)		*	*	*
Augustin (1997) (19)	The Freiburger question-naire of QoL in venous disease (German)	*	*	*	
Klyscz (1998) (20)	The Tubingen questionnaire for chronic venous insuf-ficiency (TLQ-CVI) (German)	*	*	*	*
Lamping (1998) (21)	VEINES-QoL (for chronic vascular disorders of the leg)		*	*	*
Venous thrombosis					
Mathias (1999) (23)	Health related QoL questionnaire for DVT		*	*	*
Venous leg ulceration					
Hyland (1986) (26)	Self-report QoL questionnaire for patients with leg ulcers		*	*	*
Franks (1994) (29)	Health questionnaire for leg ulcers		*	*	
Smith (2000) (14)	Charing Cross venous ulcer questionnaire	*	*	*	*
Varicose veins					
Garratt (1993) (33)	Aberdeen Varicose Vein Questionnaire (AVVQ)		*		*
Smith (2000) (14)	Aberdeen Varicose Vein Questionnaire (AVVQ)	*	*	*	*

Abbreviations: CIVIQ, chronic lower limb venous insufficiency; CVI, chronic venous insufficiency; TLQ-CVI, tubingen questionnaire for measuring quality of life in patients with chronic venous insufficiency; VEINES-QOL, venous insufficiency epidemiologic and economic study questionnaire; QoL, quality of life; DVT, deep vein thrombosis; AVVQ, aberdeen varicose vein questionnaire.

Some major areas of quality of life affected by chronic venous disease can be identified. Patients with venous thrombosis report pain and impairment of physical function with low health perceptions and high health distress. Impairment of quality of life is related to severity of symptoms and the presence of postthrombotic syndrome. Patients with venous leg ulceration report impairment in physical functioning and mobility, with negative emotions and social isolation. Patients with varicose veins have a lower health perception and real impairment of quality of life. Using the SF-36 to assess patients with varicose veins, females scored on average less (i.e., worse function and health) than controls for all eight domains of the SF-36. Significance was achieved in four of eight domains and in two of the eight domains for females and males respectively. Following surgery for varicose veins patients' quality of life improved in one domain (mental health) six weeks post surgery (14). Another study found that at six months patients who had undergone varicose vein surgery showed significant improvements in health scores using both SF-36 and EuroQol scores (15).

Similarly, recurrent varicose veins at the time of re-presentation have a greater negative influence on patients' quality of life than primary disease when measured by validated health-related quality of life and general quality of life tools (16).

CONCLUSION

Funding difficulties will be an ongoing issue in the management of venous diseases. It is paramount that health economics continues to play a vital role in the delivery of health care to patients with venous disorder, a subject some believe is a "Cinderella field of study."

Quality of life should be a standard measure in future studies in patients with venous disorders, preferably with a combination of generic and disease-specific measures. There also needs to be longitudinal research on the long-term effect of chronic venous disease on the quality of life of patients and its impact on the partners and families concerned.

KEY POINTS

- The impact of venous disorders on health services is large both in terms of time consumed and cost.
- There is no single quality of life tool that can be used to measure the impact of venous disorders on patients.

REFERENCES

1. Laing W. Chronic Venous Disease of the Legs. London: Office of Health Economics, 1992.
2. Ruckley CV. Socioeconomic impact of chronic venous insufficiency and leg ulcers. Angiology 1997; 48:67–69.
3. Moffatt CJ, Franks PJ, Oldroyd M, et al. Community clinics for leg ulcers and impact on healing. BMJ 1992; 305:1389–1392.
4. Callam MJ, Harper DR, Dale JJ, Ruckley CV. Chronic ulcer of the leg: clinical history. BMJ 1987; 294:1389–1391.
5. Franks PJ, Bosanquet N, Brown L, et al. Perceived health in a randomised trial of single and multilayer bandaging for chronic venous ulceration. Phlebology 1995; 1:17–19.
6. Brand FN, Dannenberg AL, Abbott RD, Kannel WB. The epidemiology of varicose veins: the Framingham Study. Am J Prev Med 1988; 4:96–101.
7. Bradbury A, Evans CJ, Allan P, Lee AJ, Ruckley CV, Fowkes FG. The relationship between lower limb symptoms and superficial and deep venous reflux on duplex ultrasonography: the Edinburgh Vein Study. J Vasc Surg 2000; 32:921–931.
8. Rawlins MD, Culyer AJ. National Institute for Clinical Excellence and its value judgments. BMJ 2004; 329:224–227.

9. Michaels JA, Campbell WB, Brazier JE, et al. Randomised Trial of Treatment for Uncomplicated Varicose Veins: Surgery Is Clinically and Cost-effective p. 70. The Vascular Society of Great Britain and Ireland Yearbook. Shropshire: TFM, 2004.

10. Price P. Defining and measuring quality of life. J Wound Care 1996; 5:139–140.

11. Beattie DK, Golledge J, Greenhalgh RM, Davies AH. Quality of life assessment in vascular disease: towards a consensus. Eur J Vasc Endovasc Surg 1997; 13:9–13.

12. Aaronson NK, Acquadro C, Alonso J, et al. International Quality of Life Assessment (IQOLA) Project. Qual Life Res 1992; 1:349–351.

13. van Korlaar I, Vossen C, Rosendaal F, Cameron L, Bovill E, Kaptein A. Quality of life in venous disease. Thromb Haemost 2003; 90:27–35.

14. Smith JJ, Guest MG, Greenhalgh RM, Davies AH. Measuring the quality of life in patients with venous ulcers. J Vasc Surg 2000; 31:642–649.

15. Durkin MT, Turton EP, Wijesinghe LD, Scott DJ, Berridge DC. Long saphenous vein stripping and quality of life—a randomised trial. Eur J Vasc Endovasc Surg 2001; 21:545–549.

16. Beresford T, Smith JJ, Brown L, Greenhalgh RM, Davies AH. A comparison of health-related quality of life of patients with primary and recurrent varicose veins. Phlebology 2003; 18:35–37.

17. Franks PJ, Wright DD, Fletcher AE, et al. A questionnaire to assess risk factors, quality of life, and use of health resources in patients with venous disease. Eur J Surg 1992; 158:149–155.

18. Launois R, Reboul-Marty J, Henry B. Construction and validation of a quality of life questionnaire in chronic lower limb venous insufficiency (CIVIQ). Qual Life Res 1996; 5:539–554.

19. Augustin M, Dieterle W, Zschocke I, et al. Development and validation of a disease-specific questionnaire on the quality of life of patients with chronic venous insufficiency. Vasa 1997; 26:291–301.

20. Klyscz T, Junger M, Schanz S, et al. Quality of life in chronic venous insufficiency (CVI). Results of a study with the newly developed Tubingen Questionnaire for measuring quality of life of patients with chronic venous insufficiency. Hautarzt 1998; 49:372–381.

21. Lamping DL, Abenhaim L, Kurz X, et al. Measuring quality of life and symptoms in chronic venous disorders of the leg: development and psychometric evaluation of the VEINES-QOL/VEINES-SYM questionnaire. Qual Life Res 1998; 7:621–622.

22. Beyth RJ, Cohen AM, Landefeld CS. Long-term outcomes of deep-vein thrombosis. Arch Intern Med 1995; 155:1031–1037.

23. Mathias SD, Prebil LA, Putterman CG, et al. A health-related quality of life measure in patients with deep vein thrombosis: a validation study. Drug Inf J 1999; 33:1173–1187.

24. Ziegler S, Schillinger M, Maca TH, Minar E. Post-thrombotic syndrome after primary event of deep venous thrombosis 10 to 20 yr ago. Thromb Res 2001; 101:23 33.

25. Kahn SR, Hirsch A, Shrier I. Effect of postthrombotic syndrome on health-related quality of life after deep venous thrombosis. Arch Intern Med 2002; 162:1144–1148.

26. Hyland ME, Ley A, Thomson B. Quality of life of leg ulcer patients: questionnaire and preliminary findings. J. Wound Care 1986; 3:294–298.

27. Lindholm C, Bjellerup M, Christensen OB, Zederfeldt B. Quality of life in chronic leg ulcer patients. An assessment according to the Nottingham Health Profile. Acta Derm Venereol 1993; 73:440–443.

28. Phillips T, Stanton B, Provan A, Lew R. A study of the impact of leg ulcers on quality of life: financial, social, and psychologic implications. J Am Acad Dermatol 1994; 31:49–53.

29. Franks PJ, Morrell CJ, Culyer AJ, et al. Community leg ulcer clinics: effect on quality of life. Phlebology 1994; 9:83–86.

30. Charles H. The impact of leg ulcers on patients' quality of life. Prof Nurse 1995; 10:571–574.

31. Walters SJ, Morrell CJ, Dixon S. Measuring health-related quality of life in patients with venous leg ulcers. Qual Life Res 1999; 8:327–336.

32. Franks PJ, Moffatt CJ. Health related quality of life in patients with venous ulceration: use of the Nottingham health profile. Qual Life Res 2001; 10:693–700.

33. Garratt AM, Macdonald LM, Ruta DA, Russell IT, Buckingham JK, Krukowski ZH. Towards measurement of outcome for patients with varicose veins. Qual Health Care 1993; 2:5–10.

34. Kurz X, Lamping DL, Kahn SR, Baccaglini U, Zuccarelli F, Spreafico G, et al. Do varicose veins affect quality of life? Results of an international population-based study J Vasc Surg 2001; 34:641–648.

6

Classification of Chronic Venous Disease and Outcome Assessment

Gudmundur Danielsson and Bo Eklöf
Department of Vascular Diseases, Lund University, Lund, Sweden

INTRODUCTION

The field of chronic venous disorders (CVD) previously suffered from a lack of precision in diagnosis. This deficiency led to conflicting reports in studies of the management of specific venous problems at a time when new modalities were being offered to improve treatment for simple, as well as more complicated, venous diseases. It was believed that these conflicts could be resolved by a precise diagnosis and classification of the underlying venous problem. The CEAP classification (1) (Clinical-Etiology-Anatomy-Pathophysiology) was developed by an international consensus committee organized by the American Venous Forum (AVF) in 1994 and adopted world-wide to facilitate meaningful communication about CVD and to serve as a basis for a more scientific analysis of the management alternatives. This classification, based on a correct diagnosis, was also expected to serve as a systematic guide in the daily clinical investigation of patients as an orderly documentation system and basis for decisions regarding the appropriate treatment. It is important to stress that CEAP is a descriptive classification and not a severity scoring system. A venous severity scoring system was also developed in 1994 with an improvement presented by an AVF committee on outcomes in 2000 (2). Together with patient-derived functional assessments (Quality of Life, QoL scores), the venous severity scoring system are instruments for longitudinal research to assess outcomes.

THE CREATION OF THE CEAP CLASSIFICATION

There have been several classifications of CVD in the past, the Widmer classification being the most well known (3), but all lack the completeness and objectivity needed for scientific accuracy (Table 1).

At the fifth annual meeting of the AVF in 1993, John Porter suggested using the same approach as TNM for cancer in developing a classification system for venous diseases. Following a year of intense discussions a consensus conference was held at the sixth annual

Table 1   Published Classifications of Chronic Venous Disorders

Author	Year
Widmer (3)	1978
Hach et al. (25)	1980
Partsch (26)	1980
Molokhia (27)	1981
Sytchev (28)	1985
Pierchalla and Tronnier (29)	1985
Porter et al. (30)	1988
Cornu-Thenard et al. (31)	1991
Enrici and Caldevilla (32)	1992
Miranda et al. (33)	1993

meeting of AVF in February 1994, at which an international *ad hoc* committee, chaired by Andrew Nicolaides, and with representatives from Australia, Europe, as well as the Unites States, developed the first CEAP consensus document. It contained two parts, a classification of CVD and a scoring system of the severity of CVD. The classification was based on clinical manifestations (C), etiologic factors (E), anatomic distribution of disease (A), and the underlying pathophysiological findings (P), thus the name CEAP. The severity scoring system was based on three elements: the number of anatomic segments affected, grading of symptoms and signs, and disability. The CEAP consensus statement was published in 26 journals and books in nine languages (Table 2), truly a universal document for CVD. It was endorsed by the Joint Councils of the Society for Vascular Surgery and the North American Chapter of the International Society for Cardiovascular Surgery, and its basic elements were incorporated into venous reporting standards (4). Today most published clinical papers on CVD use all or portions of the CEAP classification.

OTHER DEVELOPMENTS RELATED TO CEAP

In 1998, at an international consensus meeting in Paris, Perrin et al. (5) established a classification for recurrent varicose veins, REVAS, the evaluation of which is ongoing. In 2000, Rutherford et al. (2)—the *ad hoc* committee of AVF on Outcomes—published an upgraded version of the original venous severity scoring system. Carpentier, Cornu-Thenard and Uhl established a European Venous Registry based on CEAP and reported studies on intra- and interobserver variability showing significant discrepancies in the clinical classification of CEAP, prompting improved definitions of clinical classes C0 to C6 (6).

An international consensus meeting in Rome in 2001 suggested definitions and refinements of the clinical classification, the "C" in CEAP (7). which were published with a commentary by the first author of the current revision of the venous reporting standards (8). These did not only contribute to CEAP, but formed the basis for its ultimate modification, as recommended below.

REVISION OF CEAP

The diagnosis and treatment of CVD is developing rapidly and the need for an update of the classification logically follows. It is important to stress that CEAP is a descriptive

Table 2 Journals and Books in Which the CEAP Classification Has Been Published

Actualités Vasculaires Internationales 1995; 31:19–22
Angiologie 1995; 47:9–16
Angiology News 1996; 19:4–6
Australia and New Zealand Journal of Surgery 1995; 65:769–72
Clinica Terapeutica 1997; 148:521–6
Dermatologic Surgery 1995; 21:642–6
Elleniki Angiochirurgiki 1996; 5:12–9
European Journal of Vascular and Endovascular Surgery 1996; 12:487–91
Forum de Flebologia y Limphologia 1997; 2:67–74
Handbook of Venous Disorders 1996; 652–60
International Angiology 1995; 2:197–201
Japanese Journal of Phlebology 1995; 1:103–8
Journal of Cardiovascular Surgery 1997; 38:437–41
Journal of Vascular Surgery 1995; 21:635–45
Journal des Maladies Vasculaires 1995; 20:78–83
Mayo Clinic Proceedings 1996; 71:338–45
Minerva Cardioangiologica 1997; 45:31–6
Myakkangaku 1995; 31:1–6
Phlébologie–Annales Vasculaires 1995; 48:275–81
Phlebologie (German version) 1995; 24:125–9
Phlebology 1995; 10:42–5
Przeglad Flebologiczny 1996; 4:63–73
Scope on Phlebology and Lymphology 1996; 3:4–7
VASA 1995; 24:313–8
Vascular Surgery 1996; 30:5–11
Vensjukdomar 2004; 89–91

classification. Venous Severity Scoring was developed to allow longitudinal outcome assessment, but it became apparent that CEAP itself required updating and modification (2). In April 2002, an *ad hoc* committee on CEAP was appointed by AVF to review the classification and make recommendations for change by 2004, 10 years after its introduction (Table 3). An international ad hoc committee was also established to assure continued universal utilization (Table 4). The two held four joint meetings, with key members contributing in the interim to the revised document. The revision of the CEAP classification is published in the Journal of Vascular surgery (9).

Table 3 Members of the American Venous Forum Ad Hoc Committee on Revision of CEAP Classification

John Bergan
Bo Eklof, Chair
Peter Gloviczki
Robert Kistner
Mark Meissner, Secretary
Gregory Moneta
Frank Padberg
Robert Rutherford
Thomas Wakefield

The following passages summarize the results of these deliberations, by describing the new aspects of the revised CEAP.

The recommended changes, detailed below, include: additions to or refinements of several definitions used in describing CVD; refinement of the C-classes of CEAP; addition of the descriptor *n* (no venous abnormality identified); incorporation of the date of classification and level of clinical investigation, and the description of basic CEAP, introduced as a simpler alternative to the full (advanced) CEAP classification.

TERMINOLOGY AND NEW DEFINITIONS

The CEAP classification deals with all forms of CVD. The term *chronic venous disorder* (CVD) includes the full spectrum of morphological and functional abnormalities of the venous system from telangiectasies to venous ulcers. Some of these, like telangiectasies, are highly prevalent in the normal adult population and in many cases the use of the term "disease" is not appropriate. The term chronic venous insufficiency (CVI) implies a functional abnormality of the venous system and it is usually reserved for patients with more advanced diseases including those with edema (C3), skin changes (C4) or venous ulcers (C5–6).

Table 4   The International Ad Hoc Committee on Revision of CEAP Classification

The AVF ad hoc committee plus
Claudio Allegra, Italy
Pier Luigi Antignani, Italy
Patrick Carpentier, France[a]
Philip Coleridge Smith, UK[a]
André Cornu-Thenard, France
Ermenegildo Enrici, Argentina
Jean Jerome Guex, France
Shunichi Hoshino, Japan
Arkadiusz Jawien, Poland
Nicos Labropoulos, USA
Fedor Lurie, USA
Mark Malouf, Australia
Nick Morrison, USA
Kenneth Myers, Australia[a]
Peter Neglén, USA
Andrew Nicolaides, Cyprus
Tomo Ogawa, Japan
Hugo Partsch, Austria
Michel Perrin, France[a]
Eberhard Rabe, Germany
Seshadri Raju, USA
Vaughan Ruckley, UK[a]
Ulrich Schultz-Ehrenburg, Germany
Jean Francois Uhl, France
Martin Veller, South Africa
Yuqi Wang, China
Zhong Gao Wang, China

[a] Editorial committee.

It was agreed to maintain the present overall structure of the CEAP classification, but to add more precise definitions. The following recommended definitions apply to the clinical "C" classes in CEAP:

Telangiectasia a confluence of dilated intradermal venules of less than 1 mm in caliber. Synonyms include spider veins, hyphen webs, and thread veins.

Reticular veins dilated bluish subdermal veins usually from 1 mm in diameter to less than 3 mm in diameter. They are usually tortuous. This excludes normal visible veins in people with thin, transparent skin. Synonyms include blue veins, subdermal varices, and venulectasies.

Varicose veins subcutaneous dilated veins equal to or more than 3 mm in diameter measured in the upright position. These may involve saphenous veins, saphenous tributaries, or non-saphenous superficial leg veins. Varicose veins are usually tortuous, but tubular saphenous veins with demonstrated reflux may be classified as varicose veins. Synonyms include varix, varices, and varicosities.

Corona phlebectatica a fan-shaped pattern of numerous small intradermal veins on the medial or lateral aspects of the ankle and foot. This is commonly thought to be an early sign of advanced venous disease. Synonyms include malleolar flare and ankle flare.

Edema a perceptible increase in the volume of fluid in the skin and subcutaneous tissue, characteristically indented with pressure. Venous edema usually occurs in the ankle region, but it may extend to the leg and foot.

Pigmentation a brownish darkening of the skin resulting from extravasated blood, which usually occurs in the ankle region, but may extend to the leg and foot.

Eczema an erythematous dermatitis, which may progress to a blistering, weeping, or scaling eruption of the skin of the leg. It is most often located near varicose veins, but may be located anywhere in the leg. Eczema is usually seen in uncontrolled CVD but may reflect sensitization to local therapy.

Lipodermatosclerosis (LDS) localized chronic inflammation and fibrosis of the skin and subcutaneous tissues of the lower leg, sometimes associated with scarring or contracture of the achilles tendon. LDS is sometimes preceded by diffuse inflammatory edema of the skin, which may be painful and which is often referred to as hypodermitis. This condition must be distinguished from lymphangitis, erysipelas or cellulitis by their characteristically different local signs and systemic features. LDS is a sign of severe CVD.

Atrophie blanche or white atrophy localized, often circular whitish and atrophic skin areas surrounded by dilated capillaries and sometimes hyperpigmentation. This finding is a sign of severe CVD and not to be confused with healed ulcer scars. Scars of healed ulceration may also have atrophic skin with pigmentary changes, but are distinguishable by the history of ulceration and appearance from atrophie blanche and are excluded from this definition.

Venous ulcer full thickness defect of the skin most frequently in the ankle region that fails to heal spontaneously and is sustained by CVD.

REFINEMENT OF C-CLASSES IN CEAP

The essential change here is the division of class C4 into two subgroups, which reflect different severities of disease, and carry a different prognosis in terms of risk of ulceration:

C0 no visible or palpable signs of venous disease.

C1 telangiectasies or reticular veins.

C2 varicose veins—distinguished from reticular veins by a diameter of 3 mm or more.

C3 edema.

C4 changes in the skin and subcutaneous tissue secondary to CVD (now divided into two subclasses to better define the differing severity of venous disease):
C4a pigmentation and/or eczema;
C4b LDS and/or atrophie blanche.

C5 healed venous ulcer.

C6 active venous ulcer

Each clinical class is further characterized by a subscript for the presence of symptoms (S, symptomatic) or absence of symptoms (A, asymptomatic), e.g., $C2_A$, or $C5_S$. The symptoms include aching, pain, tightness, skin irritation, heaviness, and muscle cramps, as well as other complaints attributable to venous dysfunction.

REFINEMENT OF E, A, AND P IN CEAP

To improve the assignment of designations under the E, A, and P a new descriptor *n* is now recommended for use where no venous abnormality is identified. This *n* could be added to E (En: no venous etiology identified), A (An: no venous location identified) and P (Pn: no venous pathophysiology identified). Observer variability in assigning designations may have been contributed to by the lack of a normal option. Further definition of the A and P has also been afforded by the new venous severity scoring system (2), which was developed by the ad hoc Committee on Outcomes of the AVF to compliment CEAP. It includes not only a Clinical Severity Score, but also a Venous Segmental Score. The latter is based on imaging studies of the leg veins, e.g., duplex scan, and the degree of obstruction or reflux (P) in each major segment (A) and forms the basis for the overall score (see further below).

This same committee is also pursuing a prospective multicenter investigation of the variability in vascular diagnostic laboratory assessment of venous hemodynamics in patients with CVD. The last revision of the venous reporting standards still cites changes in ambulatory venous pressure or plethysmographically measured venous return time (VRT) as objective measures of change (4). The current multicenter study aims to establish the variability, and thus the limits, of "normal" for the VRT and the newer non invasive venous tests as an objective basis for claiming significant improvement as a result of therapy, and it will hopefully provide improved reporting standards for definitive diagnosis and results of competitive treatments in patients with CVD.

DATE OF CLASSIFICATION

CEAP is not a static classification; the patient can be reclassified at any future point in time. The classification starts with the initial visit, but can be better defined after further investigations. A final classification may not be complete until after surgery and histopathologic assessment. We therefore recommend that any CEAP classification be followed by the date, e.g., C4b, S, Ep, As, p, Pr (2003-08-21).

LEVEL OF INVESTIGATION

A precise diagnosis is the basis of correct classification of the venous problem. The diagnostic evaluation of the patient with CVD can be logically organized into one or more of three levels of testing, depending on the severity of the disease:

> Level I the office visit with history and clinical examination, which may include the use of a hand-held Doppler.
> Level II the noninvasive vascular laboratory, which now routinely includes duplex color scanning, with some plethysmographic method added as desired.
> Level III invasive investigations or more complex imaging studies including ascending and descending venography, venous pressure measurements, CT scan, venous helical scan or MRI.

We recommend that the level of investigation (L) should also be added to the classification, e.g., C2, 4b, S, Ep, As, p, Pr (2003-08-21,L II).

BASIC CEAP

A new basic CEAP is offered here. Use of all components of CEAP is still encouraged. Unfortunately, many use the C-classification *only*, which is only a modest advance beyond the previous classifications based solely on the clinical appearance. Venous disease is complex, but can be described by the use of well-defined categorical descriptions. For the practicing physician, CEAP can be a valuable instrument for correct diagnosis to guide treatment and assess prognosis. In modern phlebological practice the vast majority of patients will have a duplex scan of the venous system of the leg, which will largely define the E, A, and P categories.

Nevertheless, it is recognized that the merits of using the *full* (advanced) CEAP classification system hold primarily for the researcher and for standardized reporting in scientific journals. It allows grouping of patients so that the same types of patients can be analyzed together and such a subgroup analysis allows their treatments to be more accurately assessed. Furthermore, reports using CEAP can be compared with one another with much greater certainty. This more complex classification, for example, also allows any of the 18 named venous segments to be identified as the location of venous pathology. Take a patient with pain, varicose veins and LDS, where duplex scan confirms primary reflux of the great saphenous vein and incompetent perforators in the calf. The classification here would be C2, 4b, S, Ep, As, p, Pr2, 3, 18.

While the detailed elaboration of venous disease in this form may seem unnecessarily complex, even intimidating, to some clinicians, it provides universal understandable descriptions, which may be essential to the investigators in the field. To serve the needs of both, the full CEAP classification, as modified above, is retained as advanced CEAP and the following simplified form is offered as basic CEAP.

In essence, basic CEAP applies two simplifications:

1. In basic CEAP the single highest descriptor can be used for clinical classification. For example, a patient with varicose veins, swelling and LDS would be C4b. The more comprehensive clinical description, in advanced CEAP, would be C2, 3, 4b
2. In basic CEAP, where duplex scan is performed, E, A, and P should also be classified by using the multiple descriptors recommended, but the complexity of

applying these to the 18 possible anatomic segments is avoided in favor of applying the simple s, p, and d descriptors to denote the superficial, perforator and deep systems. Thus, using basic CEAP, the same patient cited in a previous example (painful varicosities plus LDS and duplex scan-determined reflux involving the superficial and perforator systems) would be classified as C4b, S, Ep, As, p, Pr (rather than C2,4b,S, Ep, As,p, Pr2,3,18).

REVISION OF CEAP: AN ONGOING PROCESS

With improvement in diagnostics and treatment there will be continued demands to adapt the CEAP classification to better serve future developments. There is a need to incorporate appropriate new features without too frequent disturbances of the stability of the classification. As one of the committee members (F. Padberg) stated in our deliberations: "It is critically important that recommendations for change in the CEAP standard be supported by solid research. While there is precious little that we are recommending which meets this standard, we can certainly emphasize it for the future. If we are to progress we should focus on levels of evidence for changes rather than levels of investigation. While a substantial portion of our effort will be developed from consensus opinion, we should still strive to achieve an evidence-based format."

REVISION OF CEAP: SUMMARY

CLINICAL CLASSIFICATION
C0 no visible or palpable signs of venous disease
C1 telangiectasies or reticular veins
C2 varicose veins
C3 edema
C4a pigmentation and/or eczema
C4b LDS and/or atrophie blanche
C5 healed venous ulcer
C6 active venous ulcer
S   symptoms including ache, pain, tightness, skin irritation, heaviness, muscle cramps, as well as other complaints attributable to venous dysfunction
A   asymptomatic

ETIOLOGIC CLASSIFICATION
Ec congenital
Ep primary
Es secondary (post-thrombotic)
En no venous etiology identified

ANATOMIC CLASSIFICATION
As superficial veins
Ap perforator veins
Ad deep veins
An no venous location identified.

PATHOPHYSIOLOGIC CLASSIFICATION
Basic CEAP:
Pr   reflux
Po   obstruction
Pr,o reflux and obstruction
Pn   no venous pathophysiology identifiable

Advanced CEAP—Same as Basic with the addition that any of 18 named venous segments can be utilized as locators for venous pathology:
Superficial veins
   1. telangiectasies/reticular veins
   2. great saphenous vein (GSV) above knee
   3. GSV below knee
   4. small saphenous vein
   5. nonsaphenous veins
Deep veins
   6. inferior vena cava
   7. common iliac vein
   8. internal iliac vein
   9. external iliac vein
  10. pelvic: gonadal, broad ligament veins, other
  11. common femoral vein
  12. deep femoral vein
  13. femoral vein
  14. popliteal vein
  15. crural: anterior tibial, posterior tibial, peroneal veins (all paired)
  16. muscular: gastrocnemial, soleal veins, other
  17. perforating veins, thigh
  18. perforating veins, calf

Example: A patient presents with painful swelling of the leg and varicose veins, LDS and active ulceration. Duplex scanning on May 17, 2004 showed axial reflux of GSV above and below the knee, incompetent calf perforators and axial reflux in the femoral and popliteal veins. No signs of post-thrombotic obstruction.
- Classification according to basic CEAP: C6, S, Ep, As, p, d, Pr.
- Classification according to advanced CEAP: C2,3,4b,6,S, Ep, As, p, d, Pr2, 3, 18, 13, 14 (2004-05-17, LII).

OUTCOME ASSESSMENT

For the practicing physician, CEAP is an instrument for correct diagnosis to guide treatment and assess prognosis. For the researcher and reporting standards, CEAP aids to group the patients so that we are looking at the same type of patients. It is important again to state that CEAP is a descriptive classification and a base for diagnosis and prognosis, while venous severity scoring and quality of life (QoL) estimation are instruments for longitudinal research to assess outcomes. From the introduction of CEAP classification in 1994, 138 scientific articles have been published according to medline search for CEAP and venous disease. Most of them have, though, only used the basic part of CEAP or only the clinical classification. A recently published study on 98 legs (83 patients) with open venous ulcer, using the advanced CEAP classification, showed that 86% of the legs had superficial venous incompetence that might be offered surgery and axial reflux in superficial or deep veins were present in 79% of the legs (10). A randomized controlled study comparing surgery of the superficial venous system and compression with compression alone by Barwell et al. (11) came to similar conclusion, showing that 85% of all patients with venous ulcer could be managed by simple venous surgery.

The venous severity scoring system was intended to complement the descriptive CEAP classification and consists of three parts, venous clinical severity score (VCSS), venous segmental disease score (VSDS) and venous disability score (VDS). The validity and reliability of the scoring system have not yet been confirmed although it has been validated regarding the effect of superficial venous surgery (12). VCSS was found to better reflect changes in response to superficial venous surgery than the CEAP clinical class did. It was concluded that the scoring is a valuable tool in clinical studies to quantify venous outcome rather than using only the clinical class of CEAP. Meissner et al. (13) found the score reliable with good correlation with the CEAP clinical classification. Ricci et al. (14) found the VCSS useful as a screening tool for venous disease as it has a good association with abnormalities on ultrasound scanning and it might therefore be valuable in clinical practice.

Venous Clinical Severity Score

Outcome assessment with emphasis on skin changes and ulcer is the main part of the Venous Clinical Severity Score (VCSS). Nine clinical characteristics of CVD are described and the symptoms are graded from 0–3 (absent, mild, moderate, severe). The only subjective symptom graded is the degree of pain. As the need for compression therapy is an indirect indicator for the severity of the disease it has been added as a separate factor in the VCSS. The nine clinical characteristics and the need for compression therapy make totally a 30 point-maximum flat scale. Qualifying comments, describing in detail how symptoms and grades are defined, are provided to ascertain homogeneity in the clinical judgments (Table 5).

What is the main difference in the new VCSS compared to the previous severity scoring system? In the VCSS the grading has been changed from a 3-count scale (0–2) to a 4-count scale (0–3), where 0 is none, 1 is mild, 2 is moderate and 3 is severe. In the VCSS venous claudication and ulcer recurrence have been omitted and varicose veins and induration been added instead. Compression therapy has also been added as an indirect indicator for disease severity.

Although the VCSS seems valuable for patients with venous ulcer, the value of judging the severity is limited for the majority of patients with CVD. Patients with symptomatic varicose veins without skin changes and without pain belong to this group.

Table 5 Venous Segmental Disease Score (VSDS)

	Attribute	Absent = 0	Mild = 1	Moderate = 2	Severe = 3
1.	Pain	None	Occasional, not daily, restricting activity or requiring analgesics	Moderate activity, limitation, occasional analgesics	Daily, severely limits activities, regular use of analgesics
2.	Varicose veins	None	Few, scattered: branch VV w. competent GS/LS	Multiple: single segment GS/LS reflux	Extensive: multisegment GS/LS reflux
3.	Venous edema	None	Evening ankle edema only	Afternoon edema above ankle	Morning edema above ankle requiring activity change, elevation
4.	Skin pigmentation	None or focal, low intensity (tan)	Diffuse, but limited in area and old (brown)	Diffuse over gaiter distribution (lower 1/3) or recent pigmentation (purple)	Wider distribution (above lower 1/3) and recent pigmentation
5.	Inflammation	None	Mild cellulitis, limited or marginal area around ulcer	Moderate cellulitis, involves most of gaiter area	Severe cellulitis (lower 1/3 or above) or venous eczema
6.	Induration	None	Focal, circum-areolar (<5 cm)	Medial or lateral, less than lower third	Entire lower third or more
7.	Total no. ulcers	0	1	2–4	>4
8.	Active ulceration,	None	<3 mo	>3 mo, <1 yr	Not healed >1 yr
9.	Active ulcer, size	None	<2 cm diameter	2–4 cm diameter	>4 cm diameter
10.	Compressive therapy	Not used or not compliant	Intermittent use of stockings	Wears elastic stockings most days	Full compliance stockings + elevation

Although skin changes with or without ulcer are the most severe forms of venous disorder, we cannot forget that most patients with CVD do not develop ulcer. It is also interesting to compare the treatments for these patients. The importance of pain, as the subjective parameter in the clinical score, may also be argued. Most patients with varicose veins do not experience pain, and even patients with venous ulcer do not always report pain as the main symptom. The VCSS does not take into account other symptoms as heaviness or tiredness that can be the main reason for the patient to seek medical attention. Possible alternative is to measure the most severe symptom (pain, heaviness, tiredness, night cramp, etc.) reported by the patient and follow up changes regarding this one symptom over time. An arguement against this is that most lower leg symptoms in patients with varicose veins are probably non-venous in origin (according to the Edinburgh vein study (15)) and therefore they should not be a part of a venous severity scoring system. Another issue that has not been addressed is the length of the follow-up time. Almost all venous ulcers eventually heal. The time factor is important when comparing different treatments. If the follow-up VCSS is done when the ulcer has healed, almost any treatment can be shown to be effective as regard to the VCSS. Ulcer history before treatment and ulcer recurrence after treatment are not measured in VCSS, although the main goal of the treatment is to keep the ulcer healed over time. Further modifications are probably needed before we have the optimal tool for measuring the severity of CVD in all clinical classes of the CEAP.

Venous Segmental Disease Score

The Venous Segmental Disease Score (VSDS) combines the anatomical and the pathophysiological components of CEAP. The major venous segments are graded separately both regarding the occurrence of reflux and obstruction (Table 6). This is done to highlight the importance of occlusion in the disease pattern and patients with a more severe form of CVD, as post-thrombotic changes, will therefore get a higher score than those with reflux only. Also, segments that are thought to be more important in the disease manifestation, as popliteal and crural veins get a higher score (16,17). Other anatomical segments with little or no role in CVD are excluded. Reflux in one segment is defined as all valves in that segment are incompetent. Obstruction means that there is total occlusion at some point in the segment or >50% narrowing of at least half of the segment. Points can be assigned for both obstruction and reflux in the same segment, as can be in legs

Table 6   Venous Segmental Disease Score

Reflux	Obstruction/occlusion	Reflux	Obstruction/occlusion
1. LSV	0–0.5	1. GSV	0–1
2. GSV	0–1	2. Calf veins, multiple	0–1
3. Perforating thigh	0–0.5	3. Popliteal	0–2
4. Perforating calf	0–1	4. FV	0–1
5. Calf veins, multiple	0–2	5. DFV	0–1
6. Popliteal	0–2	6. CFV	0–2
7. FV	0–1	7. Iliac vein	0–1
8. DFV	0–1	8. IVC	0–1
9. CFV	0–1		

Abbreviations: LSV, lesser saphenous vein; GSV, greater saphenous vein; FV, femoral vein; DFV, deep femoral vein; CFV, common femoral vein; IVC, inferior venal cava.

with post-thrombotic changes. The maximal scoring is 20, 10 for reflux and 10 for obstruction/occlusion.

According to the original system the anatomical score consisted of 18 venous segments with one count for each diseased segment irrespective of whether it was reflux, obstruction or both. This approach in the original system was criticized for overestimating some insignificant features of the disease. For example, occlusion of the common iliac vein adds the same weight to the severity score as reticular veins do. Scoring is also often low using the system as eight of the segments are only occasionally involved in CVD. The new VSDS grades the relative importance of each segment. The importance of occlusion in the disease pattern is highlighted with separate scoring for occlusive segments. The pathophysiological importance (weighting) of different venous segments remains though to be confirmed.

Venous Disability Score

Venous Disability Score (VDS) measures the impact of CVD on the ability to carry out usual daily activities, using a 4-point scale from 0 to 3. Patients that are symptomatic, but can carry out usual activities without support, get 1 point, patients that need compression therapy to be able to carry out usual activities get 2 points and patients that cannot carry out usual activities even with compression or limb elevation get 3 points.

Quality of Life and CVD

How to adequately evaluate QoL in patients with CVD is unclear. A number of QoL questionnaires have been used to measure the impact of CVD on the general health of patients. Some of them have been generic and others have included more disease-specific questions. The medical outcomes study, short form "health survey" (SF-36), often regarded as the "golden standard" for QoL measures, has been extensively validated. It consists of 36 item-generic measures of QoL, which measures eight health dimensions. The perceived health of patients with varicose veins, as measured by the SF-36, was significantly lower than that of samples of the general population according to a study by Garratt et al. (18). The success of varicose vein surgery has been analyzed using SF-36, including seven extra questions with more CVD-related topics (19). After six months, all dimensions except social function and health perception were improved. A specific questionnaire for venous ulcer patients was validated by Smith et al. (20) showing good reliability, as assessed by means of the internal consistency. The validity was demonstrated by means of a high correlation with all eight domains of the SF-36 and it was concluded that clinically derived measures for patients with venous ulcers have validity to measure the QoL. Another generic QoL questionnaire, the Nottingham Health Profile (NHP), was used to assess patients with chronic leg ulcer, indicating that the disease has a marked impact on the patients' subjectively perceived health, especially in men (21). NHP has been criticized for its problematic weighting scoring system and lack of sensitivity to low levels of distress. CVI Questionnaire (CIVIQ) was developed by a French group in 1996 (22). This is a 20-item self-administered questionnaire, which explores four dimensions: psychological, physical and social functioning and pain. It is simple and easy to administer. The conclusion was that the questionnaire might be used with confidence to assess QoL in clinical trials on CVI. The Aberdeen Varicose Vein Score (AVSS) was used to judge the effect of saphenous stripping on disease-specific QoL showing improvement in 87% of the patients (23). There were significant improvements in AVSS scores for as much as two years. After adjustment for recurrent disease, stripping conferred additional benefit in terms of AVSS at six months. SF-36 scores were, on the other hand, not affected by stripping. An international population-based study by Kurz et al. (24) indicated that impairment in physical QoL in patients with varicose veins is associated with concomitant venous disease, rather than with the presence of varicose veins, and therefore it could only be reliably interpreted when concomitant venous disease is taken into account. The limitation of most QoL questionnaires in CVD is that they have not been fully evaluated in terms of validity and reliability and they often focus on only one part of the disease spectrum of CVD, as just varicose veins or ulcer.

CONCLUSION

The CEAP classification of CVD was adopted world-wide to facilitate meaningful communication about CVD and serves as a basis for a more scientific analysis of management alternatives. Today most published clinical papers on CVD use all or portions of CEAP. Venous disease is complex, but can be described by the use of well-defined categorical descriptions. The revision of CEAP can be a valuable instrument for the practicing physician for correct diagnosis to guide treatment and assess prognosis. For the researcher and reporting standards, CEAP allows grouping of patients so that the same type of patients can be analyzed together and such a subgroup analysis allows their treatments to be more accurately assessed. Furthermore, reports using CEAP can be compared with one another with much greater certainty. CEAP is a descriptive classification, while venous severity scoring and QoL estimation are instruments for longitudinal research to assess outcomes. With these weapons in our hands we should be able to improve the scientific approach to CVD and introduce evidence-based medicine for the benefit of our patients.

KEY POINTS

- The CEAP classification system has been adopted worldwide.
- Accurate classification allows better analysis and patient management.
- The CEAP is continuously revised to accommodate new developments.
- Venous scoring systems are used to grade severity and disability of venous disease.
- Venous severity scoring and quality of life questionnaires are instruments for longitudinal research to assess outcomes.

REFERENCES

1. Beebe HG, Bergan JJ, Bergqvist D, et al. Classification and grading of chronic venous disease in the lower limbs. A consensus statement. Eur J Vasc Endovasc Surg 1996; 12:487–491; discussion 491-492.
2. Rutherford RB, Padberg FT, Jr., Comerota AJ, Kistner RL, Meissner MH, Moneta GL. Venous severity scoring: An adjunct to venous outcome assessment. J Vasc Surg 2000; 31:1307–1312.
3. Widmer LK, Kamber V, da Silva A, Madar G. Prevalence and socio-medical importance: observations in 4529 apparently healthy persons: Basle III study. Langenbecks Arch Chir 1978; 347:203–207.
4. Porter JM, Moneta GL. Reporting standards in venous disease: an update. International Consensus Committee on Chronic Venous Disease. J Vasc Surg 1995; 21:635–645.

5. Perrin MR, Guex JJ, Ruckley CV, et al. Recurrent varices after surgery (REVAS), a consensus document. REVAS group. Cardiovasc Surg 2000; 8:233–245.
6. Uhl J, Cornu-Thenard A, Carpentier P, Schadek M, Parpex P, Chleir F. Reproducibility of the "C" classes of the CEAP classification. J Phlebology 2001; 1:39–48.
7. Allegra C, Antignani P, Bergan JJ, et al. The "C" of CEAP: suggested definitions and refinements: An International Union of Phlebology conference of experts. J Vasc Surg 2003; 37:129–131.
8. Moneta G. Regarding the "C" of CEAP. J Vasc Surg 2003; 37:224–225.
9. Eklöf B, Rutherford R, Bergan J, et al. Revision of the CEAP classification for chronic venous disorders. A consensus statement. J Vasc Surg 2004.
10. Danielsson G, Arfvidsson B, Eklof B, Kistner RL, Masuda EM, Satoc DT. Reflux from thigh to calf, the major pathology in chronic venous ulcer disease: surgery indicated in the majority of patients. Vasc Endovascular Surg 2004; 38:209–219.
11. Barwell JR, Davies CE, Deacon J, et al. Comparison of surgery and compression with compression alone in chronic venous ulceration (ESCHAR study): randomised controlled trial. Lancet 2004; 363:1854–1859.
12. Kakkos SK, Rivera MA, Matsagas MI, et al. Validation of the new venous severity scoring system in varicose vein surgery. J Vasc Surg 2003; 38:224–228.
13. Meissner MH, Natiello C, Nicholls SC. Performance characteristics of the venous clinical severity score. J Vasc Surg 2002; 36:889–895.
14. Ricci MA, Emmerich J, Callas PW, et al. Evaluating chronic venous disease with a new venous severity scoring system. J Vasc Surg 2003; 38:909–915.
15. Bradbury AW, Evans C, Allan P, Lee A, Ruckley CV, Fowkes FG. What are the symptoms of varicose veins? Edinburgh vein study cross sectional population survey BMJ 1999; 318:353–356.
16. Rosfors S, Lamke LO, Nordstrom E, Bygdeman S. Severity and location of venous valvular insufficiency: the importance of distal valve function. Acta Chir Scand 1990; 156:689–694.
17. Nash TP. Venous ulceration: factors influencing recurrence after standard surgical procedures. Med J Aust 1991; 154:48–50.
18. Garratt AM, Macdonald LM, Ruta DA, Russell IT, Buckingham JK, Krukowski ZH. Towards measurement of outcome for patients with varicose veins. Qual Health Care 1993; 2:5–10.
19. Baker DM, Turnbull NB, Pearson JC, Makin GS. How successful is varicose vein surgery? A patient outcome study following varicose vein surgery using the SF-36 Health Assessment Questionnaire Eur J Vasc Endovasc Surg 1995; 9:299–304.
20. Smith JJ, Guest MG, Greenhalgh RM, Davies AH. Measuring the quality of life in patients with venous ulcers. J Vasc Surg 2000; 31:642–649.
21. Lindholm C, Bjellerup M, Christensen OB, Zederfeldt B. Quality of life in chronic leg ulcer patients. An assessment according to the Nottingham Health Profile. Acta Derm Venereol 1993, 73.440–443.
22. Launois R, Reboul-Marty J, Henry B. Construction and validation of a quality of life questionnaire in chronic lower limb venous insufficiency (CIVIQ). Qual Life Res 1996; 5:539–554.
23. Mackenzie RK, Lee AJ, Paisley A, et al. Patient, operative, and surgeon factors that influence the effect of superficial venous surgery on disease-specific quality of life. J Vasc Surg 2002; 36:896–902.
24. Kurz X, Lamping DL, Kahn SR, et al. Do varicose veins affect quality of life? Results of an international population-based study. J Vasc Surg 2001; 34:641–648.
25. Hach W, Schirmers U, Becker L. Veränderungen der tiefen Leitvenen bei einer Stammvaricose der Vena saphena magna. In: Muller-Wiefel H, ed. Microzirkulation und Blutrheologie. Baden, Germany: Witzstrock, 1980.
26. Partsch H. "Betterable" and "nonbetterable" chronic venous insufficiency: a proposal for a practice oriented classification. VASA 1980; 9:165–167.
27. Molokhia F. A proposal for a new classification of occlusive venous diseases of lower limbs. Alexandria Med J 1981; 27:76–81.

28. Sytchev G. Classification of chronic venous disorders of lower extremities and pelvis. Int Angiol 1985; 4:203–206.
29. Pierchalla P, Tronnier H. Diagnosis and classification of venous insufficiency of the leg. Deutsche Med Wochenschr 1985; 110:1700–1702.
30. Porter J, Rutherford RB, Clagett GP, et al. Reporting standards in venous disease. J Vasc Surg 1988; 8:172–181.
31. Cornu-Thenard A, De Vincenzi G, Maraval MJ. Evaluation of different systems for clinical quantification of varicose veins. Dermatol Surg Oncol 1991; 17:345–348.
32. Enrici E, Caldevilla H. Classification de la insuficiencia venosa cronica de los miembros inferiores. In: Insuficiencia Venosa Cronica de los Miembros Inferiores, Buenos Aires, Argentina: Editorial Celcius; 1992:107–114.
33. Miranda C, Fabre M, Meyer P, et al. Evaluation of a reference anatomo-clinical classification of varices of the lower limbs. Phlebologie 1993; 46:235–239.

7

Clinical Assessment of Venous Disease

Sriram Subramonia and Tim A. Lees
Northern Vascular Centre, Freeman Hospital, Newcastle upon Tyne, U.K.

INTRODUCTION

Varicose veins are the commonest of all the vascular disorders affecting man. Of all the earth's mobile creatures man alone is afflicted by this abnormal condition due to his penchant for maintaining an upright posture. Venous disease has interested mankind for many centuries. "Serpentine windings" on the legs have been recorded as early as 1550 B.C. in the papyrus of Ebers and the author advises against operation because it causes hemorrhage and death! Since then, the assessment and treatment of venous disease has advanced manyfold and surgery, when indicated, can be offered with acceptable risk to those affected. However, an inadequate clinical assessment can result in an unsatisfactory outcome following treatment with consequent significant patient dissatisfaction.

Diseases of the venous system cause significant morbidity and also have a major socio-economic impact on society (1–5). They are more common in the lower limb than in the upper limb. Acute presentations, the most common of which is deep vein thrombosis, usually demand urgent attention. Chronic presentations, on the other hand, rarely threaten limb or life. The past two decades have seen a greater application of physiologic principles to the assessment and treatment of venous disease and a better understanding of the pathophysiology underlying chronic venous insufficiency due to the advent of new technology for non invasive testing, such as the continuous-wave hand held Doppler and color duplex ultrasonography. Much of this chapter will focus on the clinical assessment of patients who present to an outpatient clinic with features of uncomplicated (e.g., primary varicose veins) or complicated (e.g., chronic venous insufficiency) venous disease. The authors' practice is to assess these patients in a "one-stop" venous clinic where duplex ultrasonography can be performed, when indicated, to complement the findings of clinical assessment. A sound understanding of the anatomical and physiological basis for the development of venous disease is paramount to clinical assessment.

VENOUS ANATOMY

Lower Limb

The veins of the lower limb (6–8) can be divided into the superficial venous system that lies subcutaneously, the deep veins accompanying major arteries beneath the deep fascia and the perforating veins connecting the two. All these veins have valves with the exception of soleus venous sinuses. Valves are more numerous in the deep veins and increase in number progressively from proximal to distal in keeping with greater hydrostatic pressures in the lower part of the leg. The valves prevent retrograde flow into the superficial veins, reduce the venous pressure in the superficial and deep systems in the upright posture and aid in the venous return against gravity by the calf muscle pump.

The superficial venous system consists of an extensive plexus of venules and veins beneath the skin and the long saphenous vein (LSV) and the short saphenous vein (SSV) that run *on the deep fascia*.

Long Saphenous Vein

The LSV (Fig. 1), the longest vein in the body, commences from the medial marginal vein of the foot and ascends about 2.5–3 cm anterior to the medial malleolus, crosses the distal third of the medial surface of the tibia obliquely, and runs upwards behind its medial border to the knee; here it is posteromedial to the medial tibial and femoral condyles (a hand's breadth behind the medial border of the patella) and then ascends slightly forward across the medial aspect of the thigh and passes through the cribriform fascia covering the saphenous opening to join the femoral vein. It is often duplicated, more frequently distal to the knee. The surface marking of the sapheno–femoral junction is 1–1.25 inches (2.5–3.5 cm) below and lateral to the pubic tubercle and a line drawn from this to the femoral adductor tubercle represents the LSV.

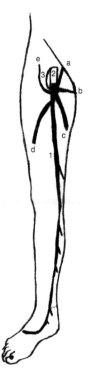

Figure 1 Long saphenous vein (LSV): (1) LSV; (2) common femoral vein; (3) saphenous opening. (**a**)–(**e**) Terminal tributaries of the LSV encountered at groin dissection.

Tributaries. The LSV drains the sole via the medial marginal veins. In the leg, it connects with the upper of the three ankle perforating veins. Just below the knee, the LSV receives a vein from the posterior calf communicating with the SSV, the anterior vein of the leg and the posterior arch vein of Dodd and Cockett formed by the union of the venous arches connecting the three ankle perforating veins (also called Leonardo's vein). Perforating veins join the LSV or its main tributaries in the upper calf (tibial tubercle or Boyd's perforator), in the distal thigh (Dodd's perforator) and in the mid thigh (Hunterian perforator). In the thigh, the LSV receives several small tributaries. Two large veins— posteromedial and anterolateral—join the LSV close to its termination. Near its termination, the LSV receives the superficial circumflex iliac, superficial epigastric, and superficial and deep external pudendal veins. The LSV is connected to the SSV via common tributaries in various segments of the leg.

Short Saphenous Vein

The SSV (Fig. 2) begins behind the lateral malleolus as a continuation of the lateral marginal vein. It ascends in the lower third of the calf lateral to tendo achilles lying on the deep fascia. In the middle third, it inclines medially to the midline and enters an intrafascial compartment in the aponeurotic investment of the gastrocnemius muscle, and in the upper third it penetrates the deep fascia passing between the heads of the gastrocnemius to enter the popliteal fossa and usually drains into the popliteal vein above the skin crease of the knee joint. Its termination however is variable, and it may terminate above, below, or at the level of the knee and may join the popliteal vein, LSV, deep posterior femoral veins, or deep sural muscular veins. The sural nerve closely follows the SSV on its lateral aspect in its lower third. At its termination in the popliteal fossa, the SSV

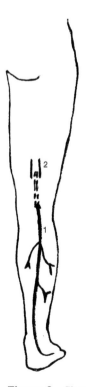

Figure 2   Short saphenous vein (SSV) (1) and popliteal vein (2).

is closely related to the medial popliteal nerve. Its deep situation renders the vein inconspicuous even when markedly varicose. The lateral or external ankle perforating vein at the junction of the lower and middle third of the calf joins the SSV to the peroneal vein and sometimes a mid-calf perforating vein connects it to the soleus sinusoids.

Deep Veins

The deep veins are those accompanying the major arteries, the gastrocnemius veins and the soleus venous arcades and sinusoids which are the main collecting chambers of the calf-muscle pump.

Perforating Veins

These connect the deep veins to the superficial veins or their tributaries and are valved such that blood flows only from the superficial to the deep veins.

Upper Limb

The superficial veins in the upper limb are the cephalic and basilic veins. The former runs along the lateral aspect of the forearm and arm and terminates in the axillary vein. The latter runs along the medial aspect of the forearm and then accompanies the brachial artery, finally joining the brachial vein to form the axillary vein. At the outer border of the first rib the axillary vein continues as the subclavian vein which joins the internal jugular vein to form the brachiocephalic vein.

VENOUS PHYSIOLOGY AND PATHOPHYSIOLOGY

Knowledge of the physiology of venous return is crucial to the understanding of the fundamental factors responsible for the development of chronic venous hypertension and the changes that accompany it. In the supine position the venous return occurs evenly along the superficial and deep veins propelled by the capillary hydrostatic pressure (about 20 mmHg). In the erect posture the main mechanism of venous return is the muscle pump or "peripheral heart" (9). The venous drainage of the superficial tissues in the erect exercising leg is inwards to the deep veins via the perforating veins.

Calf-Muscle Pump (Musculo-Venous Pump)

The valved intra- and inter-muscular deep veins constitute a series-parallel arrangement of reciprocating pumps (10). The chambers of the pump receive blood from the distal deep veins and plantar veins aided by the foot pump during walking, from the superficial veins via the ankle perforators, but the greatest supply is from the muscle capillary bed. The tight deep fascia that invests the calf muscles causes high pressure within the musculo-fascial compartment during muscle contraction, forcing the venous blood upward against the hydrostatic pressure gradient. The pump also reduces the mean hydrostatic pressure both in the superficial and deep veins which, in turn, increases the arteriovenous pressure gradient in the tissues and facilitates arterial inflow in the exercising limb. Thus the "peripheral heart" achieves a substantial increase in peripheral blood flow with a modest energy input than the alternative of a significant increase in cardiac output. During muscle relaxation, the superficial venous pressure also falls and blood is sucked in from the superficial tissues into the deep veins through the perforating veins. Thus the skin of the lower leg is protected during exercise against venous hypertension by the ability of the musculo-venous pump to lower the superficial venous pressure at the ankle and the competence of the valves in the perforating veins that maintain unidirectional flow into the deep veins.

Ambulatory Venous Hypertension and Leg Ulceration

Chronic venous insufficiency (CVI) results from venous obstruction or reflux, calf muscle pump dysfunction or a combination of these factors. The effect of venous incompetence is to prevent the fall in superficial venous pressure during exercise. This is called ambulatory venous hypertension and is the main cause of leg ulceration. Patients with an ambulatory venous pressure (AVP) of less than 40 mmHg have a minimal incidence of venous ulceration compared with an 80% incidence of ulceration in those with an AVP of greater than 80 mmHg (11). Incompetence of the deep veins has a more severe effect on the skin around the ankle than does superficial venous incompetence. Reflux in the popliteal and infrapopliteal veins is more important than proximal deep reflux to the development of advanced CVI (12). However, signs of CVI, including ulceration, can result from superficial incompetence alone (13–17).

RISK FACTORS

The most important risk factors for primary varicose veins are female sex, a family history of varicose veins and a history of phlebitis (18). Increasing age (19), Caucasian race, prolonged standing and pregnancy are also reported as risk factors. Progesterone secreted from the corpus luteum inhibits smooth muscle contractility causing relaxation of the vein wall, which may cause varicose veins to appear in the first trimester of pregnancy in the presence of inherent predisposition.

The principal risk factors for venous ulceration are age, male sex, obesity and a history of deep vein thrombosis and serious lower extremity trauma (18).

The important risk factors for deep vein thrombosis are prolonged immobilisation, recent surgery, trauma, malignancy, age, hypercoagulable states, pregnancy, oral contraceptive pill and a history of venous thromboembolism.

SYMPTOMATOLOGY

Symptoms of venous disease are usually non specific and it is often the accompanying physical signs that help to confirm the diagnosis. Symptoms do not correlate well with the presence, size or extent of varicosities. They are often worse towards the end of the day or after prolonged standing or walking and are usually relieved by elevation of the leg. This is a characteristic feature of venous disease and helps to differentiate it from other causes of leg pain arising from arterial, neurologic or musculoskeletal pathology. Relief of symptoms with compression stockings may indicate that they are of venous origin. A poor cosmetic appearance is often the only complaint. Not infrequently, complications of the disease such as superficial thrombophlebitis, haemorrhage or ulceration may be the first manifestation. Even in the presence of varicosities, many lower limb symptoms have a non venous cause and surgical treatment is unlikely to ameliorate symptoms in these patients (20). Nevertheless, a careful evaluation of the presenting symptoms may yield valuable diagnostic clues. The three most common symptoms of venous disease are pain, swelling and changes in the skin of the lower leg, particularly ulceration.

Pain

Aching pain is quite common in patients with varicose veins and is due to direct pressure of the distended veins on the adjacent somatic nerves. Hence this pain is usually localized to the site of varicosities. Symptoms such as ache, discomfort, heaviness, tightness or fatigue in the leg that are poorly localized usually result from valvular incompetence. Proximal venous outflow obstruction produces a characteristic "bursting pain" in the leg on exercise that is not relieved quickly by rest. This is due to sudden venous hypertension from exercise-induced hyperemia and outflow resistance and is called venous claudication. Apart from this claudication, severe pain is unusual in venous disease. Thrombophlebitis causes pain and tenderness along the length of the involved superficial or deep vein.

Swelling

The causes of leg swelling are outlined in Table 1. The most common cause is venous hypertension. The associated skin changes around the ankle and the pattern of distribution of the edema often help in the diagnosis. In primary uncomplicated varicose veins ankle swelling is uncommon, and when it appears is mild and more pronounced toward the end of the day. Acute onset of edema is associated with sudden venous outflow obstruction. Ankle edema is more typical of CVI and is often the first manifestation of the post-phlebitic limb. This venous edema is typically brawny, predominantly affecting the lower part of the leg and the ankle and tends to spare the feet. It is characteristically associated with skin changes of chronic venous hypertension. It usually involves one limb more than the other and is relieved by elevating the leg. Varicose veins may or may not be present.

Table 1 Causes of Leg Swelling

Local	Systemic
Venous incompetence	Hypoproteinemia
Deep veins	Secondary hyperaldosteronism
Perforating veins	Right heart failure
Superficial veins	
Venous outflow obstruction	
Intraluminal	
Extraluminal	
Calf muscle pump dysfunction	
Intrinsic muscular disease	
Neurologic disease	
Joint disease or surgery	
Lymphedema	
Primary	
Secondary	
Cellulitis	
Posture dependent	
Physiologic	
Ischemic limb	

Lymphedema usually involves the feet first and spreads proximally. It is not brawny in nature; and in advanced cases the skin is often hypertrophic, thickened, and folded over rather than atrophic, resembling an elephant hide, hence the term "elephantiasis." Failure to pinch a fold of skin at the base of the second toe is characteristic of lymphedema— Kaposi-Stemmer sign (21). The edema from systemic disease characteristically pits on pressure and the surrounding skin is normal. It is usually generalised and symmetrically affects both legs.

Ulceration

The causes of leg ulceration are outlined in Table 2. The common causes are chronic venous hypertension, ischemia or neuropathy. The underlying cause can usually be diagnosed from the site and appearance of the ulcer, i.e., from inspection. Venous ulceration typically affects the lower third of the leg, the so called "gaiter area," in the vicinity of the medial malleolus and is always associated with the skin changes of chronic venous hypertension. The ulcer is painful initially but when it becomes chronic the severity of pain subsides. It is usually shallow with its floor covered by granulation tissue and the base fixed to the deeper tissues. Long-standing ulcers may cause an equinus deformity of the ankle joint. A chronic ulcer with raised, thickened or rolled irregular edges and associated with inguinal adenopathy suggests malignant change and is known as Marjolin's *ulcer*. Ischemic ulcer on the other hand usually affects the most distal part of the extremity and is associated with continuous rest pain that is relieved by dependency. Neuropathic ulcers usually occur at pressure points and are associated with some degree of sensory deficit.

SKIN CHANGES OF CHRONIC VENOUS INSUFFICIENCY

Chronic venous hypertension induces characteristic changes in the skin and subcutaneous tissues above the ankle or the "gaiter area" (Fig. 3). The sustained high venous pressure at the ankle forces red blood cells out of the skin capillaries, where the hemoglobin is broken

Table 2 Causes of Leg Ulceration

Venous insufficiency
  Primary
  Secondary
Arterial insufficiency
Neuropathy
  Central nervous system
  Peripheral nervous system
Malignancy
  Cutaneous
  Hematologic
Miscellaneous
  Infections
  Vasculitis
  Connective tissue disorders
  Hypertension
  Hemolytic anemia
  AV malformations
  Pyoderma gangrenosum
  Traumatic

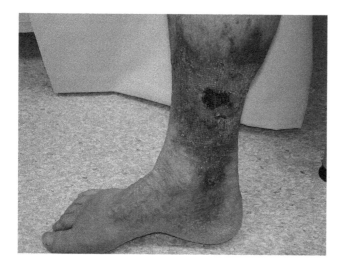

Figure 3 Chronic venous ulceration with pigmentation and lipodermatosclerosis. (*See color insert.*)

down to hemosiderin giving rise to a brown pigmentation of the skin. This is an early sign of skin injury. Eczema may develop as a dry, pigmented, scaly patch over enlarged varices or over the malleolar area. Exudation of protein-rich fluid and red blood cells sets up an inflammatory reaction in the subcutaneous tissues leading to fibrosis of the skin and subcutaneous tissues. This is called lipodermatosclerosis and may be the precursor of ulceration. The combination of a narrow ankle and prominent calf gives the appearance of an inverted "champagne bottle." Reductions in capillary numbers in areas of prior ulceration causes white patches in the skin called atrophie blanche (22). In primary uncomplicated varicose veins, eczema with pigmentation is usually confined to the skin overlying prominent varicosities.

ACUTE PRESENTATIONS OF VENOUS DISEASE

Superficial Thrombophlebitis

The affected vein is painful and is felt as a firm, palpable, tender cord with signs of localized inflammation. It may result from trauma, cellulitis, varicose veins, intravenous infusions, polycythaemia, autoimmune diseases like Behcet's syndrome, thromboangiitis obliterans, or Buerger's disease, or it may be idiopathic. Occasionally, the thrombus may extend to involve the adjacent deep vein. Episodes of thrombophlebitis that are transient and recur spontaneously at different sites is called phlebitis migrans and may indicate an occult malignancy.

Deep Vein Thrombosis

This can occur with or without demonstrable risk factors. The majority of cases of deep vein thrombosis (DVT) are clinically silent. 75% of outpatients who present with clinical features suggestive of DVT do not have the disease (23). In the majority of cases, the thrombus originates in the calf veins and either spreads proximally or remains localized to the calf. A more proximal origin of thrombus may occur following pelvic or hip surgery or trauma. The more proximal the extension of thrombosis, the more severe the symptomatology.

Clinical features cannot be relied upon to make a correct diagnosis (24,25). Pain or swelling in the leg, or low-grade pyrexia in a post-operative setting, should arouse suspicion. Pain and tenderness usually indicate significant associated inflammation. The onset is fairly sudden, and in an ambulant patient pain is severe enough to limit walking. Fullness or tightness of the calf is a common complaint. Significant outflow obstruction will cause a 'bursting' pain in the leg when attempting to walk called venous claudication. Associated pulmonary embolism may produce symptoms of pleuritic pain, dyspnea, haemoptysis or collapse. One or more of the following signs may be elicited on careful examination. However, rough manipulation can dislodge a clot with resultant embolisation.

- Swelling of the leg is the most significant and sometimes the only sign. Its distribution depends on the extent of thrombus. Ankle edema is pitting in nature.
- Dilated veins are seen over the dorsum of the foot and across the front of tibia.
- Muscles that contain the thrombosed veins feel hard and stiff and are tender.
- The entire course of the deep veins from behind the medial malleolus to the groin should be palpated for tenderness.
- Homan's sign: If the posterior tibial veins are involved, dorsiflexion of the foot exerts traction on them to produce calf pain.
- Bancroft's sign: If the posterior tibial veins are involved, tenderness can be elicited by pressing forwards the main muscle belly of the calf forwards but not from side to side.

Duplex ultrasonography is the imaging modality of choice in clinically suspected DVT. However Wells et al. have shown that DVT can be ruled out in patients with a low clinical probability of DVT and a negative d-dimer test (26). Ultrasound testing can be safely omitted in such patients.

Extensive thrombosis involving all the major venous channels in the leg is characterized by a massively swollen, painful and tender limb that is cold and pale. This condition is called phlegmasia alba dolens (white leg; milk leg). The femoral artery may go into spasm, and this, along with the overlying edema, makes it difficult to feel the femoral pulse and then it may be confused with acute ischemia especially in the initial stages. When the thrombosis extends to involve the collateral venous channels to cause complete venous outflow obstruction, the condition is called phlegmasia cerulea dolens (blue leg). Venous gangrene ensues when the thrombosis involves even the small veins and capillaries and the high venous pressure and edema significantly reduces arterial inflow into the limb (27).

Axillary vein thrombosis follows unusual and excessive use of the arm above head or extrinsic compression of the vein by pathology in the axilla or thoracic outlet. The clinical features are similar to DVT affecting the lower limb.

OUTPATIENT CLINICAL ASSESSMENT

Venous disease may result from reflux disease, outflow obstruction or both. The aim of clinical assessment is to detect and localize it and possibly identify the causative or pre-disposing factor (Table 3). Quantification of the underlying pathophysiology requires special investigations but is not necessary in all cases. The continuous wave hand-held Doppler probe has become an indispensable adjunct to clinical assessment and has largely replaced traditional examination methods using a tourniquet. Duplex ultrasonography helps to detect the underlying pathophysiology and to assess the severity and extent of the disease process, factors that are vital in choosing the most appropriate form of treatment.

Table 3 Causes of Varicose Veins

Primary—unknown cause, often familial
Secondary
  Reflux disease due to valve destruction, dysfunction or both following recanalization of deep vein
    thrombosis causing deep, perforator or superficial vein incompetence
  Nonthrombotic venous outflow obstruction
  Pelvic tumors—benign or malignant
    Pelvic lymphadenopathy
    Pregnancy
  Thrombotic venous occlusion
  Rare causes
    Arteriovenous fistulae
    Klippel-Trenaunay syndrome

History and physical examination are, however, important in clinical assessment and often help to choose the most appropriate test for further assessment.

History

A young patient with varicose veins with no history of deep vein thrombosis or positive family history usually indicates primary disease. The following points should be recorded meticulously:

- Age and sex of the patient—Varicose veins or venous ulceration in the very young suggest a congenital abnormality.
- Presenting complaint—pain, ache, heaviness of the legs, ankle swelling, night cramps, restlessness, heat or burning sensation, throbbing, itching, pins and needles or tingling sensation, cosmesis, etc.
- Duration and mode of onset—Swelling often precedes the onset of varicose veins in the post-phlebitic limb.
- Aggravating factors—prolonged standing or walking, worse towards the end of the day.
- Relieving factors—leg elevation, compression stockings.
- History of complications of the disease—thrombophlebitis, bleeding, ulceration.
- Details of previous treatment.
- History of deep vein thrombosis, swelling or significant trauma to the leg, or leg fracture.
- History of thrombophilia.
- The type of occupation, overall health status, way of life and the impact of the problem on activity and life style.
- History of abdominal or pelvic symptoms and pregnancy status if a secondary cause for varicose veins is suspected.
- Family history of varicose veins or deep vein thrombosis or thrombophilia.

Physical Examination

This is best done in the standing position. Comparison of the two limbs may be useful. Both lower limbs are exposed from the umbilicus to the toes and inspected over the front and the back. Examination is carried out methodically by *inspection*, *palpation*, *ausculation* and *insonation*.

Inspection

- Distribution of varicosities: This may indicate the superficial venous system involved. Varicosities in unusual areas such as the pubis or the lower abdominal wall or bilateral varicose veins should raise the possibility of secondary varicose veins due to deep venous obstruction. Incompetent perforating veins may produce a characteristic bulge along the varicosity.
- Presence of telangiectases (also known as thread veins or dermal flares) or reticular veins both of which can be signs of venous dysfunction.
- Ankle swelling—mild edema can be detected by comparing with the other leg.
- Skin changes of chronic venous insufficiency in the lower third of the leg, e.g., pigmentation, eczema, lipodermatosclerosis, healed or active ulceration, atrophie blanche.

Palpation

Many clinical tests to assess venous disease have been described. These include the cough impulse test and the percussion or tap sign to detect groin reflux and long saphenous vein incompetence, Brodie-Trendelenburg test using single or multiple tourniquets to detect the site or sites of superficial venous reflux, Fegan's method of seeking the sites of perforators and Perthe's test for patency of the deep veins (21,28). Although these tests are based on the anatomical and physiological principles underlying the development of venous disease, they have been largely replaced by the hand-held Doppler because of its ease of use and the accuracy and extent of information that can be obtained. The principles of testing, however, remain the same. A palpation of the leg is routinely performed prior to Doppler testing.

- Palpate the texture of the skin and subcutaneous tissues of the lower leg and for any tenderness or pitting edema.
- Palpate over the varicosities for tenderness and along the course of the long and short saphenous vein. Varicose veins may be felt lying in a subcutaneous gutter when they are not visible.
- Palpate the peripheral pulses, as venous and arterial disease of the lower limb often co-exist, especially in the elderly.
- Examine the innervation of the leg, if there is ulceration.
- Palpate for inguinal lymphadenopathy if there is chronic ulceration, particularly if there is suspicion of malignant change.
- Examination of the abdomen should be performed (including a rectal and vaginal or testicular examination when an intra-abdominal or pelvic pathology is suspected).

Auscultation

Varicosities that remain prominent on lying down may indicate an underlying arteriovenous fistula and ausculatation may reveal the characteristic "machinery" murmur.

Insonation (Hand-Held Doppler Examination)

An assessment using the hand-held Doppler probe is widely accepted as the minimum level of investigation before treatment is initiated. Its utility in the evaluation of primary and uncomplicated varicose veins is well established (29–31). With practice, it can identify flow and detect clinically significant reflux in the superficial veins reliably (32) and can also be used to exclude arterial disease.

Basic principles. The frequency of ultrasound transmitted from the transmitting crystal (T) strikes an interface (I) which is moving towards the transducer (Fig. 4). The frequency of the reflected signal is increased and is received by the receiving transducer (R). The Doppler instrument is designed to extract this frequency shift or difference. This difference is small and within the audible range and hence can be amplified by feeding into an output device such as the loudspeaker. When the angle between the ultrasound beam and the reflector is 90° there is no detectable Doppler shift frequency. Therefore, the angle between transducer and reflector should be less than 60° whenever possible (33–35).

Continuous wave hand-held Doppler is the most basic Doppler system. The transducer assembly has both a transmitter element and a receiver element so that the sound is transmitted and received continuously. A filter is used to remove large, low-frequency components from the signal. These instruments are small, inexpensive, good for superficial vessels and very sensitive to weak signals. However, they are unable to produce any form of image of the underlying vessel, or to determine from what depth or from how many vessels the Doppler signals are being received.

The technique of examination using the hand-held Doppler is simple and easily acquired. With the patient standing, the Doppler probe is placed over the saphenofemoral junction and the calf squeezed to augment forward flow through the junction which is heard as a characteristic "whoosh." This confirms good "sonic contact." The calf compression is then released. Any significant reflux through the junction would result in a second prolonged "whoosh." The probe is then placed over the LSV where it is visibly distended or otherwise just above the knee, where its location is predictable, and the calf squeezed and released to detect any reflux in the vein. A prolonged "whoosh," both at the groin and over the LSV, would indicate an incompetent saphenofemoral junction and LSV to the point of examination. Isolated truncal incompetence in the LSV may sometimes occur in the presence of a competent saphenofemoral junction. Insonation over the LSV may be repeated after occluding the LSV either digitally or with a tourniquet proximally in the thigh or at the knee level. Elimination of a previously demonstrable refluxing signal or "whoosh" would confirm superficial venous incompetence. Reflux across the saphenofemoral junction during hand-held Doppler probe testing may also be elicited by asking the patient to cough

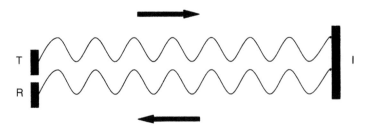

Figure 4 The Doppler effect. *Abbreviations*: T, transmitting crystal; I, interface; R, receiving transducer.

(36) or to carry out a Valsalva manoeuvre. The short saphenous system is similarly tested by placing the probe over the popliteal fossa bearing in mind the anatomical variations in the termination of the short saphenous vein (37). If the findings are inconclusive after a hand-held Doppler examination, a duplex ultrasonography should be performed.

The hand-held Doppler is also useful to estimate the ankle-brachial pressure index in suspected arterial insufficiency in patients presenting with varicose veins.

Duplex Ultrasonography

This allows direct visualization of the veins and provides anatomical and functional information. By detecting flow, they are helpful in identifying vessels that appear too small in the 2D image.

It is controversial as to whether a hand-held Doppler examination alone is sufficient for assessment of all primary long saphenous vein incompetence, especially if surgical treatment is planned. Resource constraints, perhaps more than scientific rationale, often precludes the routine use of duplex ultrasonography in all such patients. However, in the authors' opinion and experience, a limited duplex scan can be performed in clinic in patients with uncomplicated LSV incompetence in much the same time as a hand-held Doppler examination. There are instances when a more detailed examination is warranted whether or not hand-held Doppler demonstrates reflux. These include:

- Reflux in the popliteal fossa—because of variation in the position of the sapheno-popliteal junction (which needs to be surface marked prior to surgery) and to differentiate superficial venous reflux from deep vein incompetence.
- Clinical features of chronic venous insufficiency.
- Recurrent varicose veins—because of a more complex morphology (38).
- History of deep vein thrombosis, limb swelling or significant trauma or fracture to the limb—to study the flow in the deep veins and perforators. Superficial varices that develop after deep vein thrombosis may be the only route of venous outflow from the limb.
- Atypical distribution of varicose veins and uncertainty regarding sites of incompetence.
- Selection of patients for new therapies such as endovenous ablation techniques using radiofrequency energy, laser or foam sclerotherapy, and the use and follow up of these treatments.
- Varicose veins associated with arteriovenous fistulae—to study the flow pattern and extent of the lesion and for follow up after surgery or embolisation.

Duplex ultrasonography is now accepted as the gold standard in the above circumstances to precisely identify the pathophysiology and site and extent of abnormality. A systematic examination of the superficial and deep venous system is performed to obtain a comprehensive "venous" map of the leg. Duplex ultrasonography has largely replaced venography in this respect.

CLASSIFICATION OF VENOUS DISEASE

CEAP Classification

The CEAP classification (39,40) was originally devised by experts under the auspices of the American Venous Forum in 1994 to address the diagnostic needs of patients with chronic venous disease. It defines the clinical class (C) of the problem, its aetiology (E), its anatomic distribution in the veins of the extremity (A) and its underlying pathologic (P) mechanism (reflux, obstruction or both). It also provides a severity rating scale and a disability scale. The diagnostic tests are used based on the severity of venous disease. This classification provides a scientific way of categorizing the entire range of chronic venous disease with diagnoses determined by objective testing (40).

Michael's Classification

The CEAP classification is sometimes too elaborate for the purposes of a clinical trial on a specific sub-group of patient population. Michael's classification is simple and easy to use in an outpatient setting and has a direct and pragmatic bearing on treatment (41). The classification uses information obtained from physical and hand-held Doppler examination and defines groups of patients that are most likely to benefit from particular forms of intervention. Complications of varicose veins, the need for recurrent groin or popliteal surgery and factors that influence the suitability for surgery or sclerotherapy such as site, size and extent of varicosities are all taken into consideration.

Basle Classification

It is not widely used nowadays since the advent of the CEAP classification and is not suitable for use in a clinical trial (42).

KEY POINTS

- Diseases of the venous system cause significant morbidity and have a major socio–economic impact on society.
- Outpatient assessment of venous disease should be carried out by specialists ideally in a dedicated "one-stop" venous clinic. Inadequate assessment can result in poorer treatment outcome and patient dissatisfaction.
- The three most common presentations of lower limb venous disease are pain, swelling and skin changes in the lower third of the leg. Cosmesis is another significant reason for seeking medical attention.
- The aim of clinical assessment is to detect and localize the underlying pathophysiology and to identify any risk factors.
- Physical examination includes inspection, palpation, auscultation and insonation using the hand-held Doppler. The latter is an indispensable tool in clinical assessment.
- Clinical diagnosis of DVT is unreliable. However, DVT can safely be ruled out if clinical probability is low and d–dimer test is negative. Duplex ultrasonography is the imaging modality of choice in suspected cases.

REFERENCES

1. Callam MJ. Epidemiology of varicose veins. Br J Surg 1994; 81:167–173.
2. Smith JJ, Garratt AM, Guest M, et al. Evaluating and improving health-related quality of life in patients with varicose veins. J Vasc Surg 1999; 30:710–719.

3. Garratt AM, Macdonald LM, Ruta DA, et al. Towards measurement of outcome for patients with varicose veins. Qual Health Care 1993; 2:5–10.
4. Sparey C, Haddad N, Sissons G, et al. The effect of pregnancy on the lower limb venous system of women with varicose veins. Eur J Vasc Endovasc Surg 1999; 18:294–299.
5. Evans CJ, Fowkes FG, Hajivassiliou CA, et al. Epidemiology of varicose veins. A review. Int Angiol 1994; 13:263–270.
6. Sinnatamby CS. Chapter 3: Lower Limb. In: Sinnatamby CS, ed. Last's Anatomy Regional and Applied 10th ed. Edinburgh, New York: Churchill Livingstone, 1999:101–110.
7. Negus D. The Surgical Anatomy of the Veins of the Lower Limb. In: Dodd H, Cockett FB, eds. The Pathology and Surgery of the veins of the lower limb. 2nd ed. New York: Churchill Livingstone, 1976:18–49.
8. Gabella G. Veins of the lower limb. In: Bannister LH, Berry MB, Collins P et al, eds. Gray's Anatomy. 38th ed. 1995:1595–1598.
9. Scurr JH. Venous Disorders. In: Russell RCG, Williams NS, Bulstrode CJK, eds. Bailey & Love's Short Practice of Surgery. 24th ed. 2004:954–973.
10. Ludbrook J. Applied physiology of the veins. In: Dodd H, Cockett FB, eds. The Pathology and Surgery of the veins of the lower limb. 2nd ed. 1976:50–55.
11. Nicolaides AN, Zukowski AJ. The value of dynamic pressure measurements. World J Surg 1986; 10:919.
12. Hanrahan LM, Araki CT, Rodriguez AA, et al. Distribution of valvular incompetence in patients with venous stasis ulceration. J Vasc Surg 1991; 13:805.
13. Sethia KK, Darke SG. Long saphenous incompetence as a cause of venous ulceration. Br J Surg 1984; 71:754.
14. Hoare MC, Nicolaides AN, Miles CR, et al. The role of primary varicose veins in venous ulceration. Surgery 1982; 92:450.
15. Bass A, Chayen D, Weinmann EE, et al. Lateral venous ulcer and short saphenous vein insufficiency. J Vasc Surg 1997; 25:654.
16. Darke SG, Penfold C. Venous ulceration and saphenous ligation. Eur J Vasc Surg 1992; 6:4–9.
17. Lees TA, Lambert D. Patterns of venous reflux in limbs with skin changes associated with chronic venous insufficiency. Br J Surg 1993; 80:725–728.
18. Scott TE, La Morte WW, Gorin DR, et al. Risk factors for chronic venous insufficiency: A dual case-control study. J Vasc Surg 1995; 22:622.
19. Adhikari A, Criqui MH, Wooll V, et al. The epidemiology of chronic venous diseases. Phlebology 2000; 15:2–18.
20. Bradbury AW, Evans C, Allan PL, et al. What are the symptoms of varicose veins? Edinburgh Vein Study cross-sectional population survey BMJ 1999; 318:353–356.
21. Giannoukas AD. Chapter 29. Venous and lymphatic diseases. In: Lumley JSP, ed. Hamilton Bailey's Physical Signs. Demonstrations of Physical Signs in Clinical Surgery. 18th ed. Oxford: Butterworth-Heinemann, 1997:381–396.
22. Leu AJ, Leu HJ, Franzeck UK, et al. Microvascular changes in chronic venous insufficiency: A review. Cardiovasc Surg 1995; 3:237.
23. Wells PS, Hirsh J, Anderson DR, et al. Accuracy of clinical assessment of deep-vein thrombosis. Lancet 1995; 346(8973):516.
24. Cranley JJ, Canos AJ, Sull WJ. The diagnosis of deep venous thrombosis. Fallibility of clinical symptoms and signs. Arch Surg 1976; 111:34–36.
25. Donada C, Galofaro G, Maccioni A, et al. Unreliability of the clinical diagnosis in deep venous thrombosis of the lower limbs. Minerva Med 1990; 81:61–66 [Article in Italian].
26. Wells PS, Anderson DR, Rodger M, et al. Evaluation of d-Dimer in the Diagnosis of Suspected Deep-Vein Thrombosis. N Engl J Med 2003; 349:1227–1235.
27. Sumner DS. Chapter 7: Essential hemodynamic principles. In: Rutherford RB, ed. Vascular Surgery. 5th ed. Philadelphia: W.B. Saunders Company, 2000:73–120.
28. Browse NL. Chapter 7: The arteries, veins and lymphatics. In: Browse NL, ed. An Introduction to the Symptoms and Signs of Surgical Disease. 3rd ed. London: Arnold, 1997:180–195.

29. McIrvine AJ, Corbett CRR, Aston NO, et al. The demonstration of saphenofemoral incompetence: Doppler ultrasound compared with standard clinical tests. Br J Surg 1984; 71:509–510.

30. Mitchell DC, Darke SG. The assessment of primary varicose veins by doppler ultrasound; the role of sapheno-popliteal incompetence and the short saphenous system. Eur J Vasc Endovasc Surg 1987; 1:113–115.

31. Milliken JC, Dinn E, O'Connor R, et al. A simple Doppler technique for the rapid diagnosis of significant sapheno-femoral reflux. Phlebology 1986; 1:125–128.

32. Campbell WB, Niblett BM, Ridler BMF, et al. Hand-held Doppler as a screening test in primary varicose veins. Br J Surg 1997; 84:1541–1543.

33. Williamson MR. Chapter 1: Physics in ultrasound. In: Williamson MR, ed. Essentials of Ultrasound. New York: W.B. Saunders Company, 1996:1–28.

34. McDicken WN, Hoskins PR. Physics: Principles. Practice and Artefacts. In: Allan PA, Dubbins PA, Pozniak MA, McDicken WN, eds. Clinical Doppler Ultrasound. 1st ed. 2000:1–25.

35. Farrant P, Meire HB. Chapter 9: Doppler Ultrasound. In: Farrant P, Meire HB, eds. Basic Ultrasound. Chinchester: Wiley, 1995:56–67.

36. Darke SG, Vetrivel S, Foy DMA, et al. Comparison of duplex scanning and continuous wave doppler in the assessment of primary and uncomplicated varicose veins. J Vasc Endovasc Surg 1997; 14:457–461.

37. Chan A, Chisolm I, Royle JP. The use of directional ultrasound in the assessment of saphenous incompetence. Aust NZ J Surg 1983; 53:399–402.

38. Darke SG. The morphology of recurrent varicose veins. Eur J Vasc Surg 1992; 6:512–517.

39. Kistner RL, Masuda EM. Chapter 145: A practical approach to the diagnosis and classification of chronic venous disease. In: Rutherford RB, ed. Vascular Surgey. 5th ed. Philadelphia: W.B. Saunders, 2000:1990–1999.

40. Kistner RL, Eklof B, Masuda EM. Diagnosis of chronic venous disease of the lower extremities: the "CEAP" classification. Mayo Clin Proc 1996; 71:338–345.

41. Michaels JA, Campbell WB. A new pragmatic classification system for varicose veins. Phlebology 2001; 16:29–33.

42. Madar G, Widmer L, Zemp E, et al. Varicose veins and chronic venous insufficiency disorder or disease. Vasa 1986; 15:126–134.

8

Noninvasive Evaluation of Venous Disease

Ahmad Bhatti
Division of Vascular Surgery, Loyola University Medical Center, Maywood, Illinois, U.S.A.

Nicos Labropoulos
Vascular Laboratory, Division of Vascular Surgery, New Jersey Medical School, Newark, New Jersey, U.S.A.

INTRODUCTION

Anatomy, flow, valve function, and occlusion are the primary variables that are assessed non invasively. Evaluation of these parameters can be direct (e.g., doppler ultrasonography) or indirect/physiologic (e.g., plethysmography). The disease states that prompt these investigations can be broken down into reflux and obstruction. These methods have allowed us to increase our understanding on the pathophysiology of chronic venous disease (CVD). As a consequence the management of CVD has also improved.

PHYSIOLOGIC TESTS

They provide quantitative measurements of venous hemodynamics. The severity of the CVD in the limbs can be globally assessed. However, they do not provide targeted segmental evaluation and the distribution and extent of CVD is not known. Thus using them alone it is difficult to instigate appropriate treatment. They are very helpful in monitoring the effects of conservative and interventional treatment.

AIR PLETHYSMOGRAPHY

Air plethysmography involves pressure cuffs that are placed on the leg. Changes in volume are transduced to changes in pressure via the polyurethane air bladders in these cuffs. Measurements are taken in supine and standing positions and after certain maneuvers. Several measurements can be obtained: functional venous volume (VV), ejection fraction (EF), venous filling index (VFI), and residual volume fraction (RVF). These measurements, along with patient maneuvers during the exam, can help evaluate for reflux, obstruction, and calf-pump function. Reproducibility of this test in patients with venous disease has been brought into question (1,2). Additionally, these parameters are absolute and do not take limb size into account.

Reflux is evaluated with the patient in supine position and the legs are elevated in order to empty the veins. The patient is asked to stand to allow filling of the veins until a plateau is reached. VV is the amount of blood from the baseline to the plateau and is approximately 70–110 cc in normal individuals (3). VFI measures the amount of blood that fills the veins. A slow filling which is <2 ml/s indicates the absence of significant reflux. The higher the value of VFI the worse the problem. Patients with venous insufficiency may have a VV of up to 400 cc (4). VV, VFI, and RVF rise with increasing reflux (3). Venous ulcer formation is more likely with increasing VFI and RVF (5,6).

Obstructive changes may also be measured by the outflow fraction (OF). With the patient in supine position and limb elevation, a thigh tourniquet is applied and inflated to 80 mmHg. The VV volume will rise and plateau. Then the tourniquet is rapidly deflated and the veins are emptied. The slower the emptying the worse the obstruction. The OF is measured at one second and a normal value is $>40\%$. The test can also be performed with digital occlusion of the greater saphenous vein (GSV) to assess its outflow contribution.

PHOTO PLETHYSMOGRAPHY

Photo plethysmography (PPG) works on the principal of blood absorption of infrared light that is maximally absorbed by hemoglobin. These are the same principles employed in oxygen pulse oximetry. An infrared light and sensor are mounted to one another in a PPG. Infrared light is emitted from the transmitter, and the sensor detects the amount of light reflected back. Blood absorbs this infrared light, so increases in local blood volume decrease reflection to the sensor. Special algorithms and/or sensors are used to subtract out arterial artifacts when venous studies are performed. Quantitative digital PPG goes one step further and automatically calibrates itself and provides amplitude measurement. A volume-time tracing is created using this method. For reflux studies, the patient is seated and an emitter/sensor is applied to their calf. The patient then performs several tiptoes to empty the venous system. PPG records a decrease in the blood volume. All measurements are relative and qualitative. The patient then stops and the arteries refill the venous system slowly in a normal limb. In the patient with reflux, the venous system will refill faster. While the time-volume curve is important to assess, a refilling time (RT) greater than 23 seconds is normal, and less than 20 seconds is consistent with reflux (7). If a short RT is noted, the test is repeated with a narrow cuff below the knee to occlude the superficial veins. After cuff inflation and repeat testing, a repeat short RT indicates deep venous incompetence, whereas normalization indicates superficial venous incompetence. Although PPG can detect the presence of venous disease or reflux, its correlation to severity of disease is poor (8,9).

LIGHT REFLECTION RHEOGRAPHY

Light reflection rheography (LRR) is similar to PPG except that it is designed to minimize artifact from the patient's skin or surface (e.g., stockings). To assess for venous reflux, the same measurements, techniques, and limitations apply as in PPG.

STRAIN GAUGE PLETHYSMOGRAPHY

Ambulatory strain gauge plethysmography (SGP or ASGP) measures calf volume changes. Variations of the actual strain gauge device exist, but all devices essentially measure the diameter supramalleolar ankle during testing (10). This reduces artifact from calf contraction and produces more reproducible results (11). The patient then performs 20 knee bends in 40 seconds to 60 degrees. The expelled volume (EV) and refill time (RT) are calculated. Both EV and RT decrease with increasing severity of venous disease. Cuffs can be applied to occlude the superficial venous system in an attempt to attribute abnormal findings to the deep or superficial system.

FOOT VOLUMETRY

Foot volumetry employs similar principles to other plethysmographic studies. A container filled with water is equipped with a photoelectric sensor that relays the water level (volume) to a recording device. The foot is immersed after various maneuvers, and the foot volume recorded with each immersion. Foot volumes are measured initially and then after 20 knee bends. Parameters such as expelled volume (EV), expelled volume rate (EVR), and refilling flow (Q) are measured. A cuff may then be applied to occlude the superficial venous system, and the measurements repeated to differentiate between deep and superficial venous pathology. EV has been shown to correlate with venous pressure in normal and pathologic exercised limbs (12). Foot volumetry parameters have also been shown to correlate with the clinical class/severity of venous insufficiency (13).

CONTINUOUS WAVE DOPPLER

Doppler ultrasound can only detect the presence or absence of reflux in those systems being assessed. With the patient standing upright to maximize venous engorgement and reflux (if present), a Doppler probe is placed at a 45° angle to the skin in the same plane as the axial stream. Each vein segment is individually probed. Antegrade flow is elicited by brisk calf or thigh compression, and a Doppler signal is heard. If a second prolonged sound is heard after the release of the compression this is reflux. The absence of signal during the compression indicates occlusion. In areas like the popliteal fossa it can determine the presence of reflux but it will be unable to determine its origin (small saphenous versus gastrocnemial versus popliteal). Also it will be falsely negative for thrombosis in patients with partial luminal occlusion and in those with duplicated veins. Nowadays it is not commonly performed as it provides limited information. It remains a fast, simple, and inexpensive screening tool for reflux (14,15).

DUPLEX ULTRASOUND

Duplex ultrasound scanning (DUS) combines color flow imaging with B-mode and pulsed Doppler. This provides anatomic detail, visualization of flow, and flow velocity data. It is noninvasive, relatively portable, and low priced, but it is operator dependent. DUS has largely supplanted venography as a routine study for assessment of CVD. It has become the test of choice in many cases, including assessing primary and recurrent venous reflux (16,17).

A thorough history and physical exam is paramount, as this will highlight areas of importance and provide relevant information such as previous thrombosis or venous surgery. The test starts with the patient standing with support of their body weight on the contralateral limb. It has been shown that this is the best position for testing reflux and the supine position should no longer be used (18). If the patients are unable to stand for long then the sitting position may be used.

The different veins are tested for reflux by rapidly squeezing and suddenly releasing of the calf or other muscle beds. At the groin the Valsalva maneuver may also be performed. In obese patients and in those with edema a dorsi/plantar flexion may be used if the compression is unable to augment flow sufficiently (18). Automatic rapid inflation-deflation cuffs may also be used especially when precise measurements are needed. Different transducers can be changed as needed, as superficial and deep veins may require different frequencies particularly in the obese and edematous limbs. All main veins are imaged and assessed along their entire lengths. Nonsaphenous, accessory veins and tributaries should be noted and studied accordingly (19,20). The venous anatomy is complex. The examiner should be aware of the different variations such as duplications (common in popliteal and femoral, rare in the saphenous veins) hypoplasia (saphenous veins) and segmental aplasia (posterior tibial and GSV). These are important for the accurate diagnosis and may also have an impact on the management of the patient.

Throughout the exam, color flow imaging is used on top of the B-mode ultrasound. Typically, red indicates arterial flow, and blue indicates venous flow. Therefore, any red (retrograde) flow in a vein indicates reflux. Increasing venous back pressure should produce no retrograde flow. Some reflux behind competent valves is physiologic (21,22). Reflux has been recently defined as a retrograde flow lasting > 1000 ms in the femoropopliteal veins, > 500 ms in the deep calf veins, deep femoral vein and the superficial veins, and > 350 ms in the perforator veins (18). The risk for skin damage is proportional to the degree of reflux. The distribution and extent of reflux throughout the limb's venous system also correlate with clinical severity of chronic venous insufficiency (23). Reflux may exist in the superficial and/or deep system. The perforators are assessed in the ankle, calf and the thigh in their usual locations. Additionally, localized varicose veins should heighten suspicion for an underlying incompetent perforator, and that region may require further evaluation. Ulcers and other wounds should not prevent examination of the underlying veins. Covering the probe with a sterile glove, or covering the wound itself with a transparent sterile dressing, allows for adequate assessment (24).

COMPUTED TOMOGRAPHIC VENOGRAPHY

Several studies have suggested performing computed tomographic venography (CTV) of the lower extremities at the same time a CTA of the pulmonary arterial tree for suspect pulmonary embolism (PE) is performed (25,26). One study compared CTV to DUS and found CTV to be 100% sensitive and 97% specific for pelvic or thigh deep venous thrombosis (DVT) from the iliac crests to knees (26). Another study compared CTV to ultrasound for DVT in the same anatomic region and found 100% sensitivity and specificity (27). CTV is generally limited to anatomic information of veins between the iliac crest and knees, and therefore cannot assess reflux or pathology in calf veins. CTV is not currently being used to assess CVD. Its role appears to be limited to evaluate for DVT in patients as a venous thromboembolic (VTE) source. However, there is limited experience with using

CTV for anatomic evaluation of the venous system. This includes assessment of venous anatomy in post-operative varicose vein recurrence, or in evaluation for May-Thurner syndrome (28,29).

MAGNETIC RESONANCE VENOGRAPHY

Magnetic resonance venography (MRV) allows assessment of the pelvic and iliac veins. It has an advantage over venography and DUS in assessing the internal iliac veins for thrombosis (30). It has been cited as being as sensitive and specific as venography (93–100% and 95–97% respectively) (31–34). This includes, unlike CTV, assessing calf veins for DVT or anatomy (33,35). Thrombus age may also be estimated by MRV (36,37). Three-dimensional views of the venous system can be reconstructed. Lesions significant to venous pathology, such as in May-Thurner syndrome, can also be diagnosed concordantly (38). Predominate disadvantages of this technique are those that apply to MR in general: motion artifact, metallic implant and claustrophobia.

KEY POINTS

- The noninvasive tests measure the severity and anatomic extent of reflux and obstruction.
- The plethysmographic tests are good to assess venous hemodynamics of the limb but with their use alone appropriate treatment cannot be instigated.
- Duplex ultrasound has become the method of choice for assessing venous disease. It can detect reflux obstruction in individual veins and allow imaging of other pathologies.
- Computer tomography can detect pulmonary embolism and proximal vein thrombosis during the same exam.
- Magnetic resonance venography is used in detection of thrombosis and is particularly useful in the evaluation of pelvic veins.

REFERENCES

1. Yang D, Sacco P. Reproducibility of air plethysmography for the evaluation of arterial and venous function of the lower leg. Clinical Physiology & Functional Imaging 2002; 22:379–382.
2. Yang D, Vandongen YK, Stacey MC. Variability and reliability of air plethysmographic measurement for the evaluation of chronic venous disease. J Vasc Surg 1997; 26:638–642.
3. Labropoulos N, Giannoukas AD, Nicolaides AN, Veller M, Leon M, Volteas N. The role of venous reflux and calf muscle pump function in nonthrombotic chronic venous insufficiency. Correlation with severity of signs and symptoms. Arch Surg 1996; 131:403–406.
4. Nicolaides AN. Investigation of chronic venous insufficiency: A consensus statement. Circulation 2000; 102:E126–E163.
5. van Rij AM, Solomon C, Christie R. Anatomic and physiologic characteristics of venous ulceration. J Vasc Surg 1994; 20:759–764.
6. Araki CT, Back TL, Padberg FT, et al. The significance of calf muscle pump function in venous ulceration. J Vasc Surg 1994; 20:872–877.
7. Sarin S, Shields DA, Scurr JH, Coleridge Smith PD. Photoplethysmography: a valuable noninvasive tool in the assessment of venous dysfunction? J Vasc Surg 1992; 16:154–162.

8. Van Bemmelen PS, Van Ramshort B, Eikelboom BC. Photoplethysmography reexamined: lack of correlation with duplex scanning. Surgery 1992; 112:544–548.

9. Bays RA, Healy DA, Atnip RG, et al. Validation of air plethysmography, photoplethysmography, and duplex ultrasonography in the evaluation of severe venous stasis. J Vasc Surg 1994; 20:721–727.

10. Struckmann JR, Mathiesen FR. A noninvasive plethysmographic method for evaluation of the musculovenous pump in the lower extremities. Acta Chir Scand 1985; 15:235–240.

11. Struckmann JR, Vissing SF, Hjortso E. Ambulatory strain-gauge plethysmography and blood volume scintimetry for quantitative assessment of venous insufficiency. Clin Physiol 1992; 12:277–285.

12. Lawrence D, Kakkar VV. Venous pressure measurement and foot volumetry in venous disease. In: Verstraete M, ed. Techniques in Angiology. The Hague, the Netherlands: Martinus Nijhoff, NV, 1979.

13. Danielsson G, Norgren L, Jungbeck C, Peterson K. Global venous function correlates better than duplex derived reflux to clinical class in the evaluation of chronic venous disease. Int Angiol 2003; 22:177–181.

14. Darke SG, Vetrivel S, Foy DM, Smith S, Baker S. A comparison of duplex scanning and continuous wave Doppler in the assessment of primary and uncomplicated varicose veins. Eur J Vasc Endovasc Surg 1997; 14:457–461.

15. Labropoulos N, Kang SS, Mansour MA, Giannoukas AD, Buckman J, Baker WH. Primary superficial vein reflux with competent saphenous trunk. Eur J Vasc Endovasc Surg 1999; 18:201–206.

16. Labropoulos N, Touloupakis E, Giannoukas AD, Leon M, Katsamouris A, Nicolaides AN. Recurrent varicose veins: Investigation of the pattern and extent of reflux with color flow duplex imaging. Surgery 1996; 119:406–409.

17. Valentin LI, Valentin WH, Mercado S, Rosado CJ. Venous reflux localization: Comparative study of venography and DU. Phlebology 1993; 8:124–127.

18. Labropoulos N, Tiongson J, Landon P, et al. Definition of venous reflux in lower extremity veins. J Vasc Surg 2003; 38:793–798.

19. Labropoulos N, Tiongson J, Pryor L, et al. Nonsaphenous superficial vein reflux. J Vasc Surg 2001; 34:872–877.

20. Labropoulos N, Kang SS, Mansour MA, Giannoukas AD, Buckman J, Baker WH. Primary superficial vein reflux with competent saphenous trunk. Eur J Vasc Endovasc Surg 1999; 18:201–206.

21. Vasdekis SN, Clarke GH, Nicolaides AN. Quantification of venous reflux by means of DU. J Vasc Surg 1989; 10:670–677.

22. van Bemmelen PS, Bedford G, Beach K, Strandness DE. Quantitative segmental evaluation of venous valvular reflux with duplex ultrasound scanning. J Vasc Surg 1989; 10:425–431.

23. Labropoulos N, Delis K, Nicolaides AN, Leon M, Ramaswami G, Volteas N. The role of the distribution and anatomic extent of reflux in the development of signs and symptoms in chronic venous insufficiency. J Vasc Surg 1996; 23:504–510.

24. Labropoulos N, Giannoukas AD, Nicolaides AN, Ramaswami G, Leon M, Burke P. New insights into the pathophysiologic condition of venous ulceration with color-flow duplex imaging: implications for treatment? J Vasc Surg 1995; 22:45–50.

25. Katz DS, Hon M. Current DVT imaging. Tech Vasc Interv Radiol 2004; 7:55–62.

26. Begemann PG, Bonacker M, Kemper J, et al. Evaluation of the deep venous system in patients with suspected pulmonary embolism with multi-detector CT: a prospective study in comparison to Doppler sonography. J Comput Assist Tomogr 2003; 27:399–409.

27. Yoshida S, Akiba H, Tamakawa M, et al. Spiral CT venography of the lower extremities by injection via an arm vein in patients with leg swelling. Br J Radiol 2001; 74:1013–1016.

28. Uhl JF, Verdeille S, Martin-Bouyer Y. Three-dimensional spiral CT venography for the pre-operative assessment of varicose patients. Vasa 2003; 32:91–94.

29. Chung JW, Yoon CJ, Jung SI, et al. Acute iliofemoral deep vein thrombosis: evaluation of underlying anatomic abnormalities by spiral CT venography. J Vasc Interv Radiol 2004; 15:249–256.

30. Spritzer CE, Arata MA, Freed KS. Isolated pelvic deep venous thrombosis: relative frequency as detected with MR imaging. Radiology 2001; 219:521–525.

31. Aschauer M, Deutschmann HA, Stollberger R, et al. Value of a blood pool contrast agent in MR venography of the lower extremities and pelvis: preliminary results in 12 patients. Magn Reson Med 2003; 50:993–1002.

32. Carpenter JP, Holland GA, Baum RA, Owen RS, Carpenter JT, Cope C. Magnetic resonance venography for the detection of deep venous thrombosis: comparison with contrast venography and duplex Doppler ultrasonography. J Vasc Surg 1993; 18:734–741.

33. Gallix BP, Achard-Lichere C, Dauzat M, Bruel JM, Lopez FM. Flow-independent magnetic resonance venography of the calf. J Magn Reson Imaging 2003; 17:421–426.

34. Evans AJ, Sostman HD, Knelson MH, et al. Detection of deep venous thrombosis: prospective comparison of MR imaging with contrast venography. AJR Am J Roentgenol 1993; 161:131–139.

35. Sica GT, Pugach ME, Koniaris LS, et al. Isolated calf vein thrombosis: comparison of MR venography and conventional venography after initial sonography in symptomatic patients. Acad Radiol 2001; 8:856–863.

36. Froehlich JB, Prince MR, Greenfield LJ, Downing LJ, Shah NL, Wakefield TW. "Bull's-eye" sign on gadolinium-enhanced magnetic resonance venography determines thrombus presence and age: a preliminary study. J Vasc Surg 1997; 26:809–816.

37. Moody AR, Pollock JG, O'Connor AR, Bagnall M. Lower-limb deep venous thrombosis: direct MR imaging of the thrombus. Radiology 1998; 209:349–355.

38. Wolpert LM, Rahmani O, Stein B, Gallagher JJ, Drezner AD. Magnetic resonance venography in the diagnosis and management of May-Thurner syndrome. Vasc Endovascular Surg 2002; 36:51–57.

9

Invasive Tests—Radiological and Pressure Measurements

Peter Neglén and Seshadri Raju
River Oaks Hospital and University of Mississippi Medical Center, Jackson, Mississippi, U.S.A.

INTRODUCTION

Chronic venous disease is a complex disorder affecting the macro- as well as the micro-circulation. Venous function is dependant on many factors, not only reflux and obstruction, but also calf muscle pump function (ankle/knee joint status and muscle mass), venous volume, vein wall compliance and geometry. It is undoubtedly difficult to separate the contribution of these different factors to the condition of the patient by testing. It is important that the utilized test is identified as whether it measures anatomic or functional aspects of venous disorders. Invasive tests to assess venous function and morphology have been largely replaced by noninvasive tests, at least for the initial evaluation. Despite the importance of assessing sensitivity, specificity and accuracy of individual tests, these calculations are hindered by the lack of acceptable "gold standards." For decades tests such as invasive ambulatory foot venous pressure and descending venography were considered the ultimate reference tests, but presently their role as "gold standards" is in doubt. Nevertheless, invasive tests are often necessary to identify anatomic sites of disease for final invasive treatment and can, in some situations, not be replaced by noninvasive evaluation.

AMBULATORY VENOUS PRESSURE—A GLOBAL HEMODYNAMIC TEST

The only way to ascertain venous pressure is to measure it directly by cannulation or catheterization. Direct pressure measurements cannot be replaced by approximation by leg volume changes (1–4). Venous pressures may differ greatly with identical volume changes owing to variability of vein wall compliance. The most frequently used venous pressure is obtained by cannulation of a vein of the dorsum of the foot. The initial observation was made by Pollack and Woods in the 1940s (5), who observed that the foot venous pressure decreased on walking. This led to the development of the standardized ambulatory venous pressure (AVP) measurements, which many still consider the "gold standard" for testing the global

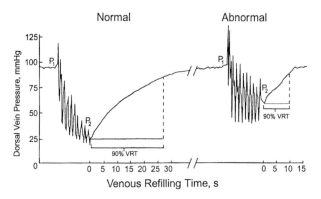

Figure 1 Foot vein pressure curve obtained in a normal limb and a limb with venous reflux. The pressure was recorded at rest and during 10-minute tiptoe movements until it returned to base line level. The percent drop of pressure ($P_1 - P_2/P_1 \times 100$, %) is markedly less in the abnormal limb and the venous refilling time (VRT, s) is shorter.

impact of venous insufficiency. The pressure is measured at rest and during and after exercise, resulting in a typical pressure curve (Fig. 1). Two parameters can be calculated: the percent decrease of pressure and the venous refilling time. Generally speaking, the smaller drop of pressure and the shorter refilling time, the worse is the venous insufficiency.

It is well known that the ulcer incidence and clinical severity of CVD increases with higher AVP (6,7). However, 15–19% of limbs will develop ulcer despite normal AVP, and, on the other hand, not all with severe venous hypertension will develop ulcer. Deep venous pressures have been measured at different levels in the leg by placing pressure-tipped catheters in the popliteal, posterior tibial and great saphenous veins simultaneously with dorsal foot vein pressure (8,9). Despite normal drop of foot venous pressure on exercise, the deep and saphenous venous pressures may increase. The post-exercise pressure and recovery times are widely different in the three veins. It appears that these veins behave hydraulically as separate compartments and changes within these compartments are not necessarily reflected in the dorsal vein pressure. Clinically significant isolated obstruction of the iliac vein is also poorly reflected by the AVP, which usually is found to be normal (10,11).

Ambulatory venous pressure is an exercise test requiring the cooperation of the patient. Stiff joints, small muscle mass, and poor coordination may also influence the result, although not being directly related to the venous function per se. This may contribute to the clinical condition of the patients, but then fails to shed any light on the venous valve function or presence of obstruction (12).

These observations indicate that a normal AVP does not necessarily exclude significant venous disease. On the other hand, high AVP in limbs which are asymptomatic indicate that all aspects of the pathophysiology, especially the impact of microcirculatory changes, are not fully understood.

ARM-FOOT VENOUS PRESSURE DIFFERENTIAL AND REACTIVE HYPEREMIA FOOT VEIN PRESSURE ELEVATION—A HEMODYNAMIC TEST FOR GLOBAL OUTFLOW OBSTRUCTION

Reliable hemodynamic tests for global measurement of venous outflow obstruction are not available. The degree of hemodynamic obstruction depends on multiple factors, e.g., the number, location, degree of narrowing, and length of the lesions, development of collaterals, and the volume flow varying at rest and during exercise. The concept of a significant vessel obstruction being a stenosis of more than 70–80% is derived from observations on the arterial system. These conclusions are probably not applicable in the venous system since there are many fundamental differences. The venous circulation is a low pressure, low velocity, large volume and low resistance vascular system as compared to the high pressure, high velocity, small volume and high resistance arterial system (13). In fact, it is not know at what degree a venous stenosis becomes "critical." Thus, there is no "gold standard" test. Ultrasound investigation may show localized segmental obstruction, but cannot assess the hemodynamic importance. Outflow fraction determinations by plethysmographic methods may indicate hemodynamic obstruction but cannot reveal the level or anatomic site of the blockage. Although the finding of low outflow fraction may suggest obstruction to the venous outflow, significant blockage may exist in the presence of normal result (14–16). In short, these noninvasive tests have insufficient accuracy and play, therefore, only a limited role in the management of obstructive disease.

Raju has described a method using venous pressure measurements to assess degree of hemodynamically significant obstruction (17,18). With the patient in the supine position, venous pressure in the dorsum of the foot and hand are simultaneously measured through venous transducers and recorded. In normal patients, the foot pressure is not more than 4 mmHg above the arm pressure. In addition, the foot pressure is continuously recorded. The arterial flow is occluded by inflating a thigh cuff to 200–300 mmHg, maintaining the pressure for three minutes, and then instantly deflate the cuff. Unfortunately, some patient experience pain and discomfort owing to the duration of the high cuff pressure. The ischemia induced reactive hyperemia leads to increased venous pressure. The increase from base level should not exceed 6 mmHg in normal limbs. Using these pressure measurements limbs with obstruction have been classified in four grades (Table 1). Simultaneous measurement of dorsal vein pressure and calf volume allows calculation of outflow resistance, which has been shown to be related to the grading of obstruction to Raju (7,16).

The pressure test described by Raju appears to be the most reliable investigation currently available for detection and grading of global obstruction (16). However, this test, like the others, has proved to be inaccurate in clinically significant outflow obstruction and is flawed by poor sensitivity (11). The hyperemia flow induced by the tourniquet ischemia may not be reproducible in repeat tests or the volume flow high enough to detect a significant stenosis in all conditions. An additional disadvantage is the inability to define the location of the most significant obstruction in multi-level disease. No correlation has been found between this method and the number and sites of obstruction or development

Table 1 Grading of Obstruction in Patients with Chronic Venous Disorder According to Raju

		Arm/foot venous pressure differential (normal ≤4 mmHg)	Reactive hyperemia foot venous pressure elevation (normal ≤6 mmHg)
Grade 1	Normal or fully compensated	≤4 mmHg	≤6 mmHg
Grade 2	Partially compensated	≤4 mmHg	>6 mmHg
Grade 3	Partially decompensated	>4 mmHg	>6 mmHg
Grade 4	Fully decompensated	>4 mmHg	≤6 mmHg

Source: From Ref. 17.

of collaterals detected by venography (10). Positive pressure tests, like positive non-invasive tests, for obstruction may support further investigation and intervention, but a negative test does not exclude clinically significant venous outflow obstruction.

FEMORAL VENOUS PRESSURE—A TEST FOR FOCAL OUTFLOW OBSTRUCTION

After cannulation, femoral resting pressure may be measured in the femoral vein either in supine position or after tilting the table 30–60 degrees feet down. For this purpose transducer-tip catheters can be used with high accuracy. The catheter may also be forwarded to the IVC and a resting pressure gradient can be obtained. This pull-through pressure differential over a lesion or a pressure increase peripherally to the lesion with augmentation of venous inflow may be indicative of a significant stenosis (19,20).

In the venous system, the venous pressure is a function of not only resistance to the flow (degree of obstruction and collateral formation), but also depends to a high degree on the flow velocity and magnitude of volume flow. It is unknown to what degree the resting venous flow has to be increased to detect a functionally significant stenosis, and the method to reproduce this flow rate consistently. The augmentation of flow may be induced by twenty forceful calf muscle contractions by an awake patient, (19,20) by injection of papaverine (30–60 mg) into the ipsilateral femoral artery, (21) or by ischemia induced by a tourniquet (300 mmHg pressure for 3 min) (17).

Pressure gradients recorded in the venous system is much lower than in the arterial system and only small pressure differentials may indicate significant obstruction. Studies suggest that a pre-stenotic pressure rise in supine position greater than 2–4 mmHg on provocation, a slow return to base level (>30 s), or a gradient compared to the contralateral femoral pressure exceeding 2–5 mmHg indicate a hemodynamically significant obstruction (19,20,22). It has been suggested that a pressure differential on exercise should be at least 5 mmHg to warrant intervention. Good clinical result has been, however, obtained treating morphologic obstruction with normal pressure findings (23). In lieu of any "gold standard" test to compare with, these pressure levels are set arbitrarily. High pressure gradients support the need for intervention. However, similar to the global invasive and noninvasive tests for obstruction, a positive hemodynamic test may indicate hemodynamic significance, but a normal test does not necessarily exclude it. Thus, it is presently impossible to detect potentially important focal obstructions by femoral pressure measurements.

POPLITEAL VENOUS PRESSURE—A TEST FOR FOCAL OBSTRUCTION

Popliteal vein pressure has been measured in patients with suspicion of popliteal vein entrapment (24). A 2F catheter with a tip-mounted pressure transducer can be inserted into the posterior tibial vein posterior to the medial malleolus, either percutaneously or through a small cutdown. The tip is advanced to the popliteal vein at the level of the joint line with fluoroscopic control. The patient is then asked to stand and perform 10 toe stands, while the popliteal pressure is recorded continuously. A popliteal pressure increase to any degree or a decrease of less than 15% was considered to be supportive of significant outflow obstruction. Patients operated with release of the venous entrapment, normalized the popliteal pressures postoperatively. This test could probably be performed to identify a significant popliteal venous obstruction of other etiology.

ASCENDING VENOGRAPHY

Ascending venography is an investigation in which contrast medium is injected into a foot vein and followed proximally. Misinterpretation due to poor technique is common. A tourniquet above the ankle should always be used to force the contrast dye deep into the system and avoid simultaneous visualization of the deep and superficial veins, which can be very confusing. The purpose of this investigation is to test patency of the deep veins, i.e., identify and localize the extent of obstruction, if present. Images of the profunda vein and all calf veins are most often not obtained. It is often difficult to achieve adequate filling of the iliac vein by the contrast medium. Then the distal contrast medium administration has to be complemented by a transfemoral injection. Duplex Doppler has replaced ascending venogram to diagnose acute deep venous thrombosis, and has in fact largely replaced venogram as the "gold standard" for this condition. In cases of recurrent thrombosis, when it may be difficult to assess by ultrasound scanning whether the clot is fresh or not, ascending venography may still play a role. In postthrombotic limbs, ascending venography may show total or partial obstruction with different degrees of collateralization. It will often identify any profunda transformation due to occlusion of the femoral vein (25). Ascending venography is entirely a morphological study and cannot show any hemodynamic impact of visualized lesions. It is mainly used today as a preoperative mapping tool.

TRANSFEMORAL DESCENDING VENOGRAPHY

Descending venography is performed by injecting a bolus of contrast medium into the common femoral vein. With the patient in a 60 degree tilt and performing a standardized Valsalva's maneuver simultaneously with the injection, reflux may be depicted as contrast flowing retrogradely into the lower extremity (26,27). Depending of the degree of the axial deep reflux, severity can be classified according to Kistner (28,29). Clinically most relevant is axial reflux reaching to below the knee (Class 3) and especially when it is cascading into the calf veins (Class 4). Noninvasive erect duplex Doppler ultrasound scanning has now replaced descending venography in diagnosis of axial deep reflux (30). Although developed for descending venography, the Kistner classification can still be applied. Descending venography is presently mainly utilized preoperatively in surgical candidates to delineate the morphology, i.e., the presence or absence of valve stations and, sometimes, the condition of valve leaflets.

TRANSFEMORAL ASCENDING (ANTEGRADE) VENOGRAPHY

Ascending or antegrade transfemoral venography is the time-honored way to describe iliofemoral venous outflow obstruction. Injection of contrast medium into the common femoral vein delineate the distribution and nature of the morphologic changes, including occlusion, stenosis and presence of collateral circulation, but like ascending venography it does not provide any information whether a significant hemodynamic obstruction is present or not. Optimally, all antegrade transfemoral venograms should be performed using arterial angiographic techniques with subtraction imaging, multiple oblique views and pressure injectors. With this technique the quality of the images will improve and the contrast medium load will be minimal.

Single-plane transfemoral venogram, the standard investigation tool in the United States, may show definite obstruction and development of collaterals. Findings on the anterio–posterior (AP) view are, however, often subtle and only suggestive of an underlying obstruction. Outside compression of the vessel in the frontal plane may on an AP-view only show widening of the iliac vein (pancaking) or "thinning" of the contrast medium resulting in a translucence of the area, while compression in the sagittal plane is readily seen in this projection. Sometimes only a partial intraluminal defect (septum), or a minimal filling of transpelvic collaterals are present. Increased accuracy may be achieved with multiple angled projections, which may reveal surprisingly tight stenosis on oblique projections, although the AP view is quite normal (Fig. 2) (31).

Although the formation of collaterals is classically regarded as a compensatory mechanism to bypass and thus alleviate an obstruction, the mechanism and inducement of collateral formation are unknown. It is doubtful that blood flow through this meandering large vessel could replace that through the straighter main vein. In fact, the collaterals are often refluxive and may carry the blood in the reverse direction (32). Collateral circulation shown prior to stenting is often not visualized following stenting of a venous stenosis (Fig. 3). The flow through the stent is obviously favored. Limbs with collateral formation have been shown to have a significantly tighter stenosis than limbs with no collaterals, as measured by IVUS (33). The rate of limbs with femoral pressure increase on intra-arterial injection of papaverine was three times more common in patients with collaterals. These observations support the concept of pelvic collateralization to be an

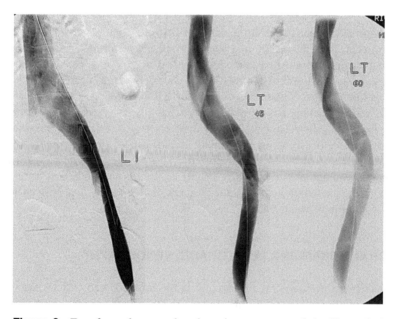

Figure 2 Transfemoral antegrade subtraction venogram of the iliac vein in multiple oblique projections (45 and 60 degrees). The right common iliac artery makes a distinct impression on the vein in the oblique projections ("cork screw" appearance), while only a slight translucency with widening is seen on the AP-view.

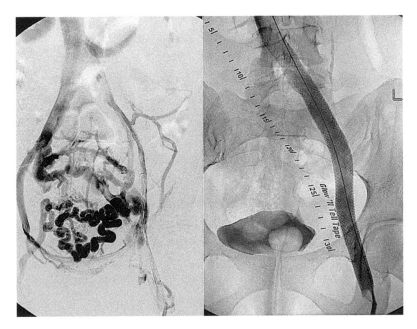

Figure 3 Left iliofemoral vein obstruction with massive collaterals before and after stent placement. Note that collaterals are not visualized after disobliteration.

indicator of obstruction and that collaterals poorly compensate for the blockage in symptomatic patients.

Transfemoral antegrade venography can not be replaced by ultrasound scanning of the iliac vein since it lacks the adequate accuracy to detect acute deep venous thrombosis, partial or complete chronic obstruction, and separate axial collaterals from main stem veins. It can be used to evaluate patency of inserted stents, but not to the degree of in-stent restenosis. Other non invasive imaging studies like magnetic resonance venography (MRV) are under evaluation and may replace transfemoral venogram for screening in the future.

INTRAVASCULAR ULTRASOUND

Intravascular ultrasound (IVUS) is superior to the single- and multi-plane venography in detection of the extent and type of morphologic lesion of the vein (33–37). Transpelvic collaterals will escape detection as IVUS can detect only axial collaterals running close to the original vessel. Several studies have shown, however, that IVUS better shows intraluminal details, e.g., trabeculations and webs, which may be hidden in the contrast medium (Fig. 4). In addition, venous wall thickness, neointimal hyperplasia and movement can be seen. An external compression with the resulting deformity of the venous lumen or postthrombotic remodeling can be directly visualized. Accurate calculations of cross-cut areas and diameters can then be made of the normal and compressed or diseased veins using the software built into the IVUS apparatus. This makes IVUS superior to venography for estimating the morphological degree of iliac vein stenosis (Fig. 5). It has been suggested that the flow through a compressed vein is inhibited as compared to a circular vessel, even if the transverse surface area is the same (38). On average, the transfemoral venogram

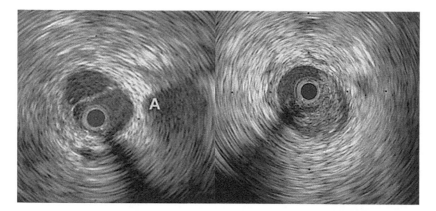

Figure 4 Intravascular ultrasound (IVUS) showing a septum not easily visualized by venogram (*left*) and partially thrombosed vein (*right*). The adjacent artery is marked with an A. The black circle within the vein is the IVUS catheter.

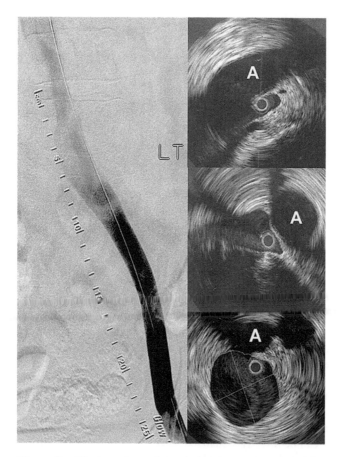

Figure 5 AP-view of transfemoral antegrade venogram, which appears normal with no obvious stenosis (*left*). IVUS of the same vein at different levels showing severe proximal common iliac vein (CIV) stenosis due to compression by transversing iliac artery, partial obstruction mid-CIV, and normal distal CIV (*right*). The adjacent artery is marked with an A. The black circle within the vein is the IVUS catheter.

significantly underestimated the degree of stenosis by 30%. The venogram was actually considered "normal" in one-fourth of limbs despite the fact that IVUS showed >50% obstruction (39). In a similar population of limbs, the stenosis was less than 50% in 42% of venograms but only in 10% of IVUS investigations (33). On the other hand, the venous stenosis was found to be greater than 70% in 32% of venograms, but twice as often with the IVUS. Using the IVUS result as the standard, the venogram had a poor sensitivity of 45% and negative predictive value of 49% in detecting an obstruction of greater than 70%.

Intravascular ultrasound is clearly superior to venography in providing adequate morphological information and is presently the best available method for diagnosing clinically significant chronic iliac vein obstruction. It is also an invaluable tool for accurate placement of iliofemoral stents ensuring stent cover of the entire diseased segment. Owing to the lack of hemodynamic tests and inability of duplex Doppler scanning to visualize accurately the iliac vein, it is insufficient to limit the workup of all patients with chronic venous disease to duplex ultrasound alone. In patients with significant signs and symptoms of CVD, transfemoral venography (preferably multi-plane) or IVUS should be utilized more often to identify patients with potentially important venous outflow obstruction.

Good clinical results have been obtained when stenosis of greater than 50%, as identified by IVUS, or occlusions have been stented. In selecting symptomatic patients for IVUS investigation, one or several of these parameters have been used: (1) single-plane venographic stenosis >30%; (2) presence of pelvic collaterals; and (3) positive invasive pressure test (35,39). Utilizing this policy, however, 10–15% of iliofemoral veins are found to be normal. An appropriate hemodynamic test needs to be developed.

CONCLUSION

There is rightly a general trend for avoidance of invasive studies owing to potential complications and discomfort for the patient. This concern should, however, not lead to complete abandonment of invasive studies, especially in the situation where they cannot be adequately replaced by a non invasive test. Although AVP is not necessary for daily clinical practice, obstruction testing may give valuable information in select patients. The importance and frequency of iliofemoral venous outflow obstruction and the lack of accurate non invasive hemodynamic tests for obstruction necessitate increasing use of invasive morphologic studies of the iliofemoral venous outflow tract. Ascending dorsal foot vein, transfemoral antegrade and descending venograms are still important for mapping of the pathologic morphology in preparation for open or endovascular surgery of the deep venous system.

KEY POINTS

- Invasive tests are often necessary to identify anatomic sites of disease for interventional treatment.
- Ascending venography is used to detect the anatomic extent of obstruction while descending venography is used to detect reflux. Both techniques are used for intervention in the deep veins.
- Ambulatory venous pressure assesses the global hemodynamics of the limbs but a normal pressure cannot exclude venous disease.

- Pressure measurements are used to detect obstruction and evaluate the significance of vein stenosis. They are also useful to assess the outcome of an intervention.
- Intravascular ultrasound is superior to venography in providing morphological information and a valuable tool for accurate placement of iliofemoral stents.

REFERENCES

1. Welkie JF, Comerota AJ, Katz ML, Aldridge SC, Kerr RP, White JV. Hemodynamic deterioration in chronic venous disease. J Vasc Surg 1992; 16:733–740.
2. Payne SP, Thrush AJ, London NJ, Bell PR, Barrie WW. Venous assessment using air plethysmography: a comparison with clinical examination, ambulatory venous pressure measurement and duplex scanning. Br J Surg 1993; 80:967–970.
3. Neglén P, Raju S. A rational approach to detection of significant reflux with duplex Doppler scanning and air plethysmography. J Vasc Surg 1993; 17:590–595.
4. Gillespie DL. Letter to the editor. J Vasc Surg 1993; 18:140.
5. Pollack AA, Wood EH. Venous pressure in teh saphenous vein in ankle in man during exercise and changes in posture. J Appl Physiol 1949; 1:649–653.
6. Raju S, Fredericks R. Hemodynamic basis of stasis ulceration—a hypothesis. J Vasc Surg 1991; 13:491–495.
7. Nicolaides AN. Outflow obstruction. Investigations of Patients with Deep Vein Thrombosis and Chronic Venous Insufficiency. Los Angeles, C.A.: Med-Orion Publishing Co, 1991 pp. 56–62.
8. Neglén P, Raju S. Differences in pressures of the popliteal, long saphenous, and dorsal foot veins. J Vasc Surg 2000; 32:894–901.
9. Neglén P, Raju S. Ambulatory venous pressure revisited. J Vasc Surg 2000; 31:1206–1213.
10. Raju S, Fredericks R. Venous obstruction: an analysis of one hundred thirty-seven cases with hemodynamic, venographic, and clinical correlations. J Vasc Surg 1991; 14:305–313.
11. Neglén P, Thrasher TL, Raju S. Venous outflow obstruction: An underestimated contributor to chronic venous disease. J Vasc Surg 2003; 38:879–885.
12. Back TL, Padberg FT, Jr., Araki CT, Thompson PN, Hobson RW, II. Limited range of motion is a significant factor in venous ulceration. J Vasc Surg 1995; 22:519–523.
13. Strandness DE, Jr., Sumner DS. The effect of geometry on arterial blood flow. Hemodynamics for Surgeons. New York: Grune&Stratton, 1975: 96–119.
14. Hurst DR, Forauer AR, Bloom JR, Greenfield LJ, Wakefield TW, Williams DM. Diagnosis and endovascular treatment of iliocaval compression syndrome. J Vasc Surg 2001; 34:106–113.
15. Labropoulos N, Volteas N, Leon M, et al. The role of venous outflow obstruction in patients with chronic venous dysfunction. Arch Surg 1997; 132:46–51.
16. Neglén P, Raju S. Detection of outflow obstruction in chronic venous insufficiency. J Vasc Surg 1993; 17:583–589.
17. Raju S. A pressure-based technique for the detection of acute and chronic venous obstruction. Phlebology 1988; 3:207–216.
18. Raju S. New approaches to the diagnosis and treatment of venous obstruction. J Vasc Surg 1986; 4:42–54.
19. Albrechtsson U, Einarsson E, Eklof B. Femoral vein pressure measurements for evaluation of venous function in patients with postthrombotic iliac veins. Cardiovasc Intervent Radiol 1981; 4:43–50.
20. Negus D, Cockett FB. Femoral vein pressures in post-phlebitic iliac vein obstruction. Br J Surg 1967; 54:522–525.
21. Illig KA, Ouriel K, DeWeese JA, Riggs P, Green RM. Increasing the sensitivity of the diagnosis of chronic venous obstruction. J Vasc Surg 1996; 24:176–178.

22. Rigas A, Vomvoyannis A, Giannoulis K, Antipas S, Tsardakas E. Measurement of the femoral vein pressure in edema of the lower extremities. Report of 50 cases. J Cardiovasc Surg (Torino) 1971; 12:411–416.

23. Raju S, Owen S, Jr., Neglén P. The clinical impact of iliac venous stents in the management of chronic venous insufficiency. J Vasc Surg 2002; 35:8–15.

24. Raju S, Neglén P. Popliteal vein entrapment: a benign venographic feature or a pathologic entity? J Vasc Surg 2000; 31:631–641.

25. Raju S, Fountain T, Neglén P, Devidas M. Axial transformation of the profunda femoris vein. J Vasc Surg 1998; 27:651–659.

26. Kistner RL, Ferris EB, Randhawa G, Kamida CA. Method of performing descending venography. J Vasc Surg 1986; 4:464–468.

27. Morano JU, Raju S. Chronic venous insufficiency: assessment with descending venography. Radiology 1990; 174:441–444.

28. Herman RJ, Neiman HL, Yao JS, Egan TJ, Bergan JJ, Malave SR. Descending venography: a method of evaluating lower extremity venous valvular function. Radiology 1980; 137:63–69.

29. Kistner RL. Transvenous repair of the incompetent femoral vein valve. In: Bergan JJ, Yao JS, eds. Venous Problems. London: Year Book Medical Publishers, 1978:493–509.

30. Neglén P, Raju S. A comparison between descending phlebography and duplex Doppler investigation in the evaluation of reflux in chronic venous insufficiency: a challenge to phlebography as the "gold standard." J Vasc Surg 1992; 16:687–693.

31. Juhan C, Hartung O, Alimi Y, Barthelemy P, Valerio N, Portier F. Treatment of nonmalignant obstructive iliocaval lesions by stent placement: mid-term results. Ann Vasc Surg 2001; 15:227–232.

32. Thomas ML, Fletcher EW, Cockett FB, Negus D. Venous collaterals in external and common iliac vein obstruction. Clin Radiol 1967; 18:403–411.

33. Neglén P, Raju S. Intravascular ultrasound scan evaluation of the obstructed vein. J Vasc Surg 2002; 35:694–700.

34. Forauer AR, Gemmete JJ, Dasika NL, Cho KJ, Williams DM. Intravascular ultrasound in the diagnosis and treatment of iliac vein compression (May-Thurner) syndrome. J Vasc Interv Radiol 2002; 13:523–527.

35. Neglén P, Raju S. Balloon dilation and stenting of chronic iliac vein obstruction: technical aspects and early clinical outcome. J Endovasc Ther 2000; 7:79–91.

36. Ahmed HK, Hagspiel KD. Intravascular ultrasonographic findings in May-Thurner syndrome (iliac vein compression syndrome). J Ultrasound Med 2001; 20:251–256.

37. Satokawa H, Hoshino S, Iwaya F, Igari T, Midorikawa H, Ogawa T. Intravascular Imaging Methods for Venous Disorders. Int J Angiol 2000; 9:117–121.

38. Brice IG, Dowsett DJ, Lowe RD. The effect of constriction on carotid blood-flow and pressure gradient. Lancet 1964; 10 04 85.

39. Neglén P, Berry MA, Raju S. Endovascular surgery in the treatment of chronic primary and post-thrombotic iliac vein obstruction. Eur J Vasc Endovasc Surg 2000; 20:560–571.

10

Diagnosis of Deep Vein Thrombosis

Luis Leon
Division of Vascular Surgery, Loyola University Medical Center, Maywood, Illinois, U.S.A.

Nicos Labropoulos
Vascular Laboratory, Division of Vascular Surgery, New Jersey Medical School, Newark, New Jersey, U.S.A.

INTRODUCTION AND MAGNITUDE OF THE PROBLEM

Deep vein thrombosis (DVT) is a serious condition that frequently occurs in the inpatient setting but may also affect otherwise healthy subjects. It is rare in the young and it is more often found in the elderly (1). Inpatients >64 years old in sub-acute care facilities have a high prevalence of DVT despite the use of prophylaxis (2).

DVT has a silent nature. About a third of patients who present with its signs and symptoms will have the disease. This, combined with the low autopsy rate in most countries, makes its real occurrence unknown. Estimated yearly figures from a community-based study in the United States revealed 170,000 new cases and 99,000 admissions for recurrent cases of symptomatic DVT and pulmonary embolism (PE), its most feared complication, in patients treated in short-stay hospitals (3).

PATHOPHYSIOLOGY

Endothelial damage, hypercoagulability, and stasis have been recognized for over 150 years to be the three elements associated with venous thromboembolism (VTE), with often two of those three factors needed for its initiation. Therefore, its etiology is multifactorial with each component having different impacts on different patients.

The vein wall has been extensively analyzed and it is no longer viewed as a mere passive conduit of blood. The endothelium and the subendothelium are key structures in the development of VTE. The endothelium is a negatively charged physical barrier that protects the blood from the thrombogenic subendothelium, produces pro- and anti-coagulant substances, inhibits thrombosis and platelet aggregation and promotes fibrinolysis. After trauma, leukocyte adhesion and transmigration disrupt the endothelium and expose the subendothelium, providing a surface for the beginning of coagulation (4,5). Circulating platelets are activated and platelet aggregation starts as the first step in the formation of a hemostatic plug.

Antithrombin III, protein C and protein S deficiencies and mutations of factor V and prothrombin genes have been recently associated with the development of venous

113

thrombosis (6). The activated protein C resistance phenotype associated with an abnormal factor V Leiden and the G20210A prothrombin gene mutations are the most common findings in patients with VTE (7). The use of oral contraceptives, pregnancy and malignancies also increase the risk for VTE (6). A pooled analysis of eight case-control studies revealed an odds ratio for VTE of 4.9 (95% CI=4.1–5.9) for factor V Leiden and 3.8 (3.0–4.9) for the factor II G20210A mutation. In double heterozygotes it increased to 20 (11.1–36.1). The overall odds ratio for VTE associated with the use of oral contraceptives was 2.29 (1.72–3.04). If oral contraceptives users were associated with a factor V Leiden carrier, the odds ratio was 10.25 (5.69–18.45) and 7.14 (3.39–15.04) for a factor II mutation carrier (8).

Thrombosis often begins in areas of blood flow stasis, usually in a vein valve or in intramuscular veins, from local factors, such as venous mechanical compression and prolonged immobility and from systemic factors such as blood sluggishness (9). Stasis determines the site of thrombosis and probably represents the most important factor in postoperative and posttrauma patients with limited activity. Together with endothelial damage, they act as cofactors in the development of VTE inducing platelet activation and blood clotting. Studies have shown that P-selectins have a role in vein wall cytokine elevation, edema and thrombosis days after stasis. Selectins are the mediators of leukocyte interaction with the endothelium and platelets. A CD 15-selectin is involved in the transfer of tissue factor from leukocytes to platelets for them to be able to initiate and propagate thrombosis. Its immunoneutralization may potentially have a clinical role in VTE (10). Large varicose veins with sluggish flow are often a place for spontaneous thrombosis. In immobilized patients, there is prolonged stasis at the calf level. Not surprisingly, it has been suggested that DVT often begins in these veins and then propagates proximally (11,12).

NATURAL HISTORY OF VENOUS THROMBOSIS

Superficial

Most thrombotic episodes of the great saphenous vein (GSV) start in the calf and are often self-limiting. When limited to the calf they are a rare cause of symptoms or of symptomatic PE. They represent a more serious condition if they extend above the knee, with a 33% prevalence of documented PE (95% confidence interval [CI] = 14.6–57) (13).

Most of the studies that deal with concomitant superficial thrombophlebitis (STP) and DVT and/or PE in the literature are of a retrospective nature and include a small number of subjects. DVT in association with saphenous thrombosis ranges from 6% to 53%. Thrombus can propagate in a contiguous and in a non contiguous manner. From 53 patients with clinical manifestations of STP and diagnosed with DVT, evidence of direct contiguous propagation was found in 75.5%, and the rest was non contiguous calf involvement at the posterior tibial and soleal levels (14). Contiguous extension has been proposed through three different routes (15). Most occur from the GSV into the femoral vein, and this route appears to be the most significant (14,15). Less common, the thrombus extends from the small saphenous vein (SSV) into the popliteal vein through the saphenopopliteal junction. Extension through perforators can also occur, either directly to involve the tibial veins or indirectly through the soleal veins (14). Thrombosis can, in theory, also extend from the deep veins to the superficial ones, but this has not been evaluated (Fig. 1). Patients with STP should have their deep veins evaluated even if we accept the lowest DVT prevalence of 5.6% reported (16).

Fifty-six patients with clinical evidence of STP underwent ascending venography (AV), and evidence of DVT was found in nine. The prevalence of DVT in patients with varicose veins was 44% in contrast with 2.6% in patients without them (p < 0.01). The site of STP did not influence the presence or absence of DVT. Another important finding was that no patients with varicose veins developed a malignancy on follow-up whereas two patients without varicosities did. Both patients had venographic evidence of DVT on initial studies (11).

Deep

Recurrent events after a first episode of DVT are not uncommon and its risk persists for many years. Three hundred fifty-five patients were followed after a first DVT and a cumulative incidence of recurrent VTE of 17.5% after two years, 24.6% after five and 30.3% after eight years was found (17). This risk was significantly higher in patients with cancer or hypercoagulable states compared to that associated with surgery or trauma (18).

After DVT, up to 79% of limbs may develop edema, pain, lipodermatosclerosis or skin ulcers, condition known as the post-thrombotic syndrome (PTS), mostly due to vein reflux. Persistent venous obstruction may also play a role but is seen less often. PTS was found in 22%, 28% and 29% after two, five and eight years, respectively (17,19). Ipsilateral recurrent DVT was strongly associated with its development (hazard ratio = 6.4). Furthermore, the eight-year survival of this cohort was 70.2% indicating a substantial mortality associated with this disease (17,19).

Untreated above-the-knee DVT has a 50% risk for PE and a 10% risk for fatal PE (20,21). However, the optimum length of anticoagulation remains unknown. Traditionally, patients are anticoagulated for three to six months. With time, re-canalization or collateral development occurs and these translate into clinical improvement. Recanalization begins within the first week from the acute episode and the thrombus load is significantly reduced

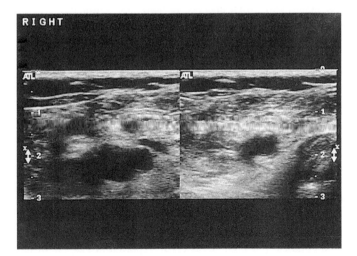

Figure 1 Normal popliteal and gastrocnemial veins. The popliteal vein is duplicated. All veins are fully compressed and free of thrombus as seen on the right screen. The popliteal artery is non-compressible under light compression and is the only vessel seen. The patient was a 60-year-old female with right knee pain for the past 15 years, complaining of difficulty getting up and down the stairs, as well as standing. She underwent an uneventful right total knee arthroplasty. Postoperatively, the patient complained of right calf pain.

mostly in the first three months. About 56% of patients have complete thrombus resolution as shown by Duplex ultrasound (DUS) (22). Thrombosis evolution after an acute event appears to be a dynamic process with spontaneous lysis of the original thrombus and further thrombosis occurring as competing processes (18). Thrombus remodeling in the acute phase occurs in 44%. This includes, ascending, descending or bidirectional propagation and lysis (23). DUS analysis of the affected veins can aid to individualize management. Residual venous thrombosis is associated with a 2.4 hazard ratio (95% CI = 1.3–4.4; p = 0.004) to develop recurrent DVT and these patients may need longer anticoagulation (24).

Children

Acute DVT in children was found to be rare after studying 1997 patients < 18 years old hospitalized for > 72 hours who had ≥ two risk factors for the development of DVT (history of DVT or PE, recent surgery, immobilization, trauma, acute neurologic deficits, cancer, sepsis, > 150% ideal body weight, hypercoagulable states and the presence of a femoral venous catheter) and had at least one screening duplex scan. Nineteen females and forty males were enrolled. Over a nine-month follow up one patient developed DVT. DVT prophylaxis and screening was deemed unnecessary in children with ≤ two risk factors for its development (25).

DIAGNOSIS

Ascending Venography

Ascending Venography is the accepted gold standard for the diagnosis of DVT. It is routinely performed with venous contrast injection in the dorsum of the foot using a 21- or 22-gauge butterfly needle. Pedal, calf, thigh and pelvic veins are outlined. To enhance detailed vision of the venous anatomy a direct popliteal or common femoral vein (CFV) puncture can be done with subsequent passage of a catheter for selective injection of contrast (Fig. 2).

An intraluminal filling defect is a definitive finding for acute DVT (26). Well-developed collaterals, linear webs and synechiae within the veins also imply vein occlusion but of an older age. Acute DVT can be overimposed showing as a more rounded and larger filling defect. Non filling veins or abrupt termination of the contrast column are considered by some to be an indirect sign of DVT. Others have debated that finding. Bjorgell et al. (27) prospectively studied the occurrence of DVT in 100 consecutive patients with isolated, non filling deep veins as seen on AV. Using DUS, they found that about one-third of patients had DVT, a third of them had concomitant incidental findings that explained the non filling and a third had no identifiable pathology. They can be due to extrinsic or intrinsic pressure changes with abnormal flow patterns that may lead to interpretation errors (26).

Reaction to iodinated contrast, postprocedural DVT (reported in 1.3–7% of cases) (28,29) and skin necrosis from extravasation are among its most important complications (26). It also has limitations with regard to costs, patient's discomfort and inability to show other conditions that may explain the patient symptomatology. Its use is currently restricted for equivocal cases after noninvasive testing, for catheter-directed thrombolysis is considered, when thrombectomy is planned, or if the information is essential to consider an intervention (26).

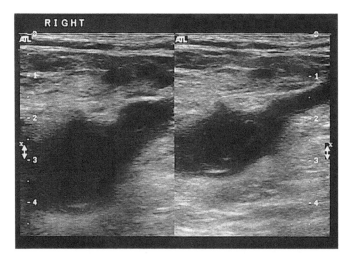

Figure 2   Acute thrombosis of the common femoral vein and the saphenofemoral junction. Both veins are distended, partially compressible and containing thrombus. The thrombus is echolucent (dark), which indicates that it is fresh. The patient is a 79-year-old male with history of congestive heart failure and mitral valve disease. He underwent cardiac catheterization five days prior to admission through a right common femoral artery approach. He stated that the right groin was slightly swollen after catheterization that worsened progressively. Doppler ultrasound of the right lower extremity demonstrated a pseudoaneurysm of the right common femoral artery and DVT of the right common femoral and iliac veins. *Abbreviation*: DVT, deep vein thrombosis.

Duplex Ultrasound Examination

DUS has clear advantages over AV with respect to its noninvasive nature, portability, lower cost, patient comfort, ability to image all the individual veins and tributaries, to differentiate acute from chronic thrombi and it can be repeated as many times as needed. Furthermore, it can detect other pathologies that may explain the patients' symptoms and potentially alter their management. Baker's cysts, enlarged hematomas, lymph nodes, musculoskeletal injuries, vascular anomalies, aneurysms and tumors are often encountered. It became the method of choice for the diagnosis of DVT (30).

The excellent sensitivity and specificity of DUS for symptomatic proximal DVT is well recognized. The results of several prospective studies including at least 40 patients in their analysis are summarized in Table 1 (31–36). However, screening for asymptomatic DVT in high-risk patients and in patients with isolated calf vein DVT is considered unwarranted by some authors (37,38) due to a sensitivity of 62% (95% CI = 54%–70%), a specificity of 97% (CI = 96%–98%), and a positive predictive value (PPV) of 66% (CI = 58%–74%) for detecting proximal thrombi. This does not reflect our experience. Such results are due to inadequate experience and training in identifying non-occlusive thrombi and those located in the calf veins. Furthermore, improved results have been possible, mainly due to intensive training and to modern and better equipment. These results were independent of thrombus size and were superior to AV in its identification (23,39,40).

DUS combines a Doppler mode that yields functional information about spontaneous and phasic vein flow and about the function of the vein valves, and a B-mode, that offers real-time anatomic information of the vein wall and lumen and can visualize intraluminal thrombus.

Table 1 Duplex Ultrasonography and Deep Vein Thrombosis

Study	Subjects	Tests	Extension	Results	Design
Baxter, 1990 (31)	40 patients with suspected lower extremity DVT	DUS and AV	Femoropopliteal and calf levels	Se = 93%, Sp = 100%	Prospective, double blind
van Ramshorst, 1991 (32)	117 patients (126 limbs) with suspected DVT or PE	DUS and AV	Femoropopliteal level	Se = 90.6%, Sp = 94.6%; DUS was more accurate in grading the anatomical extent of DVT; AV failed to visualize the PFV with sufficient accuracy in 88% vs. 8.5% with DUS	Prospective
Cogo, 1993 (33)	158 consecutive outpatients with symptomatic DVT	CUS, and AV	Femoropopliteal and calf levels	CUS Se = 100% For all thrombi (including isolated calf DVT), CUS Se = 95%. CUS was normal in all patients with normal AV (Sp = 100%; 95% CI = 95–100%)	Prospective
Lewis, 1994 (34)	101 patients (103 limbs)	DUS and AV	Femoropopliteal level	Se = 95%, Sp = 99%, PPV = 95%, NPV = 99%, Ac = 98%	Prospective
Miller, 1996 (35)	216 patients (220 limbs) suspected of DVT	DUS and AV	Femoropopliteal and tibioperoneal levels	Above-knee Se = 98.7%, Sp = 100%; below-knee Se = 85.2%, Sp = 99.2%. Excluding technically inadequate studies, below-knee Se = 93.8%	Prospective, blinded
Theodorou, 2003 (36)	106 patients (115 limbs) with suspected lower extremity DVT	DUS and AV	Femoropopliteal and calf levels	Se = 92.8%, Sp = 98%, Ac = 96.8%	Prospective

Abbreviations: Ac, accuracy; AV, ascending venography; CI, confidence intervals; CUS, compression ultrasound; DUS, Duplex ultrasound; DVT, deep vein thrombosis; NPV, negative predictive value; PE, pulmonary embolism; PFV, profunda femoral vein; PPV, positive predictive value; Se, sensitivity; Sp, specificity.

Medium frequency linear array transducers of 4–7 MHz are routinely used; obese patients, the pelvic veins and inferior vena cava (IVC) are examined with low frequency phased or curve-linear array transducers 2–3.5 MHz. The exam begins with the patient supine and the examined limb externally rotated with the knee in mild flexion.

The CFV and the sapheno-femoral junction are identified and compressed until the adjacent artery lumen is reduced on a transverse view, every 3 cm intervals. The veins should be easily collapsed. When thrombus is present there is limited compression, which increases as the thrombus ages. Flow characterization is done next in the longitudinal view, followed by distal augmentation in color mode. The limb distal to the probe is squeezed and the examined vessels should fill with color wall to wall. The maneuver is repeated with the Doppler on and tracing augmentation is verified. The proximal (femoropopliteal veins) and calf veins (posterior tibial, peroneal, gastrocnemial and soleal veins) are examined in identical manner (Fig. 3). When imaging of the calf veins is not optimal in the supine position the examination is performed with the leg in the dependent position (Fig. 4). The anterior tibial veins are examined only in the presence of local trauma or symptoms because the prevalence of isolated thrombosis is <1% (40). It is important to address the entire popliteal fossa to rule out the presence of other conditions that might be causing the patients' symptoms. The GSV and the SSV are identified next and examined similarly. The iliac veins and IVC are only examined selectively, in cases where continuous CFV flow is seen with limited phasicity by Doppler, poor distal CFV augmentation, asymmetric CFV waveforms and bilateral limb symptoms with normal lower extremity DUS. Nonocclusive thrombosis of the iliac vein or the IVC can be missed as they may not have any hemodynamic effects in the CFV. The prevalence of non-occlusive thrombi in these veins is not known. Therefore these veins should be still examined if there is strong suspicion for thrombosis. In centers that do not have experience in examining these veins by DUS and when DUS is technically difficult, ascending, computed tomography (CT) or magnetic resonance (MR) venography should be performed.

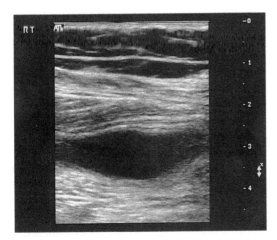

Figure 3   Acute thrombosis in the soleal vein in the midcalf. The vein is distended and contains echolucent material. It is located within the soleus muscle as it is seen by the surrounding muscle fibers. He was a 47-year-old male with a history of epilepsy status burned with hot water while having a seizure. His left leg was swollen and later was found to be painful.

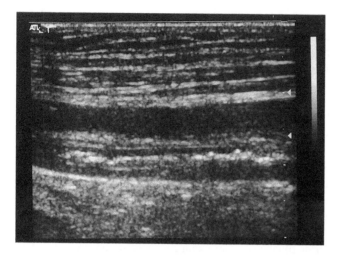

Figure 4 Chronic thrombosis in the femoral vein. He was a 76-year-old patient with swelling, varicose veins and skin changes. He had a femoropopliteal DVT 5 years ago. He recently developed pain in his calf, which was worst on standing. There was no new thrombosis but he had partially recanalized femoral and popliteal veins with reflux. The femoral vein is partially recanalized with echogenic material that has similar brightness with the surrounding tissues. *Abbreviation*: DVT, deep vein thrombosis.

DUS is negative if complete approximation of the near and far vein walls during compression or complete color filling of the lumen without defects are visualized. It is positive if a vein is partially compressible or non compressible, if echogenic material is seen within the vein, or if a filling defect on color imaging or absence of Doppler signal is identified.

Recurrent episodes are diagnosed similarly. It is relatively easy in the superficial system, given that local symptoms at the site of thrombosis indicate a new event. But the diagnosis of recurrent DVT is more difficult because the presence of old thrombus complicates the interpretation of ultrasound or AV (41). Establishing its diagnosis requires comparison of the location and size of this thrombus to those seen in a previous DUS. An increase of >2 mm in the compressed diameter of a previously thrombosed venous segment has been reported to be diagnostic of recurrent DVT (42,43). These results come from a single center that has performed this study in the femoral and popliteal veins only and need further confirmation from other centers prior to widespread acceptance.

DUS can estimate the age of the thrombus. Diagnostic criteria for acute and chronic DVT are summarized in Table 2.

Magnetic Resonance Venography

High-resolution images are produced after radio-frequency pulses are applied to a patient within complex and controlled magnetic fields. These pulses perturb protonic spins of the hydrogen nucleus (mainly in molecules of water), producing resonant radio-frequency signals, echoes of the original. Different shades of gray represent different tissues, with white being a high signal (large amount of hydrogen protons) and black indicating no signal (areas without hydrogen protons such as air or cortical bone) (44). The imaging plane is chosen by the examiner for each image sequence performed with the information always collected in three planes, which can be changed as needed. This implies that there is no secondary image manipulation that may alter imaging resolution as there is with

Table 2 Diagnostic Criteria to Differentiate Acute vs. Chronic Deep Vein Thrombosis

Criteria	Acute	Chronic
Vein size	Distended	Reduced; occasionally vein segments cannot be traced by DUS
Collateral vessels	Not usually seen	Often surrounding thrombosed segments
Thrombus echogenicity	Echolucent to intermediate echogenicity; the brightness is less than the adventitia and adjacent tissues	Bright echoes within the lumen similar to adjacent tissues
Lumen characteristics	Non- or partially compressible	Normal size or reduced; filling defects and reflux may be found
Wall characteristics	Thin and smooth	Normal, thickened or undistinguished from luminal fibrous tissue

Abbreviation: DUS, duplex ultrasound.

computed tomographic scanning. The IVC and pelvic veins can be imaged using this technology with high sensitivities and specificities. Table 3 depicts the results of several prospective studies that compared MR venography and AV or DUS (45–50).

When compared with AV it is less invasive, offers lower morbidity and may identify other soft tissue pathology (51). Its major advantage over CT and AV is the ability to depict flow and its dynamics without the use of contrast. However, it does not offer significant advantages over DUS. Due to its higher cost, cumbersome patient monitoring, inability to be used with metallic implants or claustrophobic patients, time requirements and unavailability, this technique should be used as a complimentary test to DUS. Moreover, interpretation of MR venographic studies can be difficult for those unfamiliar with the procedure and its several associated flow-related artifacts. Its use is currently limited to instances where contrast use is contraindicated, or when other diagnostic modalities cannot provide diagnostic information, especially in the abdominopelvic area (44).

Computed Tomography Venography

A computed tomography scanner is an X-ray device that yields cross sectional images in different shades of gray representing different tissues. The gray scale is similar to what we are used to when interpreting plain X rays, with black representing air and white representing bone. Tones in between represent the X-ray beam attenuation. Its images are always cross-sections, but they can be reformatted in different planes, although that manipulation results in less spatial resolution. Other reasons for low resolution include patient motion, differences in respiratory phases from one image to the next, and cardiovascular pulsation transmitted to neighboring structures. Newer scanner designs, such as the spiral CT, are faster and allow many pictures to be acquired during a single patient's breath. Motion artifact is thus reduced and contrast utilization is maximized (44).

The use of CT venography of the legs and abdominal veins is currently limited and usually performed in combination with CT angiography of the pulmonary arteries to allow a complete examination of VTE (52). Very few studies address the utility of CT venography as a sole diagnostic method for DVT. The results of those clinical trials are summarized in Table 4 (53–55). One of them correlated CT and AV findings in the

Table 3 Magnetic Resonance Imaging and Deep Vein Thrombosis

Study	Subjects	Tests	Extension	Results	Design
Erdman, 1990 (45)	36 patients with suspected upper or lower extremity DVT	MRV and AV	Acquisitions from the knee, midthigh, pubic symphysis	Se=90%; Sp=100%; Kappa agreement level=0.752 (p<0.0001)	Prospective
Carpenter, 1993 (46)	85 VA patients with suspected DVT	MRV and AV	IVC to popliteal veins	Se=100%; Sp=90%; PPV=100%; NPV=96%	Prospective
Evans, 1993 (47)	61 patients with suspected DVT	MRV and AV	Pelvis to calf	Pelvis Se=100% (95%CI=72–100%) Sp=95% (95%CI=85–99%) Thigh Se=100% (95%CI=83–100%) Sp=100% (95%CI=93–100%) Calf Se=87% (95%CI=60–98%) Sp=97% (95%CI=93–100%)	Prospective, blinded
Evans, 1996 (48)	75 patients with suspected DVT	MRV and DUS	Femoropopliteal	Se=100% (95%CI=87–100%) Sp=100% (95%CI=92–100%) Ac=83% (95%CI=72–90%)	Prospective
Fraser, 2002 (49)	101 patients with suspected DVT	MRV and AV	Iliofemoral, femoropopliteal, calf areas	Se=94–96%, Sp=90–92% overall; Se=83–92%, Sp=94–96% calf; Se=97%, Sp=100% femoro-popliteal; Se=100%, Sp=100% iliofemoral. Interobserver variability=0.89–0.98	Prospective, blinded
Fraser, 2003 (50)	55 nonconsecutive patients with suspected DVT	MRV and AV	Femoral and iliac veins	Se=100% for both femoral and iliac veins; Sp=100% for iliacs and 97% for femorals. Interobserver variability=0.85 (femoral) and 0.97 (iliac)	Prospective, blinded

Abbreviations: Ac, accuracy; AV, ascending venography; CI, confidence intervals; CT, computed tomography; DUS, Duplex ultrasonography; DVT, deep vein thrombosis; IVC, inferior vena cava; MRV, magnetic resonance venography; NPV, negative predictive value; PE, pulmonary embolism; PPV, positive predictive value; Se, sensitivity; Sp, specificity; VA, Veteran Affairs Hospital.

Table 4 Computed Tomography Imaging and Deep Vein Thrombosis

Study	Subjects	Tests	Extension	Results	Design
Baldt, 1996 (53)	52 patients with suspected DVT	CTV and AV	IVC to the ankle	Se = 100% (95%CI = 92–100%) Sp = 96% (95%CI = 84–98%); PPV = 91%; NPV = 100%	Prospective
Loud, 2001 (54)	308 patients with suspected PE	CTV (venous phase at time of CTPA), DUS	Diaphragm to upper calves	Se = 97%; Sp = 100% for femoropopliteal	Prospective, multicenter, blinded
Peterson, 2001 (55)	136 patients with suspected PE	CTV, DUS	Above-the-knee	Se = 71%; Sp = 93%; PPV = 53%; NPV = 97%, Ac = 90%	Retrospective

Abbreviations: Ac, accuracy; AV, ascending venography; CI, confidence intervals; CTPA, computed tomographic pulmonary arteriogram; CTV, computed tomographic venography; DUS, duplex ultrasound; DVT, deep vein thrombosis; NPV, negative predictive value; PE, pulmonary embolism; PPV, positive predictive value; Se, sensitivity; Sp, specificity.

Table 5 D-dimer Testing and Deep Vein Thrombosis

Study	Subjects	Tests	Results	Design
Wells, 1999 (60)	150 consecutive inpatients with suspected DVT	Dd, PTP, DUS and AV	1.8% (95%CI = 0.02–6.4%) patients considered to have DVT excluded had events in a 3-month follow-up. The Dd NPV in LPP = 96.2% (not statistically different from the NPV of a negative DUS in LPP (97.8%)	Prospective
Anderson, 2000 (61)	214 patients with suspected DVT	Dd, PTP and DUS (fingerstick SimpliRED whole blood agglutination)	Dd Se = 82.5%, Sp = 84.9%, NPV = 96.9% (95% CI = 93-99.1%) overall, and 100% (95%CI = 96.3–100%) in LPP, 94.1% (95%CI = 83.8–98.8%) in MPP and 86.7% (95% CI = 59.4–98.3%) in HPP	Prospective cohort
Kearon, 2001 (62)	445 outpatients with suspected first DVT	Dd and PTP	40% patients had both a LPP and a negative Dd. 1 of them had DVT during a 3 month follow-up (NPV = 99.4% [95% CI = 96.9–100%])	Prospective cohort
Kovacs, 2001 (63)	993 patients with suspected DVT or PE	Comparison of Accuclot, IL-Test and SimpliRED	Se = 90,87 and 79% NPV = 98, 97 and 96%	Prospective
Bates, 2003 (64)	556 consecutive outpatients with suspected first DVT	Dd, PTP and CUS	283 patients (51%) had LPP or MPP and negative Dd. 1 of them had DVT on follow-up (NLR = 0.05 [CI, 0.01–0.23]). Dd NLR overall = 0.03 (CI = 0.01–0.16)	Prospective cohort
Philbrick, 2003 (65)	6 studies using Dd	16 different Dd assays	Se = 76.6–100%, Sp = 39.5–93.9%, NPV = 78.8–100%	Meta-analysis
Schutgens, 2003 (66)	812 patients with suspected DVT.	Dd, PTP and CUS	NPV: 97.7%, Se: 98.4%	Prospective multicenter cohort
Wells, 2003 (67)	1096 outpatients with suspected DVT	Dd, PTP and DUS	LPP, NPV: 99.1% HPP, NPV: 89% Dd reduced the use of DUS, from 1.34 tests/patient (control: DUS imaging alone) to 0.78	Prospective randomized

Abbreviations: Ac, accuracy; AV, ascending venography; CI, confidence intervals; CUS, compression ultrasound; Dd, D-dimer; DUS, Duplex ultrasound; DVT, deep vein thrombosis; HPP, high probability patients; LPP, low probability patients; MPP, moderate probability patients; NLR, negative likelihood ratio; NPV, negative predictive value; PE, pulmonary embolism; PPV, positive predictive value; PTP, pretest probability; Se, sensitivity; Sp, specificity.

detection of DVT in 52 symptomatic patients. CT venography showed a 100% sensitivity (CI=0.92–1.00), 96% specificity (CI=0.84–0.98), 91% positive predictive value and 100% negative predictive value (NPV). CT venography was superior in demonstrating extension of DVT into the pelvic veins and IVC than was AV. The amount of contrast required by CT is significantly less compared to AV (53). Obvious disadvantages include its invasiveness, inability to be performed at the bedside, its cost and the need for ionizing radiation and iodinated contrast material.

D-dimer and Pretest Probability

Classification into low-, intermediate- and high-risk groups using pretest probability (PTP), empirically or using scoring systems is essential when suspecting VTE. It reduces the need for initial and supplementary testing and allows considerable refinement of the posterior likelihood of VTE following non-invasive imaging (56). The simplified Wells scores for suspected DVT and PE is the most used (57). An overview of data suggests that fewer patients tend to be classified as low PTP when assessed empirically (56).

D-dimer testing detects fibrin degeneration products. The development of monoclonal antibodies made its detection possible, using the principle of enzyme-linked immunosorbent assay (ELISA) or agglutination techniques. An increased D-dimer level is not specific for VTE. It may be seen in cancer, sepsis, kidney failure, pregnancy and trauma or in the postoperative state. Because a very low PPV has been reported in most studies (28–31%) (58,59), objective testing must be performed before instigating treatment. Therefore D-dimer testing is most appropriate in the outpatient setting. But a negative test is most accurate for exclusion of VTE, especially in patients with a low PTP (NPV=99.5%) and least accurate in patients with a high PTP (NPV=85.7%). The results of seven recent prospective trials and one meta-analysis that studied D-dimer testing and DVT are shown in Table 5 (60–67). From the socioeconomic point of view, patients with low PTP and a normal D-dimer are the largest number of outpatients referred for testing. Considerable resources may be saved if future studies confirm the utility of D-dimer testing in those patients by reducing the number of further imaging needed (68). When a patient has a high PTP, it is probably cost-effective to obtain a DUS without the need for D-dimer testing, given the high likelihood for the latter to be positive in this subgroup of patients (about 75%). This needs to be studied further before any recommendations are given.

The results from one commercially available test might not be applicable to others and different results may be obtained when using the same manufacturer's assay (69). In patients with suspected DVT, rapid ELISA tests show promise as a practical D-dimer assay. They have a similar sensitivity to that of the conventional ELISA assay. The most studied and reliable tests are the SimpliRED whole-blood assay (Agen Biomedical, Brisbane, Australia) or the Instant-IA rapid ELISA (Stago, Asnieres, France) in combination with a noninvasive test or PTP can safely rule out DVT in the outpatient setting (68,69).

KEY POINTS

- Venous thromboembolism is responsible for a large number of hospital admissions and for more than 50,000 deaths every year.
- Its etiology is multifactorial with endothelial damage, hypercoagulability and stasis having different impact on different patients.

- There is an association between superficial vein thrombosis and DVT and a questionable relationship with malignancy. Concomitant DVT should be ruled out at presentation.
- Postphlebitic syndrome occurs in over 20% of patients. Ipsilateral recurrent DVT, a combination of reflux and obstruction and popliteal vein reflux, are significantly associated with skin changes and ulceration.
- Ascending venography is rarely used for screening. It is invasive, not widely available and can produce venous thrombosis.
- Duplex ultrasound is the most frequently used test for DVT screening and surveillance. It is noninvasive, portable and relatively inexpensive. It can differentiate between acute and chronic thrombus and detect other pathologies.
- The accuracy of CT venography is comparable to duplex ultrasound. When combined with CT lung angiography, it represents a useful tool for the diagnosis of PE. Its cost, need for contrast and radiation exposure are its main limitations.
- MR scanning is mainly used as a confirmatory test or to evaluate the proximal venous systems. It has a low morbidity, does not need contrast and may diagnose additional soft tissue pathologies. Its cost and limited availability makes it a poor screening test.
- For outpatient screening a combination of clinical parameters and D-dimer testing is effective for identifying patients for venous duplex scan. A negative test is most accurate for exclusion of VTE in patients with a low pretest probability and less accurate in patients with a high pretest probability.

REFERENCES

1. Prandoni P, Mannucci PM. Deep-vein thrombosis of the lower limbs: diagnosis and management. Baillieres Best Pract Res Clin Haematol 1999; 12:533–554.
2. Bosson JL, Labarere J, Sevestre MA, et al. Deep vein thrombosis in elderly patients hospitalized in subacute care facilities: a multicenter cross-sectional study of risk factors, prophylaxis, and prevalence. Arch Intern Med 2003; 163:2613–2618.
3. Anderson FA, Jr., Wheeler HB, Goldberg RJ, et al. A population-based perspective of the hospital incidence and case-fatality rates of deep vein thrombosis and pulmonary embolism. The Worcester DVT Study. Arch Intern Med 1991; 151:933–938.
4. Stewart GJ, Ritchie WGM, Lynch PR. Venous endothelial damage produced by massive sticking and emigration of leukocytes. Am J Pathol 1974; 74:507–532.
5. Stewart GJ, Stern HS, Lynch PR, Malmud LS, Schaub RG. Responses of canine jugular veins and carotid arteries to hysterectomy: increased permeability and leukocyte adhesions and invasion. Thromb Res 1980; 20:473–489.
6. Heit JA, Silverstein MD, Mohr DN, et al. The epidemiology of venous thromboembolism in the community. Thromb Haemost 2001; 86:452–463.
7. Gouin-Thibault I, Arkam R, Nassiri S, et al. Markers of activated coagulation in patients with factor V Leiden and/or G20210A prothrombin gene mutation. Thromb Res 2002; 107:7–11.
8. Emmerich J, Rosendaal FR, Cattaneo M, et al. Combined effect of factor V Leiden and prothrombin 20210A on the risk of venous thromboembolism—pooled analysis of 8 case-control studies including 2310 cases and 3204 controls. Study Group for Pooled-Analysis in Venous Thromboembolism. Thromb Haemost 2001; 86:809–816.
9. Becattini C, Agnelli G. Pathogenesis of venous thromboembolism. Curr Opin Pulm Med 2002; 8:360–364.

10. Downing LJ, Wakefield TW, Strieter RM, et al. Anti-P-selectin antibody decreases inflammation and thrombus formation in venous thrombosis. J Vasc Surg 1997; 25:81627.

11. Lohr JM, Kerr TM, Lutter KS, et al. Lower extremity calf thrombosis-to treat or not to treat. J Vasc Surg 1991; 14:618–623.

12. White R, McGahan J, Daschbach M, Hartling R. Diagnosis of deep-vein thrombosis using duplex ultrasound. Ann Intern Med 1989; 111:297–304.

13. Verlato F, Zucchetta P, Paolo P, et al. An unexpectedly high rate of pulmonary embolism in patients with superficial thrombophlebitis of the thigh. J Vasc Surg 1999; 30:1113–1115.

14. Lutter KS, Rerr TM, Roedersheimer R, Lohr JM, Sampson MG, Cranley JJ. Superficial thrombophlebitis diagnosed by duplex scanning. Surgery 1991; 100:42–77.

15. Hafner CD, Cranley JJ, Krause RJ, Strasser ES. A method of managing superficial thrombophlebitis. Surgery 1964; 55:201–206.

16. Bounameaux H, Reber-Wasem MA. Superficial thrombophlebitis and deep vein thrombosis. A controversial association. Arch Intern Med 1997; 157:1822–1824.

17. Prandoni P, Lensing AW, Cogo A, et al. The long-term clinical course of acute deep venous thrombosis. Ann Intern Med 1996; 125:1–7.

18. Meissner MH, Caps MT, Bergelin RO, et al. Propagation, rethrombosis and new thrombus formation after acute deep vein thrombosis. J Vasc Surg 1995; 22:558–567.

19. Prandoni P. Long-term clinical course of proximal deep venous thrombosis and detection of recurrent thrombosis. Semin Thromb Hemost 2001; 27:9–13.

20. Barritt DW, Jordan SC. Anticoagulant drugs in the treatment of pulmonary embolism: a controlled trial. Lancet 1960; 1:1309–1312.

21. Anderson FA, Wheeler HB. Physician practices in the management of venous thromboembolism: a community-wide survey. J Vasc Surg 1992; 15:707–714.

22. Killewich LA, Macko RF, Cox K, et al. Regression of proximal deep venous thrombosis is associated with fibrinolytic enhancement. J Vasc Surg 1997; 26:861–868.

23. Labropoulos N, Kang SS, Mansour MA, Giannoukas AD, Moutzouros V, Baker WH. Early thrombus remodeling of isolated calf deep vein thrombosis. Eur J Vasc Endovasc Surg 2002; 23:344–348.

24. Prandoni P, Lensing AWA, Prins MHE, et al. Residual vein thrombosis as a predictive factor of recurrent venous thromboembolism. Ann Intern Med 2002; 137:955–960.

25. Rohrer MJ, Cutler BS, MacDougall E, Herrmann JB, Anderson FA, Jr., Wheeler HB. A prospective study of the incidence of deep venous thrombosis in hospitalized children. J Vasc Surg 1996; 24:46–49.

26. Kamida CB, Kistner RL, Eklof B, Masuda EM. Lower extremity ascending and descending phlebography. In: Gloviczki P, Yao JST, eds. Handbook Of Venous Disorders. London, UK: Arnold Publishers, 2001:132–139.

27. Bjorgell O, Nilsson PE, Jarenros H. Isolated nonfilling of contrast in deep leg vein segments seen on phlebography, and a comparison with color Doppler ultrasound, to assess the incidence of deep leg vein thrombosis. Angiology 2000; 51:451–461.

28. Hull R, Hirsh J, Sackett DL, et al. Clinical validity of a negative venogram in patients with clinically suspected venous thrombosis. Circulation 1981; 64:622–625.

29. Albrechtsson U, Olsson CG. Thrombotic side-effects of lower-limb phlebography. Lancet 1976; 1:723–724.

30. Wheeler HB, Hirsh J, Wells P, Anderson FA, Jr. Diagnostic tests for deep vein thrombosis. Clinical usefulness depends on probability of disease. Arch Intern Med 1994; 154:1921–1928.

31. Baxter GM, McKechnie S, Duffy P. Colour Doppler ultrasound in deep venous thrombosis: a comparison with venography. Clin Radiol 1990; 42:32–36.

32. van Ramshorst B, Legemate DA, Verzijlbergen JF, et al. Duplex scanning in the diagnosis of acute deep vein thrombosis of the lower extremity. Eur J Vasc Surg 1991; 5:255–260.

33. Cogo A, Lensing AW, Prandoni P, Buller HR, Girolami A, ten Cate JW. Comparison of real-time B-mode ultrasonography and Doppler ultrasound with contrast venography in the diagnosis of venous thrombosis in symptomatic outpatients. Thromb Haemost 1993; 70:404–407.

34. Lewis BD, James EM, Welch TJ, Joyce JW, Hallett JW, Weaver AL. Diagnosis of acute deep venous thrombosis of the lower extremities: prospective evaluation of color Doppler flow imaging versus venography. Radiology 1994; 192:651–655.

35. Miller N, Satin R, Tousignant L, Sheiner NM. A prospective study comparing duplex scan and venography for diagnosis of lower extremity deep vein thrombosis. Cardiovasc Surg 1996; 4:505–508.

36. Theodorou SJ, Theodorou DJ, Kakitsubata Y. Sonography and venography of the lower extremities for diagnosing deep vein thrombosis in symptomatic patients. Clin Imaging 2003; 27:180–183.

37. Zierler BK. Screening for acute DVT: optimal utilization of the vascular diagnostic laboratory. Semin Vasc Surg 2001; 14:206–214.

38. Wells PS, Lensing AW, Davidson BL, Prins MH, Hirsh J. Accuracy of ultrasound for the diagnosis of deep venous thrombosis in asymptomatic patients after orthopedic surgery. A meta-analysis. Ann Intern Med 1995; 122:47–53.

39. Labropoulos N, Leon M, Kalodiki E, al Kutoubi A, Chan P, Nicolaides AN. Colour flow duplex scanning in suspected acute deep vein thrombosis; experience with routine use. Eur J Vasc Endovasc Surg 1995; 9:49–52.

40. Labropoulos N, Webb KM, Kang SS, et al. Patterns and distribution of isolated calf deep vein thrombosis. J Vasc Surg 1999; 30:787–791.

41. Hirsh J, Lee AY. How we diagnose and treat deep vein thrombosis. Blood 2002; 99:3102–3110.

42. Prandoni P, Lensing AW, Bernardi E, Villalta S, Bagatella P, Girolami A. DERECUS Investigators Group. The diagnostic value of compression ultrasonography in patients with suspected recurrent deep vein thrombosis. Thromb Haemost 2002; 88:402–406.

43. Prandoni P, Cogo A, Bernardi E, et al. A simple ultrasound approach for detection of recurrent proximal-vein thrombosis. Circulation 1993; 88:1730–1735.

44. Stanson AW, Breen JF. Computed tomography and magnetic resonance imaging in venous disorders. In: Gloviczki P, Yao JST, eds. Handbook Of Venous Disorders. London, UK: Arnold Publishers, 2001:132–139.

45. Erdman WA, Jayson HT, Redman HC, Miller GL, Parkey RW, Peshock RW. Deep venous thrombosis of extremities: role of MR imaging in the diagnosis. Radiology 1990; 174:425–431.

46. Carpenter JP, Holland GA, Baum RA, Owen RS, Carpenter JT, Cope C. Magnetic resonance venography for the detection of deep venous thrombosis: comparison with contrast venography and duplex Doppler ultrasonography. J Vasc Surg 1993; 18:734–741.

47. Evans AJ, Sostman HD, Knelson MH, et al. 1992 ARRS Executive Council Award. Detection of deep venous thrombosis: prospective comparison of MR imaging with contrast venography. AJR Am J Roentgenol 1993; 161:131–139.

48. Evans AJ, Sostman HD, Witty LA, et al. Detection of deep venous thrombosis: prospective comparison of MR imaging and sonography. J Magn Reson Imaging 1996; 6:44–51.

49. Fraser DGW, Moody AR, Morgan PS, Martel AL, Davidson I. Diagnosis of lower-limb deep venous thrombosis: a prospective blinded study of magnetic resonance direct thrombus imaging. Ann Intern Med 2002; 136:89–98.

50. Fraser DGW, Moody AR, Davidson AR, Martel AL, Morgan PS. Deep venous thrombosis: diagnosis by using venous enhanced subtracted peak arterial MR venography versus conventional venography. Radiology 2003; 226:812–820.

51. Froelich JB. Magnetic resonance phlebography. In: Ernst CB, Stanley JC, eds. Current Therapy in Vascular Surgery. 4th ed. St Louis, Missouri: Mosby, 2001:822–824.

52. Begermann PG, Bonacker M, Kemper J, et al. Evaluation of the deep venous system in patients with suspected pulmonary embolism with multi-detector CT: a prospective study in comparison to Doppler ultrasonography. J Comput Assist Tomogr 2003; 27:399–409.

53. Baldt MM, Zontsich T, Stumpflen A, et al. Deep venous thrombosis of the lower extremity: efficacy of spiral CT venography compared with conventional venography in diagnosis. Radiology 1996; 200:423–428.

54. Loud PA, Katz DS, Bruce DA, Klippenstein DL, Grossman ZD. Deep venous thrombosis with suspected pulmonary embolism: detection with combined CT venography and pulmonary angiography. Radiology 2001; 219:498–502.

55. Peterson DA, Kazerooni EA, Wakefield TW, et al. Computed tomographic venography is specific but not sensitive for diagnosis of acute lower-extremity deep venous thrombosis in patients with suspected pulmonary embolus. J Vasc Surg 2001; 34:798–804.

56. Kelly J, Hunt BJ. The utility of pretest probability assessment in patients with clinically suspected venous thromboembolism. J Thromb Haemost 2003; 1:1888–1896.

57. Wells PS, Anderson DR, Bormanis J, et al. Value of assessment of pretest probability of deep-vein thrombosis in clinical management. Lancet 1997; 350:1795–1798.

58. Bounameaux H, Schneider PA, Reber G, de Moerloose P, Krahenbuhl B. Measurement of plasma D-dimer for diagnosis of deep venous thrombosis. Am J Clin Pathol 1989; 91:82–85.

59. Kroneman H, Van Bergen PF, Knot EA, Jonker JJ, de Maat MP. Diagnostic value of D-dimer for deep venous thrombosis in outpatients. Haemostasis 1991; 21:286–292.

60. Wells PS, Anderson DR, Bormanis J, et al. Application of a diagnostic clinical model for the management of hospitalized patients with suspected deep-vein thrombosis. Thromb Haemost 1999; 81:493–497.

61. Anderson DR, Wells PS, Stiell I, et al. Management of patients with suspected deep vein thrombosis in the emergency department: combining use of a clinical diagnosis model with D-dimer testing. J Emerg Med 2000; 19:225–230.

62. Kearon C, Ginsberg JS, Douketis J, et al. Management of suspected deep venous thrombosis in outpatients by using clinical assessment and D-dimer testing. Ann Intern Med 2001; 135:108–111.

63. Kovacs MJ, MacKinnon KM, Anderson D, et al. A comparison of three rapid D-dimer methods for the diagnosis of venous thromboembolism. Br J Haematol 2001; 115:140–144.

64. Bates SM, Kearon C, Crowther M, et al. A diagnostic strategy involving a quantitative latex D-dimer assay reliably excludes deep venous thrombosis. Ann Intern Med 2003; 138:787–794.

65. Philbrick JT, Heim S. The D-dimer test for deep venous thrombosis: gold standards and bias in negative predictive value. Clinical Chemistry 2003; 49:570–574.

66. Schutgens RE, Ackermark P, Haas FJ, et al. Combination of a normal D-dimer concentration and a non-high pretest clinical probability score is a safe strategy to exclude deep venous thrombosis. Circulation 2003; 107:593–597.

67. Wells PS, Anderson DR, Rodger M, et al. Evaluation of D-dimer in the diagnosis of suspected deep-vein thrombosis. N Engl J Med 2003; 349:1227–1235.

68. Brill-Edwards P, Lee A. D-dimer testing in the diagnosis of acute venous thromboembolism. Thromb Haemost 1999; 82:688–694.

69. Lee AY, Ginsberg JS. Laboratory diagnosis of venous thromboembolism. Baillieres Clin Haematol 1998; 11:587–604.

11

The Pathophysiology of Deep Venous Thrombosis

Ahmad Bhatti
Division of Vascular Surgery, Loyola University Medical Center, Maywood, Illinois, U.S.A.

Nicos Labropoulos
Vascular Laboratory, Division of Vascular Surgery, New Jersey Medical School, Newark, New Jersey, U.S.A.

BACKGROUND

Venous thromboembolism (VTE) is a common event. It may be asymptomatic or lead to pulmonary embolism (PE), which may be fatal. In the eighteenth and nineteenth centuries, pulmonary arterial thrombosis was first recognized as an entity. While some attributed death and causality to this finding on autopsy, others merely commented on it incidentally. The fact that pulmonary arterial thrombosis may occur from a venous VTE, an extra-pulmonary source, was not entertained. In 1858, Rudolf Virchow recognized that the aforementioned phenomenon might occur from a pulmonary, or an extra-pulmonary source. He stated the importance of thrombi in remote venous systems that may dislodge and cause secondary occlusion such as PE. It is during this time that he postulated the etiologies of deep vein thrombosis (DVT) and proposed what is today called "Virchow's triad" as follows: hypercoagulability, blood stasis, and vessel injury(1).

In most patients, the etiology of DVT is multifactorial. It is important to recognize which of these etiologic factors are transient (e.g., immobility) and which are long-standing (e.g., malignancy). The anatomic location, extent and type of symptomatology of DVT increase the risk of VTE or PE to varying degrees (2). Many, if not all, of the pathophysiologic factors for DVT exert their effect through one or more of Virchow's triad. Hence, in every DVT there exists at least one of these factors as an initiating event.

STASIS

Venous stasis has received the most attention as the main reason for causing DVT (3). Although it may be simplistic to view stasis as the leading or sole cause in DVT formation, its contribution is substantial. Conditions of stasis are common and often are transient: immobility (e.g., cessation of calf-pump mechanism), outflow compression (e.g., pregnancy), or vasodilation/decreased flow (e.g., general anesthesia). Various randomized controlled studies have shown that simple intermittent pneumatic compression devices that prevent or reduce stasis reduce the incidence of DVT (4–8). There is a belief that these devices also act via stimulation of the endogenous fibrinolytic system. Research in this area is inconclusive, as there are studies in the literature to argue for and against this theory (9–12).

While it is well accepted and intuitive that blood stasis leads to thrombosis, the basic mechanisms are poorly understood. It is felt that cessation of flow causes upregulation of cell adhesion molecules (CAMs) by endothelial cells (ECs). This upregulation of CAMs increases leukocyte and platelet adherence, while the decreasing flow limits the hemodynamic clearance of adherent leukocytes or platelets (13). Animal models have demonstrated such adherence and accumulation of leukocytes and platelets with simple venous stasis in a time-dependent manner. Adhesion, accumulation, and transmigration result in EC sloughing and exposure of the highly thrombogenic basement membrane. Leukocytes are thought to play the primary role in this series of events, and regulation of these CAMs could, in theory, modulate damage to ECs, prevent basement membrane exposure, and/or thrombosis formation (13–15). Animal models have also shown that leukocyte adherence, EC sloughing, and thrombus formation first occurs behind valve cusps (13,14). While this may or may not be macroscopically apparent, this series of events occurs shortly after stasis. Contrast venography studies have shown delayed clearance of contrast in valve sinuses/cusps in non-excercised limbs (16). Even with normal flow in a vein, there may be local stasis that occurs behind the valve cusps. This local stasis is a result of eddy currents or vortices that occur behind these cusps, and these are known to increase the risk of thrombus formation (17,18).

Major causes of stasis include excessive bed rest (e.g., hospitalization), paralysis, long air-travel times and prolonged sitting. DVT associated with air-travel has a variable incidence with case reports of sudden death from PE after trans-atlantics flights (19,20). One large extensive prospective study showing the incidence to be zero regardless of the class of travel (business versus economy), once hyper-coaguable patients were excluded (21). This study did, however, demonstrate an elevation of D-dimers, compared with pre-flight levels, in 10% of travelers, suggesting activation of the thrombolytic system. With an increasingly technologically advanced society requiring less physical demand, case reports of DVT from prolonged sitting at computer terminals (work, recreational, or personal), and the like, are now being reported. The term "eThrombosis" has been used to describe this etiology (22). Stasis can also result from position independent factors by varying degrees of venous obstruction. Common examples would include pregnancy, with the gravid uterus impinging on the iliac veins, or pelvic tumors by a similar mechanism. Low hemodynamic flow rates can also result in a relative stasis of venous blood such as in hypotension or congestive heart failure (CHF). One outpatient study of patients with CHF showed an inverse ratio between cardiac ejection fraction and DVT/VTE rates (23). Although inherently intuitive, these in vivo flow and DVT correlations have not been well studied clinically. Venodilation that occurs with epidural or spinal analgesia or spinal trauma may also predispose to stasis and thereby to DVT formation. This potential cause of stasis has been acknowledged and attempts to modulate it clinically have been reported (24).

HYPERCOAGULABILITY

This condition occurs when the coagulation is promoted or anticoagulation is impaired. Acquired or inherited clotting cascade mutations, imbalances, or activation produce hypercoaguable states (Table 1). While there are many specific factors that may be implicated, a small subset has been established and their relationships with DVT formation have been well studied.

Table 1 Factors that Promote Coagulation or Impair Anticoagulation

Factor	Prevalence in patients with DVT or VTE	Prevalence in general population	Risk for DVT or VTE	Comments
Factor V Leiden (APCR)	20–60% (40)	5% (61)	Hetero: 3×; Homo 50–80×(29)	Most common heritable thrombophilia in DVT/VTE patients; majority of APCR is from Factor V Leiden
Malignancy	30–35% (62)	U.S.: 9.6 million current cases (63)	2–3× (38)	Risk varies with type of malignancy
Factor VIII	17–25% (48,49)	10%[a]	5–7× (45–47)	For increased (idiopathic) levels: >90th percentile
Plasminogen activator inhibitor (PAI)	22% (64)	7.6–44.8% (65)	Unclear (43,61,62)	Lowest in African Americans, highest in Caucasians and Japanese
Prothrombin 202-0A (Factor IIA)	4–20% (26)	2% (37)	Hetero: 2–3× (31,32)	Homozygotes rare (case reports); 2nd most common heritable thrombophilia in DVT/VTE patients
Antiphospolipid Antibodies (LA, ACA, etc.)	15% (36)	Unknown (37)	1/3 lifetime VTE risk (36)	May exist without SLE
Protein C&S deficiency	5–10% (38,40,66)	0.2–0.7% (37)	Hetero: 50% risk of VTE by age 50 (37)	Protein S deficiency more common
Hyperhomocysteinemia	10%(67)	5%[a]	2.5× (38)	For increased levels: >95th percentile
Antithrombin III deficiency	0.5–5% (38)	0.02 (37)	85% VTE risk by age 50 (38)	
Factor XI	Low (38)	10%[a]	2.5× (38)	For increased levels: >90th percentile
Factor IX	Low (38)	10%[a]	2.5× (38)	For increased levels: >90th percentile
Polycythemia vera	Low	1.9 per 100,000 (68)	3.4%/yr (arterial and venous) (69)	Risk felt to be related to cell volume
Dysfibrinogenemias	Rare (0.8%) (70)	Case reports	Unclear (42,65)	

[a] By definition.

The two most common factors for hypercoagulability in the veins are the mutations of factor V and the Prothrombin 20210A (25,26). A large risk for DVT formation occurs with activated protein C resistance (APCR) (27,28). Factor Va acts as a co-factor for the prothrombin activating complex. Activated protein C (APC) neutralizes Factor Va thereby inhibiting prothrombin activation. An abnormal/mutated factor Va called Factor V Leiden will resist APC resulting in sustained prothrombin activation and increased thrombotic risk (29). In patients with venous thrombosis 20–60% are positive for this mutation (40). Factor V heterozygotes are at three times the risk of venous thrombosis compared with the normal population, and homozygotes are at $50–80\times$ higher risk (30). In addition to DVT formation, Factor V and prothrombin gene mutations are also associated with a high risk for VTE recurrence (31). The Prothrombin 20210A mutation results in hypercoagulability via increased prothrombin levels. This is the second most common genetic mutation (Factor V Leiden being the first) in patients with venous thrombosis (32). It increases the risk of a DVT two to threefold (31,33). Most cases are heterozygous for this mutation, and homozygous patients are rare but have been reported (34,35).

Antiphospholipid antibodies, hyperhomocysteinemia and deficiencies of anti-thrombin III are also major risk factors for DVT formation. Antiphospolipid antibodies are a broad class of reactive autoimmune antibodies that include anticardiolipin antibody (ACA) and lupus anticoagulant (LA). ACA and LA were first recognized in patients with systemic lupus erythematosus (SLE). These antibodies can exist without the presence of SLE (36). Up to 15% of DVT may involve antiphospholipid antibodies and one third of patients with antiphoshpolipid antibodies will have a thromboembolic event (37).

Protein C and Protein S are two anticoagulant proteins that are implicated in DVT formation (38,39). Deficiency in either may produce a procoagualant state. This deficiency may be functional, as may be in the case of mutations, or it may be relative as with induction of warfarin anticoagulation. In patients with venous thrombosis 10% have inherited deficiencies of Protein C or Protein S (40).

Malignancy is associated with an increased incidence of DVT. Certain malignancies, such as gastric or pancreatic cancer may have a higher association with DVT (41). The mechanisms by which procoagulant states are created vary from tumor to tumor. These mechanisms are variable, but examples include tumors creating cysteine protease proco-agulants (which activate Factor X), or tumors activating the extrinsic pathway, or altering EC anticoagulant activity. In some patients, idiopathic VTE or DVT may be the presenting symptom for an undiagnosed malignancy (37).

Thrombus formation and degradation are the result of an ongoing balance of coagulation and fibrinolysis. Alterations may occur to form procoagulant states as discussed above, or in fibrinolysis leading to impairments of thrombus degradation. Imbalances in, or dysfunction of, tissue plasminogen activator and inhibitor, Factor XIIa (Hageman factor), and prekallikrein defeciences may upset this balance of thrombus formation and degradation (42–44). The association between impairments of the fibrinolytic system and symptomatic thrombosis remain controversial, with one critical review of the literature showing no association (45). Increased Factor VIII levels increase the risk of DVT, with various studies showing a five times to seven times higher recurrence rate of VTE for with patients with elevated (in or $>$ than the 90th percentile) factor VIII levels (46–48). The incidence of elevated FVIII has been reported in the range from 17–25%, making this an important contributor to DVT and VTE in the population (49,50).

Other contributors to hypercoaguability exist. Factors that increase viscosity, such as polycythemia vera, have been implicated in DVT formation (51). Polymorphisms that allow over expression of plasminogen activator inhibitor (PAI) inhibit fibrinolysis and are associated with higher DVT rates (52,53). The significance (statistical and otherwise) of this has not been well established, as reported in several studies (43,54,55). Platelet dysfunction or thrombocytosis, however have little association with venous thrombosis (56). HIV also predisposes patients to venous thrombosis, however the mechanism remains unclear (57). Dysfibrinogenemia is a rare cause of venous thrombosis, accounting for 0.8% of patients with DVTs (58). It should, however, be considered in the differential diagnosis in patients that are young or have familial histories of DVTs, as with all potentially heritable thrombophilias. Oral contraceptives (OCs) have been well known to increase the incidence of DVT in patients who take them. The mechanisms are multifactorial, but with regards to thrombophilic states, this may occur via reduction in ATIII, reduction in Protein S, or induction of APCR (50,59,60). While both estrogens and progesterones in OCs contribute to DVT formation, it is felt that the latter may have a larger role.

VESSEL INJURY

Various degrees of gross or microscopic trauma and/or disruption to the vein's architecture may produce DVT. ECs act as a physical barrier by covering the prothrombogenic basement membrane. They also actively participate in thrombus formation and degradation (71). As mentioned earlier, CAMs are expressed with stasis or EC injury and induce leukocyte adhesion, migration, and eventual EC sloughing (13–15). This exposes the collagen rich thrombogenic basement membrane inducing thrombus formation via platelet activation (72). ECs also express plasminogen activators thereby inducing thrombus lysis (43). Focal vessel injury should not impair fibrinolysis. This is because ECs and plasminogen activators may locally/remotely act upon distant thrombi. Focal vessel injury will, however, produce thrombi, for the aforementioned reasons. Any exogenous or endogenous agent that may cause EC and/or basement membrane damage, irritation, injury, or simple exposure of the basement membrane can result in thrombosis. This includes physical injury (e.g., blast, thermal, or shear), anoxia, stasis, mechanical injury (e.g., catheters, venoplasty, or stents), exposure to non-iso-osmolar agents hyperlipidemia, and hyperhomocysteinemia (58,73–78). Extravascular tissues and vessel adventitia all contain varying degrees of tissue factor (TF). TF binds factor VIIa (FVIIa) to activate the clotting cascade. Vessel injury exposes TF to flowing blood thereby inducing thrombus formation (79). This TF/FVIIa complex is postulated to be formed and released during surgery (cutting through tissue and vessels). It exerts effects at remote sites causing DVT. Pharmacologic inhibitors of TF/FVIIa complexes have been used clinically to reduce post-operative DVT rates with initial success (80–82).

OTHER CAUSES

Estrogens, OCs, and hormonal therapies exert their influence by creating a hypercoaguable state, increasing calf venous volume, and decreasing venous velocity (50,56,57). Obesity, possibly from decreased mobility and increased hormonal production, increases the risk of DVT formation two-fold, and is a co-morbidity in 27% of patients with DVT (83,84). It is difficult to separate the effects of anesthesia and surgery on DVT formation. Several studies are suggestive that anesthetic induction alone results in venous distension, decreased muscle tone, increased stasis, or decreased venous flow (85–88). There is data to suggest that general anesthesia may be a greater risk factor than regional anesthesia (74,75). Surgery or incision itself activate the extrinsic coagulation cascade or inhibit such factors as fibrinolysis, thereby making the patient hypercoaguable (89–91). These cascade of events during surgery result in a peak period of hypercoagulability from 24 to 48 hours postoperatively. Prolonged immobility may also occur during surgery, resulting in increased risk for DVT. Increasing age is a risk factor for DVT. One prospective cohort followed from age 50 to 80 years found that the incidence of DVT 0.5% at 50 years of age, and 10.7% at 80 years of age (92,93). This has been confirmed in other cross-sectional studies. Pregnancy and puerperium also predispose to venous thrombosis. This may occur from increased pelvic pressure on iliac and pelvic veins, increased hormonal levels/ hypercoaguability, and possibly decreased ambulation (94,95). Blood surface antigens (ABO blood-grouping) have been implicated as a risk factor, with Type O being protective, although there are some conflicting reports (96,97). Spinal fractures or cord injuries increase the risk of DVT 2–3× (98). This may be the result of immobility, venodilation, and venous stasis that occurs with these conditions. Previous history of DVT or VTE is a known risk factor as well. Recurrent episodes may or may not have similar etiology (85). Inflammatory bowel disease (IBD) has also been shown to have an association with venous thrombosis, the exact mechanism, however, remains unclear (99,100). Superficial venous thrombosis (SVT) and varicose veins (VVs) are additional risk factors for DVT and probably share similar etiology (101). Venous malformations such as Klippel–Trenaunay and possibly venous angiomas have a higher incidence of DVT/VTE than the general population but the etiology is unclear (102–104).

NATURAL HISTORY OF DVT

The natural history of a DVT consists of thrombus formation, propagation, and recanalization that may be partial or complete. In 1978 Aschoff et al. described the histopathology of venous thrombi (105). Thrombus typically starts by amorphous platelet adhesions to the vessel wall. This is then covered by coralline (corral like) thrombus, which is laminar. Layers of fibrin and blood cells alternate with layers of platelets. These layers form visible lines that are called the "lines of Zahn" after the man who discovered them in 1872 (92). As the thrombus extends, it alters the blood flow which reciprocally shapes the thrombus formation. This causes the lines of Zahn to form bending and swirling in the direction of the blood flow. Once the vessel becomes occluded, the static column of blood turns into a red amorphous jelly-like thrombus consisting of fibrin and red blood cells. This then propagates to the nearest tributary to where flow may be sufficient enough to prevent stasis and clotting. At this point, the thrombus becomes adherent to the vessel wall. Recanalization occurs in the majority of cases within three months (106). Resolution then ensues with thrombus resorption/lysis, but up to 50% of limbs still may have some degree of partial occlusion at three years (94). Propagation of thrombus, in this same study, occurred in 15% of cases regardless of anticoagulation status. This was limited to one or two adjacent segments (94). Propagation can occur distally and proximally. In one study of isolated calf DVT, proximal propagation occurred in 13% of limbs, and distal propagation occurred in 4%, and both directions in 10% (107). Different segments of thrombus may propagate and lyse at the same time. Resolution occurs at an exponential rate, regardless of the vein segment. Recanalization rate and thrombus resolution rate, through endogenous fibrinolysis, are proportional with initial thrombus load (108). Calf DVT tend to have small thrombus loads, and therefore resolve faster, and this has been shown clinically (95). This remodeling and resorption of thrombus can destroy the valves involved and lead to reflux. Reflux or residual obstruction, along with pain, edema, and pigmentation changes are features of post-thrombotic syndrome (PTS). One study reported PTS at two years from DVT formation and found that 50% of patients had sonographic obstruction or reflux

(109). Only 27% of post-DVT limbs were asymptomatic at two years, and subjective findings were common: pain 62%, edema 46%, and pigmentation 35%. Another study found the incidence of phelobrgraphically proven PTS to be 56% at one year (110). The actual incidence is not well documented, with rates varying in the literature from 17% to 56% at one year (98,111).

Recurrence of DVT, with or without a specific etiology, should be considered as part of the natural history of DVT. One study cites the incidence of VTE in patients with thrombophilia (Protein C, Proteins S, and antithrombin deficiencies) at 1.4% per year with anticoagulation, and 2.7% per year without (112). Another study of a prospective cohort of 528 patients with a first episode of DVT from any etiology was followed for eight years. The study found the cumulative incidence of DVT 17.2%, 24.3%, and 29.7% at two, five, and eight years, respectively (113). In this same study, the incidence of PTS was 22.8% and 28% at two and five years respectively. The incidence of PTS increased by six times after a recurrent ipsilateral DVT. These contrasting studies, and many others, provide arguments for and against life-long or long-term anticoagulation for various DVT etiologies. Symptomatic DVT itself is a risk factor for recurrent VTE (114). The incidence of PE, symptomatic, or subclinical, with DVT is quite high, with studies citing rates of 40%–50% (115,116).

KEY POINTS

- Deep venous thrombosis is an inflammatory process, that occurs from hypercoagulability, blood stasis, and vessel injury.
- Factors may be transient (e.g., stasis due to bed rest) or permanent (e.g., inherited coagulapathies).
- Stasis, which is a common, contributes by initiating a cellular prothrombotic state.
- Hypercoaguability is largely a permanent factor, with most hypercoagulable states being inherited (e.g., Factor V Leiden), while others are transient (e.g., oral contraceptive use).
- Vessel injury is usually transient and may occur as a result of many factors including stasis, mechanical, or chemical injury.
- Deep venous thrombosis is multifactorial.
- The natural history consists of thrombus formation, propagation, embolization and recanalization.

REFERENCES

1. Virchow R. Die Cellularpathologie in ihrer Begrundung auf physiologische und pathologische Gewebelehre. From the Library of the Netherlands Journal of Medicine. 1858.
2. Kearon C. Natural history of venous thromboembolism. Circulation 2003; 107:I22–I30.
3. Browse N, et al. In: Diseases of the Veins. Great Britain: Hodder & Stoughton, 1988:448.
4. Ginzburg E, et al. Randomized clinical trial of intermittent pneumatic compression and low molecular weight heparin in trauma. Br J Surg 2003; 90:1338–1344.
5. Maxwell GL. Pneumatic compression versus low molecular weight heparin in gynecologic oncology surgery: a randomized trial. J Vasc Surg 2002; 36:953–958.

6. Schwenk W, et al. Intermittent pneumatic sequential compression (ISC) of the lower extremities prevents venous stasis during laparoscopic cholecystectomy. A prospective randomized study. J Surg Res 1998; 74:96–101.

7. Stannard JP, et al. Prophylaxis of deep venous thrombosis after total hip arthroplasty by using intermittent compression of the plantar venous plexus. Am J Orthop 1996; 25:127–134.

8. Clarke-Pearson DL, et al. A randomized trial of low-dose heparin and intermittent pneumatic calf compression for the prevention of deep venous thrombosis after gynecologic oncology surgery. Am J Obstet Gynecol 1993; 168:1146–1153.

9. Comerota AJ, et al. The fibrinolytic effects of intermittent pneumatic compression: mechanism of enhanced fibrinolysis. Ann Surg 1997; 226:306–313.

10. Kosir MA, et al. Prospective double-arm study of fibrinolysis in surgical patients. J Surg Res 1998; 74:96–101.

11. Murakami M, et al. External pneumatic compression does not increase urokinase plasminogen activator after abdominal surgery. J Vasc Surg 2002; 36:917–921.

12. Killewich LA, et al. The effect of external pneumatic compression on regional fibrinolysis in a prospective randomized trial. J Vasc Surg 2002; 36:953–958.

13. Eppihimer MJ, Schaub RG. P-Selectin-dependent inhibition of thrombosis during venous stasis. Arterioscler Thromb Vasc Biol 2000; 20:2483–2488.

14. Schaub RG, et al. Early events in the formation of a venous thrombus following local trauma and stasis. Lab Invest 1984; 51:218–224.

15. Myers DD. P-selectin antagonism causes dose-dependent venous thrombosis inhibition. Thromb Haemost 2001; 85:423–429.

16. McLachlin AD, et al. Venous stasis in the lower extremeties. Ann Surg 1960; 152:678.

17. Browse N, et al. In: Diseases of the Veins. Great Britain: Hodder & Stoughton, 1988:452.

18. Cotton LT, Clarke C. Anatomical localization of venous thrombosis. Ann R Coll Surg Engl 1965; 36:214.

19. Milne R. Venous thromboembolism and travel: Is there an association? J R Coll Physicians London 1992; 26:47–49.

20. Sahiar F, Mohler SR. Economy class syndrome. Aviat Space Environ Med 1994; 65:957–960.

21. Jacobson BF, et al. The BEST study—a prospective study to compare business class versus economy class air travel as a cause of thrombosis. S Afr Med J 2003; 93:522–528.

22. Beasley R, et al. eThrombosis: the 21st century variant of venous thromboembolism associated with immobility. Eur Respir J 2003; 21:374–376.

23. Howell MD, et al. Congestive heart failure and outpatient risk of venous thromboembolism: a retrospective, case-control study. J Clin Epidemiol 2001; 54:810–816.

24. Comerota AJ. Operative venodilation: a previously unsuspected factor in the cause of postoperative deep vein thrombosis. Surgery 1989; 106:301–308.

25. Goldhaber SZ. Epidemiology of pulmonary embolism. Semin Vasc Med 2001; 1:139–146.

26. Margaglione M, Brancaccio V, Ciampa A, et al. Inherited thrombophilic risk factors in a large cohort of individuals referred to Italian thrombophilia centers: distinct roles in different clinical settings. Haematologica 2001; 86:634–639.

27. Nojima J, et al. Acquired activated protein C resistance associated with anti-protein S antibody as a strong risk factor for DVT in non-SLE patients. Thromb Haemost 2002; 88:716–722.

28. Heinemann LA, et al. The association between extrinsic activated protein C resistance and venous thromboembolism in women. Contraception 2002; 66:297–304.

29. Kalafatis M, Mann KG. Factor V: Jeckyll. Hyde. Adv Exp Med Biol 2001; 489:31–43.

30. Caprini JA, et al. Laboratory markers in the diagnosis of venous thromboembolism. Circulation 2004; 30:109.

31. Simioni P, Prandoni P, Lensing AW, et al. Risk for subsequent venous thromboembolic complications in carriers of the prothrombin or the factor V gene mutation with a first episode of deep-vein thrombosis. Blood 2000; 96:3329–3333.

32. Perez-Ceballos E, Corral J, Alberca I, et al. Prothrombin A19911G and G20210A polymorphisms' role in thrombosis. Br J Haematol 2002; 118:610–614.

33. Ceelie H, Bertina RM, van Hylckama Vlieg A, et al. Polymorphisms in the prothrombin gene and their association with plasma prothrombin levels. Thromb Haemost 2001; 85:1066–1070.

34. Ventura P, Cobelli M, Marietta M, Panini R, Rosa MC, Salvioli G. Hyperhomocysteinemia and other newly recognized inherited coagulation disorders (factor V Leiden and prothrombin gene mutation) in patients with idiopathic cerebral vein thrombosis. Cerebrovasc Dis 2004; 17:153–159.

35. Kurkowska-Jastrzebska I, Wicha W, Dowzenko A, et al. Concomitant heterozygous factor V Leiden mutation and homozygous prothrombin gene variant (G20210A) in patient with cerebral venous thrombosis. Med Sci Monit 2003; 9:CS41–CS45.

36. Grattan CE, Burton JL. Antiphospholipid syndrome and cutaneous vasoocclusive disorders. Semin Dermatol 1991; 10:152–159.

37. Triplett DA. Antiphospholipid antibodies. Arch Pathol Lab Med 2002; 126:1424–1429.

38. Tsay W, Shen MC. R147W mutation of PROC gene is common in venous thrombotic patients in Taiwanese Chinese. Am J Hematol 2004; 76:8–13.

39. Sekiyama K, et al. Successful management of a pregnant woman with heterozygous protein C deficiency using activated protein C concentrate. J Obstet Gynaecol Res 2003; 29:412–415.

40. Simkova M, Simko F, Kovacs L. Resistance to activated protein C—frequent etiologic factor for venous thrombosis. Bratisl Lek Listy 2001; 102:240–247.

41. Sutherland DE, Weitz IC, Liebman HA. Thromboembolic complications of cancer: epidemiology, pathogenesis, diagnosis, and treatment. Am J Hematol 2003; 72:43–52.

42. Mammen EF. Pathophysiology of thrombophilic states. Folia Haematol Int Mag Klin Morphol Blutforsch 1988; 115:243–252.

43. Wiman B. Plasminogen activator inhibitor 1 in thrombotic disease. Curr Opin Hematol 1996; 3:372–378.

44. Booth NA, Bennett B. Fibrinolysis and thrombosis. Baillieres Clin Haematol 1994; 7:559–572.

45. Prins MH, Hirsh J. A critical review of the evidence supporting a relationship between impaired fibrinolytic activity and venous thromboembolism. Arch Intern Med 1991; 151:1721–1731.

46. Cristina L, Benilde C, Michela C, Mirella F, Giuliana G, Gualtiero P. High plasma levels of factor VIII and risk of recurrence of venous thromboembolism. Br J Haematol 2004; 124:504–510.

47. Kyrle PA, Minar E, Hirschl M, et al. High plasma levels of factor VIII and the risk of recurrent venous thromboembolism. N Engl J Med 2000; 343:457–462.

48. Kyrle PA. High factor VIII and the risk of venous thromboembolism. Hamostaseologie 2003; 23:41–44.

49. Bloemenkamp KW, Helmerhorst FM, Rosendaal FR, Vandenbroucke JP. Venous thrombosis, oral contraceptives and high factor VIII levels. Thromb Haemost 1999; 82:1024–1027.

50. O'Donnell J, Laffan M. Elevated plasma factor VIII levels—a novel risk factor for venous thromboembolism. Clin Lab 2001; 47:1–6.

51. Smith BD, La Celle PL. Blood viscosity and thrombosis: clinical considerations. Prog Hemost Thromb 1982; 6:179–201.

52. Segui R, Estelles A, Mira Y, Espana F, et al. PAI-1 promoter 4G/5G genotype as an additional risk factor for venous thrombosis in subjects with genetic thrombophilic defects. Br J Haematol 2000; 111:122–128.

53. Tassies D, Espinosa G, Munoz-Rodriguez FJ, et al. The 4G/5G polymorphism of the type 1 plasminogen activator inhibitor gene and thrombosis in patients with antiphospholipid syndrome. Arthritis Rheum 2000; 43:2349–2358.

54. Vaya A, Mira Y, Martinez M, et al. Biological risk factors for deep vein trombosis. [sic]. Clin Hemorheol Microcirc 2002; 26:41–53.

55. Sartori MT, Wiman B, Vettore S, et al. 4G/5G polymorphism of PAI-1 gene promoter and fibrinolytic capacity in patients with deep vein thrombosis. Thromb Haemost 1998; 80:956–960.

56. Browse N, et al. In: Diseases of the Veins. Great Britain: Hodder & Stoughton, 1988:456.

57. Saif MW, Bona R, Greenberg B. AIDS and thrombosis: retrospective study of 131 HIV-infected patients. AIDS Patient Care STDS 2001; 15:311–320.

58. Haverkate F, Samama M. Familial dysfibrinogenemia and thrombophilia. Report on a study of the SSC Subcommittee on Fibrinogen. Thromb Haemost 1995; 73:151–161.

59. Carter CJ. Oral contraceptives and thrombosis. Curr Opin Pulm Med 2000; 6:296–300.

60. Alving BM, Comp PC. Recent advances in understanding clotting and evaluating patients with recurrent thrombosis. Am J Obstet Gynecol 1992; 167:1184–1191.

61. Joffe HV, Goldhaber SZ. Laboratory thrombophilias and venous thromboembolism. Vasc Med 2002; 7:93–102.

62. Goldhaber SZ, Tapson VF. A prospective registry of 5,451 patients with ultrasound-confirmed deep vein thrombosis. Am J Cardiol 2004; 93:259–262.

63. Eyre H, Kahn R, Robertson RM, Clark NG, et al. Preventing cancer, cardiovascular disease, and diabetes: a common agenda for the American Cancer Society, the American Diabetes Association, and the American Heart Association. Stroke 2004; 35:1999–2010.

64. Varela ML, Adamczuk YP, Forastiero RR, et al. Major and potential prothrombotic genotypes in a cohort of patients with venous thromboembolism. Thromb Res 2001; 104:317–324.

65. Lanfear DE, Marsh S, Cresci S, et al. Genotypes associated with myocardial infarction risk are more common in African Americans than in European Americans. J Am Coll Cardiol 2004; 44:165–167.

66. Nicolaides A.N. Investigation of chronic venous insufficiency: a consensus statement (France. March. 5–9, 1997).

67. Anderson DA, Jr., Spencer FA. Risk factors for venous thromboembolism. Circulation 2003; 107:I9–I16.

68. Ania BJ, Suman VJ, Sobell JL, et al. Trends in the incidence of polycythemia vera among Olmsted County. Minnesota residents, 1935–1989. Am J Hematol 1994; 47:89–93.

69. Perea G, Remacha A, Besses C, et al. Polycythemia vera: the natural history of 1213 patients followed for 20 years. Gruppo Italiano Studio Policitemia. Ann Intern Med 1995;123:656–664.

70. Haverkate F, Samama M. Familial dysfibrinogenemia and thrombophilia. Report on a study of the SSC Subcommittee on Fibrinogen. Thromb Haemost 1995; 73:151–161.

71. Stanger O, et al. Vascular dysfunction in hyperhomocyst(e)inemia. Implications for atherothrombotic disease. Clin Chem Lab Med 2001; 39:725–733.

72. Leon C, Platelet ADP. receptors contribute to the initiation of intravascular coagulation. Blood 2004; 103:594–600.

73. Yan SF, Mackman N, Kisiel W, Stern DM, Pinsky DJ. Hypoxia/Hypoxemia-Induced activation of the procoagulant pathways and the pathogenesis of ischemia associated thrombosis. Arterioscler Thromb Vasc Biol 1999; 19:2029–2035.

74. Herbert JM, Corseaux D, Lale A, Bernat A. Hypoxia primes endotoxin-induced tissue factor expression in human monocytes and endothelial cells by a PAF-dependent mechanism. J Cell Physiol 1996; 169:290–299.

75. Ray JG. Dyslipidemia, statins, and venous thromboembolism: a potential risk factor and a potential treatment. Curr Opin Pulm Med 2003; 9:378–384.

76. Vaya A, et al. Hyperlipidaemia and venous thromboembolism in patients lacking thrombophilic risk factors. Br J Haematol 2002; 118:255–259.

77. Kawasaki T, Kambayashi J, Sakon M. Hyperlipidemia: a novel etiologic factor in deep vein thrombosis. Thromb Res 1999; 95:353–354.

78. Khajuria A, Houston DS. Induction of monocyte tissue factor expression by homocysteine: a possible mechanism for thrombosis. Blood 2000; 96:966–972.

79. Hathcock J. Vascular biology-the role of tissue factor. Semin Hematol 2004; 41:30–34.

80. Moons AH, Peters RJ, Bijsterveld NR, et al. Recombinant nematode anticoagulant protein c2, an inhibitor of the tissue factor/factor VIIa complex, in patients undergoing elective coronary angioplasty. J Am Coll Cardiol 2003; 41:2147–2153.

81. Lee A, Agnelli G, Buller H, Ginsberg J, et al. Dose-response study of recombinant factor VIIa/tissue factor inhibitor recombinant nematode anticoagulant protein c2 in prevention of postoperative venous thromboembolism in patients undergoing total knee replacement. Circulation 2001; 104:74–78.

82. Vlasuk GP, Rote WE. Inhibition of factor VIIa/tissue factor with nematode anticoagulant protein c2: from unique mechanism to a promising new clinical anticoagulant. Trends Cardiovasc Med 2002; 12:325–331.

83. Abdollahi M, Cushman M, Rosendaal FR. Obesity: risk of venous thrombosis and the interaction with coagulation factor levels and oral contraceptive use. Thromb Haemost 2003; 89:493–498.

84. Goldhaber SZ, Tapson VF. A prospective registry of 5,451 patients with ultrasound-confirmed deep vein thrombosis. Am J Cardiol 2004; 93:259–262.

85. Coleridge-Smith PD, Hasty JH, Scurr JH. Venous stasis and vein lumen changes during surgery. Br J Surg 1990; 77:1055–1059.

86. Tiedt N. Disorders of venous blood flow during surgery and the postoperative period as a pathomechanism of venous thrombosis of the legs. Z Gesamte Inn Med 1984; 39:406–414.

87. Poikolainen E, Hendolin H. Effects of lumbar epidural analgesia and general anaesthesia on flow velocity in the femoral vein and postoperative deep vein thrombosis. Acta Chir Scand 1983; 149:361–364.

88. Modig J. Influence of regional anesthesia, local anesthetics, and sympathicomimetics on the pathophysiology of deep vein thrombosis. Acta Chir Scand Suppl 1989; 550:119–124.

89. Samama CM. Perioperative activation of hemostasis in vascular surgery patients. Anesthesiology 2001; 94:74–78.

90. Weiss HJ, Lages B. Evidence for tissue factor-dependent activation of the classic extrinsic coagulation mechanism in blood obtained from bleeding time wounds. Blood 1988; 71:629–635.

91. Pike GK. Changes in fibrinogen levels in patients undergoing open and laparoscopic Nissen fundoplication. Aust N Z J Surg 1996; 66:94–96.

92. Hansson PO, Welin L, Tibblin G, Eriksson H. Deep vein thrombosis and pulmonary embolism in the general population. 'The Study of Men Born in 1913'. Arch Intern Med 1997; 157:1665–1670.

93. Alikhan R, et al. Risk factors for venous thromboembolism in hospitalized patients with acute medical illness: analysis of the MEDENOX Study. Arch Intern Med 2004; 164:963–968.

94. Greer IA. The special case of venous thromboembolism in pregnancy. Haemostasis ;28l 1998; 3:22–34.

95. Adachi T, Hashiguchi K, Arai Y, Ohta H. Clinical study of venous thromboembolism during pregnancy and puerperium. Semin Thromb Hemost 2001; 27:149–153.

96. Carter YM, Caps MT, Meissner MH. Deep venous thrombosis and ABO blood group are unrelated in trauma patients. J Trauma 2002; 52:112–116.

97. Robinson WM, Roisenberg I. Venous thromboembolism and ABO blood groups in a Brazilian population. Hum Genet 1980; 55:129–131.

98. Velmahos GC. Prevention of venous thromboembolism after injury: an evidence-based report—part II: analysis of risk factors and evaluation of the role of vena caval filters. J Trauma 2000; 49:140–144.

99. Solem CA, et al. Venous thromboembolism in inflammatory bowel disease. Am J Gastroenterol 2004; 99:97–101.

100. Miehsler W, et al. Is inflammatory bowel disease an independent and disease specific risk factor for thromboembolism? Gut 2004; 53:542–548.

101. Gorty S, et al. Superficial venous thrombosis of the lower extremities: analysis of risk factors, and recurrence and role of anticoagulation. Vasc Med 2004; 9:1–6.

102. Browse N. In: Diseases of the Veins. Great Britain: Hodder & Stoughton, 1988:459.

103. Gianlupi A, Harper RW, Dwyre DM, Marelich GP. Recurrent pulmonary embolism associated with Klippel–Trenaunay–Weber syndrome. Chest 1999; 115:1199–1201.

104. Aggarwal K, et al. Klippel–Trenaunay syndrome with a life-threatening thromboembolic event. J Dermatol 2003; 30:236–240.

105. Browse N. Diseases of the Veins. Great Britain: Hodder & Stoughton, 1988:459.

106. Markel A. Deep venous thrombosis: rate of spontaneous lysis and thrombus extension. Int Angiol 2003; 22:376–382.

107. Labropoulos N, Kang SS, Mansour MA, Giannoukas AD, Moutzouros V, Baker WH. Early thrombus remodelling of isolated calf deep vein thrombosis. Eur J Vasc Endovasc Surg 2002; 23:344–348.

108. van Ramshorst B, van Bemmelen PS, Hoeneveld H, et al. Thrombus regression in deep venous thrombosis. Quantification of spontaneous thrombolysis with duplex scanning. Circulation 1992; 86:414–419.

109. Saarinen J, Kallio T, Lehto M, et al. The occurrence of the post-thrombotic changes after an acute deep venous thrombosis. A prospective two-year follow-up study. J Cardiovasc Surg 2000; 41:441–446.

110. Gabriel F, Labios M, Portoles O, et al. Incidence of post-thrombotic syndrome and its association with various risk factors in a cohort of Spanish patients after one year of follow-up following acute deep venous thrombosis. Thromb Haemost 2004; 92:328–336.

111. Botella FG, Labios Gomez M, et al. New advances in the knowledge on post-thrombotic syndrome. An Med Interna 2003; 20:483–492.

112. van den Belt AG, Sanson BJ, Simioni P, Prandoni P, et al. Recurrence of venous thromboembolism in patients with familial thrombophilia. Arch Intern Med 1997; 157:2227–2232.

113. Prandoni P, Villalta S, Bagatella P. The clinical course of deep-vein thrombosis. Prospective long-term follow-up of 528 symptomatic patients. Haematologica 1997; 82:423–428.

114. Prandoni P, Lensing AW, Prins MR. The natural history of deep-vein thrombosis. Semin Thromb Hemost 1997; 23:185–188.

115. Hull RD, Raskob GE, Brant RF, et al. Low-molecular-weight heparin vs heparin in the treatment of patients with pulmonary embolism. American-Canadian Thrombosis Study Group. Arch Intern Med 2000; 160:229–236.

116. Meignan M, Rosso J, Gauthier H, et al. Systematic lung scans reveal a high frequency of silent pulmonary embolism in patients with proximal deep venous thrombosis. Arch Intern Med 2000; 160:159–164.

12

Epidemiology of Venous Thrombosis

Patrick Kesteven
Department of Haematology, Freeman Hospital, Newcastle upon Tyne, U.K.

INTRODUCTION

Venous thromboembolic disease (VTE), which includes both deep vein thrombosis (DVT) and pulmonary embolism (PE), is estimated to affect approximately 10:10,000 of the population of northern Europe annually. It has been recognized for over a century that the incidence of DVT increases dramatically with age and is linked with malignancy and pregnancy. Similar links have become apparent with surgery, medical in-patients and long-haul travel. But it is only with the recent identification of prothrombotic plasma abnormalities and physiological variations that the mechanisms involved in these links are beginning to be understood. The challenge, for workers in this field, is to better define these links and to determine the relevant interactions to improve prediction and prevention of VTE.

HISTORICAL PERSPECTIVE

Virchov proposed a triad to explain the possible aetiologies in the establishment of all thromboses: abnormality of blood flow, of blood constituents, or of vessel wall. It is now known that the mechanisms involved in venous thromboses differ markedly from those in arterial thromboses. Rheological factors, in particular sheer stress, activate platelets and are an important precipitator of arterial thromboses, as shown by the effectiveness of anti-platelet agents in prevention. Conversely, platelets play little part in venous thromboses and the mechanisms involved are mainly stasis and a pro-thrombotic coagulant state.

Because the risk factors and responses to treatment are similar, it is widely assumed that DVT and PE are the same disease. However, it should be noted that in either situation recurrences tend to mimic the original thrombosis, suggesting that there may be a particular propensity for one site or the other in the individual.

PATHOPHYSIOLOGY

The pathophysiology of DVT is discussed in chapter 11, but it is important to distinguish between subclinical and overt DVT. Subclinical DVT are frequently initiated in the

143

retro-valvular region of calf veins. Such clots may be detected by I^{131}-labeled fibrinogen scanning or high resolution ultrasound. It is possible that only 10% of these asymptomatic clots progress to a clinical DVT in surgical patients (1).

Similar subclinical DVTs may also occur in up to 10% of people, aged over 50 years age, undertaking long-haul flights (>8 hr) (2). Indeed, 1% of the population may have these events during the course of their every day life (3). The rate of progression from the transient subclinical thrombus to a clinically relevant event is unknown, but differentiation between these two states is crucial to avoid confusion in the interpretation of VTE incidence rates.

INCIDENCE

A large number of studies have reported on the incidence of DVT in the general population. Results have ranged from 5 to 12 per 10,000 patients. Three important explanations for this variation should be considered. The first involves the methodology of the survey. Prospective reports (4,5) are likely to be more accurate than retrospective hospital record or discharge data reviews (6–8). The age of the studied population (see below) and whether autopsies were included in the diagnostic methods are also factors. This last factor is likely to be highly influential as many elderly patients who die in hospitals or nursing homes are found to have pulmonary emboli at postmortem, undiagnosed before death. Indeed, PE is reported in a median of 15% of all postmortem series (9). Consequently, those studies that include such reports are likely to overestimate the true incidence of VTE while those that rely on clinical diagnoses are likely to underestimate it.

A meta-analysis of these studies was performed by Fowkes et al. (10) who reported a weighted mean incidence of first time DVT in the general population of 5.04 (95% CI 4.70–5.38) per 10,000 person years. Weighting was required to compensate for differences between studies in DVT categories and population age structures (10). Taking all cases of VTE, including recurrent DVTs and clinically apparent PEs, the true incidence is likely to be closer to Rosendaal's estimate of 10 per 10,000 person years (11).

Age

All studies have noted a sharply exponential increase in the incidence of DVT with age. Venous thrombosis is most unusual in children (<15 yr) with an incidence of <0.5 per 10,000 patients (9). Almost invariably children with DVTs carry one or more major risk factors for venous thrombosis. By early middle age the incidence rises to approximately 2–3 per 10,000 patients in those aged 30–49 years (10). Incidence rates climb sharply thereafter: in the next decade (50–59 years of age) rates of between 6.2 and 14.7 per 10,000 patients have been reported, and for the 70–79 years age range, to between 31.6 and 76.5 per 10,000 patients (Table 1).

It seems reasonable to assume that some of this increased incidence probably relates to the influence of accumulated risk factors with age, including immobility and malignancy. However, the increase in incidence in the elderly is so dramatic that some related patho/physiological process may be taking place, such as a reduction in endothelial fibrinolytic activity or reduced coagulation inhibitory potential.

Sex

There is no consistent difference in incidence of DVT between the sexes. This indicates the importance of patient selection and its influence on observed incidence rates. Some studies

Table 1 Reported Incidence of DVT in Various Age Brackets (per 10,000 Person Years)

	50–59 Yr	70–79 Yr
Anderson et al. (6)	6.2	31.6
Silverstein et al. (7)	12.2 (females)	44
	14.7 (males)	
Kniffin et al. (8)	–	44.2
Hansson et al. (4)	13.2	52.2
Nordstrom et al. (5)	–	76.5

have shown a slight preponderance of females in the 20- to 40-years-old age bracket, possibly explained by the use of estrogen hormonal medications and pregnancy. In an over 60-year-old population, male VTE disease was in excess. One study showed a slight increased incidence among females aged over 18 years (7.8 vs. 6.3 per 10,000 patients) and attributed this to a higher incidence of women aged > 80 years in the study population (9).

Race

All studies examining the influence of race on the incidence of DVT have shown marked and consistent differences. This is most easily demonstrated in areas with mixed populations. In the west coast of the United States, White et al. reported an annual incidence of idiopathic VTE (> 18 yr of age; per 10,000 persons) of 2.3 among Caucasians; 2.9 among African Americans; 1.4 among Hispanics; and only 0.6 among Asians and Pacific Islanders (12). The same relationship was noted by Klatsky et al. who calculated the relative risk of VTE for the Hispanic population, compared to Caucasians, to be 0.7 (95% CI 0.3–1.5); and for Asians, 0.2 (95% CI 0.1–0.5) (13). In a comparison of VTE rates in 600 autopsies (patients aged > 40 yr) in North America compared to an equal number in Japan, Hirst et al. noted a much higher incidence of PE in the U.S. group (15%) compared to the Japanese group (0.7%) (14).

These differences are possibly due to innate biochemical variations in the coagulation (both pro-coagulant and inhibitory processes) and fibrinolytic systems. For instance, the factor V Leiden mutation is found in ~5% of Caucasians, but only in ~0.5% Asians, ~2% Hispanics, and <1% African Americans (15–17). It should be noted that these figures do not correlate with the DVT incidence figures reported above in these populations, indicating that other factors must be involved. In the plethora of papers examining thromboprophylaxis in orthopaedic surgery, there are reports of a similar incidence of venographically demonstrated post-operative *asymptomatic* vein clots in Thais (18), British Asians (19), and Chinese (20) as compared to Caucasians. This suggests that there may be racial variations in fibrinolytic activity and ability to modify the clot extension process.

Season

Several authors have noted an increased incidence of DVTs in winter (21). This is almost certainly related to other factors, such as reduced physical activity, increased septic episodes, and acute hospital admissions, for all reasons are increased over the winter period.

RISK FACTORS

Two issues need to be considered when examining risk factors for VTE. The first relates to the numerous studies reporting associations between VTE and various clinical conditions or treatments. Such studies are useful in identifying patient groups at risk but do not necessarily point to a specific cause and effect. Consequently, this information may be useful when formulating evidence-based guidelines and policies, but less useful when deciding treatment for an individual patient. We are, therefore, not much further forward than Virchov's triad in understanding the cause and effect of the various factors.

The second issue concerns the fact that VTE behaves as a multi-causal disease, as first proposed by Rosendaal (11). Many patients with VTE carry several risk factors, both long-term, pro-thrombotic tendencies and short-term, thrombosis-precipitating events, which have interacted to cause the venous clot. In some situations, for example long-haul travel, the risk of VTE appears to be moderate when applied to the whole population, but disproportionately significant to those carrying other VTE risk factors.

Thrombophilia

It has long been recognized that an important risk factor for venous thrombosis is the personal or family history of thrombosis and that this condition tended to run in some kindred. In 1965, Egeberg et al. reported a family with antithrombin deficiency, of whom approximately half of affected members suffered a VTE before the age of 25 years (22). Over the next two decades further inherited thrombophilic abnormalities were identified, including Protein C and Protein S deficiency. Despite being potent pro-thrombotic risks, these conditions were found to be relatively rare in the population and had little impact on the incidence of VTE, being found in less than 5% of all VTE cases. However, in 1992 Factor V Leiden was identified, which changed the whole outlook of VTE epidemiology. This mutation is present in 5% of populations of northern European ancestry and is found in approximately 25% of all patients from this population with VTE. The presence of a single Factor V Leiden gene mutation (heterozygote) imparts a seven-fold relative risk of venous thrombosis.

The antibodies found in the anti-phospholipid syndrome may be strongly pro-thrombotic, in both the arterial and venous systems. These are detected as either a lupus anticoagulant (LA—an inhibitor of in-vitro coagulation tests) or anticardiolipin antibodies (aCL). These antibodies may occur in asymptomatic patients and may be transient, especially after viral infections. When associated with thrombosis, thrombocytopenia or foetal loss they form part of the antiphospholipid syndrome which may be primary (idiopathic) or secondary to auto-immune disorders such as SLE (23).

Recently, further plasma derived pro-thrombotic tendencies have been identified including high concentrations of homocysteine, fibrinogen, Factor VIII, Factor IX and prothrombin. Using the cut-off reported in the literature, these physiological variants have a high prevalence in the population, but individually are associated with only a small relative risk of VTE (Table 2) (24). Tables such as these are very powerful epidemiological tools, indicating that a pro-thrombotic coagulation system appears to underlie, and interact with, all other risk factors for VTE. When there is a fuller understanding of these complex plasma factors, and how they interact with clinical risks, it may be possible to determine an individual's absolute risk of VTE.

The high prevalence of these abnormalities in the population gives rise to a problem in definitions. In Europe the term "thrombophilia" is sometimes defined as "disorders of

Table 2 Prevalence (in Controls) and Thrombotic Risk of Various Thrombophilic Abnormalities

	Prevalence	RR
Antithrombin deficiency	0.2	5.0
Protein C deficiency	1	6.5
Prothrombin mutation	2.3	2.8
Protein S deficiency	2.1	1.6
FVLeiden (heterozygote)	5	6.6
FVLeiden (homozygote)	0.1	80
Prothrombin activity (>1.15 U/ml)	20	2.1
FVIIIc activity(>125 iu/ml)	>15	3.0
VWF activity(>125 iu/ml)	>15	1.2

Abbreviations: FVIIIc, Factor VIII clotting activity; VWF, von Willebrand Factor.
Source: From Ref. 24.

the hemostatic mechanisms which are likely to predispose to thrombosis" (Laboratory Thrombophilia). However, it is clear that many of those carrying the Factor V Leiden mutation never suffer any thrombotic event. Furthermore, a thrombophilic abnormality is usually detected in only 50%–60% of VTE patients. In North America the term "thrombophilia" is often reserved for patients who have suffered a spontaneous VTE (i.e., no identifiable risk factors), those who suffer a VTE at an early age, or those with a personal or family history of VTE (clinical thrombophilia). Both definitions have their uses but should be clearly stated: Laboratory thrombophilia is an essential and objective set of criteria and part of the current thinking concerning VTE epidemiology, while clinical thrombophilia may be more useful when considering individual treatment plans.

Cancer

Trousseau noted an association between cancer and thrombosis in 1865 and in himself a few years later. Many epidemiological studies have confirmed this association with reports of 15–25% of patients presenting with an acute idiopathic VTE having cancer. Prospective clinical studies to establish the absolute risk are difficult due to the heterogeneity of cancer type and disease stage. Although venous thrombosis was reported in 30% of pancreatic cancer patients at autopsy (25) the incidence of clinically detectable cases is probably much lower. For instance, in patients with early breast cancer the reported incidence of VTE, in numerous studies, ranged from 0.2 to 9.6% (26). Prandoni has estimated the overall risk of DVT in cancer patients to be double that in non-cancer patients (27).

Due to the strength of the cancer-VTE association, venous thrombosis may frequently be present before the malignancy is clinically apparent. Recent estimates of this occurrence, in cases of idiopathic VTE, ranged from 2.7% to 8.6% (26), to as high as 10% (28). A series of 200 patients presenting with idiopathic VTE were randomized to an extensive search for occult malignancy, or no further investigation. In the investigated group, occult cancer was identified in 13.1% of patients, with a single further case presenting in the 2 years follow-up. In the control group 9.8% developed symptomatic malignancy in the following 2 years. Although the cancers tended to be diagnosed at an earlier stage in the extensively investigated group, there was no evidence that this influenced prognosis. Consequently, it is not common practice to search for occult malignancy in elderly patients with idiopathic VTE, other than by routine, non-invasive measures (28).

One of the problems confronting researchers in this field is the variety of risk factors at play in these cases: advanced age, surgery, immobility, the presence of central venous lines and sepsis are all independent risk factors for DVT. However, different types of cancer are associated with different VTE incidence rates, suggesting that the malignant cells may be having a direct effect. Early reports suggested that the cancers most frequently associated with DVT were lung and pancreas in males and gynaecologic, colorectal and pancreatic tumours in females. This led to the view that mucin-producing tumours were most likely to be responsible (29) and work has subsequently taken place attempting to identify mechanisms. It is known that when monocytes interact with malignant cells, various factors including tissue necrosis factor, interleukin-1 and interleukin-6 may be released. These cause endothelial cell damage, sloughing and produce a pro-thrombotic surface (30). In addition, several cancer cells constituents are known to be pro-thrombotic, such as tissue factor and cysteine proteases. However, more recently it has been suggested that the true incidence of cancer-associated DVT merely parallels the incidence of the specific cancer type itself (26).

Many chemotherapeutic agents are pro-thrombotic. Tamoxifen undoubtedly increases the risk of VTE, although the mechanism is unknown. Regimes containing platinum, asparaginase, high dose fluorouracil and mitomycin are associated with VTE. It is thought these may also act by direct endothelial cell damage. Thalidomide, used for multiple myeloma, is also associated with an increased incidence of VTE. This drug has been shown to affect endothelial cell function as reflected by changes in thrombomodulin levels (an endothelial anticoagulant mechanism) (31). Hormones and cytokines (G-CSF and estrogens) increase the risk of VTE disease.

Surgery

The association between surgery and thrombosis is the most extensively researched. The Worcester DVT study reported that 19% of patients with a first episode VTE had surgery as a predisposing event (6). Similarly, Nordstrom et al. reported surgery within 30 days to be a predisposing factor in 15% of confirmed DVT cases (5). The risk of postoperative VTE is increased by pre-existing risk factors (i.e., age, malignancy, personal or family history of VTE, thrombophilia or obesity). Surgery in the following circumstances was most frequently involved: trauma, orthopaedic, abdominal and genitourinary. This has led to the hypothesis that direct trauma to the veins may be the precipitating event, aggravated by immobility induced by anesthesia. Although local factors may be implicated in some cases, it should be noted that approximately one-third of DVTs after hip replacement occur in the contra-lateral limb. Furthermore, a high incidence of DVTs have been reported 3 weeks after discharge from hospital, in hip replacement patients who were venogram negative at discharge (32). Not surprisingly, these data suggest a continuing pro-thrombotic change to the clotting system, and that this risk may continue for up to three months. The greatest period of risk is during the first week, and the thrombus is thought to be precipitated by the combination of immobility and surgery-related trauma.

Obstetrics

VTE is the leading cause of maternal death in western communities (33). The rate of non-fatal VTE is difficult to determine, as many cases remain undiagnosed. However, the ante-natal incidence of obstetric VTE, in women younger than 35 years of age, has been reported as 0.6 per 1000 pregnancies and double this figure (1.2/1000 pregnancies) in those aged more than 35 years. The incidence of post-natal VTE, in these two age ranges was 0.3/1000 pregnancies and 0.7/1000 pregnancies, respectively (34). Although ante-natal VTE is more frequent, it is the post-natal period, due to its relative brevity, which carries the greatest risk.

There are some important differences between pregnancy associated VTE and other forms of this disorder. Almost 90% of DVT cases in pregnancy occur in the left leg, compared to 55% in other situations (35,36). This is thought to be due to compression of the left iliac vein by the right iliac artery which crosses it, and further occluded by the gravid uterus. Furthermore, approximately 70% of pregnancy associated DVTs are ileo-femoral, compared to only 9% in non pregnant cases (37). This is likely to have major importance clinically as these proximal DVTs embolise more frequently.

DVTs associated with pregnancy fulfill all of Virchov's triad of venous stasis, hypercoaguability and endothelial damage. In normal pregnancy there are increases in the procoagulant factors F VIII, von Willebrand factor, and fibrinogen concentration; a reduction in fibrinolytic activity due to increased levels of placental plasminogen activator inhibitors; and an acquired resistance to activated protein C, a natural anticoagulant. These changes are thought to be a physiological preparation for the hemostatic challenge of delivery and are detectable by the twelfth week of gestation. These pro-coagulant changes increase gradually throughout pregnancy, reaching a peak immediately prior to the onset of labor and taking approximately 6 weeks to return to non pregnant levels (38). The timing of pregnancy-associated VTE appears to parallel these changes with 52% of ante-partum DVTs occurring in the third trimester (39). Damage to the venous endothelium may occur during vaginal delivery or caesarian section, the latter associated with further increase in the incidence of VTE.

Additional risk factors for pregnancy-related VTE are similar to the non pregnant state. These include obesity, family or personal history of thrombosis, and thrombophilia.

Hormone Therapy

The relative risk of VTE associated with the use of oral contraceptives containing > 50 μg estradiol (first and second generation OC) has been estimated to be four-fold (40,41). It was assumed that reducing the concentration of estrogens would reduce this incidence (third generation oral contraceptive tablets), but this has not been observed. Several case control studies have indicated a similar risk with OC containing 30-40 μg estradiol (42,43).

Oral contraceptives containing the progestins levonorgestrel and gestodene are similarly associated with an increased risk of venous thrombosis, although some publications on this issue have been conflicting. Nevertheless, a survey of such reports indicated a six- to nine-fold increased risk compared to non users (44).

Hormone replacement therapy has also been shown to be associated with VTE (45). A large number of studies have shown a relative risk, compared to non-users, of between 3- and 4-fold, irrespective of the type of estrogen or progestin used, or whether taken orally or transdermally. This risk is similar to that observed with oral contraception, despite a much lower dose of estrogens administered, raising further doubts as to whether a dose relationship exists between the estrogen and the risk of VTE. With both oral contraception and hormone replacement therapy, the risk of VTE appears to be greatest over the first one to two years of administration and to take at least three months to abate.

Travel

The link between seated immobility and venous thrombosis was first suggested by Simpson in1940 who examined cases of fatal PE in those who had spent the night in air-raid shelter deck chairs during the blitz (46). The issue was raised again 14 years later by Homans who published five case reports of DVT after prolonged sitting: four of these had traveled (2 by car and 2 by plane), while the fifth case had been to the theater (47). Various case series, of increasing size, were published over the next two decades, including one which introduced the completely erroneous name of "economy class syndrome" (48). Sarvesvaran, who performed autopsies on sudden death cases at Heathrow airport, was able to demonstrate a highly significant difference in rates of PE between those who had recently disembarked, compared to those who were waiting to board (49). In a similar study, Lapostolle, working at Charles de Gaulle Airport, but with PE cases who survived, was able to correlate the incidence of cases with distance traveled (50). All of these studies helped to confirm the existence of this association, but not the strength or magnitude.

Since then, the issue has been clarified by two types of studies. First, prospective studies of travelers, undergoing some kind of VTE diagnostic test both prior to and following long haul flights. These have demonstrated a surprisingly high incidence of sub-clinical DVT in this group, ranging from 1% (51) to 10% (2).

Second, large case-control studies comparing groups with VTE and controls for recent travel (52–54). Although control groups have differed, and sometimes been criticised, these studies have tended to show a small increased relative risk ($\sim$2-fold) of VTE in long-haul travelers, when taking the whole traveling population into account. A much higher RR ($\sim$15-fold) was observed when other risk factors (such as thrombo-philia, past or family history of venous thrombosis, malignancy or estrogen use) were also present.

This is an extremely interesting and important area of research as it is a risk which applies to a very large proportion of the general population. It is estimated that 1.7 million passengers board a plane in the United States daily, and approximately 5 billion world-wide, annually. This population does not usually carry the co-morbidities associated with hospital patients.

Medicine

Medical patients have been shown to be at risk of venous thrombosis (55). The highest incidence of post-mortem PE (in patients dying in the hospital) was found in medical patients (56). It is clear that these medical patients are frequently subject to an accumulation of other risk factors, mentioned above: increasing age, immobility, malignancy (either overt or occult), and inflammation. To this list may be added categories in which the threat of VTE is even greater. Not surprisingly, patients with enforced immobility, such as the very ill or following strokes or spinal cord injury, are included. Approximately 5% of early deaths in stroke patients are attributed to PE (57). Many studies have shown that heart failure is also frequently associated with VTE. Ferrari reported a 28% incidence of congestive cardiac failure in DVT patients in whom no other cause was found (58). Not only are VTE frequently found in medically ill patients, but the strength of the pro-thrombotic risk is also high. The Medenox trial, examining the use of low-molecular weight heparin as thromboprophylaxis in this group of patients, found that the standard surgical thromboprophylactic dose (enoxaparin 20 mg daily) was ineffective. A higher dose (40 mg), used in orthopaedic surgery was required to show benefit (59).

ROSENDAAL'S MULTICAUSAL MODEL AND RECURRENCES

In 1996 Prandoni et al. reported a 30.3% recurrence rate of DVTs over an eight years follow-up (60). Kearon et al. selecting only patients without clear precipitating causes for their VTE, found a recurrence rate of 27.4% per patient year (61). Subsequent studies have confirmed these findings, demonstrating a cumulative recurrence rate of approximately 6% per annum, extending for at least five years.

All of the individual risk factors described above have demonstrated an additive effect if yet other risk factors are present. For instance, long-haul travelers taking the oral contraceptive, cancer patients with central lines, pregnancy and obesity, almost any risk and Factor V Leiden mutation. These examples confirm the value of Rosendaal's multicausal model, which describes the often seen accumulation of multiple risk factors to the point when a clinically apparent VTE develops (11). The usefulness of this model is in the assistance it gives in deciding degrees of thrombo-prophylaxis required, or duration of treatment, in individual cases. In those instances in which a VTE was precipitated by an obvious and potent factor (i.e., caesarean section, hip replacement surgery or long-haul travel) the risk of recurrence appears to be low once the precipitating factor has been removed (62). The corollary also appears to be true. In those patients who suffer a VTE with no apparent risk factors (sometimes called "spontaneous") the multicausal model predicts that there must exist underlying risk factors (probably in the coagulation system and probably long-term). This is reflected in clinical practice with a very high incidence of recurrence in these patients.

The challenge is to determine the strength of the associations discussed above, the mechanisms of action, and most importantly, the interactions between such risks. Various authors have discussed a risk scoring system. Unfortunately this requires a better understanding of the clotting system, as well as an array of expensive laboratory testing.

KEY POINTS

- Many of the causes of VTE may be anticipated from Virchov's triad, which attributed intra vascular thrombosis to an abnormality of blood flow, blood constituent, or vessel wall.
- It is important to distinguish subclinical DVT from clinically overt cases when considering the epidemiology of VTE.
- The incidence of VTE in the whole population has been estimated to be 10 per 10,000 per annum.
- The incidence of VTE increases exponentially with age, and there are ethnic variations in this incidence.
- VTE acts as a multicausal phenomenon, often requiring several risk factors to coincide for a clinically significant venous thrombosis to occur.
- The plasma thrombophilic abnormalities appear to interact with all other clinical risk factors for VTE.

REFERENCES

1. Kakkar VV, Howe CT, Flanc C, et al. Natural history of postoperative deep-vein thrombosis. Lancet 1969; 7614:230–232.
2. Scurr JH, Machin SJ, Bailey-King S, et al. Frequency and prevention of symptomless deep-vein thrombosis in long-haul flights: a randomised trial. Lancet 2001; 357:1485–1489.
3. Schwartz T, Siegert G, Oettler W, et al. Venous thrombosis after long-haul flights. Arch Intern Med 2003; 163:2759–2764.
4. Hansson PO, Welin L, Tibblin G, et al. Deep vein thrombosis and pulmonary embolism in the general population. "The study of men born in 1913." Arch Intern Med 1997; 157:1665–1670.
5. Nordstrom M, Lindblad B, Bergqvist D, et al. A prospective study of the incidence of deep-vein thrombosis within a defined urban population. J Intern Med 1992; 232:155–160.
6. Anderson FA, Jr., Wheeler HB, Goldberg RJ, et al. A population-based perspective of the hospital incidence and case-fatality rates of deep vein thrombosis and pulmonary embolism. The Worcester DVT Study. Arch Intern Med 1991; 151:933–938.
7. Silverstein MD, Heit JA, Mohr DN, et al. Trends in the incidence of deep vein thrombosis and pulmonary embolism: a 25-year population-based study. Arch Intern Med 1998; 158:585–593.
8. Kniffin WD, Jr., Baron JA, Barrett J, et al. The epidemiology of diagnosed pulmonary embolism and deep vein thrombosis in the elderly. Arch Intern Med 1994; 154:861–866.
9. White RH. The Epidemiology of Venous Thromboembolism. Circulation 2003; 107:1–4.
10. Fowkes FJ, Price JF, Fowkes FG. Incidence of diagnosed deep vein thrombosis in the general population: systematic review. Eur J Vasc Endovasc Surg 2003; 25:1–5.
11. Rosendaal FR. Thrombosis series: Venous thrombosis: a multicausal disease. Lancet 1993; 353:1167–1173.
12. White RH, Zhou H, Romano PS, et al. Incidence of idiopathic deep venous thrombosis and secondary thromboembolism among ethnic groups in California. Ann Intern Med 1998; 128:737–740.
13. Klatsky AL, Armstrong MA, Poggi J. Risk of pulmonary embolism and/or deep venous thrombosis in Asian-Americans. Am J Cardiol 2000; 85:1334–1337.
14. Hirst AE, Gore I, Tanaka K, et al. Myocardial infarction and pulmonary embolism. Arch Pathol 1965; 80:365–370.
15. Ridker PM, Miletich JP, Hennekens CH, et al. Ethnic distribution of factor V Leiden in 4047 men and women. Implications for venous thromboembolism screening. JAMA 1997; 277:1305–1307.
16. Gregg JP, Yamane AJ, Grody WW. Prevalence of the factor V-Leiden mutation in four distinct American ethnic populations. Am J Med Genet 1997, 73:334–336.
17. Angchaisuksiri P, Pingsuthiwong S, Aryuchai K, et al. Prevalence of the G1691A mutation in the factor V gene (factor V Leiden) and the G20210A prothrombin gene mutation in the Thai population. Am J Haematol 2000; 65:119–122.
18. Atichartakarn V, Pathepchotiwong K, Keorochan S, et al. Deep vein thrombosis after hip surgery among Thai. Arch Intern Med 1988; 148:1349–1353.
19. Dhillon KS, Askander A, Doraismay S. Postoperative deep-vein thrombosis in Asian patients is not a rarity: a prospective study of 88 patients with no prophylaxis. J Bone Joint Surg Br 1996; 78:427–430.
20. Mok K, Hoaglund FT, Rogoff SM, et al. The incidence of deep vein thrombosis in Hong Kong Chinese after hip surgery for fracture of the proximal femur. Br J Surg 1979; 66:640–642.
21. Gallerani M, Boari B, de Toma D, et al. Seasonal variation in the occurrence of deep vein thrombosis. Med Sci Monit 2004; 10:191–196.
22. Egeberg O. Inherited antithrombin deficiency causing Thrombophilia. Thromb Diathesis Haemorrhagica 1965; 13:516–530.

23. Proven A, Bartlett R, Moder K, et al. Clinical importance of positive test results for lupus anticoagulant and anticardiolipin antibodies. Mayo Clinic Proc 2004; 79:467–476.

24. Van der Meer F, Koster T, Vandenbroucke E, et al. The Leiden Thrombophilia Study (LETS). Thromb Haemostas 1997; 78:631–635.

25. Sproul EE. Carcinoma and venous thrombosis: the frequency of association of carcinoma in the body or tail of the pancreas with multiple venous thrombosis. Am J Cancer 1938; 34:566–585.

26. Lee AY, Levine MN. Venous thromboembolism and cancer: risks and outcomes. Circulation 2003; 107:1–17.

27. Prandoni P. Cancer and thromboembolic disease: how important is the risk of thrombosis. Cancer Treat Rev 2002; 28:133–136.

28. Piccioli A, Lensing AW, Prins MH, et al. Extensive screening for occult malignant disease in idiopathic venous thromboembolism: a prospective randomized clinical trial. J Thromb Haemostas 2004; 2:884–889.

29. Lieberman JS, Borrero J, Urdanetam E, et al. Thrombophlebitis and cancer. JAMA 1961; 177:542–545.

30. Bick RL. Cancer-associated thrombosis. NEJM 2003; 349:109–111.

31. Corso A, Lorenzi A, Terulla V, et al. Modification of thrombomodulin plasma levels in refractory myeloma patients during treatment with thalidomide and dexamethosone. Ann Hematol 2004; 83:588–591.

32. Planes A, Vochelle M, Darmon JY, et al. Risk of deep venous thrombosis after hospital discharge in patients having undergone total hip replacement. Double-blind randomised comparison of enoxaparin versus placebo. Lancet 1996; 348:224–228.

33. Greer IA. Thrombosis in pregnancy: maternal and fetal issues. Lancet 1999; 353:1258–1265.

34. Macklon NS, Greer IA, Bowman AW. An ultrasound study of gestational and postural changes in the deep venous system of the leg in pregnancy. Br J Obstet Gynaecol 1997; 104:191–197.

35. McColl M, Ramsay JE, Tait RC, et al. Risk factors for pregnancy associated venous thromboembolism. Thromb Haemostas 1997; 78:1183–1188.

36. Lindhagen A, Bergqvist A, Bergqvist D, et al. Late venous function in the leg after deep venous thrombosis occuring in relation to pregnancy. Br J Obstet Gynaecol 1986; 93:348–352.

37. Greer IA. The acute management of venous thromboembolism in pregnancy. Curr Opin Obstet Gynecol 2001; 13:569–575.

38. Macklon NS, Greer IA. Venous thromboembolic disease in obstetrics and gynaecology: the Scottish experience. Scot Med J. 1996; 41:8386.

39. Gerhardt A, Scharf RE, Beckman MW, et al. Prothrombin and Factor V mutations in women with a history of thrombosis during pregnancy and the puerperium. N Engl J Med 2000; 342:374 380.

40. Stadel V. Oral contraceptives and cardiovascular disease. N Engl J Med 1981; 305:612–618.

41. Helmrich SP, Rosenberg L, Kaufman DW, et al. Venous thromboembolism in relation to oral contraceptive use. Obstet Gynecol 1987; 69:91–95.

42. Venous WHO. Thromboembolic disease and combined oral contraceptives: results of an international multicentre case-control study. World Health Organization Collaborative Study of Cardiovascular Disease and Steroid Hormone Contraception. Lancet 1995; 346:1575–1582.

43. Vandenbroucke JP, Rosing J, Bloemenkamp KW, et al. Oral contraceptives and the risk of venous thrombosis. N Engl J Med 2001; 344:1527–1535.

44. Brenner BR, Nowak-Gottl U, Kosch A, et al. Diagnostic studies for Thrombophilia in women on hormonal therapy and during pregnancy, and in children. Arch Path Lab Med 2002; 126:1296–1304.

45. Kim V, Spandorfer J. Epidemiology of Venous Thromboembolic Disease. Emerg Med Clin North Am 2001; 19:839–859.

46. Simpson K. Shelter deaths from pulmonary embolism. Lancet 1940; 11:744–745.

47. Homans J. Thrombosis of the deep leg veins due to prolonged sitting. New Engl J Med 1954; 250:148–149.
48. Cruickshank JM, Gorlin R, Jennett B. Air travel and thrombotic episodes: the economy class syndrome. Lancet 1988; ii:497–498.
49. Sarvesvaran R. Sudden natural deaths associated with commercial air travel. Med Sci Law 1986; 26:35–38.
50. Lapostolle F, Surget V, Borron SW, et al. Severe pulmonary embolism associated with air travel. New Engl J Med 2001; 345:779–783.
51. Hughes RJ, Hopkins RJ, Hill S, et al. Frequency of venous thromboembolism in low to moderate risk long distance air travellers: the New Zealand Air Traveller's Thrombosis (NZATT) study. Lancet 2003; 362:2039–2044.
52. Ferrari E, Chevallier T, Chapelier A, et al. Travel as a risk factor for venous thromboembolic disease: a case-control study. Chest 1999; 115:440–444.
53. Martinelli I, Taioli E, Battaolioli T, et al. Risk of venous thromboembolism after air travel: interaction with thrombophilia and oral contraceptives. Arch Intern Med 2003; 163:2771–2774.
54. Kraaijenhagen R, Haverkamp D, Koopman M, et al. Travel and risk of venous thrombosis. Lancet 2000; 356:1492–1493.
55. Bouthier J. The venous thrombotic risk in nonsurgical patients. Drugs 1996; 52:16–29.
56. Lindblad B, Sternby N, Bergqvist D. Incidence of venous thromboembolism verified by necropsy over 30 yr. Brit Med J 1991; 302:709–771.
57. Clagett GP, Anderson FA, Geerts W, et al. Prevention on venous thromboembolism (Fifth ACCP Consensus Conference on Antithrombotic Therapy). Chest 1998; 114:531–560.
58. Ferrari E, Baodouy M, Cerboni P, et al. Clinical epidemiology of venous thromboembolic disease: Results of a French multicentre registry. Eur Heart j 1997; 18:685–691.
59. Samama MM, Cohen AT, Darmon JY, et al. A comparison of enoxaparin with placebo for the prevention of venous thromboembolism in acutely ill medical patients. Prophylaxis in medical patients with enoxaparin study group. N Engl J Med 1999; 341:793–800.
60. Prandoni P, Lensing A, Cogo A, et al. The long-term clinical course of acute deep venous thrombosis. Ann Int Med 1996; 125:1–7.
61. Kearon C, Gent M, Weitz J, et al. A comparison of three months of anticoagulation with extended anticoagulation for a first episode of idiopathic venous thromboembolism. NEJM 1999; 340:901–907.
62. Palareti G, Cosmi B. Predicting the risk of recurrence of venous thromboembolism. Curr Opin Hematol 2004; 11:192–197.

13

Venous Thromboembolism and Malignant Diseases

Paolo Prandoni and Andrea Piccioli
Department of Medical and Surgical Sciences, University of Padua, Padua, Italy

Anna Falanga
Department of Haematology–Oncology, Ospedali Riuniti, Bergamo, Italy

Thromboembolism is a well-recognized complication of malignant disease. Clinical manifestations vary from venous thromboembolism (VTE) to disseminated intravascular coagulation, more commonly observed in patients with haematological malignancies and those with widespread metastatic cancer, to arterial embolism, more commonly observed in patients undergoing chemotherapy and in those with non-bacterial thrombotic endocarditis. This overview will focus on the relationship between cancer and VTE.

PATHOGENESIS OF THROMBOSIS IN CANCER

Cancer growth is associated with the development of a hypercoagulable state in the host. Patients with malignancy without thrombosis commonly present with abnormalities in laboratory coagulation tests, demonstrating an ongoing process of fibrin formation and removal at different rates (1). Importantly, fibrin and other clot components play a role not only in thrombogenesis but also in tumor spread and metastasis (2). Histopathology studies have long demonstrated the presence of fibrin or platelet plugs in and around many types of tumors (3), suggesting a local activation of blood coagulation and an involvement of clotting mechanisms in the growth of malignant tissues.

Prothrombotic Mechanisms

The activation of blood coagulation in patients with cancer is complex and multifactorial (4). General prothrombotic mechanisms are related to the host response to cancer and include the acute-phase reaction, paraprotein production, inflammation, necrosis, and hemodynamic disorders. Procoagulant effects are also exerted by anticancer therapies (i.e., chemo or radiotherapy). However, a prominent role is played by tumor-specific clot promoting mechanisms represented by the prothrombotic properties expressed by tumor cells themselves. These properties are unique to the malignant state.

Malignant cells are able to activate blood coagulation in multiple ways, as follows: (1) producing procoagulant, fibrinolytic, and proaggregating activities; (2) releasing proinflammatory and proangiogenic cytokines; and (3) interacting directly with host vascular and blood cells, i.e., endothelial cells, leukocytes, and platelets, by means of adhesion molecules.

Procoagulant, Fibrinolytic, and Proaggregating Activities

Tumor cell produce their own procoagulant factors, among which the most studied are Tissue Factor (TF) and Cancer Procoagulant (CP) (5). TF, the primary activator of normal blood coagulation, forms a complex with Factor VII to proteolytically activate Factors X and IX. In normal vascular cells, TF expression is tightly controlled, so it normally is not expressed, but is induced by inflammatory stimuli, such as the cytokines interleukin-1β (IL-1β), tumor necrosis factor-α (TNF-α), and bacterial lipopolysaccharides. In malignant cells, however, TF is constitutively expressed. Differently, CP is a cysteine proteinase that directly activates Factor X independently of FVII, and has been found in tumor cells and in amnion-chorion tissues but not in normal differentiated cells. TF and CP have been identified in several human and animal tumor tissues (6). The evidence that the resolution by all-trans-retinoic acid of the severe coagulopathy of patients with acute promyelocytic leukemia is associated to a parallel loss of cellular procoagulants from bone marrow blast cells, strongly supports a role for tumor procoagulants in the clotting complications of malignancy (7).

Tumor cells can express all proteins regulating the fibrinolytic system, including the urokinase-type and tissue-type plasminogen activators (u-PA and t-PA), PA inhibitors (PAI-1 and PAI-2), and PA receptor (u-PAR) (8). The increase in plasma levels of PA inhibitors and impairment in plasma fibrinolytic activity in patients with solid tumors represent another tumor-associated prothrombotic mechanisms.

Tumor cells induce platelet activation and aggregation by a direct cell–cell contact or by releasing soluble factors, such as ADP, thrombin and other proteases (9). Circulating activated platelets expose on their surface the activation-dependent antigens P-selectin and CD63, and upon aggregation release their granule contents. Further, they increase their capacity to interact through specific adhesive mechanisms with endothelial cells, leukocytes, and blood borne tumor cells.

Tumor Cell-Derived Cytokines

Tumor cells produce and release various cytokines, including TNF-α, IL-1β and vascular endothelial growth factor (VEGF), which can be involved in the onset of thrombotic disorders of cancer patients (10). The major targets of tumor-derived cytokines are the vascular endothelium and leukocytes. TNF-α and IL-1β induce the expression of endothelial TF, and down-regulate the expression of thrombomodulin, the endothelial surface high-affinity receptor for thrombin, that complex thrombin to activate the protein C anticoagulant system. Taken together, TF up-regulation and thrombomodulin down-regulation lead to a prothrombotic condition of the vascular wall. The same cytokines highly stimulate the production of fibrinolysis inhibitor PAI-1, thus impairing the endothelial antithrombotic response. Tumor-derived VEGF also induces TF expression by endothelial cells, with implications for TF in tumor neovascularization (11). Finally, cytokines induce changes in endothelial cell adhesion molecule expression, increasing the capacity of the vessel wall to attract leukocyte and platelets and promoting localized clotting activation and fibrin formation.

Similar to endothelial cells, monocytes are activated by tumor cells and/or tumor cell products to express TF on their surface (12). Tumor-associated macrophages harvested from experimental and human tumors express significantly more TF than control cells, and circulating monocytes from patients with different types of cancer show increased TF activity. Tumor cytokines also attract and activate polymorphonuclear leukocytes (PMN), which release reactive oxygen species and intracellular proteases that possess several activities on endothelial cells and platelets, modifying the hemostatic balance towards a prothrombotic state (13).

Cell–Cell Interactions

The presence of cell adhesion molecules on the surface of tumor cells warranties the possibility to directly interact with the host cell. During the hematogenous spread, this interaction occurs with endothelial cells, platelets, and leukocytes. The tumor cell capacity to adhere to both resting and cytokine-stimulated endothelium is well described and adhesion molecule pathways specific to different tumor cell types have been identified (2,4). Malignant cells attached to the vessel wall promote localized clotting activation and thrombus formation, and favour the adhesion and arrest of leukocytes and platelets by releasing their cytokine content. Cancer cells also directly activate platelets, adhere and migrate through the vessel wall and are assisted by PMN in their interaction with endothelial cells.

Prothrombotic Mechanisms and Tumor Progression

Tumor-specific prothrombotic properties may contribute to the process of tumor growth and dissemination. The formation of thrombin, the final effector enzyme of the clotting cascade, and fibrin, the final product of the activation of blood coagulation, represent coagulation-dependent mechanisms of tumor progression. In addition to that, tumor prothrombotic properties can interfere with the malignant process by coagulation-independent mechanisms. Relevant in this setting is the emerging role of the non-coagulant activities of TF (2), particularly TF capacity to modulate VEGF expression by malignant cells and normal vascular cells. This property regulates tumor neo-vascularization and provides an important link in cancer patients between activation of coagulation, inflammation, thrombosis and cancer growth and metastasis (14).

EPIDEMIOLOGY AND RISK FACTORS OF THROMBOEMBOLISM IN CANCER PATIENTS

Since the initial observation by Armand Trousseau in 1865, numerous studies have addressed the relationship between cancer and venous VTE. VTE is either a frequent complication in cancer patients, or sometimes acts as an epiphenomenon of a hidden cancer, in such a way offering opportunities for anticipated cancer diagnosis and treatment (15). In patients with malignancy VTE represents an important cause of morbidity and mortality. It has been calculated that one of every seven hospitalized cancer patients dies due to pulmonary embolism (PE) (16). Of these patients, 60% have localized cancer or limited metastatic disease, which would have allowed for longer survival in the absence of a fatal PE. According to the Medicare Provider Analysis and Review Record database that records the primary discharge diagnosis and an additional four discharge diagnoses in the United States, the rate of initial or recurrent thromboembolism in patients with cancer exceeds by far that recorded in those without malignancy, and affects with similar frequency virtually all body systems (17).

Although the true rate of VTE in cancer patients is virtually unknown, because of the surprising lack of information in almost all studies dealing with the natural history of malignant diseases, the majority of thrombotic episodes occur spontaneously, i.e., in the absence of triggering factors commonly accounting for thromboembolic complications in subjects without cancer. This is confirmed by the high frequency of patients with known malignancy referred to clinicians for the development of VTE (18). The most common situations that make cancer patients at higher risk of VTE include immobilization, surgery, chemotherapy with or without adjuvant therapy, and the insertion of central venous catheters (19).

Immobilization

One of the most important triggering factors for VTE is prolonged immobilization, especially during hospital stay. This pattern was clearly confirmed by Shen and Pollack, who reported that as many as 14% of cancer patients admitted to the hospital died of autopsy-confirmed PE, compared with 8% of those who were free from cancer (20).

Surgery

In the absence of adequate prophylaxis, patients with active malignancy face a markedly high risk of developing postoperative VTE. In the absence of thromboprophylaxis, the overall incidence of postoperative deep vein thrombosis (DVT) in patients with cancer is about twice as high as that in patients free from malignancy (Table 1) (15,21).

Many factors can account for this high frequency, including advanced age, long and complicated surgical procedures, and late mobilization with long postoperative course due to patient's poor condition. If thromboprophylaxis is not prolonged beyond the hospital stay, cancer patients remain at risk of developing late VTE complications (29,30).

Chemotherapy, Radiotherapy, and Adjuvant Hormone Therapy

Cancer patients also face a particularly high risk of developing both venous and arterial thrombosis when they receive chemotherapy (31). In patients with high-grade glioma

Table 1   Postoperative DVT in Patients With and Without Cancer

Authors	Patients with cancer	Patients without cancer
Kakkar et al. (1970) (22)	24/59 (41%)	38/144 (26%)
Walsh et al. (1974) (23)	16/45 (35%)	22/217 (10%)
Rosenberg et al. (1975) (24)	28/66 (42%)	29/128 (23%)
Sue-Ling et al. (1986) (25)	12/23 (52%)	16/62 (26%)
Allan et al. (1983) (26)	31/100 (31%)	21/100 (21%)
Multicentre Trial et al. (1984) (27)	9/37 (22%)	13/53 (24%)
Hills et al. (1972) (28)	8/16 (50%)	7/34 (21%)
Overall	128/346 (37%)	146/738 (20%)

undergoing chemotherapy, the incidence of thromboembolic complications may be as high as 12%–16% (32–34). In a small series of patients with nonresectable or metastatic colonic tumor, the incidence of chemotherapy-induced thromboembolic complications has been reported as high as 17% (35). In a recent retrospective study conducted in a wide series of cancer patients who had been administered chemotherapy, the rate of thrombo-embolic complications arising within the first three months was unexpectedly high, yielding to an annual incidence of 11% (36).

The most reliable estimate of thromboembolic complications in patients undergoing chemotherapy comes from breast cancer patients. The incidence of chemotherapy-induced thromboembolic complications in women with stage II breast cancer undergoing chemo-therapy was found to be on average 7% in a wide series of studies dealing with this risk (Table 2) (37). Among patients with stage IV breast cancer this risk was found to be even higher (49). Adjuvant hormone therapy, alone or in combination with chemotherapy, cancer stage, and postmenopausal state further increases the incidence of thromboembo-lism in women with breast cancer (50,51).

Although radiotherapy is often advocated as a risk factor of VTE in cancer patients, no study has as yet properly evaluated its role.

Central Venous Catheters

Long-term central venous catheters have considerably improved the management of cancer patients. However, their use has been associated with the occurrence of upper limb DVT, especially in those patients who require the administration of chemotherapy (52).

The true incidence of DVT in patients with central venous lines is difficult to estimate, since data from literature are somehow conflicting. In absence of thromboprophylaxis, Bern et al. found an incidence of DVT, as shown by phlebography, of 37% (53). Monreal et al. found an even higher incidence (54). Conversely, in recent case series that adopted ultrasonography or other non-invasive methods to detect upper limb DVT, a much lower rate of this thrombotic disorder has been reported (52,55). Along with the lower sensitivity of objective non invasive methods in comparison with phlebography, the introduction of new texture and coating of catheters, as well as of new procedures to reduce their invasiveness, is likely to account for discrepancies between older and more recent studies.

Table 2 Thromboembolism in Breast Cancer Patients Undergoing Chemotherapy

Authors	Patients	Stage	Thrombosis	Type
Weiss et al. (1981) (38)	433	II	5%	V
Goodnough et al. (1984) (39)	159	IV	17.6%	V + A
Levine et al. (1988) (40)	205	II	7%	V + A
Wall et al. (1989) (41)	1014	Variable	1.3%	A
Fisher et al. (1989) (42)	383	II	3%	V
Saphner et al. (1991) (43)	2352	Variable	5%	V + A
Clahsen et al. (1994) (44)	1292	Variable	2%	V
Rifkin et al. (1994) (45)	603	II	2.5%	V + A
Pritchard et al. (1996) (46)	353	II	9.6%	V + A
Tempelhoff et al. (1996) (47)	50	II	10%	V
Orlando et al. (2000) (48)	182	Variable	7.7%	V

Abbreviations: V, venous; A, arterial.

THROMBOPROPHYLAXIS

The principal objective of thromboprophylaxis in the cancer patients is to reduce the incidence of fatal PE. Indeed, most of these patients do not live long enough to develop postthrombotic sequelae.

Although patients with active cancer often develop thrombotic complications spontaneously, i.e., in the absence of additional risk factors, there is probably little rationale behind providing thromboprophylaxis to all cancer patients who are not receiving surgical or medical therapy. However, a history of thromboembolism places cancer patients at such a high risk of recurrences that the systematic use of either mechanical or pharmacological prophylaxis may be considered even outside the common risk factors of thrombosis.

Prevention of VTE in cancer patients represents an important challenge since cancer patients experiencing a thrombotic episode have a poor outcome with greater probability of death.

Surgical Interventions

According to widely accepted guidelines, low-molecular-weight heparin (LMWH) in low doses, low-dose unfractionated heparin or physical measures should be adopted in cancer patients who require prolonged immobilization or undergo low-risk surgical procedures (56). Extensive surgery places cancer patients at a remarkably high risk of post-operative VTE. Accordingly, these patients require more intensive prophylactic regimens such as higher doses of LMWHs (on average, twice as high as those suggested for low-risk procedures), adjusted-dose heparin, or oral anticoagulants (56).

Once daily injections of LMWH are at least as effective and safe as multiple injections of unfractionated heparin for prevention of postoperative VTE in cancer patients (57–59). In this setting, fondaparinux (a short-acting pentasaccharide) shows promise. In a recent trial addressing the value of fondaparinux, 2.5 mg o.i.d., for prevention of postoperative VTE in patients requiring major abdominal surgery, in the subgroup of patients with cancer fondaparinux was shown to be significantly more effective than dalteparin without increasing the hemorrhagic risk (60).

Of interest, recent trials suggest that prolonging the administration of LMWH until the completion of the first four weeks after surgical intervention provides an additional thromboprophylactic effect without increasing the hemorrhagic risk (30,61).

In patients with ongoing bleeding or those who are at high risk for it, physical measures such as graduated compression stockings or external pneumatic compression should be used in the substitution for pharmacological prophylaxis (62).

According to the results of two recent randomized trials in cancer patients undergoing elective neurosurgery, the combination of LMWH (starting within 24 hr after surgery) with graduated compression stockings is more effective than, and as safe as, elastic stockings alone for prevention of postoperative VTE (63,64).

Chemotherapy and Radiotherapy

In the only available study, fixed low-dose warfarin (1 mg/day) for six weeks, followed by doses that maintained the INR at 1.3 to 1.9, was an effective and safe method for prevention of chemotherapy-induced thromboembolism in women with metastatic breast cancer (65). Whether this strategy or strategies that involve LMWHs are effective and safe, as well in other oncologic patterns, remains to be demonstrated.

Unfortunately, no proper study has been performed as yet to assess the preventive value of antithrombotic strategies in patients undergoing radiotherapy.

Central Venous Catheters

Two randomized, controlled studies documented the benefit of fixed low-dose warfarin (1 mg o.i.d.) in decreasing the incidence of arm vein thrombosis related to indwelling central venous catheters (53,66). The subcutaneous administration of dalteparin (2500 IU o.i.d.) for 90 days was also shown to be highly beneficial for prevention of upper extremity thrombosis in cancer patients with venous access devices (54). However, three recent clinical trials failed to show any benefit from a 1 mg daily dose of warfarin (67,68) or 5000 daily units of dalteparin (69), respectively, compared to no prophylaxis. Thus, neither mini-dose warfarin nor prophylactic LMWH can be recommended on a routine basis as prophylaxis for cancer patients with indwelling central venous lines (56). Either thromboprophylactic regimen, however, is likely to be effective whenever central venous catheters are used for administration of chemotherapy (70).

TREATMENT OF ESTABLISHED VENOUS THROMBOEMBOLISM

Initial Treatment

In general, the same therapeutic approaches that are used in non cancer patients are also used in patients with malignant diseases. Except for selected patients requiring aggressive treatments, the large majority of cancer patients should receive the subcutaneous injection of therapeutic doses (adjusted to body weight) of a LMWH in once or twice daily administrations. Alternatively, a proper course of full-dose unfractionated heparin, i.e., a heparin regimen that prolongs the APTT up to 1.5 to 3.0 times the control value, can be employed (56). Whenever possible, (LMW) heparin should be administered as soon as there is a reasonable possibility that venous thrombosis exists, and should be overlapped and followed by oral anticoagulant therapy (56). Thrombolytic drugs are rarely indicated. The limited cases in which thrombolysis may be considered include massive pulmonary embolism, extension of venous thrombosis despite extensive anticoagulation, and upper-extremity thrombosis in patients who have an indwelling central venous catheter, which must be kept patent (56). Finally, the insertion of an inferior vena cava filter should be considered whenever a full-dose anticoagulation is contraindicated or unsuccessful.

There are many unique issues in cancer patients that often make treatment more difficult. Chemotherapy, hormonal agents, invasive procedures and the presence of long-term venous catheters not only increase the risk of thrombosis but also create complex clinical situations that make anticoagulation particularly problematic. For example, temporary cessation of anticoagulant therapy may be needed to accommodate chemotherapy-induced thrombocytopenia and invasive procedures, while poor nutrition, infection, concomitant medication and impaired liver function can cause unpredictable changes in the dose response of oral anticoagulants.

Long-Term Anticoagulation

What are the main questions clinicians confront when facing cancer patients with an episode of venous thrombosis? The main controversies deal with the most appropriate duration and intensity of anticoagulation; the risk of extension and/or recurrence of VTE during anticoagulation; and the potential for an increased risk of bleeding during the course of proper anticoagulant therapy.

According to the results of recent prospective cohort and population-based studies (71–73), after discontinuation of warfarin cancer patients with venous thrombosis present a risk for recurrences that is almost twice as high as that observed in patients free from malignancies. In view of the persistently high risk of recurrent thrombotic events and the acceptable risk of bleeding, prolongation of warfarin should be considered for as long as the malignant disorder is active. The suggested policy is to administer warfarin to maintain the INR between 2.0 and 3.0.

Of interest, cancer patients have a three- to four-fold higher risk of recurrent VTE while on anticoagulation (74–76). This risk correlates with the extent of cancer. Accordingly, more aggressive initial or long-term treatment has the potential to reduce the risk of recurrent thrombosis. However, a complicating factor in improving anticoagulant therapy in cancer patients is the occurrence of excess bleeding in combination with excess recurrent thromboembolism. Although some improvements can be expected from optimizing laboratory monitoring of anticoagulant therapy, most bleeding and thrombotic complications occur in patients with anticoagulant parameters within the therapeutic range. Possibilities for improvement using the current paradigms of anticoagulation seem, therefore, limited.

According to the results of recent randomized clinical trials, LMWH in full doses for the first month followed by three-fourth of the initial regimen has the potential to provide a more effective antithrombotic regimen in cancer patients with venous thrombosis than the conventional treatment, and is not associated with an increased hemorrhagic risk (77,78). Although LMWHs are more expensive than oral anticoagulants, they provide an anticoagulation that is easier to administer, more convenient and flexible, and not influenced by nutrition problems or liver impairment.

The anticoagulation strategy in the treatment of patients with recurrent VTE during oral anticoagulation is not rigidly standardized. A patient who develops a recurrent VTE while the INR is subtherapeutic can be retreated with unfractionated or LMWH for a few days, and oral anticoagulant therapy can be continued with the INR kept between 2.0 and 3.0. For those who experience warfarin failure and develop a recurrence while the INR is therapeutic, the long-term management is less clear. Three options are acceptable after initial re-treatment with unfractionated or LMWH: continue with oral anticoagulant therapy aiming for a higher target INR of 3.0 to 3.5, switch to adjusted-dose twice daily subcutaneous standard heparin to maintain a therapeutic APTT, or use once daily weight-dose LMWH For patients with a high risk of pulmonary embolism, or who are hemodynamically unstable, an inferior vena cava filter can be inserted in addition to any one of the above options.

IMPACT OF ANTITHROMBOTIC DRUGS ON CANCER EVOLUTION AND DEVELOPMENT

Anticoagulant treatment of cancer patients, particularly those with lung cancer, has been reported to improve survival (79). These interesting, albeit preliminary, results of controlled trials lent some support to the argument that activation of blood coagulation plays a role in the natural history of tumor growth.

Numerous studies have been performed in recent years that have addressed the value of LMWH in comparison with standard heparin in the treatment of VTE, and an updated meta-analysis of the most adequate reports has been published in 2000 (80). In eight of the nine studies reporting on the long-term follow-up of enrolled patients, the analysis of total mortality exhibited a surprising trend in favour of LMWH. In the five studies that provided subgroups analysis, this effect was entirely attributable to the differences in the subgroup of patients with cancer.

Which is the rationale for the antitumor effect of anticoagulant drugs? In the last decades, strategies to impair the hemostatic system of the host in order to affect the growth and the dissemination of malignant tumors have been explored (81). The biological mechanisms of coumarins mainly rely on the inhibition of blood coagulation (coagulation-dependent mechanisms). Instead the biological mechanisms of heparins, particularly LMWH, in addition to clotting inhibition, involve coagulation-independent activities able to affect: (1) tumor cell growth by binding to growth factors, (2) tumor cell invasion by heparin-inhibitable enzyme systems, (3) tumor cell metastasis by binding to cell surface selectins (presumably by competing with these ligands), (4) tumor-induced angiogenesis by interacting with angiogenic growth factor, (5) tumor matrix formation related to deposition of fibrinogen/fibrin, and (6) tumor cell invasion of the vascular basement membrane by inhibiting tumor cell heparanase (82).

The evidence of lowered cancer mortality in patients on LMWH has stimulated renewed interest in these agents as antineoplastic drugs. Three small randomized studies have recently compared the long-term survival of cancer patients receiving conventional treatment with that of patients receiving a supplementary dose of LMWH in therapeutic or prophylactic doses (83–85). All three studies showed a favorable impact of the tested heparin on patients' survival. This result was particularly evident in patients with better prognosis. Further studies on wider samples of patients are needed before LMWH can be implemented in the routine treatment of patients with cancer.

Of interest, in a recent trial addressing the value of different durations of warfarin for prevention of recurrent thromboembolism in patients with the first episode of VTE, the development of late malignancies was recorded much more frequently in patients allocated to six weeks than in those allocated to six months of anticoagulation (86). Although these results have not been confirmed by those of a subsequent similar study (87), they prospect the distinct possibility that cancer and thrombosis share common mechanisms, and that antithrombotic drugs may interfere with cancer development.

RISK OF CANCER IN PATIENTS WITH VENOUS THROMBOEMBOLISM

The strong association between cancer and VTE is further emphasized by the high rate of current detection or development in patients with VTE.

In patients presenting with VTE, the prevalence of concomitant cancer, defined as cancer not known before VTE and discovered by routine investigation (history taking, physical examination, urinanalysis, routine blood tests, and chest X-ray) varies considerably between the studies, this variation being related to the depth of the routine examinations and to the characteristics of the included patients (18). The risk of concomitant cancer was increased among patients with idiopathic VTE by a factor of 3–19, while the prevalence of concomitant cancer disease in patients with secondary VTE from detectable risk factors was low and, in general, comparable with the 2%–3% prevalence expected in the general population after middle age (88). According to the results of a recent retrospective study, the values of D-dimer at presentation can help predict the presence of concomitant cancer disease (88). Using a quantitative latex test, these authors were able to detect cancer much more frequently in patients with values exceeding 1000 ng/ml than in those with lower values. These findings require confirmation from prospective studies.

As far as the risk of developing subsequent overt malignancy, this risk was found across prospective studies to be consistently higher (4 to 5 times) in patients with idiopathic VTE than in those with secondary thrombosis (Table 3) (15). Newly discovered malignancies, whose incidence in idiopathic VTE is consistently around 10%, involve virtually all body systems. The risk of cancer is even higher in patients with recurrent thromboembolism (90) and in those with bilateral VTE (95).

These findings have been confirmed by those of three large, population-based studies conducted in Denmark, Sweden and Scotland, respectively (96–98). By examining data from both cancer and thromboembolic disease national registries, in all three studies the authors found a significantly increased risk for developing cancer in patients discharged with thromboembolism, particularly in the first year following VTE diagnosis. Of interest, in two of these studies a significant effect persisted for up to 10 years, suggesting that either a malignant disorder can induce hypercoagulability many years prior to its overt clinical development, or, more likely, cancer and thrombosis may share common pathogenetic mechanisms (96,97).

Despite the conclusive evidence of a strong relationship between idiopathic VTE and the risk for hidden cancer, whether extensive screening for occult malignancy in patients with idiopathic VTE is appropriate is still controversial. Since extensive screening procedures are associated with high costs and themselves carry some morbidity, they are only acceptable if they prove to be cost-effective and have an impact on cancer related mortality.

A recent publication has raised some concern about the utility of screening for occult malignancy all patients with idiopathic thromboembolism (99). By assessing the survival rate in patients with cancer diagnosed in the first year following the thrombotic episode in comparison with that of matched cancer patients without thrombosis, Sorensen and co-workers found increased mortality in the former group.

The same was true of cancers diagnosed at the time of hospitalisation for VTE. Results seem discouraging, as it appears that whenever a cancer disease is preceded by a clinical manifestation of thrombosis, its prognosis is far worse. However, due to the retrospective nature of the study design, we suppose that the large majority of identified cancers were already symptomatic at the time of detection. The early detection of occult cancers at the time they are totally asymptomatic might still lead to a more favorable clinical outcome. Two adequate studies have recently addressed this issue (100,101).

Monreal and colleagues published the results of a prospective cohort follow-up study in consecutive patients with acute VTE (100). All patients underwent a routine clinical

Table 3 Incidence of Occult Cancer After VTE Diagnosis

Authors	Cancer		
	All VTE	Secondary VTE	Idiopathic VTE
Aderka et al. (1986) (89)	11/83 (13.3%)	2/48 (4.2%)	9/35 (25.7%)
Prandoni et al. (1992) (90)	13/250 (5.2%)	2/105 (1.9%)	11/145 (7.6%)
Ahmed and Mohuddin (1996) (91)	3/196 (1.5%)	0/83 (0%)	3/113 (2.7%)
Monreal et al. (1997) (92)	8/659 (1.2%)	4/563 (0.7%)	4/96 (4.2%)
Hettiarachchi et al. (1998) (93)	13/326 (4.0%)	3/171 (1.8%)	10/155 (6.5%)
Rajan et al. (1998) (94)	21/264 (8.0%)	8/112 (7.1%)	13/152 (8.6%)
Schulman (2000) (95)	111/854 (13.0%)	18/320 (5.6%)	93/534 (17.4%)

evaluation for malignancy, if negative followed by a limited diagnostic work-up consisting of abdominal and pelvic ultrasound and laboratory markers for malignancy. The routine clinical evaluation was performed in 864 patients and revealed malignancy in 34 (3.9%) of them. Among the remaining 830 patients the limited diagnostic work-up revealed 13 further malignancies. During follow-up, cancer became symptomatic in 14 patients who were negative for cancer at screening (sensitivity of limited diagnostic work-up, 48%). Malignancies that were identified by the limited diagnostic work-up were early stage in 61% of cases versus 14% in cases occurring during follow-up. Most patients with occult cancer had idiopathic VTE and were older than 70 years. According to these study results, a limited diagnostic work-up for occult cancer in patients with VTE has the capacity to identify approximately one-half of the malignancies, predominantly in an early stage.

We have recently conducted a multicenter randomized clinical trial (the SOMIT study) in apparently cancer-free patients with acute idiopathic venous thrombosis or pulmonary embolism (101). Of 201 patients with a first episode of idiopathic VTE, after initial negative routine battery tests, 99 were randomized to undergo either extensive screening (Table 4), and 102 no further testing for malignancy. All patients were followed until the completion of two years of follow-up. Of the 14 malignancies that occurred in the extensive screening group, the screening was able to detect 13 (mostly detected by CT scanning), resulting in sensitivity higher than 90%. The risk for occult cancer was higher among elderly patients and in those without thrombophilic abnormalities. Ten malignancies developed in the follow-up of patients allocated to the control group. Overall, malignancies identified in the extensive screening group were at an earlier stage and the mean delay to diagnosis was reduced from 11 months to one month. The earlier discovery and subsequent treatment resulted in a slightly improved cancer related mortality (2.0% vs. 3.9%) and cancer-free survival (5.1 vs. 7.9) of the patients in the extensive screening group. Although these differences were not statistically significant, the reductions observed are in line with the hypothesis and would translate into a number needed to screen of only 50 patients to prevent one cancer-related death at two years.

Although data from either study do not conclusively demonstrate that early diagnosis ultimately prolongs life, the collective observations make such a beneficial effect likely. The earlier discovery of cancer, which might mean identification of the disease at an attackable state, may be crucial in an unpredictable rate of patients, especially nowadays when continuous protocol innovations are providing growing chances of success and eradication of malignancies.

Table 4 Extensive Screening Procedure According to the SOMT Study

Procedures
    Ultrasound of abdomen/pelvis
    CT scanning of abdomen and pelvis
    Gastroscopy or double contrast barium swallowing
    Flexible sigmoidoscopy or rectoscopy followed by barium enema or colonoscopy
    Hemoccult, sputum citology, tumor markers (CEA, αFP, CA125)
    Mammography and Pap-smear in women
    Transadbominal ultrasound of the prostate and PSA in men

KEY POINTS

- Malignancy produces a prothrombotic state.
- Venous thromboembolism (VTE) is a well-recognized complication of malignant disease.
- VTE may the first sign of an occult malignancy.
- Screening for occult malignancy in VTE patients remains controversial.
- Thromboprophylaxis should be used in immobile cancer patients or those undergoing surgery.
- Caval filters may be used in those with recurrent disease or if anticoagulation is contraindicated.

REFERENCES

1. Falanga A, Barbui T, Rickles FR, Levine MN. Guidelines for clotting studies in cancer patients. Thromb Haemost 1993; 70:343–350.
2. Rickles FR, Falanga A. Molecular basis for the relationship between thrombosis and cancer. Thromb Res 2001; 102:V215–V224.
3. Costantini V, Zacharski LR. Fibrin and cancer. Thromb Haemost 1993; 69:406–414.
4. Falanga A, Donati MB. Pathogenesis of thrombosis in patients with malignancy. Int J Hematol 2001; 73:137–144.
5. Gale AJ, Gordon SG. Update on tumor cell procoagulant factors. Acta Haematol 2001; 106:25–32.
6. Falanga A, Marchetti M, Vignoli A, Balducci D. Clotting mechanism and cancer: implications in thrombus formation and tumor progression. Clin Adv Hematol Oncol 2003; 1:673–678.
7. Falanga A, Iacoviello L, Evangelista V, et al. Loss of blast cell procoagulant activity and improvement of hemostatic variables in patients with acute promyelocytic leukemia given all-trans-retinoic acid. Blood 1995; 86:1072–1084.
8. Kwaan HC, Keer HN. Fibrinolysis and cancer. Semin Thromb Haemost 1990; 16:230–235.
9. Varon D, Brill A. Platelets cross-talk with tumor cells. Haemostasis 2001; 31:64–66.
10. Grignani G, Maiolo A. Cytokines and hemostasis. Haematologica 2000; 85:967–972.
11. Contrino J, Hair G, Kreutzer DL, Rickles FR. In situ detection of tissue factor in vascular endothelial cells: Correlation with the malignant phenotype of human breast disease. Nat Med 1996; 2:209–215,
12. Semeraro N, Colucci M. Tissue factor in health and disease. Thromb Haemost 1997; 78:759–764.
13. Falanga A, Marchetti M, Evangelista V, et al. Polymorphonuclear leukocyte activation and hemostasis in patients with essential thrombocythemia and polycythemia vera. Blood 2000; 96:4261–4266.
14. Shoji M, Hancock WW, Abe K, et al. Activation of coagulation and angiogenesis in cancer. Immunohistochemical localization in situ of clotting proteins and VEGF in human cancers. Am J Pathol 1998; 152:399–411.
15. Prandoni P, Piccioli A, Girolami A. Cancer and venous thromboembolism: an overview. Haematologica 1999; 84:437–445.
16. Kakkar AK, Levine M, Pinedo HM, Wolff R, Wong J. Venous thrombosis in cancer patients: insights from a frontline survey. The Oncologist 2003; 8:381–388.
17. Levitan N, Dowlati A, Remick SC, et al. Rates of initial and recurrent thromboembolic disease among patients with malignancy versus those without malignancy. Risk analysis using Medicare claims data. Medicine (Baltimore) 1999; 78:285–291.

18. Otten HM, Prins MH. Venous thromboembolism and occult malignancy. Thromb Res 2001; 102:V187–V194.

19. Piccioli A, Prandoni P, Ewenstein BM, Goldhaber SZ. Cancer and venous thromboembolism. Am Heart J 1996; 132:850–855.

20. Shen VS, Pollak EW. Fatal pulmonary embolism in cancer patients: is heparin prophylaxis justified? South Med J 1980; 73:841–843.

21. Levine MN, Lee AY. Risk assessment and primary VTE prevention in the cancer patient. Pathophysiol Thromb Haemost 2003; 33:36–41.

22. Kakkar VV, Howe CT, Nicolaides AN, Renney JTG, Clarke MB. Deep vein thrombosis of the leg. Is there a "high risk" group? Am J Surg 1970; 120:527–530.

23. Walsh JJ, Bonnar J, Wright FW. A study of pulmonary embolism and deep vein thrombosis after major gynaecological surgery using labelled fibrinogen-phlebography and lung scanning. J Obstet Gynaecol Br Commonw 1974; 81:311–316.

24. Rosemberg IL, Evans M, Pollock AV. Prophylaxis of postoperative leg vein thrombosis by low dose subcutaneous heparin or peroperative calf muscles stimulation: a controlled clinical trial. Br Med J 1975; 1:649–651.

25. Sue-Ling HM, Johnston D, McMahon MU, Philips PR, Davies JA. Preoperative identification of patients at high risk of deep venous thrombosis after elective major abdominal surgery. Lancet 1986; 1:1173–1176.

26. Allan A, Williams JT, Bolton JP, Le Quesne LP. The use of graduated compression stockings in the prevention of postoperative deep vein thrombosis. Br J Surg 1983; 70:172–174.

27. Multicentre Trial Committee. Dihydroergotamine-heparin prophylaxis of postoperative deep vein thrombosis: a multicentre trial. JAMA 1984; 251:2960–2966.

28. Hills NH, Pflug JJ, Jeyasingh K, Boardman L, Calnan JS. Prevention of deep vein thrombosis by intermittent pneumatic compression of calf. Br Med J 1972; 1:131–135.

29. Huber O, Bounameaux H, Borst F, Rohner A. Postoperative pulmonary embolism after hospital discharge. An underestimated risk. Arch Surg 1992; 127:310–313.

30. Bergqvist D, Agnelli G, Cohen AT, et al. Duration of prophylaxis against venous thromboembolism with enoxaparin after surgery for cancer. N Engl J Med 2002; 346:975–980.

31. Levine MN. Prevention of thrombotic disorders in cancer patients undergoing chemotherapy. Thromb Haemost 1997; 78:133–136.

32. Brandes AA, Scelzi E, Salmistraro G, et al. Incidence of risk of thromboembolism during treatment of high-grade gliomas: a prospective study. Eur J Cancer 1997; 33:1592–1596.

33. Cheruku R, Tapazoglou E, Ensley J, Kish JA, Cummings GD, Al-Sarraf M. The incidence and significance of thromboembolic complications in patients with high-grade gliomas. Cancer 1991; 68:2621–2624.

34. Marras LC, Geerts WH, Perry JR. The risk of venous thromboembolism is increased throughout the course of malignant glioma: an evidence based review. Cancer 2000; 89:640–646.

35. Grem JL, McAtee N, Murphy RF, et al. Phase I and pharmacokinetic study of recombinant human granulocyte-macrophage colony stimulating factor given in combination with fluorouracil plus calcium leucovorin in metastatic gastrointestinal adenocarcinoma. J Clin Oncol 1994; 12:560–588.

36. Otten HMMB, Mathijssen J, ten Cate H, et al. Symptomatic venous thromboembolism in cancer patients treated with chemotherapy. An underestimated phenomenon. Arch Intern Med 2004; 164:190–194.

37. Levine MN. Prevention of thrombotic disorders in cancer patients undergoing chemotherapy. Thromb Haemost 1997; 78:133–136.

38. Weiss RB, Tormey DC, Holland JF, Weinberg VE. Venous thrombosis during multinodal treatment of primary breast carcinoma. Cancer Treat Rep 1981; 65:677–679.

39. Goodnough LT, Saito H, Manni A, Jones PK, Pearson OH. Increased incidence of thromboembolism in stage IV breast cancer patients treated with a five drug chemotherapy regimen: a study of 159 patients. Cancer 1984; 54:1264–1268.

40. Levine MN, Gent M, Hirsh J, et al. The thrombogenic effect of anticancer drug therapy in women with stage II breast cancer. N Engl J Med 1988; 318:404–407.

41. Wall JG, Weiss RB, Norton L, et al. Arterial thrombosis associated with adjuvant chemotherapy for breast cancer: a cancer and leukemia group B study. Am J Med 1989; 87:501–504.

42. Fisher B, Redmond C, Legault-Poisson S, et al. Postoperative chemotherapy and tamoxifen compared with tamoxifen alone in the treatment of positive node breast cancer patients aged 50 years and older with tumours responsive to tamoxifen: results from the national surgical adjuvant breast and bowel project B16. J Clin Oncol 1990; 8:1005–1018.

43. Saphner T, Tormey DC, Gray R. Venous and arterial thrombosis in patients who received adjuvant therapy for breast cancer. J Clin Oncol 1991; 9:286–294.

44. Clahsen PC, Van de Velde CJH, Julien JP, Floiras JL, Mignolet RH. Thromboembolic complications after perioperative chemotherapy in women with early breast cancer: a European Organization for Research and Treatment of breast cancer cooperative group study. J Clin Oncol 1994; 12:1266–1271.

45. Rifkin SE, Green S, Metch B, et al. Adjuvant CMFVP versus tamoxifen versus concurrent CMFVP and tamoxifen for postmenopausal node positive and estrogen receptor positive breast cancer patients: a Southwest Oncology group study. J Clin Oncol 1994; 12:2078–2085.

46. Pritchard KI, Paterson AH, Paul NA, Zee B, Fine S, Pater J. Increased thromboembolic complications with concurrent tamoxifen and chemotherapy in a randomized trial of adjuvant therapy for women with breast cancer. J Clin Oncol 1996; 14:2731–2737.

47. Tempelhoff GF, Dietrich M, Hommel G, Heilmann L. Blood coagulation during adjuvant epirubicin/cyclophosphamide chemotherapy in patients with primary operable breast cancer. J Clin Oncol 1996; 14:2560–2568.

48. Orlando L, Colleoni M, Nole F, et al. Incidence of venous thromboembolism in breast cancer patients during chemotherapy with vinorelbine, cisplatin, 5-fluorouracil as continuous infusion (ViFuP regimen): is prophylaxis required? Ann Oncol 2000; 11:117–118.

49. Goodnough LT, Saito A, Manni A, Jones PK, Pearson OH. Increased incidence of thromboembolism in stage IV breast cancer patients treated with a five-drug chemotherapy regimen: a study of 159 patients. Cancer 1984; 54:1264–1268.

50. Pritchard KI, Paterson AH, Paul NA, Zee B, Fine S, Pater J. Increased thromboembolic complication with concurrent tamoxifen and chemotherapy in a randomized trial of adjuvant therapy for women with breast cancer. J Clin Oncol 1996; 14:2731–2737.

51. Deitcher SR, Gomes MPV. The risk of venous thromboembolic disease associated with adjuvant hormone therapy for breast carcinoma. Cancer 2004; 101:439–449.

52. Verso M, Agnelli G. Venous thromboembolism associated with long-term use of central venous catheters in cancer patients. J Clin Oncol 2003; 21:3665–3675.

53. Bern MM, Lokich JJ, Wallach SR, et al. Very low dose of warfarin can prevent thrombosis in central venous catheters. A prospective trial. Ann Intern Med 1990; 112:423–428.

54. Monreal M, Alastrue A, Rull M, et al. Upper extremity deep venous thrombosis in cancer patients with venous access devices- prophylaxis with a low molecular weight heparin (fragmin). Thromb Haemost 1996; 75:251–253.

55. Levine MN, Lee AY, Kakkar AK. From Trousseau to targeted therapy: new insights and innovations in thrombosis and cancer. J Thromb Haemost 2003; 1:1456–1463.

56. Geerts WH, Pineo GF, Heit JA, et al. Prevention of venous thromboembolism: the Seventh ACCP Conference on Antithrombotic and Thrombolytic Therapy. Chest 2004; 126:338S–400S.

57. Bergqvist D, Burmark US, Flordal PA, et al. Low molecular weight heparin started before surgery as prophylaxis against deep vein thrombosis: 2500 versus 5000 XaI units in 2070 patients. Br J Surg 1995; 82:496–501.

58. Enoxacan Study Group. Efficacy and safety of enoxaparin versus unfractionated heparin for prevention of deep vein thrombosis in elective cancer surgery: a double-blind randomized multicentre trial with venographic assessment. Br J Surg 1997; 84:1099–1103.

59. McLeod RS, Geerts WH, Sniderman KW, et al. Subcutaneous heparin versus low-molecular-weight heparin as thromboprophylaxis in patients undergoing colorectal DVT prophylaxis trial: a randomized, double-blind trial. Ann Surg 2001; 233:438–444.

60. Agnelli G, Bergqvist D, Cohen AT, Gallus AS, Gent M. Randomized clinical trial of postoperative fondaparinux versus perioperative dalteparin for prevention of venous thromboembolism in high-risk abdominal surgery. Br J Surg 2005; 92:1212–1220.

61. Rasmussen MS, Jorgensen LN, Wille-Jorgensen JP, et al. Prolonged prophylaxis with low molecular weight heparin (dalteparin) after major abdominal surgery: the Fame study. Programs and Abstracts of the XIX Congress of the International Society on Thrombosis and Haemostasis, Birmingham, England, July 12–18, 2003. Malden, Mass: Blackwell Publishing, 2003, abstract (computer disk).

62. Wells PS, Lensing AWA, Hirsh J. Graduated compression stockings in the prevention of postoperative venous thromboembolism: a meta-analysis. Arch Intern Med 1994; 154:67–72.

63. Nurmohamed MT, van Riel AM, Henkens CM, et al. Low molecular weight heparin and compression stockings in the prevention of venous thromboembolism in neurosurgery. Thromb Haemost 1996; 75:233–238.

64. Agnelli G, Piovella F, Buoncristiani P, et al. Enoxaparin plus compression stockings compared with compression stockings alone in the prevention of venous thromboembolism after elective neurosurgery. N Engl J Med 1998; 339:80–85.

65. Levine MN, Hirsh J, Gent M, et al. Double-blind randomized trial of very-low-dose warfarin for prevention of thromboembolism in stage IV breast cancer. Lancet 1994; 343:886–889.

66. Bern MM, Bothe A, Jr., Bistrian B, Champagne CD, Keane MS, Blackburn GL. Prophylaxis against central vein thrombosis with low-dose warfarin. Surgery 1986; 99:216–221.

67. Couban S, Goodyear M, Burnell M, et al. A randomized, double-blind, placebo-controlled study of low-dose warfarin for the prevention of symptomatic central venous catheter-associated thrombosis in patients with cancer. Blood 2002; 100:70a.

68. Heaton DC, Han DY, Inder A. Minidose warfarin as prophylaxis for central vein catheter thrombosis. Intern Med 2002; 32:84–88.

69. Reichardt P, Kretzschrnar A, Biakhov M, et al. A phase III double-blind,.placebo-controlled study evaluating the efficacy and safety of daily low-molecular-weight heparin (dalteparin) in preventing catheter-related complications in cancer patients with central venous catheters. Clin Oncol 2002; 21:1474a.

70. Klerk CP, Smorenburg SM, Buller HR. Thrombosis prophylaxis in patient populations with a central venous catheter. A systematic review. Arch Intern Med 2003; 163:1913–1921.

71. Prandoni P, Lensing AWA, Cogo A, et al. The long-term clinical course of acute deep venous thrombosis. Ann Intern Med 1996; 125:1–7.

72. Hansson PO, Sorbo J, Eriksson H. Recurrent venous thromboembolism after deep vein thrombosis. Incidence and risk factors. Arch Intern Med 2000; 1260:769–774.

73. Heit JA, Mohr DN, Silverstein MD, Petterson TM, O'Fallon WM, Melton LJ, III. Predictors of recurrence after deep vein thrombosis and pulmonary embolism. A population-based cohort study. Arch Intern Med 2000; 160:761–768.

74. Hutten B, Prins M, Gent M, Ginsberg J, Tijsen JGP, Buller HR. Incidence of recurrent thromboembolic and bleeding complications among patients with venous thromboembolism in relation to both malignancy and achieved international normalized ratio: a retrospective analysis. J Clin Oncol 2000; 18:3078–3083.

75. Palareti G, Legnani C, Agnes L, et al. A comparison of the safety and efficacy of oral anticoagulation for the treatment of venous thromboembolic disease in patients with or without malignancy. Thromb Haemost 2000; 84:805–810.

76. Prandoni P, Lensing AWA, Piccioli A, et al. Recurrent venous thromboembolism and bleeding complications during anticoagulant treatment in patients with cancer and venous thrombosis. Blood 2002; 100:3484–3488.

77. Lee AY, Levine MN, Baker RI, et al. Low-molecular-weight heparin versus a coumarin for the prevention of recurrent venous thromboembolism in patients with cancer. N Engl J Med 2003; 349:146–153.

78. Meyer G, Marjanovic Z, Valcke J, et al. Comparison of low-molecular-weight heparin and warfarin for the secondary prevention of venous thromboembolism in patients with cancer. Arch Intern Med 2002; 162:1729–1735.

79. Zacharski LR, Henderson WG, Rickles FR, et al. Effect of warfarin anticoagulation on survival in carcinoma of the lung, colon, head and neck, and prostate. Cancer 1984; 53:2046–2052.

80. Dolovich LR, Ginsberg JS, Douketis JD, Holbrook AM, Cheah G. A meta-analysis comparing low-molecular-weight heparins with unfractionated heparin in the treatment of venous thromboembolism. Arch Intern Med 2000; 160:181–188.

81. Zacharski LR. Anticoagulants in cancer treatment: malignancy as a solid phase coagulopathy. Cancer Lett 2002; 186:1–9.

82. Klerk CPW, Smorenburg SM, Buller HR. Antimalignant properties of antithrombotic agents. In: Lugassy G, Falanga A, Kakkar AK, Rickles FR, eds. Thrombosis and Cancer. London: Taylor & Francis Group, 2004:207–222.

83. Kakkar AK, Levine MN, Kadziola Z, et al. Low molecular weight heparin, therapy with dalteparin, and survival in advanced cancer: The Fragmin Advanced Malignancy Outcome Study. J Clin Oncol 2004; 22:1944–1948.

84. Klerk CPW, Smorenburg, SM, Otten, HYM, et al. The effect of low-molecular-weight heparin on survival in patients with advanced malignancy. J Clin Oncol 2005; 23:2130–2135.

85. Altinbas M, Coskun HS, Er O, et al. A randomized clinical trial of combination chemotherapy with and without low-molecular-weight heparin in small cell lung cancer. J Thromb Haemost 2004; 2:1266–1271.

86. Schulman S, Lindmarker P. Incidence of cancer after prophylaxis with warfarin against recurrent venous thromboembolism. N Engl J Med 2000; 342:1953–1958.

87. Taliani MR, Agnelli G, Prandoni P, et al. Incidence of cancer after a first episode of idiopathic venous thromboembolism treated with 3 months or 1 year of oral anticoagulation. J Thromb Haemost 2003; 1:1730–1733.

88. Rege KP, Jones S, Day J, Hoggarth CE. In proven deep vein thrombosis, a low positive D-Dimer score is a strong negative predictor for associated malignancy. Thromb Haemost 2004; 91:1219–1222.

89. Aderka D, Brown A, Zelikovski A, Pinkhas J. Idiopathic deep vein thrombosis in an apparently healthy patient as a premonitory sign of occult cancer. Cancer 1986; 57:1846–1849.

90. Prandoni P, Lensing AWA, Büller HR, et al. Deep-vein thrombosis and the incidence of subsequent symptomatic cancer. N Engl J Med 1992; 327:1128–1133.

91. Ahmed Z, Mohuddin Z. Deep vein thrombosis as a predictor of cancer. Angiology 1996; 47:261–265.

92. Monreal M, Fernandez-Llamazares J, Perandreu J, Urrutia A, Sahuquillo JC, Contel E. Occult cancer in patients with venous thromboembolism: which patients, which cancers. Thromb Haemost 1997; 78:1316–1318.

93. Hettiarachchi RJK, Lok J, Prins MH, Büller HR, Prandoni P. Undiagnosed malignancy in patients with deep vein thrombosis. Cancer 1998; 83:180–185.

94. Rajan R, Levine M, Gent M, et al. The occurrence of subsequent malignancy in patients presenting with deep vein thrombosis: results from a historical cohort study. Thromb Haemost 1998; 79:19–22.

95. Bura A, Cailleux N, Bienvenu B, et al. Incidence and prognosis of cancer associated with bilateral venous thrombosis: a prospective study of 103 patients. J Thromb Haemost 2004; 2:441–444.

96. Sorensen HT, Mellemkjaer L, Steffensen H, Olsen JH, Nielsen GL. The risk of a diagnosis of cancer after primary deep-venous thrombosis or pulmonary embolism. N Engl J Med 1998; 338:1169–1173.

97. Baron JA, Gridley G, Weiderpass E, Nyren G, Linet M. Venous thromboembolism and cancer. Lancet 1998; 351:1077–1080.

98. Murchison JT, Wylie L, Stockton DL. Excess risk of cancer in patients with primary venous thromboembolism: a national, population-based cohort study. Br J Cancer 2004; 91:92–95.

99. Sorensen HT, Mellemkjaer L, Olsen JH, Baron JA. Prognosis of cancers associated with venous thromboembolism. N Engl J Med 2000; 343:1846–1850.

100. Monreal M, Lensing AWA, Prins MH, et al. Screening for occult cancer in patients with acute deep vein thrombosis or pulmonary embolism. J Thromb Haemost 2004; 2:876–881.

101. Piccioli A, Lensing AWA, Prins MH, et al. Extensive screening for occult malignant disease in idiopathic venous thromboembolism. J Thromb Haemost 2004; 2:884–889.

14

Venous Thrombosis Prophylaxis

Joseph A. Caprini
Feinberg School of Medicine, Northwestern University, Chicago, Illinois;
Evanston Northwestern Healthcare, Evanston, Illinois; and
Glenbrook Hospital, Glenview, Illinois, U.S.A.

Dereck W. Wentworth
U.S. Medical Affairs, New York, New York, U.S.A.

INCIDENCE AND MAGNITUDE OF THE PROBLEM

Venous thromboembolism (VTE) is a leading cause of mortality in the United States and causes more deaths than AIDS, breast cancer, and motor vehicle crashes combined. Pulmonary embolism (PE) is responsible for up to 200,000 fatalities annually in the United States, while in 2002 AIDS-related deaths were seen in 14,095 individuals (1). Breast cancer-related fatalities for the year 2002 were estimated to be 41,883 patients (2), while U.S. highway fatalities that same year were 44,065 individuals (3). The in-hospital case fatality rate attributed to venous thromboembolic disease is 10–25% in the United States. Elderly patients suffering pulmonary emboli have a case fatality rate of 15% at 28 days, while cancer patients have a 25% fatality rate at 28 days. By one year elderly VTE victims suffered a mortality rate of 21% and cancer patients 39% (1,4,5). Most of these studies underestimate the incidence of VTE because of low autopsy rates of 10–20%, outpatient cases were not counted, and long-term care facility data were not considered. The actual mortality from VTE is probably higher, but unfortunately, unlike breast cancer and AIDS, the National Center for Health Statistics does not track deaths due to VTE.

Surgical patients have been well studied and their risk for VTE is known. In patients undergoing total hip replacement who do not have additional risk factors and do not receive prophylaxis, the incidence of fatal PE is 0.2% to 0.5%. Patients who undergo surgery for fractured hips and do not receive prophylaxis may suffer a 2.5% to 7.5% incidence of fatal PE (6). Risk factors associated with acute inpatient mortality following orthopedic surgery were evaluated in 43,215 patients. Conditions identified preoperatively related to mortality included chronic renal failure, congestive heart failure, cancer with bone metastasis, COPD, atrial fibrillation, and age over 70 years. Procedural factors influencing mortality were found to be surgery for trauma or hip fracture, with a mortality rate five times higher than other procedures. Mortality rates from postoperative complications were 27.6% from renal failure, 19.3% from pulmonary embolus, 19.3% from myocardial infarction, and 8.6% each for cerebrovascular accidents and pneumonia (7). One of the important lessons learned from this study is that mortality from surgical procedures is frequently caused by pulmonary embolism, certain surgical procedures are higher risk than others, and preoperative patient factors also affect risk of VTE. This indicates that the choice of VTE prophylaxis should take into account all of these factors.

Surgical patients are not the only ones at risk for VTE. The incidence of thrombosis in patients admitted to the hospital on the medical service averages 10% to 20% overall. Patients admitted with stroke have up to a 56% incidence of DVT and those admitted to the medical intensive care unit have a rate of DVT between 28% and 33% (8–10). Patients at risk are those who have COPD, CHF, pneumonia, and inflammatory bowel disease. Large randomized prospective trials in the medical population have been done and consistently demonstrate an incidence of DVT between 10% to 20% in patients who receive no prophylaxis (11,12).

Patients undergoing colorectal surgery have a high incidence of VTE due in part to the long duration of surgery, pelvic resection, and the presence of cancer and/or inflammatory bowel disease. In a series of 20,000 patients in this category, 1.8% died of fatal pulmonary embolism despite receiving low-dose unfractionated heparin prophylaxis. The risk of PE in untreated patients is approximately 5% (13). The incidence of DVT in 12 general surgical trials was 22% in untreated surgical subjects, while it was seen in 29% of patients undergoing colorectal procedures (14).

There are a number of important reasons to provide thrombosis prophylaxis to patients who are at risk for VTE, as seen in Table 1. Prandoni and others have provided data regarding the long-term clinical course of acute DVT. In approximately 5% of patients, DVT will recur within three months, in 18% at two years, and by eight years following the acute event, about 30% of individuals will suffer a second DVT (15–17).

The post-thrombotic syndrome (PTS) is estimated to occur in about 25% of patients following a first episode of DVT. This syndrome is characterized by the development of leg swelling, skin pigmentation, rashes, and in approximately 4% of individuals, an open ulcer. PTS can develop in patients with asymptomatic DVT, while recurrent ipsilateral DVT and proximal DVT will increase the risk of developing the syndrome. PTS also takes time to develop, with only 23% of post-thrombotic cases presenting within two years of the acute DVT (16). After such a long time, symptoms of recurrent VTE and PTS are not often attributed to a previous operative procedure or hospitalization for illness. One startling fact about the post-thrombotic syndrome is that 7% of patients are disabled by this condition and if a person develops recurrent DVT, the risk of the post-thrombotic syndrome is increased by six-fold (18).

Table 1 Rationale for VTE Prophylaxis

Prevent fatal pulmonary emboli
1–5% incidence in patients with >4 risk factors
16.7% mortality at 3 months
Prevent clinical venous thromboembolism
Morbidity—months of anticoagulation, tests, hose, changes in lifestyle
Prevent silent venous thromboembolism
Risk of subsequent event double that of control population (Borrow)
Prevent embolic stroke in those with patent foramen ovale
20–30% PFO rate; 50% disabled; 20% die; 30% recover
Prevent the post-thrombotic syndrome
25% incidence following DVT and 7% severe
May not be evident for 2–5 years

Abbreviations: VTE, venous thromboembolism; PFO, patent foramen ovaie; DVT, deep vein thrombosis.

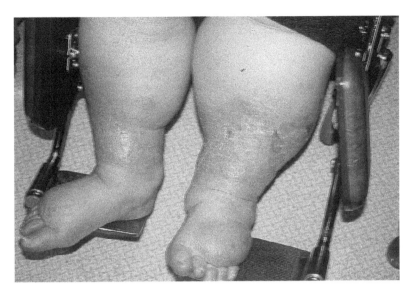

Figure 1 An example of severe post-thrombotic syndrome (PTS) post–hip arthroplasty. This woman demonstrates lymphedema, discoloration, pain, ulceration, and obviously is severely debilitated by her condition. *Source:* Adapted from Ref. 34. (*See color insert.*)

The American Venous Forum has published an excellent classification of venous problems called the CEAP score, which helps classify the severity of changes in individual patients. Figure 1 shows a woman with severe post-thrombotic changes combined with lymphedema. This is a very difficult picture as far as treatment is concerned and is definitely a permanent problem. It has been estimated that in the United States 2 million workdays are lost annually and 15 million Americans suffer from this problem (19). The cost of care for these problems in the United Kingdom is estimated at 400 million pounds annually and $300 million in the United States (8). The syndrome represents one of the most compelling arguments for effective thrombosis prophylaxis in all medical and surgical patients at risk, as it is much easier to prevent VTE than it is to treat PTS.

Another problem that is poorly recognized and very difficult to assess is the incidence of recurrent thromboembolism in patients who have had a subclinical event and later are at risk because of an operation or medical illness. Borow reported on 500 patients who underwent surgical procedures lasting an hour or more, were over the age of 40 years, and were studied postoperatively with fibrinogen scans and confirmed with contrast venography (20). He found that 66% of patients who had a history of venous thrombosis developed thrombosis postoperatively. He also reported that 50% of the patients with a significant medical history, including previous abdominal or leg surgery, trauma to the lower abdomen, or long bone fracture, developed postoperative venous thrombosis. Table 2 is a list of various signs, symptoms and clinical findings that may be associated with a venous thromboembolic event. Obviously, all of these problems do not end with a fatality but that does not diminish the importance of the presence of these abnormalities as a clue to signal a possible VTE event.

We frequently encounter successful, busy clinicians who dispute the above data, usually saying that "in our practice we just don't see these problems." We would emphasize that in this modern era, autopsies are difficult to obtain; without them, the true incidence of venous thromboembolic problems associated with clinical fatalities is impossible to calculate. Another modern problem in the United States is delivery of health

Table 2   Nonspecific Signs and Symptoms of VTE

Leg pain	Leg swelling
Chest pain	Shortness of breath
Transient orthostatic hypotension	Narcotic excess
Fainting spell	Hypoxia
Patient readmission 90 days postoperatively	Postoperative pneumonia
Patient death 90 days postoperatively	Sudden death
Suspected MI	Death without autopsy
Patent foramen ovale	Post-thrombotic syndrome 5 years postoperatively
Postoperative stroke	Failure to thrive

Abbreviations: VTE, venous thromboembolism; MI, myocardial infarction.

care. When patients are discharged from the hospital after surgery or acute medical illness, they often may not be readmitted to the same hospital to treat a post-discharge VTE event. If these people develop venous thromboembolic complications, how is the busy clinical practitioner able to find out about these problems unless the patients' activities and whereabouts following discharge are carefully documented? We would remind those clinicians who are skeptical about the incidence and clinical significance of venous thromboembolic problems that the data are real and have been derived from hundreds of references. The thrombosis prophylaxis chapter in the latest Chest Consensus Conference on Antithrombotic Therapy contains 797 references that are the scientific basis for the incidence, morbidity and mortality associated with venous thromboembolic disease (6).

RISK ASSESSMENT

Some of us feel that the single most important aspect of thrombosis prophylaxis in medical and surgical patients is a careful, detailed risk analysis of each individual patient, being careful not to miss any important risk factors. One might say that this process is the medical equivalent of the preflight cockpit checklist for a commercial airliner. It would be unthinkable to fly without checking every possible item on the list to ensure the safety of the passengers and crew. We are indebted to the Chest Consensus Conference Guidelines that now have been published for the seventh time and give us clear direction regarding risk factors and their importance in the prevention of VTE. A number of formal risk assessment models are available for this purpose (21,22). Many feel that these are cumbersome and have not been adequately validated (6). Furthermore, clinicians find them cumbersome to implement in their routine practice. The consensus group suggests a simplified approach, categorizing patients into four different categories depending on their age, type of surgery, and presence of additional risk factors (Table 3). This is intended to provide a uniform approach to a population of patients; however, we encounter daily situations where a low-risk procedure is performed on a patient at very high risk for VTE. It is true that in these very-high-risk individuals maximum prophylaxis will be used, so one could ask why all risk factors must be listed. There is considerable literature to suggest that patients with large numbers of risk factors may be at enormous risk for developing a postoperative venous thromboembolic event (6,8,23,24). If the patient is undergoing a quality-of-life procedure and falls into this category, we feel that part of the preoperative informed consent process should be to advise the patient of the degree of risk so the patient can decide on the importance of the procedure given the risks involved as assessed.

Table 3 Risk of VTE and Therapy Recommendations

Level of patient risk	DVT (%)		PE (%)		Recommended therapy
	Calf	Proximal	Symptomatic	Fatal	
Low					
Age under 40 yr	2	0.4	0.2	0.002	Aggressive mobilization
Minor surgery No other RF					
Moderate					
Minor surgery and additional RF	10–20	2–4	1–2	0.1–0.4	LDUFH q12 h, LMWH, GCS, IPC
Minor surgery, 40–60 yr and no additional RF					
Major surgery, <40 yr with no additional RF					
High					
Minor surgery in patients >60 yr or w/additional RF	20–40	4–8	2–4	0.4–1.0	LMWH, LDUFH q8 h, IPC
Major surgery in patients >40 yr or w/additional RF					
Very high					
Major surgery in patients >40 yr plus prior VTE, cancer, or hypercoaguable state	40–80	10–20	4–10	0.2–5	LMWH, fondaparinux, oral VKA, adjusted UFH, IPC/GCS + LDUFH/LMWH
Hip or knee arthroplasty, hip fracture surgery					
Major trauma, spinal cord injury					

Abbreviations: GCS, graduated compression stockings; IPC, intermittent pneumatic compression; LDUFH, low dose unfractionated heparin; LMWH, low molecular weight heparin; RF, risk factors; VKA, Vitamin K antagonists.
Source: Adapted from Ref. 6.

For example, if a patient with a heterozygous Factor V Leiden defect also has a protein C or S defect, the incidence of thrombosis may be as high as 70% to 90% (25). That may be too much of a chance to take for an elective quality-of-life procedure. Even with proper prophylaxis, VTE may still occur (the event rate is not zero), or they might experience excessive bleeding requiring withdrawal of prophylaxis, thus exposing the patient to a high risk of severe or fatal events. Without a complete preoperative risk assessment, how would one know which patients are in this category and need this extra counseling and decision-making analysis preoperatively?

We have developed a risk assessment form that has been used in our clinic for more than 15 years and is provided in Table 4. It consists of a point system linking the patient to the risk factor schema proposed by the Chest Consensus Guidelines (see Table 3). The use

Table 4 Recommendations for Therapy Based on Full Patient Risk Assessment

Thrombosis Risk Factor Assessment

≡ENH EVANSTON
NORTHWESTERN
HEALTHCARE

Joseph A. Caprini, MD, MS, FACS, RVT
Louis W. Biegler Professor of Surgery,
Northwestern University
The Feinberg School of Medicine
Professor of Biomedical Engineering
Northwestern University,
Director of Surgical Research,
Evanston Northwestern Healthcare
Email: j-caprini@northwestern.edu
Website: venousdisease.com

Patient's Name:_____ Age: ____ Sex: ____ Wgt:____lbs

Choose All That Apply

Each Risk Factor Represents 1 Point
❑ Age 41-60 years
❑ Minor surgery planned
❑ History of prior major surgery (< 1 month)
❑ Varicose veins
❑ History of inflammatory bowel disease
❑ Swollen legs (current)
❑ Obesity (BMI > 25)
❑ Acute myocardial infarction
❑ Congestive heart failure (< 1 month)
❑ Sepsis (< 1 month)
❑ Serious lung disease incl. pneumonia (< 1 month)
❑ Abnormal pulmonary function (COPD)
❑ Medical patient currently at bed rest
❑ Other risk factors_____

Each Risk Factor Represents 2 Points
❑ Age 60-74 years
❑ Arthroscopic surgery
❑ Malignancy (present or previous)
❑ Major surgery (> 45 minutes)
❑ Laparoscopic surgery (> 45 minutes)
❑ Patient confined to bed (> 72 hours)
❑ Immobilizing plaster cast (< 1 month)
❑ Central venous access

Each Risk Factor Represents 5 Points
❑ Elective major lower extremity arthroplasty
❑ Hip, pelvis or leg fracture (< 1 month)
❑ Stroke (< 1 month)
❑ Multiple trauma (< 1 month)
❑ Acute spinal cord injury (paralysis)(< 1 month)

Each Risk Factor Represents 3 Points
❑ Age over 75 years
❑ History of DVT/PE
❑ **Family history of thrombosis***
❑ Positive Factor V Leiden
❑ Positive Prothrombin 20210A
❑ Elevated serum homocysteine
❑ Positive Lupus anticoagulant
❑ Elevated anticardiolipin antibodies
❑ Heparin-induced thrombocytopenia (HIT)
❑ Other congenital or acquired thrombophilia
If yes:
Type_____
most frequently missed risk factor

For Women Only (Each Represents 1 Point)
❑ Oral contraceptives or hormone replacement therapy
❑ Pregnancy or postpartum (<1 month)
❑ History of unexplained stillborn infant, recurrent spontaneous abortion (≥ 3), premature birth with toxemia or growth-restricted infant

Total Risk Factor Score [   ]

Prophylaxis Safety Considerations: Check box if answer is 'YES'

Anticoagulants: Factors Associated with Increased Bleeding
❑ Is patient experiencing any active bleeding?
❑ Does patient have (or has had history of) heparin-induced thrombocytopenia?
❑ Is patient's platelet count <100,000/mm³?
❑ Is patient taking oral anticoagulants, platelet inhibitors (e.g. NSAIDS, Clopidigrel, Salicylates)?
❑ Is patient's creatinine clearance abnormal? If yes, please indicate value _____
If any of the above boxes are checked, the patient may not be a candidate for anticoagulant therapy and should consider alternative prophylactic measures.

Intermittent Pneumatic Compression (IPC)
❑ Does patient have severe peripheral arterial disease?
❑ Does patient have congestive heart failure?
❑ Does patient have an acute superficial/deep vein thrombosis?
If any of the above boxes are checked, then patient may not be a candidate for intermittent compression therapy and should consider alternative prophylactic measures.

Total risk-factor score	Incidence of DVT	Risk level	Prophylactic regimen
0–1	<10%	Low	No specific measures, early ambulation
2	10–20%	Moderate	GCS, IPC, LDUFH or LMWH
3–4	20–40%	High	IPC, LDUFH or LMWH
5	40–80%	Highest	Pharmacological: LDUFH, LMWH[a], warfarin[a], or Factor Xa inhibitor[a] alone or combined with GCS/IPC

[a] For use in patients undergoing hip or knee arthroplasty or hip fracture repair.
Abbreviations: DVT, deep vein thrombosis; GCS, graduated compression stockings, IPC, intermittent pneumatic compression; LDUFH, low dose unfractionated heparin; LMWH, low molecular weight heparin.
Source: Adapted from Refs. 6, 8, 22, 108, 124, 125.

of this form allows one to go beyond the Guidelines since randomized, prospective data and appropriate clinical trials are not available for every circumstance the clinician sees in daily practice. As a result of this problem, one must take the available literature, incorporate the results of individual clinical trials when available, and assess an individual patient's risk for VTE to reach a tentative conclusion regarding the degree of thrombosis risk. In addition, one must apply a certain amount of logic, emotion, and experience to the overall clinical scenario in order to develop the best approach for each individual patient. This method is very conservative and has two dominant characteristics; namely, almost everyone gets prophylaxis, and the choice for each patient represents the best balance between efficacy and safety. We were a bit disappointed with the Consensus Guidelines when the statement was made that in orthopedic situations, the emphasis was on prevention of bleeding more than the prevention of thrombosis. Some of us would have a different view. Depending on the overall degree of risk of the patient, the selection of prophylaxis and intensity may carry more risk for bleeding; however, the intention is to prevent a fatal pulmonary embolus or disabling stroke. In today's world we feel that the patient should be a part of this discussion and decision-making process.

The most common pitfall we see in assessing risk in clinical practice is failure of the clinician to inquire about a past history of thrombosis or a family history of thrombosis. Some feel that the family history of thrombosis is not that important; however, we differ with this view based on results from our thrombosis referral clinic. We conducted a study where markers of probability were obtained in approximately 175 patients over a three-year period. Individuals who had a history of DVT were found to have a marker of thrombophilia 56% of the time. Those with a family history of thrombosis were found to have at least one abnormality at least 42% of the time. These defects included factor V Leiden, prothrombin 20210A, protein C and S, antithrombin deficiency, and antiphospholipid antibodies. We have seen examples of serious or fatal outcomes in our clinical practice when this history is not obtained and investigated thoroughly. We are always careful to assess the obstetrical history of every female in order to determine if a past stillborn infant, toxemia, recurrent spontaneous abortions, or placental insufficiency has occurred. These events may be clinical manifestations of the antiphospholipid antibody syndrome, including a lupus anticoagulant, which are severe risk factors for the development of postoperative VTE. We also investigate personal and family history of stroke and assess homocysteine levels. We believe that elevated levels should be treated with preventive doses of vitamin B6, B12 and folic acid in order to minimize the chance of endothelial damage from the elevated homocysteine levels that may produce a stroke, DVT or myocardial infarction. We realize that conflicting data exist in the literature regarding this principle (26), but until we see data that show there is some harm in this approach, we prefer to prescribe this therapy (27).

An example of our approach to risk assessment is our use of thrombosis prophylaxis in laparoscopic surgical patients, since this approach is not solely procedure-dependent but also based on the individual risk factors involved. Some investigators have reported that laparoscopic cholecystectomy is a low-risk procedure not requiring thrombosis prophylaxis (28). One study in 700 patients showed a VTE incidence of 1%. On further examination, the patients in this study all had fewer than three risk factors (29). We caution clinicians about translating these studies into routine clinical practice without first considering whether the individual patient might have a very high risk of developing a VTE. Patients undergoing laparoscopic surgery are like any other surgical patient in that the incidence of DVT is directly related to the risk factor score. This fact is well documented in the Chest Consensus Guidelines, as is seen in Table 3. The presence of pneumoperitoneum as well as reverse Trendelenburg position introduces additional

Table 5 Recommended Duration of VTE Prophylaxis for Various Indications

Indication	Duration of prophylaxis
Abdominal surgery	7–10 days (Ref. 6)
Abdominal surgery involving cancer	29 days (Ref. 32)
Hip fracture repair	4 weeks (Ref. 93)
Hip arthroplasty	4–6 weeks (Refs. 30–31,63,87,88)
Knee arthroplasty	10–14 days (Ref. 89)
Bariatric surgery	3 week (Ref. 125)
Medical prophylaxis	10–14 days (Ref. 11)

elements of risk. These include decreased venous return resulting in venous stasis and venous dilatation that can produce endothelial cracks that serve as the nidus for development of postoperative venous thrombosis. Take, for example, the patient with acute cholecystitis, over the age of 60, with obesity, and a past history of successful treatment for cancer. We would classify this individual in the highest risk group (Table 4) with a score of eight to nine points. We would provide this patient with stockings and intermittent pneumatic compression devices during and following surgery, and low molecular weight heparin (LMWH) postoperatively for 10 to 30 days.

The duration of prophylaxis after surgery or hospitalization is important as well. It has been demonstrated that DVT prophylaxis should be continued for the duration the patient is at risk (30–33). These studies demonstrate that different durations of prophylaxis are appropriate for specific patients as shown in Table 5. When patients demonstrate several to many risk factors, it seems logical that multiple methods of DVT prevention may be used to further decrease the patient's risk (8). Considering all of these factors, our risk assessment schema accounts for many sources of risk (patient history, duration of protection needed, known prior VTE events, and clinical events not always recognized as related to VTE) not just the procedure itself. Only in this fashion may a selection for the appropriate prophylaxis be made that will fully protect the patient.

Physical Methods of Prophylaxis

Physical methods of prophylaxis may be divided into several categories, including graduated compression stockings (GCS), intermittent pneumatic compression devices (IPC), foot pumps, and combinations of foot and leg compression devices. GCS are stockings that have a higher pressure at the ankle than in the calf or thigh in order to provide a pressure profile that encourages blood flow out of the leg. The average pressure at the ankle is approximately 18 mmHg, which gradually decreases to approximately 8 mmHg in the thigh. These devices have been shown to decrease venous diameter slightly, which helps prevent venous distention, particularly when the limb is in the dependent position (34). Data to show the effectiveness of GCS appeared many years ago when it was legitimate to have a placebo group in thrombosis prophylaxis trials (20,35,36). Compared to doing nothing, these stockings improved results and lowered the incidence of venous thromboembolism. A summary of these results may be found in the 2000 Cochran analysis, which analyzed the results of a number of randomized clinical trials showing that the placebo incidence of DVT was 27% and was reduced to 13% utilizing GCS (37). Of even greater importance was the fact that when GCS was combined with another physical or pharmacologic method, the incidence of DVT was reduced from 15% using stockings alone to 2% in the combined modality group.

The IPC devices have been compared to placebo in 11 general surgery studies and demonstrated an impressive 74% reduction in DVT from 26% to 6.8% (8). We were disappointed that the Seventh Chest Consensus Guidelines contain very little discussion regarding these modalities and the editors do not clearly delineate between the differences in trials using stockings versus pneumatic compression devices. If one looks at the International Consensus statement published in 2001, it summarizes a number of landmark trials which show the effectiveness of IPC and differentiates them from graduated elastic compression stockings (8). In general, IPCs are more effective, but GCS remain useful. One real advantage of stockings is that they provide some protection when the patient is sitting in a chair. The pneumatic devices are normally disconnected when a patient is placed in a chair and, if no other form of prophylaxis is being used, the stockings become an important modality. Some clinicians would comment that moving surgical patients into a chair in the early postoperative period does not represent early *ambulation* but rather early *angulation*. Stockings also have a role when the patient is being transported for tests and, due to shortages in personnel, pneumatic devices may not be reconnected in a timely fashion when the patient returns to bed. Additionally, pneumatic devices may feel uncomfortable to the patient as perspiration collects next to the skin. The obstructive qualities of stockings underneath these devices may increase patient comfort and compliance. We feel that it is important for the reader to understand that IPC's are clearly different from GCS and that there are a number of advantages to using the combination of both modalities for greatest patient comfort and effectiveness.

Many investigators feel that although IPC's are effective, it is very difficult to obtain a high degree of patient compliance. This view has been expressed by Comerota who reported approximately a 35% compliance rate utilizing the devices in a university setting (38). We have employed IPC's in our hospitals for over 30 years with great success and have developed techniques to maximize compliance. Our technique involves both patient and nursing staff education. By utilizing these methods, we achieved an 85% compliance rate in a recent study involving total knee replacement patients (39). Teaching the patient that these devices are important to prevent blood clots and should be on at all times when they are not ambulating is the most important factor in our successful program.

The question of which device within each group (long or short GCS, or various IPC methods) is superior to another cannot be answered due to lack of appropriate randomized head-to-head trials. One recent study examined the added benefit of GCS compared to IPC when applied to patients receiving prophylaxis with low molecular weight heparin (LMWH) after arthroplasty. The authors discovered that the IPC group had 0% VTE rate compared to the 28.6% rate in the GCS group (40). This trial demonstrates further that a combination of modalities can improve the effectiveness of VTE prophylaxis.

In our opinion, there are three main indications for the use of the physical devices, the most obvious being in those patients where anticoagulants are contraindicated. Examples would be patients with active bleeding, patients with bleeding tumors or hematologic defects, and in operations upon the central nervous system including both neoplasms and vascular malformations (Table 6). The second very strong indication for use of these physical methods is in the highest risk patients where the clinician attempts to reduce the incidence of VTE as much as possible. The study by Ramos involving 2551 patients undergoing cardiac surgery over a 10-years period is a good example of the value of combining anticoagulants and physical modalities to lower the incidence of PE (41). This trial represents the single best large example of how pneumatic devices can prevent pulmonary emboli and are more effective when combined with unfractionated heparin (UFH) than the use of unfractionated heparin alone. Another study by Kamran, although

Table 6 Many Uses for Pneumatic Compression

Hemostatic defects—hemophilia, von Willebrand's disease, platelet functional defects, heparin-induced thrombocytopenia, etc.	History of venous thromboembolism, used in combination with pharmacologic prophylaxis
Post-cardiopulmonary bypass (CABG) procedures (along with heparin or LMWH)	Ruptured vessels—bleeding ulcers, bleeding from colitis or ileitis
Pelvic hematomas, and/or other complex trauma situations	Craniotomy or spinal cord surgery
Complex cancer operations—pancreatoduodenectomy, major hepatic resection, extensive pelvic resection, etc.[a]	Patients with stroke in the acute phase, and in combination with heparin or LMWH later, particularly those who cannot ambulate
In selected THR replacement patients at lower risk	All total knee replacements along with LMWH
Low risk of VTE, avoids anticoagulant bleeding[b]	

[a] Used alone until it is safe to start anticoagulants.
[b] In patients with only two risk factors.
Abbreviations: CABG, coronary artery bypass; LMWH, low molecular weight heparin; THR, total hip replacement; VTE, venous thromboembolism.

not a randomized prospective study, clearly shows the benefits of adding pneumatic compression stockings and UFH for the prevention of DVT in stroke patients (42). The third indication for the use of physical methods is in patients with two risk factors where the incidence of DVT is 10–20% (see Table 3). The use of anticoagulants has never been shown to be better than using GCS and IPC combined for the prevention of venous thrombosis in this low-risk group of patients. Finally, as one who has used these devices for many years, I re-emphasize that, when using physical methods, combining IPC and GCS produces the best results. This opinion is based on 29 years of experience with IPC, observing many occasions during hospitalization where IPC devices were removed and their reapplication was delayed because of nursing personnel shortages (e.g., sending patients for diagnostic tests, getting them up in a reclining chair or to ambulate, wash or go to the bathroom). If the patient has GCS on, at least some degree of protection from venous stasis and overdistention of the venous system in the legs is afforded (34). If the patient cannot receive anticoagulants, we feel that the use of GCS alone is inadequate and will produce higher rates of venous thrombosis.

Unfractionated Heparin

The use of this drug for thrombosis prophylaxis in surgical patients can be traced to the pioneering work of Kakkar who, in 1977, reported a trial involving 28 hospitals and 4000 patients comparing small doses of UFH to placebo given to surgical patients postoperatively (43). The study clearly showed that UFH statistically significantly prevents all DVT compared to placebo and the incidence of fatal PE was reduced by 50% in the treated group (43). Table 7 shows these data, as well as the remarkable finding by Collins in 1988. He conducted a meta-analysis of all the trials that could be compared to the original Kakkar trial. This involved another 70 centers and 16,000 patients over a 15-years period. The results were exactly the same as the original trial (44). Once these data were available, the knowledge that UFH could lower the morbidity and mortality from thromboembolic disease after surgical procedures was unquestioned. For the next

Table 7 Early Use of Unfractionated Heparin for the Prevention of VTE in Surgical Patients

Group	Kakkar Trial[a]		Collins Trial[b]	
	Control (%)	Heparin (%)	Control (%)	Heparin (%)
DVT	29.6	9.40	27.4	10.6
Fatal PE	1.7	0.9	3.4	1.7
Bleeding	5.80	8.80	1.80	3.10

[a] 4,000 patients, 28 centers. Ref. 42.
[b] 16,000 patients, 70 centers. Ref. 43.
Abbreviations: DVT, deep vein thrombosis; PE, pulmonary embolism; VTE, venous thromboembolism.

decade this drug became the standard for prevention of venous thromboembolism in these surgical groups. As a matter of fact, UFH continues today to be the most widely used thrombosis prophylaxis modality in medical and surgical patients (45,46). This drug is very popular because it is inexpensive, has a half-life of under one hour, can be measured with the APTT, can be reversed easily with protamine, and is very familiar to generations of physicians.

The results of trials in general surgery involving UFH versus LMWH show varying results for thrombosis prophylaxis, with meta-analyses demonstrating either no difference between UFH and LMWH or improved VTE protection and lower bleeding complications with LMWH (47,48). One of the most recent trials by McLeod, a double-blind, randomized trial of 5000 units of UFH t.i.d. versus 40 mg QD of the LMWH enoxaparin, showed no significant differences in outcomes using UFH compared to LMWH in general surgical patients and the authors state that they prefer UFH due to its lower cost (49).

There are some disadvantages of unfractionated heparin, including the dreaded complication of heparin-induced thrombocytopenia (HIT). In susceptible patients heparin attaches to platelet Factor IV and stimulates an immune reaction which leads to platelet activation, clumping and thrombus formation. The syndrome usually develops after seven to ten days of heparin therapy and can recur in patients previously exposed to heparin (50,51). In this scenario the patient develops paradoxical clotting, most commonly manifested clinically as thrombotic episodes. At times, severe, disabling and often life-threatening strokes, pulmonary emboli, or thrombosis of the major arteries that are limb-threatening can result from HIT. This complication occurs in approximately 1% of patients receiving prophylactic or therapeutic doses of heparin (52). If one accounts for the cost of these complications, the economic advantage of UFH over LMWH is not so great (53). In addition, UFH inhibits platelet function to a greater degree than LMWH, which may produce more bleeding (47). Although both of these drugs are highly effective in general surgical patients, often neither one of them is used for fear of bleeding. Patients undergoing general, vascular, urologic, gynecologic and thoracic surgical procedures are often protected against thrombosis with stockings and/or IPC. Unfortunately, these modalities alone are only good for lower-risk surgical patients and not nearly as effective when patients have additional risk factors. In a study in our university academic setting, 70% of patients who were at very high risk did not receive appropriate thrombosis prophylaxis according to Consensus Conference Guidelines. The most commonly used form of prophylaxis in these individuals was a combination of stockings and pneumatic compression devices (54). Although long-term outcomes were not done as a part of this study, overall, patients on the surgical services had a higher than expected incidence of venous thrombosis compared to other hospitals (55). These data further illustrate that detailed individual risk assessment coupled with adherence to guidelines based on the risk factor point total is the key to reducing the incidence of thrombosis to the lowest possible level.

The under-use of thrombosis prophylaxis is not limited to surgical patients. One of the greatest needs in the medical community is to use appropriate thrombosis prophylaxis in patients at risk according to Consensus Conference Guidelines. Three large clinical trials which were randomized and prospective clearly showed that 10 to 15% of medical patients admitted to hospital with additional risk factors can be expected to develop venous thrombosis without appropriate prophylaxis (11,56,57). Two of these three trails were done with newer anti-thrombotic agents and the results will be described in subsequent sections of the text.

A common practice on both medical and surgical services is to administer UFH 5000 units b.i.d. as primary thrombosis prophylaxis. Bergmann, in a study of geriatric patients, showed that UFH 5000 units b.i.d. and 20 mg of enoxaparin were equivalent in preventing venous thrombosis (58). This dose of enoxaparin was subsequently found to be ineffective in reducing DVT in high-risk medical patients (11). There is good evidence in both the medical and surgical literature, however, that the use of 5000 units of UFH t.i.d. is superior to the b.i.d. dosing schedule (49,59). In fact, there is no large, randomized, prospective trial that shows the value of UFH 5000 units b.i.d. in medical patients. Three randomized, prospective trials in high-risk medical patients showed no differences between the b.i.d. heparin dosing and placebo (60–62). Goldhaber has commented on this problem, stating that "new onset VTE is more often caused by prophylaxis failure than lack of prophylaxis use" (63). In his series, patients readmitted to hospital with recurrent DVT most often had been given GCS or UFH b.i.d. alone as prophylactic modalities during the previous hospitalization. Many of these patients had multiple risk factors, with 80% having more than two risk factors. The majority of these patients were on medical services, not surgical services (where it is common for GCS, IPC and pharmacologic prophylaxis to be used together). These data indicate that GCS or UFH b.i.d. should not be used alone in patients at high risk for VTE.

Low-Molecular-Weight Heparin

This class of drugs was developed in the 1970s by chemical or enzymatic degradation of unfractionated heparin. In an attempt to isolate the part of the heparin molecule responsible for anticoagulant properties, a 19-saccharide chain was isolated from the original 50 saccharide units in unfractionated heparin. Low Molecular Weight Heparin (LMWH) solves many of the problems associated with UFH. Table 8 compares some of the more important characteristics of both compounds. The improved bio-availability, longer half-life and freedom from routine monitoring were important characteristics, along with the lower incidence of HIT and heparin-induced osteoporosis. The most fascinating property of this class of drugs is the improved patient survival seen in cancer patients in studies comparing UFH and LMWH in patients with venous thromboembolism.

Dr. David Bergqvist from Uppsala, Sweden pioneered the use of low molecular weight heparin for thrombosis prophylaxis in surgical patients. His original observations found that LMWH had less influence on primary hemostasis than UFH in the animal model (64). Unfortunately, this initially led to too high dosing in early clinical prophylaxis studies. He performed the first pharmacokinetic and pharmacodynamic studies on LMWH, as well as extensive clinical studies using this drug in a variety of clinical scenarios over the next 20 years (28,65–71). He was also first to show the long-term benefits of LMWH for extended prophylaxis (72). Bergqvist also showed that larger prophylactic doses of LMWH were more effective than smaller prophylactic doses both in cancer and benign

Table 8 Advantages of LMWH Compared to UFH

UFH	LMWH
Nonspecific binding to plasma proteins, endothelial cells, and macrophages	More specific binding to ATIII
Variable anticoagulant effect, requires anticoagulant monitoring high-risk patients	Consistent and predictable anticoagulant effect
Monitoring required for high-risk patients	No anticoagulant monitoring required
Dosed Q8h in high-risk patients	Most situations once daily dosing
Relatively poor bioavailability, especially low dose	Better bioavailability at low doses
Heparin resistance may occur	No heparin resistance
Short half-life	Longer half-life
	Redudced incidence of HIT and heparin-indudced osteoporosis
	Improved patient survival in patients with cancer

Abbreviations: LMWH, low molecular weight heparin; UFH, unfractionated heparin; ATIII, antithrombin; Q8h, every eight hours; HIT, heparin induced thrombocytopenia.

disease (73). He also demonstrated equal efficacy of several low molecular weight heparins compared to UFH in general surgical patients (65). One of his most important contributions was the recently completed Enoxacan II trial, which showed that 30 days of LMWH statistically significantly lowers the venographic incidence of venous thrombosis compared to seven days of LMWH prophylaxis. This study was done in abdominal surgery patients undergoing operations for cancer. For many of us who believe in extended outpatient prophylaxis, this study provided some guidelines as to the appropriate length of prophylaxis (66). However, if after 30 days the patient is still not ambulatory, then continued prophylaxis may be necessary because of the patient's continued VTE risk from immobilization, usually in a reclining chair.

Another fascinating property of LMWH was discovered in thrombosis treatment trials in patients with cancer who were randomized to receive either LMWH or UFH as initial treatment for their venous thrombosis. The patients in the LMWH group had a longer survival than did their counterparts who received UFH. This is a very complex association which is not well understood and has also been seen in some prophylaxis trials, most notably the work of von Tempelhof (74). This trial involved the administration of only seven days of LMWH or UFH for prophylaxis following gynecologic oncology debulking pelvic procedures. 650 days later, patients who had received LMWH only at the time of their surgery (seven days) had a statistically significantly better survival compared to their counterparts in the UFH group. Subsequent studies in cancer patients suggest that the administration of LMWH for one year in good-prognosis cancer patients without DVT prolonged their survival compared to those not receiving the drug (75,76). Additionally, other researchers have postulated that warfarin is not as effective as LMWH in cancer VTE prevention (77–79). While further studies are necessary to determine the effects on tumor biology, the authors would urge clinicians to prescribe LMWH whenever possible for prophylaxis or treatment of venous thromboembolic disease in patients with cancer, based on these studies.

Patients who present with multiple trauma suffer from a high incidence of VTE, which is seen over 70% of the time when long bone fractures are part of the clinical picture (80). Data have emerged to suggest that the administration of LMWH as prophylaxis in these trauma patients statistically significantly lowers the incidence of VTE compared to UFH prophylaxis (81). It is not always possible to employ anticoagulants in some of these patients, particularly those with closed head injury, pelvic fractures, or when lacerations of the liver or spleen are observed. Depending upon the risk of the patient, it is sometimes necessary to introduce prophylactic vena cava filters, especially when the patient has a strong past history of venous thromboembolism, multiple markers of thrombophilia, the post-thrombotic syndrome, or severe chronic venous insufficiency. Duplex scan screening of these individuals has also been used as a strategy, but the sensitivity and specificity of this noninvasive modality in patients without symptoms of deep vein thrombosis varies widely among institutions (82,83).

A great many studies have been carried out in the orthopedic population using LMWH, particularly following total joint replacement. It has been nearly 20 years since the first trials employing LMWH compared to UFH following total hip replacement showed a statistically significant superiority in favor of LMWH (84,85). Initially this drug was administered close to the time of surgery or in the early postoperative period, which resulted in excessive bleeding (86,87). Subsequent studies have demonstrated that the administration of enoxaparin at 12 hr, or later postoperatively, is associated with a less than 0.5% incidence of bleeding. That percentage rises to 5.3% if the drug is administered eight hours postoperatively (88). The question of pre- or postoperative initiation of LMWH has not been completely settled. The European community tends to use a preoperative dose given 12 hours prior to surgery, while North American clinicians favor starting the drug 12 to 24 hours postoperatively. One recent trial involved the use of dalteparin given in two regimes which were prospectively randomized and analyzed with respect to both efficacy and bleeding risk (89). In one limb of the study, the drug was administered 12 hours preoperatively, given in a reduced dose 6 hours postoperatively, and then a full dose every 24 hours thereafter for a total of seven to 10 days. In the other limb of the study, the preoperative dose was omitted. The results showed that the efficacy of postoperative dosing compared to pre- and postoperative dosing was not statistically different, while those patients who received LMWH preoperatively suffered a higher incidence of bleeding complications. For many North American clinicians, this settled the question, although many of us recognize that further research needs to be completed.

Should LMWH prophylaxis be continued following discharge in total hip replacement patients? Borgqvist first demonstrated a 54% risk reduction with 30 days of LMWH prophylaxis compared to seven to 10 days postoperatively (30). A number of other authors subsequently confirmed these findings in this high-risk orthopedic population (31,66,90,91). The clinical and venographic incidence of VTE is statistically reduced following this extended prophylaxis in hip replacement surgery, hip fracture surgery, and in cancer patients who have endured surgery.

LMWH is also widely used following total knee replacement and is usually administered for seven to 10 days (92). Extended prophylaxis in this group of patients has not been shown to be necessary in prospective clinical trials (31). It has been our personal observation that many times these patients will be relatively immobile for four to six weeks following surgery, spending long periods of time in the recliner. These patients may require continued prophylaxis until they are fully ambulatory.

In the United States the use of oral anticoagulants following total joint replacement has been popular and approximately half of all patients are treated in this fashion. Many clinicians favor this approach because bleeding problems are minimal and the clinical incidence of VTE appears low. While prospective, randomized clinical trials such as the one by Hull showed venographic superiority in the prevention of VTE using LMWH compared to oral anticoagulants, warfarin still remains popular among clinicians (89,93). One reason for using the oral approach can be traced to the work of Colwell. This trial collected data from 156 centers and involved 3000 patients who were followed for 90 days following total hip replacement and randomly assigned to warfarin or enoxaparin. There was no statistically significant difference in the incidence of symptomatic VTE at 90 days between the two groups (94). LMWH enthusiasts would be quick to point out that there was a statistically significantly higher incidence of clinical VTE during hospitalization in the patients receiving oral anticoagulants. Only 1.1% of the patients had VTE and this was reduced to 0.3% in the LMWH group. Most clinicians did not consider this tiny reduction in incidence to be worth the potential increased bleeding and cost of LMWH. Additionally, both agents were given for 10–14 days, which is a shorter duration than what is recommended today. Some of us feel that looking only at a clinical endpoint is a very one-dimensional philosophy that does not address the overall advantages of LMWH to statistically significantly reduce the overall incidence of VTE. We are bothered by those who do not pay attention to venographic endpoints, arguing that they are artificial laboratory results that have little clinical significance. Kakkar demonstrated decades ago that delayed diagnosis of a clot led to damaged venous valves and to PTS (43). It would follow that inadequate prevention leads to asymptomatic clots that may not cause PE early in the course, but would lead to PTS and recurrent thrombosis. To those individuals, we point out that there are now several trials that demonstrate that venographic endpoints are surrogate markers for clinical events (95,96). We feel that in patients at extremely high risk for VTE, the use of a drug that provides the best efficacy should be selected.

LMWH prophylaxis has been used in medically ill patients in a number of studies, including the Medenox trial, which compared placebo, enoxaparin 20 mg/day, and enoxaparin 40 mg/day, in medical patients with one additional risk factor such as infection, heart failure, or pulmonary disease (11). The higher enoxaparin dose produced statistically significant improvement in the incidence of all VTE from 14.9% in the placebo group to 5.5% in the treated group. Interestingly, the lower-dose enoxaparin group had a 15% incidence of VTE compared to 14.9% in the placebo group. This study clearly illustrated that one must use not only the right drug, but also the right dose for a specific thrombosis prophylaxis indication. A second trial called the PREVENT trial involved dalteparin 5000 units a day in 3706 medically ill patients and showed a statistically significant reduction in the incidence of VTE from 4.96% to 2.77% (12).

The question of cost-effectiveness was first addressed by Bergqvist when he showed how patients who self-administered LMWH avoided clinical DVT (97,98). A number of other authors have studied the cost-effectiveness of using LMWH compared to UFH in both prophylactic and therapeutic studies. They conclude that the higher initial cost of the LMWH compared to UFH is justified because of the savings attributed to improved efficacy and reduced side-effects, particularly the dreaded HIT (99–102).

Fondaparinux

As the first synthetic Factor Xa inhibitor, fondaparinux further refines the quest for a specific inhibitor of clotting. Even with their successful use, LMWH still have limitations: b.i.d. dosing with many indications, cannot be used in HIT, and they are derived from animal sources. Many years of research during the 1980s led to the realization that only a 5-sugar sequence was required for antithrombotic activity. In collaboration, the Institute of Choay, Sanofi-Synthelabo, and Organon synthesized a 5-sugar molecule, fondapairnux, which would bind to antithrombin 94% and increase antithrombin affinity for Factor Xa by 300-fold (103–105). The specific binding and small size of fondaparinux also results in a lack of cross-reactivity with platelet Factor IV, resulting in a substantially reduced ability to promote HIT (51,106). Early research demonstrated its effectiveness in prevention of DVT in hip and knee replacement with a fixed, once-daily subcutaneous injection (107). A large study program in hip replacement, knee replacement, and hip fracture repair introduced fondaparinux to orthopedic care. Fondaparinux was compared to both the European and North American conventional doses of enoxaparin in a randomized, double-blind fashion. Fondaparinux reduced the occurrence of venographically detected venous thrombosis over 50% better than did enoxaparin (108). Patients undergoing knee replacement experienced a higher bleeding rate in the fondaparinux group (109). An analysis of the timing of dosage initiation demonstrated that excess bleeding risk was attributable to drug administration less than four hours after surgery, similar to the LMWH trial by Hull (89). The researchers found that the preferred administration time for fondaparinux came six to eight hours after surgery (108,110). Subsequently it was found that next-day (<24 hr) administration maintained efficacy but reduced bleeding in patients following total hip or knee replacement (111). Pharmacoeconomic studies have demonstrated that fondaparinux is more cost-effective when chosen instead of enoxaparin in several models in the United States and Europe (112–116).

With regard to extended prophylaxis in orthopedic surgery, Eriksson pursued the ability of fondaparinux to reduce VTE events in patients undergoing hip fracture repair. Compared to seven days of prophylaxis, 30 days of fondaparinux prophylaxis reduced the event rate from 35% to 1.4%. Additionally, the symptomatic event rate was significantly reduced from 2.7% to 0.3%, nearly eliminating VTE (96). This trial is a significant contribution to patient care. First, it confirmed the ability of a venogram to accurately predict the effects on clinical VTE events; both were prevented by 90%. Second, unlike previous studies, this study was able to identify beneficial effects on symptomatic events alone in only 656 patients, confirming the benefit of fondaparinux prophylaxis. Additionally, with four weeks of fondaparinux treatment, major bleeding was no different from placebo.

With its success in DVT prevention after orthopedic surgery, fondaparinux was studied in other indications as well. Abdominal surgery patients at risk for postoperative DVT were assigned to fondaparinux or a pre-op/post-op dosage of dalteparin in a double-blind fashion. Both drugs reduced the VTE rate similarly; however, unexpectedly, fondaparinux reduced the VTE rate in the cancer cohort significantly compared to dalteparin. Major bleeding was low for both agents (117). This is the first study comparing fondaparinux to LMWH in a cancer cohort. These interesting results await larger, more specific trials in cancer patients receiving surgical treatment as well as DVT prevention in patients being medically treated for cancer.

A European placebo-controlled trial was undertaken to determine the effect of fondaparinux in the prevention of VTE in patients hospitalized for medical illness. This was possible due to the low rate of heparin or LMWH utilization in medical patients at the time the trial was conducted. Fondaparinux significantly reduced the VTE rate in medical patients compared to placebo from 10.5% to 5.6%, with no significant difference in major bleeding. Additionally, fondaparinux reduced the rate of death due to PE from 1.5% to 0% (57). This was the first time a single study demonstrated reduced mortality in medical prophylaxis patients. Previous meta-analysis of many LMWH studies demonstrated reduced mortality in medical and cancer patients receiving prophylaxis as described earlier.

Fondaparinux is undergoing evaluation by the FDA for prophylaxis after abdominal surgery and in medical prophylaxis. Its place in therapy has been addressed for its current indications in orthopedics by the Consensus Conference Guidelines (6). It has been given FDA approval in hip fracture patients for both standard and extended prophylaxis, is a useful prophylactic agent in high-risk patients, and can prevent VTE better than LMWH. Proper administration time after surgery, and avoidance in patients with severe renal dysfunction (creatinine clearance < 30 ml/min), will optimize its safety. This agent demonstrates again that patient-specific risk assessment is needed in order to enjoy the benefits and minimize the risk of thrombosis prophylaxis.

Ximelagatran

For many years warfarin was the only oral anticoagulant available for long-term thrombosis prophylaxis in patients with chronic atrial fibrillation and mechanical heart valves, and as primary treatment after an initial period of heparin therapy in patients with VTE. Warfarin has also been the mainstay of long-term prophylaxis in VTE. It has been widely used as primary thrombosis prophylaxis after major orthopedic surgery, particularly in joint replacements and following hip fracture surgery. However, warfarin has a slow onset of action and is inconvenient because it requires frequent coagulation monitoring and dose adjustments. In addition, the anticoagulant properties of warfarin can be affected by certain foods, alcoholic beverages, and a wide variety of medications. The logistics of managing warfarin may be cumbersome in certain clinical situations, particularly in those individuals who do not have access to coagulation clinics or other advanced health-care management systems that specialize in patient monitoring. A small subset of patients exists in whom maintaining appropriate levels of anticoagulation is a difficult chore due to warfarin resistance or other factors (118).

Over the past few years a new oral anticoagulant called ximelagatran has been developed. Taken orally, this drug undergoes a rapid biotransformation in the GI tract to melagatran. It directly inhibits thrombin, both clot-bound and circulating in plasma. Melagatran is not metabolized, and 80% of the drug is excreted renally. It is not bound to plasma proteins and has a low potential for food or drug interactions. This drug does not require routine anticoagulant monitoring; however, it does require liver enzyme tests (AST, ALT, bilirubin) monthly. Fixed dosing produces a predictable dose response and it must be taken twice daily. Melagatran reaches a peak concentration in the blood in two hours and has a four-to-five-hours half-life. It has a pharmacokinetic profile comparable to LMWH. This drug has undergone an extensive clinical trial program involving nearly 30,000 patients. The clinical areas involved in these studies include DVT prophylaxis after orthopedic surgery and in medically ill patients, DVT treatment both primary and extended prophylaxis, atrial fibrillation, and in patients with certain acute coronary syndromes (119–122). This clinical program has been very successful regarding efficacy endpoints; however, at the present time, concern over liver function test elevations has prevented this drug from achieving FDA approval in the United States (123). The drug has been approved for short-term use in a number of European countries and has been used in about 50,000 patients. To date, no serious liver-related problems have been observed.

KEY POINTS

- Venous thromboembolism (VTE) is a major cause of mortality particularly in the elderly, in those undergoing surgery and in those with cancer.
- Longer term the post-thrombotic syndrome occurs in 25% of those with a DVT.

- All patients should undergo a formal risk assessment for VTE.
- Physical measures such as graduated compression stockings and intermittent pneumatic compression are effective.
- Physical measures should be particularly considered in those where anticoagulants are contraindicated or where there is high risk.
- Pharmacological prophylaxis includes unfractionated heparin and low-molecular weight heparin.
- Newer agents including direct factor Xa inhibitors are being developed and introduced.

REFERENCES

1. Cushman M, Tsai AW, White RH, et al. Deep vein thrombosis and pulmonary embolism in two cohorts: the longitudinal investigation of thromboembolism etiology. Am J Med 2004; 117:19–25.
2. National Center for Health Statistics Fast Facts Web site. (Accessed December 15, 2004, at www.cdc.gov/nchs/fastfacts/mamogram.htm.).
3. National Center for Health Statistics Report 2002; 53:1–116. (Accessed December 15, 2004, at www.cdc.gov/nchs/data/nvsr/nvsr53/nvsr53_05.pdf.).
4. Kniffin WD, Jr., Baron JA, Barrett J, et al. The epidemiology of diagnosed pulmonary embolism and deep venous thrombosis in the elderly. Arch Intern Med 1994; 154:861–866.
5. Anderson FA, Jr., Wheeler HB, Goldberg RJ, et al. A population-based perspective of the hospital incidence and case-fatality rates of deep vein thrombosis and pulmonary embolism. The Worcester DVT Study. Arch Intern Med 1991; 151:933–938.
6. Geerts WH, Pineo GF, Heit JA, et al. Prevention of venous thromboembolism: the seventh ACCP conference on antithrombotic and thrombolytic therapy. Chest 2004; 126:338S–400S.
7. Bhattacharyya T, Iorio R, Healy WL. Rate of and risk factors for acute inpatient mortality after orthopaedic surgery. J Bone Joint Surg Am 2002; 84:562–572.
8. Nicolaides AN, Breddin HK, Fareed J, et al. Prevention of venous thromboembolism. International Consensus Statement. Guidelines compiled in accordance with the scientific evidence. Int Angiol 2001; 20:1–37.
9. Hirsch DR, Ingenito EP, Goldhaber SZ. Prevalence of deep venous thrombosis among patients in medical intensive care. JAMA 1995; 274:335–337.
10. Fraisse F, Holzapfel L, Couland JM, et al. Nadroparin in the prevention of deep vein thrombosis in acute decompensated COPD. The Association of Non-University Affiliated Intensive Care Specialist Physicians of France. Am J Respir Crit Care Med 2000; 161:1109–1114.
11. Samama MM, Cohen AT, Darmon JY, et al. A comparison of enoxaparin with placebo for the prevention of venous thromboembolism in acutely ill medical patients. Prophylaxis in Medical Patients with Enoxaparin Study Group. N Engl J Med 1999; 341:793–800.
12. Leizorovicz A, Mismetti P. Preventing venous thromboembolism in medical patients. Circulation 2004; 110:IV13–IV19.
13. Kakkar AK, Williamson RC. Prevention of venous thromboembolism in cancer patients. Semin Thromb Hemost 1999; 25:239–243.
14. Clagett GP, Reisch JS. Prevention of venous thromboembolism in general surgical patients. Results of meta-analysis. Ann Surg 1988; 208:227–240.
15. Prandoni P, Lensing AW, Cogo A, et al. The long-term clinical course of acute deep venous thrombosis. Ann Intern Med 1996; 125:1–7.
16. Prandoni P, Lensing AW, Prins MR. The natural history of deep-vein thrombosis. Semin Thromb Hemost 1997; 23:185–188.

17. Prandoni P, Villalta S, Bagatella P, et al. The clinical course of deep-vein thrombosis. Prospective long-term follow-up of 528 symptomatic patients. Haematologica 1997; 82:423–428.

18. Siragusa S, Beltrametti C, Barone M, et al. Clinical course and incidence of post-thrombophlebitic syndrome after profound asymptomatic deep vein thrombosis. Results of a transverse epidemiologic study. Minerva Cardioangiol 1997; 45:57–66.

19. Kahn SR. Venous thrombosis in long-haul travelers. Arch Intern Med 2004; 164:1699–1700.

20. Borow M, Goldson H. Postoperative venous thrombosis. Evaluation of five methods of treatment. Am J Surg 1981; 141:245–251.

21. Brandjes DP, ten Cate JW, Buller HR. Pre-surgical identification of the patient at risk for developing venous thromboembolism post-operatively. Acta Chir Scand Suppl 1990; 556:18–21.

22. Caprini JA, Arcelus JI, Traverso CI, et al. Low molecular weight heparins and external pneumatic compression as options for venous thromboembolism prophylaxis: a surgeon's perspective. Semin Thromb Hemost 1991; 17:356–366.

23. Geerts WH, Heit JA, Clagett GP, et al. Prevention of venous thromboembolism. Chest 2001; 119:132S–175S.

24. Clagett GP, Anderson FA, Jr., Geerts W, et al. Prevention of venous thromboembolism. Chest 1998; 114:531S–560S.

25. Kessler CM. Propensity for hemorrhage and thrombosis in chronic myeloproliferative disorders. Semin Hematol 2004; 41:10–14.

26. Peeters AC, van der Molen EF, Blom HJ, et al. The effect of homocysteine reduction by B-vitamin supplementation on markers of endothelial dysfunction. Thromb Haemost 2004; 92:1086–1091.

27. Stanger O, Herrmann W, Pietrzik K, et al. Clinical use and rational management of homocysteine, folic acid, and B vitamins in cardiovascular and thrombotic diseases. Z Kardiol 2004; 93:439–453.

28. Bergqvist D, Lowe G. Venous thromboembolism in patients undergoing laparoscopic and arthroscopic surgery and in leg casts. Arch Intern Med 2002; 162:2173–2176.

29. Baca I, Schneider B, Kohler T, et al. Prevention of thromboembolism in minimal invasive interventions and brief inpatient treatment. Results of a multicenter, prospective, randomized, controlled study with a low molecular weight heparin. Chirurg 1997; 68:1275–1280.

30. Bergqvist D, Benoni G, Bjorgell O, et al. Low-molecular-weight heparin (enoxaparin) as prophylaxis against venous thromboembolism after total hip replacement. N Engl J Med 1996; 335:696–700.

31. Comp PC, Spiro TE, Friedman RJ, et al. Prolonged enoxaparin therapy to prevent venous thromboembolism after primary hip or knee replacement. Enoxaparin Clinical Trial Group. J Bone Joint Surg Am 2001; 83:336–345.

32. Efficacy and safety of enoxaparin versus unfractionated heparin for prevention of deep vein thrombosis in elective cancer surgery: a double-blind randomized multicentre trial with venographic assessment. ENOXACAN Study Group. Br J Surg, 1997; 84:1099–1103.

33. Eriksson BI, Bauer KA, Lassen MR, et al. Fondaparinux compared with enoxaparin for the prevention of venous thromboembolism after hip-fracture surgery. N Engl J Med 2001; 345:1298–1304.

34. Arcelus JI, Caprini JA, Sehgal LR, et al. Home use of impulse compression of the foot and compression stockings in the treatment of chronic venous insufficiency. J Vasc Surg 2001; 34:805–811.

35. Turner GM, Cole SE, Brooks JH. The efficacy of graduated compression stockings in the prevention of deep vein thrombosis after major gynaecological surgery. Br J Obstet Gynaecol 1984; 91:588–591.

36. Holford CP. Graded compression for preventing deep venous thrombosis. Br Med J 1976; 2:969–970.

37. Amarigiri SV, Lees TA. Elastic compression stockings for prevention of deep vein thrombosis. Cochrane Database Syst Rev 2000; CD001484.
38. Comerota AJ, Katz ML, White JV. Why does prophylaxis with external pneumatic compression for deep vein thrombosis fail? Am J Surg 1992; 164:265–268.
39. Caprini JA OM, Robb WJ. Thrombosis phophylaxis following total knee replacement. Poster presentation. American Venous Forum, San Diego, CA, February. 2005:9–13.
40. Silbersack Y, Taute BM, Hein W, et al. Prevention of deep-vein thrombosis after total hip and knee replacement. Low-molecular-weight heparin in combination with intermittent pneumatic compression. J Bone Joint Surg Br 2004; 86:809–812.
41. Ramos R, Salem BI, De Pawlikowski MP, et al. The efficacy of pneumatic compression stockings in the prevention of pulmonary embolism after cardiac surgery. Chest 1996; 109:82–85.
42. Kamran SI, Downey D, Ruff RL. Pneumatic sequential compression reduces the risk of deep vein thrombosis in stroke patients. Neurology 1998; 50:1683–1688.
43. Kakkar VV, Corrigan TP, Fossard DP, et al. Prevention of Fatal Postoperative pulmonary embolism by low doses of heparin. Reappraisal of results of international multicentre trial. Lancet 1977; 1:567–569.
44. Collins R, Scrimgeour A, Yusuf S, et al. Reduction in fatal pulmonary embolism and venous thrombosis by perioperative administration of subcutaneous heparin. Overview of results of randomized trials in general, orthopedic, and urologic surgery. N Engl J Med 1988; 318:1162–1173.
45. Caprini JA, Arcelus J, Sehgal LR, et al. The use of low molecular weight heparins for the prevention of postoperative venous thromboembolism in general surgery. A survey of practice in the United States. Int Angiol 2002; 21:78–85.
46. Caprini JA, Arcelus JI, Hoffman K, et al. Prevention of venous thromboembolism in North America: results of a survey among general surgeons. J Vasc Surg 1994; 20:751–758.
47. Mismetti P, Laporte S, Darmon JY, et al. Meta-analysis of low molecular weight heparin in the prevention of venous thromboembolism in general surgery. Br J Surg 2001; 88:913–930.
48. Koch A, Bouges S, Ziegler S, et al. Low molecular weight heparin and unfractionated heparin in thrombosis prophylaxis after major surgical intervention: update of previous meta-analyses. Br J Surg 1997; 84:750–759.
49. McLeod RS, Geerts WH, Sniderman KW, et al. Subcutaneous heparin versus low-molecular-weight heparin as thromboprophylaxis in patients undergoing colorectal surgery: results of the canadian colorectal DVT prophylaxis trial: a randomized, double-blind trial. Ann Surg 2001; 233:438–444.
50. Warkentin TE. Clinical presentation of heparin-induced thrombocytopenia. Semin Hematol 1998; 35:9–16; discussion 35–36.
51. Warkentin TE, Greinacher A. Heparin-induced thrombocytopenia: recognition, treatment, and prevention: the Seventh ACCP Conference on Antithrombotic and Thrombolytic Therapy. Chest 2004; 126:311S–337S.
52. Warkentin TE, Levine MN, Hirsh J, et al. Heparin-induced thrombocytopenia in patients treated with low-molecular-weight heparin or unfractionated heparin. N Engl J Med 1995; 332:1330–1335.
53. Weinberg M, Lichtig LK, Caprini JA, et al. Implications of heparin utilization for medical at-risk patients. Submitted for publication.
54. Caprini JA, Glase C, Martchev D. Thrombosis risk factor assessment in surgical patients: compliance with chest consensus guidelines. Poster presentation. American Venous Forum, Cancun, Mexico, February. 2003:20–23
55. Personal communication, Solucent Database, 2004.
56. Turpie AG. Thrombosis prophylaxis in the acutely ill medical patient: insights from the prophylaxis in MEDical patients with ENOXaparin (MEDENOX) trial. Am J Cardiol 2000; 86:48M–52M.
57. Cohen AT, Gallus AS, Lassen MR, et al. Fondaparinux vs. placebo for the prevention of venous throboembolism in acutely ill meidcla patients (artemis). J Thromb Haemost 2003; 1:2046.

58. Bergmann JF, Neuhart E. A multicenter randomized double-blind study of enoxaparin compared with unfractionated heparin in the prevention of venous thromboembolic disease in elderly in-patients bedridden for an acute medical illness. The Enoxaparin in Medicine Study Group. Thromb Haemost 1996; 76:529–534.

59. Kleber FX, Witt C, Vogel G, et al. Randomized comparison of enoxaparin with unfractionated heparin for the prevention of venous thromboembolism in medical patients with heart failure or severe respiratory disease. Am Heart J 2003; 145:614–621.

60. Gardlund B. Randomised, controlled trial of low-dose heparin for prevention of fatal pulmonary embolism in patients with infectious diseases. The Heparin Prophylaxis Study Group. Lancet 1996; 347:1357–1361.

61. Cade JF, Andrews JT, Stubbs AE. Comparison of sodium and calcium heparin in prevention of venous thromboembolism. Aust NZ J Med 1982; 12:501–504.

62. Halkin H, Goldberg J, Modan M, et al. Reduction of mortality in general medical in-patients by low-dose heparin prophylaxis. Ann Intern Med 1982; 96:561–565.

63. Goldhaber SZ, Dunn K, MacDougall RC. New onset of venous thromboembolism among hospitalized patients at Brigham and Women's Hospital is caused more often by prophylaxis failure than by withholding treatment. Chest 2000; 118:1680–1684.

64. Holmer E, Soderberg K, Bergqvist D, et al. Heparin and its low molecular weight derivatives: anticoagulant and antithrombotic properties. Haemostasis 1986; 16:1–7.

65. Bergqvist D. Prophylaxis of postoperative deep vein thrombosis in general surgery: experiences with Fragmin. Acta Chir Scand Suppl 1988; 543:87–89.

66. Bergqvist D, Agnelli G, Cohen AT, et al. Duration of prophylaxis against venous thrombo-embolism with enoxaparin after surgery for cancer. N Engl J Med 2002; 346:975–980.

67. Bergqvist D, Burmark US, Frisell J, et al. Thromboprophylactic effect of low molecular weight heparin started in the evening before elective general abdominal surgery: a comparison with low-dose heparin. Semin Thromb Hemost 1990; 16:19–24.

68. Bergqvist D, Flordal PA, Friberg B, et al. Thromboprophylaxis with a low molecular weight heparin (tinzaparin) in emergency abdominal surgery. A double-blind multicenter trial. Vasa 1996; 25:156–160.

69. Bergqvist D, Lindblad B, Matzsch T. Low molecular weight heparin for thromboprophylaxis and epidural/spinal anaesthesia—is there a risk? Acta Anaesthesiol Scand 1992; 36:605–609.

70. Bergqvist D, Matzsch T, Burmark US, et al. Low molecular weight heparin given the evening before surgery compared with conventional low-dose heparin in prevention of thrombosis. Br J Surg 1988; 75:888–891.

71. Bergqvist D, Nilsson B. The influence of low molecular weight heparin in combination with dihydroergotamine on experimental thrombosis and haemostasis. Thromb Haemost 1987; 58:893–895.

72. Bergqvist D. Prolonged prophylaxis against postoperative venous thromboembolism. Haemostasis 1996; 26:379–387.

73. Bergqvist D, Burmark US, Flordal PA, et al. Low molecular weight heparin started before surgery as prophylaxis against deep vein thrombosis: 2500 versus 5000 XaI units in 2070 patients. Br J Surg 1995; 82:496–501.

74. von Tempelhoff GF, Harenberg J, Niemann F, et al. Effect of low molecular weight heparin (Certoparin) versus unfractionated heparin on cancer survival following breast and pelvic cancer surgery: a prospective randomized double-blind trial. Int J Oncol 2000; 16:815–824.

75. Kakkar AK, Levine MN, Kadziola Z, et al. Low molecular weight heparin, therapy with dalteparin, and survival in advanced cancer: the fragmin advanced malignancy outcome study (FAMOUS). J Clin Oncol 2004; 22:1944–1948.

76. Altinbas M, Coskun HS, Er O, et al. A randomized clinical trial of combination chemotherapy with and without low-molecular-weight heparin in small cell lung cancer. J Thromb Haemost 2004; 2:1266–1271.

77. Lee AY. Epidemiology and management of venous thromboembolism in patients with cancer. Thromb Res 2003; 110:167–172.

78. Lee AY. The role of low-molecular-weight heparins in the prevention and treatment of venous thromboembolism in cancer patients. Curr Opin Pulm Med 2003; 9:351–355.

79. Cosmi B, Palareti G. Oral anticoagulant therapy in venous thromboembolism. Semin Vasc Med 2003; 3:303–314.

80. Geerts WH, Code KI, Jay RM, et al. A prospective study of venous thromboembolism after major trauma. N Engl J Med 1994; 331:1601–1606.

81. Geerts WH, Jay RM, Code KI, et al. A comparison of low-dose heparin with low-molecular-weight heparin as prophylaxis against venous thromboembolism after major trauma. N Engl J Med 1996; 335:701–707.

82. Cipolle MD, Wojcik R, Seislove E, et al. The role of surveillance duplex scanning in preventing venous thromboembolism in trauma patients. J Trauma 2002; 52:453–462.

83. Kadyan V, Clinchot DM, Mitchell GL, et al. Surveillance with duplex ultrasound in traumatic spinal cord injury on initial admission to rehabilitation. J Spinal Cord Med 2003; 26:231–235.

84. Planes A, Vochelle N, Ferru J, et al. Enoxaparine low molecular weight heparin: its use in the prevention of deep venous thrombosis following total hip replacement. Haemostasis 1986; 16:152–158.

85. Turpie AG, Levine MN, Hirsh J, et al. A randomized controlled trial of a low-molecular-weight heparin (enoxaparin) to prevent deep-vein thrombosis in patients undergoing elective hip surgery. N Engl J Med 1986; 315:925–929.

86. Spiro TE, Johnson GJ, Christie MJ, et al. Efficacy and safety of enoxaparin to prevent deep venous thrombosis after hip replacement surgery. Enoxaparin Clinical Trial Group. Ann Intern Med 1994; 121:81–89.

87. Colwell CW, Jr., Spiro TE, Trowbridge AA, et al. Use of enoxaparin, a low-molecular-weight heparin, and unfractionated heparin for the prevention of deep venous thrombosis after elective hip replacement. A clinical trial comparing efficacy and safety. Enoxaparin Clinical Trial Group. J Bone Joint Surg Am 1994; 76:3–14.

88. Fitzgerald RH, Jr., Spiro TE, Trowbridge AA, et al. Prevention of venous thromboembolic disease following primary total knee arthroplasty. A randomized, multicenter, open-label, parallel-group comparison of enoxaparin and warfarin. J Bone Joint Surg Am 2001; 83:900–906.

89. Hull RD, Pineo GF, Francis C, et al. Low-molecular-weight heparin prophylaxis using dalteparin in close proximity to surgery vs warfarin in hip arthroplasty patients: a double-blind, randomized comparison. The North American Fragmin Trial Investigators. Arch Intern Med 2000; 160:2199–2207.

90. Dahl OE, Andreassen G, Aspelin T, et al. Prolonged thromboprophylaxis following hip replacement surgery–results of a double-blind, prospective, randomised, placebo-controlled study with dalteparin (Fragmin). Thromb Haemost 1997; 77:26–31.

91. Dahl OE, Pleil AM. Investment in prolonged thromboprophylaxis with dalteparin improves clinical outcomes after hip replacement. J Thromb Haemost 2003; 1:896–906.

92. Leclerc JR, Geerts WH, Desjardins L, et al. Prevention of deep vein thrombosis after major knee surgery—a randomized, double-blind trial comparing a low molecular weight heparin fragment (enoxaparin) to placebo. Thromb Haemost 1992; 67:417–423.

93. Hull RD, Raskob GE, Pineo GF, et al. Subcutaneous low-molecular-weight heparin vs warfarin for prophylaxis of deep vein thrombosis after hip or knee implantation. An economic perspective. Arch Intern Med 1997; 157:298–303.

94. Colwell CW, Jr., Collis DK, Paulson R, et al. Comparison of enoxaparin and warfarin for the prevention of venous thromboembolic disease after total hip arthroplasty. Evaluation during hospitalization and three months after discharge. J Bone Joint Surg Am 1999; 81:932–940.

95. Eriksson BI, Bauer KA, Lassen MR, et al. Influence of the duration of fondaparinux (Arixtra) prophylaxis in preventing venous thromboembolism following major orthopedic surgery. J Thromb Haemost 2003; 1:383–384.

96. Eriksson BI, Lassen MR. Duration of prophylaxis against venous thromboembolism with fondaparinux after hip fracture surgery: a multicenter, randomized, placebo-controlled, double-blind study. Arch Intern Med 2003; 163:1337–1342.

97. Bergqvist D, Matzsch T. Cost/benefit aspects on thromboprophylaxis. Haemostasis 1993; 23:15–19.

98. Bergqvist D, Lindgren B, Matzsch T. Comparison of the cost of preventing postoperative deep vein thrombosis with either unfractionated or low molecular weight heparin. Br J Surg 1996; 83:1548–1552.

99. McGarry LJ, Thompson D. Retrospective database analysis of the prevention of venous thromboembolism with low-molecular-weight heparin in acutely III medical inpatients in community practice. Clin Ther 2004; 26:419–430.

100. de Lissovoy G, Subedi P. Economic evaluation of enoxaparin as prophylaxis against venous thromboembolism in seriously ill medical patients: a U.S. perspective. Am J Manag Care 2002; 8:1082–1088.

101. Botteman MF, Caprini J, Stephens JM, et al. Results of an economic model to assess the cost-effectiveness of enoxaparin, a low-molecular-weight heparin, versus warfarin for the prophylaxis of deep vein thrombosis and associated long-term complications in total hip replacement surgery in the United States. Clin Ther 2002; 24:1960–1986; discussion 1938.

102. Nerurkar J, Wade WE, Martin BC. Cost/death averted with venous thromboembolism prophylaxis in patients undergoing total knee replacement or knee arthroplasty. Pharmaco-therapy 2002; 22:990–1000.

103. Walenga JM, Bara L, Petitou M, et al. The inhibition of the generation of thrombin and the antithrombotic effect of a pentasaccharide with sole anti-factor Xa activity. Thromb Res 1988; 51:23–33.

104. Petitou M, Duchaussoy P, Lederman I, et al. Synthesis of heparin fragments. A chemical synthesis of the pentasaccharide O-(2-deoxy-2-sulfamido-6-O-sulfo-alpha-D-glucopyrano-syl)-(1-4)-O-(beta-D-glucopyranosyluronic acid)-(1-4)-O-(2-deoxy-2-sulfamido-3,6-di-O-sulfo-alpha-D-glu copyranosyl)-(1-4)-O-(2-O-sulfo-alpha-L-idopyranosyluronic acid)-(1-4)-2-deoxy-2-sulfamido-6-O-sulfo-D-glucopyranose decasodium salt, a heparin fragment having high affinity for antithrombin III. Carbohydr Res 1986; 147:221–236.

105. Choay J, Petitou M, Lormeau JC, et al. Structure-activity relationship in heparin: a synthetic pentasaccharide with high affinity for antithrombin III and eliciting high anti-factor Xa activity. Biochem Biophys Res Commun 1983; 116:492–499.

106. Savi P, Chong BH, Greinacher A, et al. Effect of fondaparinux on platelet activation in the presence of heparin-dependent antibodies. A blinded comparative multicenter study with unfractionated heparin. Blood 2004.

107. Turpie AG, Gallus AS, Hoek JA. A synthetic pentasaccharide for the prevention of deep-vein thrombosis after total hip replacement. N Engl J Med 2001; 344:619–625.

108. Turpie AG, Bauer KA, Eriksson BI, et al. Fondaparinux vs enoxaparin for the prevention of venous thromboembolism in major orthopedic surgery: a meta-analysis of 4 randomized double blind studies. Arch Intern Med 2002; 162:1833–1840.

109. Bauer KA, Eriksson BI, Lassen MR, et al. Fondaparinux compared with enoxaparin for the prevention of venous thromboembolism after elective major knee surgery. N Engl J Med 2001; 345:1305–1310.

110. Bauer KA, Eriksson BI, Lassen MR, et al. Factor Xa inhibition in the prevention of venous thromboembolism and treatment of patients with venous thromboembolism. Curr Opin Pulm Med 2002; 8:398–404.

111. Pineo GF, Hull RD. Dalteparin sodium. Expert Opin Pharmacother 2001; 2:1325–1337.

112. Sullivan SD, Davidson BL, Kahn SR, et al. A cost-effectiveness analysis of fondaparinux sodium compared with enoxaparin sodium as prophylaxis against venous thromboembolism: use in patients undergoing major orthopaedic surgery. Pharmacoeconomics 2004; 22:605–620.

113. Gordois A, Posnett J, Borris L, et al. The cost-effectiveness of fondaparinux compared with enoxaparin as prophylaxis against thromboembolism following major orthopedic surgery. J Thromb Haemost 2003; 1:2167–2174.

114. Spruill WJ, Wade WE, Leslie RB. A cost analysis of fondaparinux versus enoxaparin in total knee arthroplasty. Am J Ther 2004; 11:3–8.

115. Spruill WJ, Wade WE, Leslie RB. Cost analysis of fondaparinux versus enoxaparin as venous thromboembolism prophylaxis in elective hip replacement surgery. Blood Coagul Fibrinolysis 2004; 15:539–543.

116. Dranitsaris G, Kahn SR, Stumpo C, et al. Pharmacoeconomic analysis of fondaparinux versus enoxaparin for the prevention of thromboembolic events in orthopedic surgery patients. Am J Cardiovasc Drugs 2004; 4:325–333.

117. Agnelli G, Bergqvist D, Cohen A, Gallus A, Gent M. A randomized double-blind study to compare the efficacy and safety of fondaparinux with dalteparin in the prevention of venous thromboembolism after high-risk abdominal surgery: the Pegasus study. J Thromb Haemost 2003; 1:OC006.

118. Hirsh J. Current anticoagulant therapy–unmet clinical needs. Thromb Res 2003; 109:S1–S8.

119. Colwell CW, Jr., Berkowitz SD, Davidson BL, et al. Comparison of ximelagatran, an oral direct thrombin inhibitor, with enoxaparin for the prevention of venous thromboembolism following total hip replacement. A randomized, double-blind study. J Thromb Haemost 2003; 1:2119–2130.

120. Eriksson BI. Clinical experience of melagatran/ximelagatran in major orthopaedic surgery. Thromb Res 2003; 109:S23–S29.

121. Schulman S, Wahlander K, Lundstrom T, et al. Secondary prevention of venous thromboembolism with the oral direct thrombin inhibitor ximelagatran. N Engl J Med 2003; 349:1713–1721.

122. Halperin JL. Ximelagatran compared with warfarin for prevention of thromboembolism in patients with nonvalvular atrial fibrillation: rationale, objectives, and design of a pair of clinical studies and baseline patient characteristics (SPORTIF III and V). Am Heart J 2003; 146:431–438.

123. FDA Cardiovascular and Renal Drugs Advisory Committee Board, Septmeber 10, 2004 (Accessed Decmeber 15, 2004, at http://www.fda.gov/ohrms/dockets/ac/04/briefing/2004-4069b1.htm.)

124. Morris RJ, Woodcock JP. Effects of supine intermittent compression on arterial inflow to the lower limb. Arch Surg 2002; 137:1269–1273.

125. Ringley CD, Johanning JM, Gruenberg JC, et al. Evaluation of pulmonary arterial catheter parameters utilizing intermittent pneumatic compression boots in congestive heart failure. Am Surg 2002; 68:286–289 discussion 289–290.

15
Venous Thrombolysis of the Extremities

Ahmad Bhatti
Division of Vascular Surgery, Loyola University Medical Center, Maywood, Illinois, U.S.A.

Nicos Labropoulos
Vascular Laboratory, Division of Vascular Surgery, New Jersey Medical School, Newark, New Jersey, U.S.A.

Marc Borge
Interventional Radiology, Department of Radiology, Loyola University Medical Center, Maywood, Illinois, U.S.A.

INTRODUCTION

Thrombolysis first gained popularity in the 1960s when it was used systemically for pulmonary emboli (PE). Dotter et al. advanced thrombolytic treatment in 1974 when they introduced catheter directed thrombolysis. Extremity venous thrombosis can confer significant morbidity and mortality, and thrombolysis has been increasingly employed in an attempt to curb these. Deep venous thrombosis (DVT) can cause outflow obstruction producing venous hypertension, which may result in signs and symptoms of chronic venous disease (CVD) (1–4). Additionally, proximal DVT may result in more severe forms of CVD such as limb-threatening venous gangrene (e.g., phlegmasia) due to significant impairment of venous outflow (5,6). Various treatments, including anticoagulation, thrombolysis, surgery, and endovascular modalities are in use in attempts to reduce acute and long-term morbidity from DVT.

INDICATIONS

The indications for thrombolysis in DVT remain controversial (7). Acutely, patients can develop limb swelling, pain, and edema. Rarely, phlegmasia can develop with severe acute venous obstruction. Thrombolytic treatment in phlegmasia has been described, and is probably the least controversial indication (8–12). Conservative treatment of DVT with anticoagulation may help retard progression of thrombosis and help ameliorate acute symptoms. However, conclusive data showing a reduction of PTS with anticoagulation is lacking (13,14). The inflammatory process caused by the deep venous thrombosis often causes extensive permanent damage to the vein walls and valves. In the legs the lack of valve function can leave patients with long-term sequela of venous insufficiency. In the upper extremities DVT can result in chronic venous obstruction. Patients may develop

197

collateral flow around occluded segments in the chest or arm; however, the chronically obstructed vein segments may make further central venous access more complicated. In an effort to prevent these long-term sequelae of DVT, the concept of DVT thrombolysis to eradicate the clot has been developed. The theory is that heparin will stabilize the thrombotic process, but vein damage may continue to evolve. With thrombolysis there is the possibility to eradicate the clot and minimize damage to vein walls and vein valves. Therefore, thrombolysis may be considered in all patients with significant DVT who do not have contraindications (cerebral metastasis, recent surgery, etc.). Patients with acute DVT less than 10 days old without a prior history of DVT are most likely to benefit from thrombolysis (15).

TECHNIQUE

Many investigators have explored aggressive techniques to accelerate thrombolysis in the belief that eradicating clots quickly will minimize vein damage and maximize vein wall integrity and valve function, thereby minimizing long-term post-phlebitic syndrome. Initial attempts at systemic thrombolysis proved relatively ineffective probably due to shunting of blood past the area of obstruction resulting in poor penetration of thrombolytic agents into the clot. It is possible that systemic (peripheral IV) administration of thrombolytic agents shows some efficacy for pulmonary embolus dissolution due to the flow pattern where systemic venous drainage has to flow through the pulmonary arterial circulation. In contrast, in peripheral extremity flowing blood may not deliver drug to an obstructed venous segment in the limb.

FLOW-DIRECTED THROMBOLYSIS

Specially designed tourniquets have been used to manipulate venous flow patterns in order to drive flow of blood and drug into thrombosed venous segments. Pedal venography is used to delineate flow patterns in the foot, calf and thigh. Tourniquets are then placed with pressure pads specifically located to occlude superficial venous drainage and drive flow into the deep system. This often includes a tourniquet at the malleolar level with compression of the saphenous vein at the ankle. Thrombolytic agents are then infused into the pedal catheter. The tourniquets are released for 15 minutes every hour during infusion to prevent compressive complications. This is a slow technique and the treatment will often last up to 48 hours. Periodic venography is performed at least daily to assess response. Patients may often experience significant symptomatic improvement with in four to twelve hours. The goal of treatment with this method is not complete eradication of thrombus but, rather, improvement in symptoms and flow. This technique can be particularly helpful for large clot burden in the calf in addition to more proximal thrombi.

CATHETER-DIRECTED THROMBOLYSIS

If a catheter is embedded directly into thrombus the potential exists to deliver higher concentrations of thrombolytic agents to the clot than can be achieved with a peripheral infusion.

The preferred method for catheter directed ileo-femoral DVT thrombolysis is to access the popliteal vein with the patient in prone position. Ultrasound guidance should be used to achieve single wall puncture and minimize the risk of popliteal artery injury.

A micropuncture set with a 22-gauge needle can also be used to minimize potential for bleeding complications. Once access to the popliteal vein is achieved venography can be performed to further assess the extent of clot burden and flow. A steerable catheter and guidewire can be used to traverse the thrombosed segments of femoral/iliac vein and achieve access through the clot to the level of patent vein cephalad. Access from the popliteal vein facilitates catheter passage to the IVC because the catheter traverses venous valves in the direction of flow. Occasionally, additional catheter access is required from jugular or contralateral approaches. These routes present the difficulty of traversing valve leaflets, which may be closed. Finding the orifice of a closed valve in a thrombosed vein segment can present a considerable challenge. Sometimes these retrograde access sites are necessary, particularly if there is considerable popliteal/trifurcation thrombus and below the knee thrombolysis is necessary. Alternatively, the pedal infusion method can be used simultaneously with catheter directed technique to treat clots in the calf and thigh. With this combination the infusion dose should be split between the two sites.

When access across the thrombosed segment is achieved, a system of variable length multi-side hole infusion catheter and infusion guide wires can be used to deliver thrombolytic drugs throughout the length of the clot. Often a 40–50 cm multi-side hole infusion catheter such as the Cragg-McNamara valved infusion catheter (Microtherapeutics, Inc, Irvine, CA) is sufficient to traverse the ileo-femoral length. A 12 cm infusion length Katzen wire (Boston Scientific, Miami, FL) can be used coaxially to extend the infusion length.

Various infusion regimens have been advocated with little data to support a specific method. In general we lace the thrombus with 1–2 mg of tPA mixed in 10 cc of normal saline. This is delivered over several minutes in a pulse-spray fashion to mechanically disrupt the clot and drive the drug into the interstices of the thrombus to maximize drug-clot contact. We then continue tPA infusion at 0.5–1 mg/hour infusion.

The patient is closely monitored in the ICU setting for signs of bleeding. CBC, fibrinogen and coagulation parameters should be monitored every four to eight hours. Follow-up imaging is performed in 12–24 hours or sooner if the patient's clinical exam changes significantly. Depending on the follow-up venography, catheter position can be changed to optimize drug delivery to residual thrombus. Lytic infusion can be continued for several days with interval imaging to assess progress. The infusion is continued as long as the clot remains and progress is being demonstrated (Fig. 1). Lytic infusion should be stopped if venography demonstrates, "lytic stagnation" where clot burden remains unchanged despite continued infusion.

MECHANICAL THROMBECTOMY

Several methods have been utilized to accelerate the declotting process. Mechanical devices can be used to decrease clot burden and to increase distribution of the thrombolytic agent in the clot. Devices such as the Possis Angiojet Rheolytic Thrombectomy System (Possis Medical, Inc, Minneapolis, MN), the Treretola Percutaneous Thrombolytic Device (Arrow International, Inc, Reading PA), the Prolumen Rotational Thrombectomy System (Datascope, Mahwah, NJ), or simple balloon maceration have been used as adjuncts to thrombolytic therapy. It is possible to accelerate the declotting process and restore flow to the ileo-femoral segment in one setting or one day rather than a two to four day infusion using mechanical devices in conjunction with thrombolytic agents. Care should be taken with these devices to avoid additional trauma to the vein wall and the valve complex.

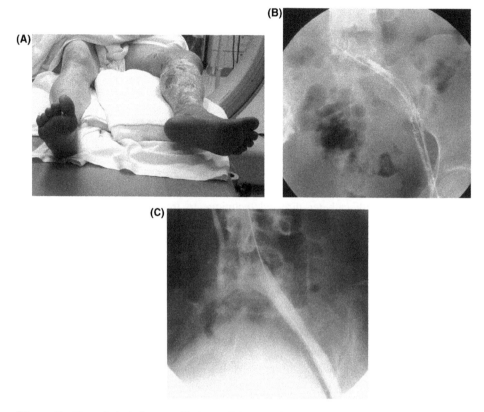

Figure 1 Thrombolysis in acute iliofemoral thrombosis. (**A**) The left lower extremity had acute swelling for five days that became progressively worse. After the ultrasound demonstrated thrombosis, thrombolysis was performed. The catheter was inserted through the popliteal vein. (**B**) The venogram shows acute thrombus in the iliofemoral veins. (**C**) After 36 hours most of the thrombus was lysed and a stent was placed in the left common iliac vein for a residual stenosis.

In particular, the wall-contact devices may cause additional valve trauma defeating the potential benefit of thrombolysis.

We do not routinely place IVC filters prior to catheter direct thrombolysis because the thrombus usually lyses from the outside in without significant embolization. With aggressive use of mechanical declotting devices the risk of embolization may be greater and use of IVC filtration may be more of a consideration. The retrievable filters, Gunther Tulip (Cook, Inc, Bloomington, IN) and Recovery (Bard Inc, Tempe, AZ) are attractive options for protection from pulmonary embolus.

PHARMACOLOGIC ADJUNCTS

Various drugs may also help accelerate the thrombolytic process. Antiplatelet agents (abciximab, tirofiban, eftifibatide) may have a synergistic effect with thrombolytic agents and accelerate the catheter directed thrombolytic process. In addition the newer thrombolytic agents may accelerate the lytic process. These include Reteplase (r-PA, Retavase, Centocor/Johnson and Johnson, Malvern, PA), which is a recombinant derivative of rt-PA with less fibrin affinity and increased half-life; Tenecteplase (TNK-tPA, Genentech, INC), which is a triple mutated version of the parent molecule rt-PA. It has enhanced fibrin specificity, a longer half-life, increased resistance to plasminogen activator inhibitor-1 and an enhanced safety profile compared to rt-PA. These are areas of investigation without conclusive data to form definite conclusions.

OUTCOME

Technical success rates have been reported ranging from 74–100% (16–18,31,34). The type of thrombolytic does not appear to change acute or long-term outcome, and a lot of thrombolytic agents have been used (19,20,30). While many short-term outcome studies exist, few long-term studies have been performed. Of the long-term studies, most comment on clinical outcome and few comment or study actual venous patency. Studies with long-term venous patency data are listed in Tables 1 and 2.

With regards to clinical outcome, many studies have shown superior outcome with thrombolysis. There is decreased long-term valvular incompetence, reflux, and CEAP categorization in patients with having received thrombolysis (21). Additionally, long-term follow-up of those patients treated with thrombolysis or anticoagulation reveals significantly improved quality of life for the former (22).

Whether better results are achieved with thrombolysis delivered locally or systemically is not clear. One prospective randomized study found high-dose systemic thrombolysis to be superior to local thrombolysis or anticoagulation alone with regards to acute outcome and CVD (20). Combination open/surgical thrombectomy and thrombolysis has been described, but comparative studies are lacking (23). One such study did demonstrate 100% patency and no CVD in 33 such patients at one-year (23). Animal models comparing thrombectomy to thrombolysis have shown that thrombolysis preserves more structural integrity and endothelial function, and this may explain why patients undergoing thrombolysis fare better (24). Mewissen showed that those patients with initial complete lysis had higher patency rates at one-year than those with incomplete lysis (<50%), 75% versus 32%, respectively (36). The same large multicenter registry

Table 1 Upper Extremity DVT

Author	Year	Patients	Mean follow-up	Primary patency	Comments
Schneider (31)	2004	21	1 year	92%	TOS, multi-modality treatment
Sabeti (32)	2002	33	3.3 years	52%	Systemic lysis for axillo-subclavian DVT
Kreienberg (33)	2001	14	3.5 years	64%	TOS, multi-modality treatment
Machleder (34)	1993	43	3.1 years	93%	TOS, multi-modality treatment

Abbreviations: TOS, thoracic outlet obstruction; DVT, deep venous thrombosis.

Table 2 Lower Extremity DVT

Author	Year	Patients	Mean follow-up	Primary patency	Comments
Elsharawy (35)	2002	18	6 months	72%	Prospective randomized
Mewissen (36)	1999	287	1 year	60%	Multicenter registry
Bjarnason (37)	1997	75	1 year	63% iliac 40% femoral	Consecutive review of 5 years

Abbreviation: DVT, deep venous thrombosis.

showed that proximal thrombi had more favorable outcomes, with the ileo-femoral veins having a patency of 64% and the femoro-popliteal of 48% at one year.

Most studies with long-term venous patency outcome from upper extremity DVT thrombolysis relate to thoracic outlet obstruction (TOS). The etiology of DVT in TOS and the multimodality treatments employed in these studies makes drawing conclusions with regards to thrombolysis and DVT difficult at best. Though thrombolysis may be superior in axillo-subclavian thrombosis (25).

There is no level 1 data in the literature comparing thrombolysis to other treatment arms (anticoagulation, surgical, endovascular, etc.). Thrombolysis does confer morbidity of which major bleeding is the most common with a reported incidence of 11–25% (15,26,34). One series reported puncture site bleeding as accounting for 39% of major bleeding complications (36). The incidence of PE has been variably reported at 1% and that of death less than 0.5% (15,36). The relative risk conferred by thrombolysis for major bleed has been reported as three-fold (27). Fibrinogen degradation products increasing to >200 mg/L after two hours of thrombolysis initiation have an associated odds ratio of 4.95 for parenchymal bleed (28). The risk of bleeding is not felt to increase if fibrinogen levels remain >20% of normal levels (29). The risk of bleeding or cerebrovascular accident has been shown to be significant (30,35). Bearing these risks in mind, with appropriate patient and pathology selection, treatment with thrombolysis should result in short- and long-term favorable outcome.

KEY POINTS

- Thrombolysis is an acceptable treatment for extremity venous thrombosis.
- Long-term level-1 evidence is lacking as to whether thrombolysis is superior to other modalities. However, several studies suggest short- and long-term clinical benefits in favor of thrombolysis.
- Proximal acute thrombi fare better with thrombolysis. Complete initial thrombolysis is favorably prognostic of long-term patency.
- Techniques, lytic agents, and protocols vary widely. None of these variables have been shown to be superior.
- Complication rates and specifically bleeding are higher with thrombolysis when compared to anticoagulation alone.
- Appropriate patient and pathology selection are paramount for success, patient benefit, and for reducing adverse outcome.

REFERENCES

1. O'Shaughnessy AM, Fitzgerald DE. Underlying factors influencing the development of the post-thrombotic limb. J Vasc Surg. 2001; 34:247–253.
2. Johnson BF, Manzo RA, Bergelin RO, Strandness DE, Jr. Relationship between changes in the deep venous system and the development of the postthrombotic syndrome after an acute episode of lower limb deep vein thrombosis: a one- to six-year follow-up. J Vasc Surg 1995; 21:307–312.
3. Haenen JH, Wollersheim H, Janssen MC, et al. Evolution of deep venous thrombosis: a 2-year follow-up using duplex ultrasound scan and strain-gauge plethysmography. J Vasc Surg 2001; 34:649–655.
4. Ziegler S, Schillinger M, Maca TH, Minar E. Post-thrombotic syndrome after primary event of deep venous thrombosis 10 to 20 years ago. Thromb Res 2001; 101:23–33.
5. Asbeutah AM, Riha AZ, Cameron JD, McGrath BP. Five-year outcome study of deep vein thrombosis in the lower limbs. J Vasc Surg 2004; 40:1184–1189.
6. Neglen P, Thrasher TL, Raju S. Venous outflow obstruction: an underestimated contributor to chronic venous disease. J Vasc Surg 2003; 38:879–885.
7. Kessel DO, Patel JV. Current trends in thrombolysis: implications for diagnostic and interventional radiology. Clin Radiol 2005; 60:413–424.
8. Patel NH, Plorde JJ, Meissner M. Catheter-directed thrombolysis in the treatment of phlegmasia cerulea dolens. Ann Vasc Surg 1998; 12:471–475.
9. Sciolaro C, Hunter GC, McIntyre KE, Bull DA, Parent FN, III, Bernhard VM. Thrombectomy and isolated limb perfusion with urokinase in the treatment of phlegmasia cerulea dolens. Cardiovasc Surg 1993; 1:56–60.
10. Hood DB, Weaver FA, Modrall JG, Yellin AE. Advances in the treatment of phlegmasia cerulea dolens. Am J Surg 1993; 166:206–210.
11. Centeno RF, Nguyen AH, Ketterer C, Stiller G, Chait A, Fallahnejad M. An alternative approach: antegrade catheter-directed thrombolysis in a case of phlegmasia cerulea dolens. Am Surg 1999; 65:229–231.
12. Robinson DL, Teitelbaum GP. Phlegmasia cerulea dolens: treatment by pulse-spray and infusion thrombolysis. AJR Am J Roentgenol 1993; 160:1288–1290.
13. Gutt CN, Oniu T, Wolkener F, Mehrabi A, Mistry S, Buchler MW. Prophylaxis and treatment of deep vein thrombosis in general surgery. Am J Surg 2005; 189:14–22.
14. Wells PS, Forster AJ. Thrombolysis in deep vein thrombosis: is there still an indication? Thromb Haemost 2001; 86:499–508.
15. Meissner MH. Thrombolytic therapy for acute deep vein thrombosis and the venous registry. Rev Cardiovasc Med 2002; 3S2:S53–S60.
16. Meissner MH. Axillary-subclavian venous thrombosis. Rev Cardiovasc Med 2002; 3:S33–S76.
17. Vedantham S, Vesely TM, Sicard GA, et al. Pharmacomechanical thrombolysis and early stent placement for iliofemoral deep vein thrombosis. J Vasc Interv Radiol 2004; 15:565–574.
18. Semba CP, Dake MD. Iliofemoral deep venous thrombosis: aggressive therapy with catheter-directed thrombolysis. Radiology 1994; 191:487–494.
19. Castaneda F, Li R, Young K, Swischuk JL, Smouse B, Brady T. Catheter-directed thrombolysis in deep venous thrombosis with use of reteplase: immediate results and complications from a pilot study. J Vasc Interv Radiol 2002; 13:577–580.
20. Schweizer J, Kirch W, Koch R, et al. Short- and long-term results after thrombolytic treatment of deep venous thrombosis. J Am Coll Cardiol 2000; 36:1336–1343.
21. Laiho MK, Oinonen A, Sugano N, et al. Preservation of venous valve function after catheter-directed and systemic thrombolysis for deep venous thrombosis. Eur J Vasc Endovasc Surg 2004; 28:391–396.
22. Comerota AJ, Throm RC, Mathias SD, Haughton S, Mewissen M. Catheter-directed thrombolysis for iliofemoral deep venous thrombosis improves health-related quality of life. J Vasc Surg 2000; 32:130–137.

23. Blattler W, Heller G, Largiader J, Savolainen H, Gloor B, Schmidli J. Combined regional thrombolysis and surgical thrombectomy for treatment of iliofemoral vein thrombosis. J Vasc Surg 2004; 40:620–625.

24. Rhodes JM, Cho JS, Gloviczki P, Mozes G, Rolle R, Miller VM. Thrombolysis for experimental deep venous thrombosis maintains valvular competence and vasoreactivity. J Vasc Surg 2000; 31:1193–1205.

25. AbuRahma AF, Sadler D, Stuart P, Khan MZ, Boland JP. Conventional versus thrombolytic therapy in spontaneous (effort) axillary-subclavian vein thrombosis. Am J Surg 1991; 161:459–465.

26. Watson LI, Armon MP. Thrombolysis for acute deep vein thrombosis. Cochrane Database Syst Rev 2004;CD002783.

27. Hirsh J, Lee AY. How we diagnose and treat deep vein thrombosis. Blood 2002; 99:3102–3110.

28. Trouillas P, Derex L, Philippeau F, et al. Early fibrinogen degradation coagulopathy is predictive of parenchymal hematomas in cerebral rt-PA thrombolysis: a study of 157 cases. Stroke 2004; 35:1323–1328.

29. Stewart D, Kong M, Novokhatny V, Jesmok G, Marder VJ. Distinct dose-dependent effects of plasmin and TPA on coagulation and hemorrhage. Blood 2003; 101:3002–3007.

30. Goldhaber SZ, Buring JE, Lipnick RJ, Hennekens CH. Pooled analyses of randomized trials of streptokinase and heparin in phlebographically documented acute deep venous thrombosis. Am J Med 1984; 76:393–397.

31. Schneider DB, Dimuzio PJ, Martin ND, et al. Combination treatment of venous thoracic outlet syndrome: open surgical decompression and intraoperative angioplasty. J Vasc Surg 2004; 40:599–603.

32. Sabeti S, Schillinger M, Mlekusch W, Haumer M, Ahmadi R, Minar E. Treatment of subclavian-axillary vein thrombosis: long-term outcome of anticoagulation versus systemic thrombolysis. Thromb Res 2002; 108:279–285.

33. Kreienberg PB, Chang BB, Darling RC, III, et al. Long-term results in patients treated with thrombolysis, thoracic inlet decompression, and subclavian vein stenting for Paget-Schroetter syndrome. J Vasc Surg 2001; 33:S100–S105.

34. Machleder HI. Evaluation of a new treatment strategy for Paget-Schroetter syndrome: spontaneous thrombosis of the axillary-subclavian vein. J Vasc Surg 1993; 17:305–315.

35. Elsharawy M, Elzayat E. Early results of thrombolysis vs anticoagulation in iliofemoral venous thrombosis. A randomised clinical trial. Eur J Vasc Endovasc Surg 2002; 24:209–214.

36. Mewissen MW, Seabrook GR, Meissner MH, Cynamon J, Labropoulos N, Haughton SH. Catheter-directed thrombolysis for lower extremity deep venous thrombosis: report of a national multicenter registry. Radiology 1999; 211:39–49.

37. Bjarnason H, Kruse JR, Asinger DA, et al. Iliofemoral deep venous thrombosis: safety and efficacy outcome during 5 years of catheter directed thrombolytic therapy. J Vasc Interv Radiol 1997; 8:405–418.

16

Role of Surgery and Endovascular Therapies in Lower Limb Deep Venous Thrombosis

Olivier Hartung, Yues S. Alimi, and Claude Juhan
Service de Chirurgie Vasculaire, Centre Hospitalier Universitaire Nord, Marseille, France

Deep venous thrombosis (DVT) is an acute condition of which the main serious complications are phlegmasia cerulea, pulmonary embolism (PE), and in the long term venous insuffiency. Heparin was the first efficient treatment of DVT, and Bauer was the first to demonstrate the properties and the efficiency of heparin in 1950 (1). However, as medical treatments are not completely able to avoid the main complications, interventional therapies have a place in the therapeutic arsenal, mainly in the case of iliocaval DVT.

Surgical venous thrombectomy was first reported by Läwen in 1938 (2), and during the 1950s and 1960s, its use spread in France as well in the United States accompanied by many encouraging reports (3,4) along with the introduction of the Fogarty catheter (5). But enthusiasm was reduced after the study of Lansing in 1968 who reported high rates of rethrombosis (6). Despite this, some teams continued to use surgical thrombectomy with some refinements like the use of an arteriovenous fistula as proposed by Kunlin (7). At the same time, by the early 1970s systemic thrombolysis had been introduced (8), and its use poorly spread until the report of Semba (9) who emphasized the advantages of catheter directed thrombolysis.

At present, when aggressive treatment of ileofemoral DVT is used, at least in selected cases, different modalities are available. These techniques will be described, results will be analyzed, and their specific advantages and complications will be discussed.

AIMS OF THE TREATMENT

The treatment of DVT should ideally avoid progression of the disease with proximal extension, prevent PE and later postthrombotic syndrome by preserving the venous outflow and functional valves. In order to accomplish this a treatment needs to make the clot disappear without causing its fragmentation and embolization and without damaging venous valves. The risk for developing such complications increases with the proximity of the thrombus in the veins.

The goal of heparin therapy is to avoid thrombus extension but it does not remove it and lysis performed by the endogenous fibrinolytic response requires weeks to months. Killewich reported a 14% rate of early extension (10). Moreover it does not protect against PE (4% in case of iliofemoral thrombosis, 18% when the inferior vena cuva is involved) (11) and the development of post thrombotic syndrome (74% of incompetent valves in the femoropopliteal veins six months after iliofemoral DVT) (12). Despite these data heparin remains the basis of treatment and is complementary to all the other modalities whatever the form of heparin used (unfractionned or low molecular weight heparin) in the absence of contra indications (13). Heparin treatment must be used in association with compressive therapy using elastic stockings or non-elastic devices when applicable. This combination does not completely avoid complications. For example, while treating iliofemoral DVT, Akesson (14) showed that at five years, 50% of the iliac veins are still occluded with less than 5% of preserved valvular function, and Johnson (15) that at three years, 88% of the patients had a postthrombotic syndrome.

Clearly there is a need for techniques resulting in clot removal without embolization while preserving valvular function. To date, two modalities have been developed to do this: surgical thrombectomy and percutaneous techniques (thrombolysis and/or thrombectomy).

SURGICAL THROMBECTOMY

Since Läwen's initial report (2), many technical refinements have been added leading to improvement in the results (e.g., use of heparin, Fogarty catheters, arterio-venous (AV), fistula, positive end expiratory pressure (PEEP), stenting, etc.).

Technique of Surgical Thrombectomy

All patients should have preoperatively (16):

- a complete physical examination
- chest radiography
- an ECG
- a blood work up including thrombosis profile
- a thoraco-abdomino-pelvic angio-CT scan (contraindicated in pregnant patients) which will have two main goals:

  1. Delineate the thrombosis: determine the cephalad extension, search for anatomic variation and for underlying chronic lesions (e.g., May-Thurner syndrome, postthrombotic lesions, etc.) (Fig. 1) and also for PE; in our practice there are currently no indications for preoperative phlebography
  2. Exclude contraindication to the technique, mainly the presence of malignant or inflammatory disease.

When such a procedure is considered for DVT, this work up should be rapidly performed, preferably within a few hours. During this time, intravenous heparin should be given. Before surgery, the patient should be cautiously moved and shaved in order to avoid clot fragmentation and migration which could cause PE. Thus, calf compression, tight flexion, and inguinal pressure should be avoided.

The procedure is performed under general anesthesia with the patient in dorsal decubitus and prophylactic antibiotics are given. A cell saver device must be used.

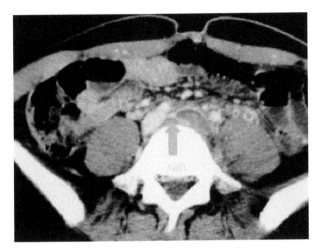

Figure 1   CT scan of a patient presenting a left ilio-femoral deep venous thrombosis (DVT) with May-Thurner syndrome.

The operative field should include the whole abdomen, both inguinal regions and the involved leg(s).

Iliofemoral Thrombectomy

Surgical approach to the common femoral vein (CFV) is performed through a vertical incision located just medial to the femoral pulse. The great saphenous vein leads to the sapheno–femoral junction. The CFV is exposed over a short length cephalad. Dissection must be cautious and gently performed. It is preferable to dissect away the surrounding structures without compressing, grasping or manipulating it. Surgical loops are passed around the great saphenous vein and the CVF proximal and distal to it. A fourth tape is used the same way to the second and the third to control the deep femoral veins without dissecting them (Fig. 2A). Only the anterior aspect of the deep veins should be exposed and this over the shortest length possible. A fifth tape is placed around the superficial femoral artery.

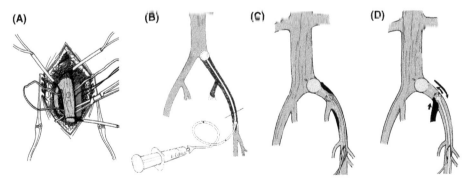

Figure 2   Technique of iliofemoral thrombectomy: (**A**) Surgical approach, (**B**) thrombectomy with a Fogarty catheter, (**C**) retrieval of the adherent clot using Vollmar rings, (**D**) thrombectomy of the internal iliac vein with a suction device while the Fogarty catheter is inflated in the common iliac vein.

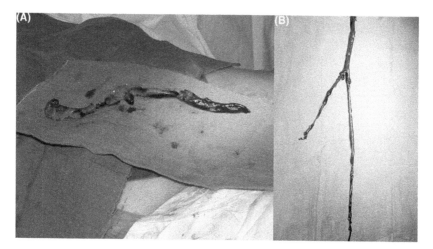

Figure 3 Operative view of the thrombus after venous thrombectomy: (**A**) iliac thrombus; (**B**) femoro-popliteal thrombus. (*See color insert.*)

Then an intravenous bolus of heparin is given and a 1.5 cm long venotomy is performed at the inferior and lateral side of the sapheno–femoral junction. At this moment, the anesthesiologists are asked to use a PEEP of 10 cm H_2O during the whole thrombectomy time in order to prevent from pulmonary embolism.

A large Fogarty catheter is then introduced cephalad between the venous wall and the clot to the IVC. It should be inserted easily to 40 cm long to avoid ascending lumbar vein catheterization. Then the balloon is inflated and the catheter is cautiously withdrawn (Fig. 2B) to remove the clot (Fig. 3A). When performed on the left side it can need deflation at 20 cm in order to pass under the right common iliac artery in cases of May-Thurner syndrome. The Fogarty catheter should be used until no more clot is retrieved.

Then the catheter is passed through a large Vollmar ring before their introduction into the CFV and is inflated into the iliocaval junction. The Vollmar ring is used to unstick the adherent clot (Fig. 2C). Moreover a suction canula is inserted to remove the clot at the internal iliac vein ostium (Fig. 2D). Then the catheter can be retrieved and the tape is tightened around the common femoral vein after infusion of heparined serum.

Limb, popliteal and femoral veins thrombectomy is then performed without using any endovenous instrumentation. All the tapes are tightened and sturdy massage of the limb is performed, starting at the foot to unstick the clot. The tapes are briefly untightened to release the clot (Fig. 3B) and the maneuver is repeated until no more clot is retrieved. Blood loss must be controlled during this time. Then an Esmarch bandage is put around the limb from the ankle to the thigh for one or two minutes before a last flush. The great saphenous vein must be thrombectomised also.

The venotomy is then closed using a 6/0 polypropylene running suture which is tied only after unclamping all the veins to prevent stricture.

The great saphenous vein is sectioned at 10 cm from the sapheno–femoral junction in order to be used for construction of an AVF. A 7F sheath is inserted through it and completion ilio-cavography is performed. If it shows persisting clot or venous stenosis, angioplasty and stenting should be performed at this time. The AVF is performed with a latero-terminal anastomosis between the superficial femoral artery and the saphenous vein using a 7/0 polypropylene running suture. The site of the anastomosis is chosen while the

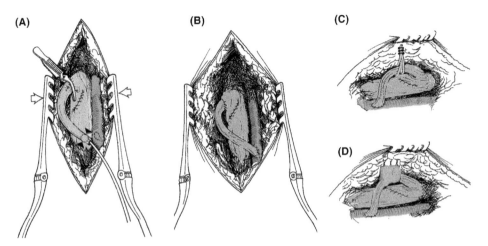

Figure 4 Confection of an arterio-venous fistula (AVF). (**A**) the implantation site of the saphenous vein on the superficial femoral artery is chosen with the retractor released, (**B**) view after performance of the AVF, (**C**) location of the AVF with a silastic tape, (**D**) or with a piece of PTFE. (*See color insert.*)

saphenous vein is under tension and the retractor is removed (Fig. 4A). In case of an unsuitable saphenous vein, a short 5 mm Plolytetrafluoro ethylene graft can be used. A good thrill must be felt on the AVF and common femoral vein on completion (Fig. 4B).

Before wound closure, the AVF is located in order to facilitate its surgical closure after six weeks. A PTFE patch (Fig. 4D) or a silastic loop (Fig. 4C) is put around it and closed with metallic clips, its extremity lying in the subcutaneous plane. A suction drain must be applied next to the CFV.

Inferior Vena Cava Thrombectomy

Thrombectomy is performed through a direct approach to the IVC. It preferentially uses a right transperitoneal subcostal route deflecting the duodenum and the ascending colon medially. The IVC can be exposed for 8 cm caudally to the renocaval confluence. Two tapes are put around the IVC, one just under the renal veins and another one 6 cm caudally. Lumbar and genital veins must be controlled by threads. Two 6/0 polypropylene stay sutures are placed on the IVC between the two tapes, at each extremity of the planned cavotomy.

If the clot reaches the renal vein or is more extensive, a Fogarty catheter is introduced cephalad in the IVC once a 2 mm cavotomy has been performed in the center of a purse string suture (Fig. 5A,B). The balloon is inflated cephalad to the superior pole of the clot and the cavotomy is extended (Fig. 5C). Then the Fogarty catheter is retrieved and the superior tape is tightened once the catheter is down to it (Fig. 5D). Then the lower part of the IVC is thrombectomized as previously described and the cavotomy is closed with a 6/0 polypropylene running suture.

If thrombosis does not reach the superior third of the infrarenal IVC, the cephalad tape is tightened and the iliac clot is massaged in order to mobilized it. Then the cavotomy is performed and the clot is removed with a large Fogarty catheter while taking great care to limit blood loss (Fig. 5D).

A median laparotomy should be used only if abdominopelvic exploration is needed, if there is a doubt about the age of the thrombosis or if an IVC filter is to be removed.

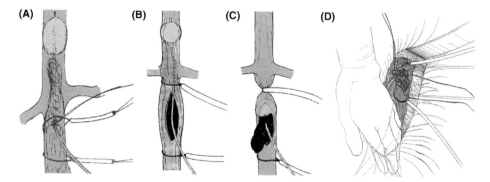

Figure 5 IVC thrombectomy. A, B, C: when the clot reach the renal veins, a purse-string is performed on the infra-renal IVC and a Fogarty is inserted between the venous wall and the clot then inflated above it (**A**). A cavotomy is performed and the Fogarty catheter is retrieved (**B**) until it is below the superior tape which is used to clamp the distal IVC (**C**). (**D**): proximal IVC thrombectomy.

A suction drain is applied next to the IVC before closure. In cases of phlegmasia cerulea dolens, the procedure should begin by fasciotomy.

Postoperative Period

Elastic stockings are on both limbs applied and an intravenous heparin infusion is continued. As soon as the patient is awake, active mobilization must be performed. The patient should be walking from day one.

Long-term anticoagulation with fluindion is started the first postoperative day for at least six months, but the AVF should be closed at six weeks with performance of ilio-cavography. This procedure can be performed through a surgical approach following the locating device or by an endovascular procedure (detachable balloons, coils) (17).

Indications for Surgical Thrombectomy

This technique should be considered for recent and proximal (iliofemoral with or without IVC involvement) DVT in patients with life expectation up to five years. This means that:

- the thrombosis should be less than seven days old. Dating is given by the first onset of symptoms. Moreover, the characteristics of the thrombosis at Duplex scan (hypoechogenic and nonadherent clot with dilatation of the vein) and CT scan (hypodense clot with peripheral enhancement) can help to confirm this.
- the thrombosis should reach at least the common femoral vein (CFV), most of them reaching the common iliac vein (CIV) or the inferior vena cava (IVC).
- patients should be in good health, less than 70 years old and should not have cancer, infectious or inflammatory disease, and no severe cardiorespiratory disease. Moreover, they should be able to walk the day after the procedure.

Pregnancy, postdelivery, and thrombolytic treatment failure are not contra indications to venous thrombectomy. In pregnant women, thrombus extension can be evaluated by Duplex scan or iliocavography, but no completion angiography is performed even if a stenosis was felt while retrieving the Fogarty catheter. AVF closure should be performed one to three months after delivery with angiography; significant residual lesions should be stented at this time if needed (18,19).

Surgical thrombectomy can be also used in cases of femoral extension of great saphenous vein thrombosis and in case of IVC thrombosis in presence of an IVC filter or clip.

Adjunctive Techniques

IVC Clip and Filters

Their goal is to avoid PE. Since the introduction of PEEP, which avoids peroperative severe PE, and of stenting for treatment of residual clot there are no more routine indications for their use during venous thrombectomy.

Angioplasty and Stenting

Stenting is used to treat lesions that could compromise patency after thrombectomy or thrombolysis. It is indicated in cases of May-Thurner syndrome after left CIV thrombectomy (Fig. 6) but also in cases of residual clot, postthrombotic occlusive disease, extrinsic stenosis (retroperitoneale fibrosis) (20). Indeed, Mickley (21) showed that if the underlying lesions are left untreated, rethrombosis rate is 73% versus only 13% after stenting. Stenting should be systematically performed because recoil is very important. If not stented, the vein would restenose quickly and the benefit of the procedure would not be durable.

After insertion of a sheath in the common femoral vein, catheterization is performed with a Terumo guidewire. Angioplasty is performed, generally using a 12 mm diameter balloon. Then stent(s) is(are) deployed. Self-expanding metallic and retrievable stents (Wallstent) should be used because balloon expandable stents can be crushed (22). These stents need to be stabilized otherwise jumping can occur (23). This is achieved by using long stents leaning on both sides of the stenosis. Raju (24) has shown that the stent must lie on the right flank of the IVC when treating May-Thurner syndrome. In such cases 16 mm diameter and at least 60 mm long stents should be used. Table 1 reviews the experience of stenting during surgical thrombectomy (18,21,25–29).

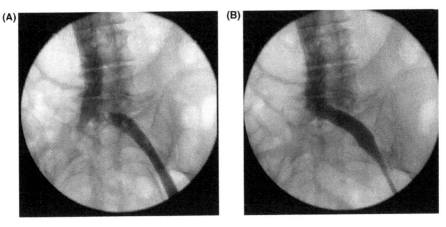

Figure 6   Iliocavography during surgical thrombectomy: (**A**) May-Thurner syndrome; associated with residual clot into the common iliac vein. (**B**) After angioplasty and stenting, no residual stenosis.

Table 1 Results of Interventional Therapy with Stenting of Underlying Iliocaval Lesions for Femoroiliac Venous Thrombosis

Study	Technique	N	Technical success	PP at 1 year	Late PP	Late SP
O'Sullivan	TL	19		93.1% (stented)		
Mewissen	TL					
Without stent		122		53%		
With stent		99		74%		
Vedantham	TL	23	100%			
Mickley	ST	20	95%		M60:72%	M60:88%
Wohlgemuth	ST	35	97%			M48:69%
Schwarzbach	ST	21	100%		M21:80%	M21:90%
Hartung	ST	20	100%	76%	M36:76%	M36:81%

Abbreviations: PP, primary patency rate; SP, secondary patency rate; ST+AVF, surgical thrombectomy and arteriovenous fistula; TL, thrombolysis.
Source: From Refs. 6, 15–18.

Contraindications to stenting are septic condition and pregnancy. In this last case, iterative thrombectomy and stenting should be considered only in case of early rethrombosis (22).

Venous Bypass

Bypasses were previously used in cases of rethrombosis after venous thrombectomy or if major occlusive lesions were found at preoperative ilio-cavography. The Palma procedure was the technique of choice in cases of iliac lesions compromising its patency. It had to be associated to the AVF.

At present stenting is the preferred technique and bypass should be reserved for cases of stenting failure without correctable remaining lesions or in case of contraindication for stenting. Since 1995, such a procedure was needed twice and both of them were performed more than four months after the surgical thrombectomy (18).

Regional Thrombolysis

Blätter (30) reported the combination of surgical thrombectomy with regional thrombolysis. 50,0000–30,00,000 UI of urokinase are infused through a 12-gauge catheter introduced in a foot vein at the beginning of the procedure. The aim is to allow the thrombolytic drug to act during 30 minutes (approach of the CVF and iliac thrombectomy) in order to facilitate the clearance of the clot in the limb.

Results

Mortality is very low in recent series reported by experienced groups. We had no death in our department in our late experience (75 patients) (31) and no more deaths since the introduction of stenting (20 patients) (18). Eklöf reported a 1% mortality rate on 203 consecutive patients (32); both deaths were not related to the thrombosis.

PE is also rarely severe. As Blättler (30), we (18,27) had no symptomatic postoperative PE in our experience, but Plate (11) reported 45% of positive perfusion scan at the admission and 20% of additional defects postoperatively, but none when an AVF was constructed.

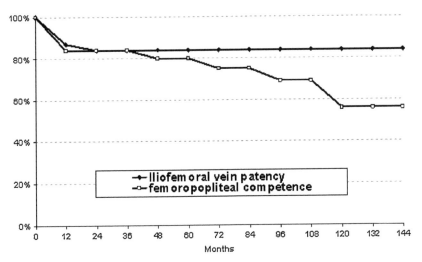

Figure 7 Cumulative iliofemoral vein patency after surgical thrombectomy and femoropopliteal venous competence curve after successful iliofemoral venous thrombectomy according to Juhan (31).

The main other complication is rethrombosis. It is commonly due to underlying venous lesions like in May-Thurner syndrome, incomplete thrombectomy, inappropriate indication, failure of the AVF or to inadequate anticoagulation. Use of an AVF has been shown to reduce the rethrombosis rate: Hutschenreiter (33) had 83% of iliac patency with AVF versus 54% without it. According to this technique, primary patency rate was 87% at three months in a metaanalysis performed by Eklöf while reviewing 527 cases (28). Residual lesions on the iliac veins and IVC represented a major cause for rethrombosis. In our experience, it occurred in 7% of the cases in absence of stenosis, 26% in case of mild stenosis and 56% in case of tight stenosis (31). Obstruction was treated by cross pubic venous bypass until Mickley (21) showed that while leaving iliac lesions untreated reocclusion rate was 73% versus 13% after stenting. Table 1 summarizes the results of the published reports (18,21,25–29). In a group of 21 consecutive patients who had surgical thrombectomy with stenting, our primary patency rate was 85.7% at one month (18).

In a report with a mean follow up of more than eight years, we reported patency and valvular competence rates of respectively 84% and 80% at five years and 84% and 56% at 13 years (Fig. 7) (31). These results are consistent with the literature review of Eklöf (32).

The association of regional thrombolysis with surgical thrombectomy (26) gave 100% primary success without recurrence or deep venous reflux at one year. After a six to 10 years follow-up, 16 legs were asymptomatic without compression therapy.

Pillny (19) reported 97 cases of venous thrombectomy during pregnancy or after delivery without maternal death and one postoperative fetal death. After a mean follow up of six years, patency rate was 89.5%, and 56.3% of the patients had no post-thrombotic syndrome, while only 3.5% had leg ulceration.

Timing

It is generally agreed that the thrombosis should be less than seven days old. Despite this some patients were operated on after larger delay, up to 16 days in our experience (31).

We were unable to draw correlations between the age of the clot and the patency of the iliofemoral vein. Nevertheless it does not seem advisable to recommend such delay because the goal of the treatment is not only the iliac patency but also preservation of valvular competence.

IVC INTERRUPTION AND FILTERS

The indications for such techniques are quite rare if strict indications are followed.

Techniques

This can be performed by different approaches, the endovascular being the only one commonly used at present.

Surgical Techniques

The approach is commonly performed through a right transperitoneal subcostal route as previously described. Once the IVC dissected free it can be ligated, plicated with transfixion polypropylene sutures or an Adam-De Weese clip can be inserted around the IVC (no longer available in France).

Endovascular Procedures

Since Greenfield's report in 1973 (34), the use of IVC filters has became the gold standard technique. Many filters are commercially available at present. Designs have been improved, and most of them can be inserted percutaneously by femoral or jugular approaches through 6 to 12 French sheaths. Moreover, temporary and retrievable filters are available. Measurement of the IVC must be performed before filter deployment. Indeed, only the Birds Nest filter (Cook) is suitable for IVC larger than 28 mm in diameter. Moreover, venous anomalies must be identified before implantation (35).

Filter placement can be performed under fluoroscopic guidance after cavography to visualize the level of the renal veins or by means of transabdominal duplex ultrasound (36) or intravascular ultrasound (IVUS) guidance (37).

Indications

Categorical Indications

Documented DVT and/or PE with

- absolute contra indication to anticoagulation
- documented progression of DVT or recurrent PE while well anticoagulated
- complication of anticoagulation therapy requiring its termination
- massive PE.

Relative Indications

Documented DVT and/or PE with

- large free floating IVC/iliac vein thrombus (unless surgical thrombectomy is performed)

Table 2 Complication Rates Depending on the Model of Filter According to Streiff

Filter	PE	Lethal PE	DVT	IVCT	PTS	AST
Greenfield	2.6%	0.9%	5.9%	3.6%	19%	23%
Greenfield Ti	3.1%	1.7%	22.7%	6.5%	14.4%	28%
Bird nest	2.9%	0.9%	6%	3.9%	14%	23%
Simon	3.8%	1.9%	8.9%	7.7%	12.9%	31%
LGM	3.4%	0.3%	32%	11.2%	41%	36%

Abbreviations: Ti, titanium; PE, pulmonary embolism; DVT, deep venous thrombosis; IVCT, inferior vena cava thrombosis; PTS, postthrombotic syndrome; AST, access site thrombosis.
Source: From Ref. 35.

- limited cardiac reserve
- high risk of complications of anticoagulation.

Indications for surgical approaches were considerably decreased by percutaneous filters. Remaining indications are the absence or impossibility of percutaneous access and in case of surgical approach of the IVC for another reason.

Placement in the suprarenal IVC can be performed in case of thrombosis of the infrarenal IVC, mostly if an infrarenal filter is thrombosed.

Results

The different devices are not free of secondary complications. The main ones are IVC thrombosis and migration.

Two main articles have reviewed the results of IVC filters: one reports the experience of one center on 1765 filters implanted over 26 years (38), and another analyzes the published results (39). The PE rate was 5.6% including 3.7% of fatal PE and no filter gave superior results compared to the others (38). According to Athanasoulis, the filter migration rate is 0.1% but Streiff (39) reported a higher rate ranging from 2.2% with the Simon filter to 12.8% with the Greenfield titanium filter. These migrations justify the performance of abdominal radiography after implantation and in case of PE or cardiac arrhythmia. The perforation rate ranged between 0 and 14.1% depending on the filter (39). Thrombosis of the access site is very frequent (30%) (39) and depends on the size of the sheath. Filter thrombosis is a more problematic complication which exposes the patient to the risk of major PE. Its rate is ranging between 3.6% and 11.2% (39). Table 2 reviews these complications. A randomized prospective study (42) showed at 8 years that filters reduce the risk of pulmonary embolism but increase that of deep-vein thrombosis and had no effect on survival.

Bedside placement under duplex scan guidance has been shown to be safe and cost-effective (36) but inadequate imaging of the IVC is reported to be 8–13% mostly in critically ill patients (36,40,41). IVUS placement technical success rate is about 92% (33) and can be done with single-puncture venous access. The main potential drawback of these techniques is missed venous anomalies.

ENDOVASCULAR TECHNIQUES

Percutaneous techniques have the theorical advantage of being less invasive than surgical thrombectomy.

Thrombolysis

Indication

According to the Venous registry (28), thrombolysis should be performed for acute (<10 days) or chronic (>10 days) femoro-popliteal or iliofemoral DVT.

More over, such patients should be healthy and active with a normal life expectancy (42).

Contraindications

In this study (28) patients were excluded with:

- contraindications to the use of anticoagulants and contrast media
- contraindications to thrombolytic agents: active internal bleeding, recent cerebro-vascular accident, allergy to thrombolytic agents, recent major surgery, recent serious gastrointestinal bleeding, recent serious trauma, severe hypertension, pregnancy, bacterial endocarditis, possibility of intracardiac thrombus, coagulopathy.

Technique

Catheterization access approach can be performed on internal jugular vein, common femoral vein, or popliteal vein, but this last vein has became the site of choice. It is recommended to perform it under ultrasonographic guidance with a 21G needle in order to reduce the risk of bleeding due to arterial puncture. Infusion is commonly performed through a multiple-side-hole catheter embedded in the thrombus and lysis is monitored at venography. The procedure should be ended when no additional lysis is achieved within the last 12 hours. Intravenous heparin therapy must be administrated during and after the procedure (100–500 IU/hr).

Adjunctive techniques can include angioplasty and stenting to treat underlying lesions (9,27,28,43) and IVC filter placement to prevent from PE in case of recurrent PE despite anticoagulation or free floating IVC or iliac thrombus (43).

Laboratory parameters of surveillance are hematocrit level, fibrinogen level, prothrombin time, activated thromboplastin time and INR. The patients should be monitored in an intensive care unit.

Results

Experimental studies have demonstrated that thrombolysis can restore venous patency while preserving valvular competence (44,45).

Since the 1970s, this technique was used to treat acute DVT first via a systemic route. Comerota pooled the results of 13 studies in 1993 (46). He showed that while anticoagulation alone gave 82% of no thrombus clearing or worsening, 45% of significant or complete clearing of the clot and 18% of partial clearing was obtained with thrombolysis. But general thrombolysis was shown to have high complication rates mainly due to bleeding and pulmonary embolism (47,48).

Catheter directed thrombolysis (CDT) was then introduced, and the first major report was published in 1994 by Semba (9). Grossman (49) pointed out in a review in 1999 the lack of data from the literature on follow-up and the absence of control groups. Technical venographic success was 84% and 4.9% of the patients needed transfusion for bleeding (49).

The Venous Registry is the most important database reporting this treatment (28). It reported the results on 303 limbs in 287 patients in 63 centers with 71% of iliofemoral

DVT including 21% of IVC involvement. Mean infusion time was 53.4 hours (2–47 hours) using a mean 7.8 million IU of urokinase. Stenting was needed in 33% of the limbs. Grade III (complete) and grade II (50–99%) lysis were respectively achieved in 31% and 52% of the patients [19% grade III in chronic patients (>10 days)]. Primary patency rates were 64% for iliofemoral DVT at 12 months versus 47% for femoral-popliteal DVT. The results were better if the DVT was acute, the patient had no history of previous ipsilateral DVT, the thrombolysis was complete, the DVT involved the iliac veins and if stenting was performed in iliac veins. Major bleeding occurred in 11% of the patients, mostly at the puncture site (39%) and in the retroperitonal space (13%) and minor bleeding in 16%. Mortality, PE and major neurologic complication rates were respectively 0.4%, 1% and 0.4%.

Quality of life after CDT was evaluated by Comerota (50). Patients receiving CDT reported significantly better overall physical functioning, less stigma and fewer post-thrombotic symptoms compared with patients who received anticoagulation alone.

Laiho (48) reported 44% of valve competence preservation with CDT versus 13% with systemic thrombolysis with less deep (44% vs. 81%) and superficial (25% vs. 63%) reflux but the clinical disability score did not differ significantly.

The Cochrane PVD group (51) reviewed all the publications describing randomized controlled trials of thrombolysis versus anticoagulation for acute DVT. Complete clot lysis and improvement in venous patency occurred significantly more often with thrombolysis at early and late follow-up. Significantly less post-thrombotic syndrome and less leg ulceration occurred in those receiving thrombolysis. Venous function was improved at late follow up, but not significantly. Out of 668 patients, those receiving thrombolysis had significantly more bleeding complications but their incidence reduced over time with introduction of stricter selection criteria. There was no effect on mortality but no conclusions can be drawn on PE and DVT recurrence rates.

Thrombolysis appears to offer advantages in terms of reducing post-thrombotic syndrome and maintaining venous patency after DVT, but optimum drug dose (none has the FDA approval in this indication) and route of administration have yet to be determined. Moreover, multiple issues such as cost, safety, reporting standards, and practice guidelines need to be studied.

Mechanical Thrombolysis

This technique was first reported for DVT by Uflacker (52). It has the potential advantages of faster vein recanalization and relief of the symptoms with reduced bleeding complication rates and cost. Main concerns are the potential risks of wall and valve injury and haemolysis.

Devices

Many devices are available, and none is perfect. Moreover, while some have FDA approval for hemodialysis graft thrombosis, none have it for DVT. The ideal device should allow complete thrombus removal without causing venous wall and valve trauma and without using thrombolytic agents. Moreover, it should prevent bleeding, hemolysis and PE. The actually available catheters can be classified depending on two major properties: complete vessel wall contact and possibility of thrombus aspiration (Table 3).

Table 3 Devices Used for Mechanical Thrombolysis

Incomplete wall contact	Complete wall contact
Angiojet	Arrow trerotola
Oasis	Cragg brush
Gelbfish endovac	MTI-castaneda brush
Thrombex PMT	Prolumen
Amplatz thrombectomy device	Solera/Fino
Hydrolyser	Cleaner
X-Sizer	Prolumen
Rotarex	
Trellis reserve	

Technique

Access is obtained through popliteal vein puncture under ultrasound guidance and the device is advanced through the thrombosed veins to unclot them. Most catheters are used in association with chemical thrombolytic agents.

One of the technical aspects is the need for IVC filter. This technique has a risk of PE due to intrathrombus maneuvers and particulate embolization, mainly in the absence of thrombus aspiration. Thus retrievable filters are commonly used while performing mechanical thrombolysis.

Results

So far, published reports are few and are summarized in Table 4 (29,53–56).

Table 4 Published Results of Percutaneous Mechanical Thrombectomy for DVT

Study	Thrombus removal	Adjunctive techniques	Complication rate	Results
Gandini	75% complete	Filter 100%	Death 12.5%	75% patency at 24 months
	12.5% partial			
Kasirajan	24% >90%	TL. 55%		Improvement 82%
	35% 50–90%			
Delomez	83% partial	Filter 100%	Death 6%	91% minimal sequelae at 30 months
		Stent 11%		
Bush	65% complete	Filter 35%	Death 0%	Improvement 74% at D1
	35% partial	TL: 35%	Bleeding 13%	
		Stent 61%		
Vedantham	83% >50%	TL: 100%	Bleeding 6%	Improvement 96%

Abbreviations: DVT, deep venous thrombosis; TL, thrombolysis.
Source: From Refs. 50–54.

Indications

These are the same as for thrombolysis due to the fact that use of thrombolytic agents is commonly associated with the technique.

RESPECTIVE INDICATIONS

To date, mechanical thrombectomy has yet to be proven effective and no device has FDA approval in the treatment of DVT.

According to the literature, thrombolysis should be the preferred method due to its lower invasiveness compare to surgical thrombectomy.

In cases of femoral-popliteal DVT, thrombolysis should be performed whenever there is no contraindication.

In case of iliofemoral DVT, an algorithm was proposed by the American Venous Forum guidelines (13). According to this, thrombolysis should be the method of choice. Nevertheless, thrombolysis has non negligible rates of complications mainly due to bleeding. Moreover, contraindications are limiting its applicability (75% in our experience), and long term patency and valve preservation rates are unknown, but mid-term results do not reach those of surgical thrombectomy. Thus, we believed that venous thrombectomy with AVF and stenting in case of residual lesions remains the best option to treat iliofemoral DVT when performed by trained teams and while respecting strict indications.

KEY POINTS

- The primary aim of DVT treatment is to avoid progression and prevent pulmonary embolism and the postthrombotic syndrome.
- Heparin prevents progression but does not remove thrombus.
- Surgical thrombectomy should be considered for recent and proximal DVT in patients with a good life expectancy.
- The thrombosis should be less than 7 days old.
- Pregnancy, post-delivery, and thrombolytic treatment failure are not contraindications to venous thrombectomy.
- CT angiography is the investigation of choice to delineate the thrombus and exclude malignancy.
- At completion of surgical thrombectomy, an arterio-venous fistula is constructed to aid patency.
- Thrombolysis can be considered in patients with normal life expectancy and thrombosis of <10 days duration.
- Major bleeding occurs in 11% of patients, mostly at the puncture site.
- Thrombolysis offers advantages in reducing postthrombotic syndrome and maintaining venous patency.
- Adjunctive techniques to both surgical thrombectomy and thrombolysis include venous angioplasty +/− stenting for residual stenoses.
- Surgical insertion of IVC filters or interruption of the IVC is rarely required since the development of percutaneous filters.

REFERENCES

1. Bauer G. Nine years' experience with heparin in acute venous thrombosis. Angiology 1950; 1:161–169.
2. Läwen A. Weitere Ehrfahung über operative Thrombenentfernung bei Venenthrombose. Zentrabl Chir 1938; 64:961–968.
3. Fontaine R, Tuchmann L. The role of thrombectomy in deep venous thrombosis. J Cardiovasc Surg 1964; 5:298–312.
4. Haller JA, Abrams BL. Use of thrombectomy in the treatment of acute iliofemoral venous thrombosis in forty-five patients. Ann Surg 1963; 158:561–569.
5. Fogarty TJ, Dennis D, Krippaehne WW. Surgical management of iliofemoral venous thrombosis. Am J Surg 1966; 112:211–217.
6. Lansing AM, Davis WM. Five year follow-up study of iliofemoral venous thrombectomy. Ann Surg 1968; 168:620–628.
7. Kunlin J. Les greffes veineuses. 15 Congress of International Surgical Society. Lisbon 1953; 15:875–907.
8. Porter JM, Seaman AJ, Common HH, Rosch J, Eidemiller LR, Calhoun AD. Comparison of heparin and streptokinase in the treatment of venous thrombosis. Am Surg 1975; 41:511–519.
9. Semba CP, Dake MD. Iliofemoral deep venous thrombosis: aggressive therapy with catheter-directed thrombolysis. Radiology 1994; 191:487–494.
10. Killewich LA, Bedford GR, Beach KW, Strandness DE, Jr. Spontaneous lysis of deep venous thrombi: rate and outcome. J Vasc Surg 1989; 9:89–97.
11. Plate G, Ohlin P, Eklöf B. Pulmonary embolism in acute iliofemoral venous thrombosis. Br J Surg 1985; 72:912–915.
12. Plate G, Einarsson E, Ohlin P, Jensen R, Qvarfordt P, Eklof B. Thrombectomy with temporary arteriovenous fistula: the treatment of choice in acute iliofemoral venous thrombosis. J Vasc Surg 1984; 1:867–876.
13. Comerota AJ. Acute deep venous thrombosis. In: Gloviczki P, Yao JST, eds. Hand book of venous disorders, guidelines of the American Venous Forum. London, UK: Chapmann & Hall Medical, 1996:243–259.
14. Akesson H, Brudin L, Dahlstrom JA, Eklof B, Ohlin P, Plate G. Venous function assessed during a 5 yr period after acute ilio-femoral venous thrombosis treated with anticoagulation. Eur J Vasc Surg 1990; 4:43–8.
15. Johnson BF, Manzo RA, Bergelin RO, Strandness DE, Jr. Relationship between changes in the deep venous system and the development of the postthrombotic syndrome after an acute episode of lower limb deep vein thrombosis: a one- to six-year follow-up. J Vasc Surg 1995, 21:307–312 discussion 313.
16. Juhan C, Eklöf B. Thrombectomie veineuse ilio-fémorale et cave inférieure. Editions Techniques, Encycl Med Chir (Paris, France), Techniques Chirurgicales, chirurgie Vasculaire, 43165 1990: 16p.
17. Endrys J, Eklöf B, Neglén P, Zyka I, Peregrin J. Percutaneous closure of femoral arteriovenous fistula after venous thrombectomy. J Cardiovasc Intervent Radiol 1989; 12:226–229.
18. Hartung O, Alimi YS. Venous stenting: for which patients? In: Becquemin JP, Alimi YS, Watelet J, eds. Controversies and updates in vascular surgery. Torino: Minerva Medica, 2005:159–168.
19. Pillny M, Sandmann W, Luther B, Gerhardt A, Zotz RB, et al. Deep venous thrombosis during pregnancy and after delivery: indications for and results of thrombectomy. J Vasc Surg 2003; 37:528–532.
20. Hartung O, Alimi YS, Di Mauro P, Portier F, Juhan C. Endovascular treatment of iliocaval occlusion caused by retroperitoneal fibrosis: late results in two cases. J Vasc Surg 2002; 36:849–552.
21. Mickley V, Schwagierek R, Schutz A, Sunder-Plassmann L. Stent implantation after thrombectomy of pelvic veins. Indications, results. Zentralbl Chir 1999; 124:7–12.

22. Juhan C, Hartung O, Alimi Y, Barthelemy P, Valerio N, Portier F. Treatment of nonmalignant obstructive iliocaval lesions by stent placement: mid-term results. Ann Vasc Surg 2001; 15:227–232.

23. Hartung O, Otero A, Boufi M, Decaridi G, Barthelemy P, Juhan C, Alimi YS, Mid-term results of endovascular treatment for symptomatic chronic nonmalignant iliocaval venous occlusive disease. J Vasc Surg 2005; 42:1138–144.

24. Raju S, Owen S, Jr., Neglen P. The clinical impact of iliac venous stents in the management of chronic venous insufficiency. J Vasc Surg 2002; 35:8–15.

25. Wohlgemuth WA, Weber H, Loeprecht H, Tietze W, Bohndorf K. PTA and stenting of benign venous stenoses in the pelvis: long-term results. Cardiovasc Intervent Radiol 2000; 23:9–16.

26. Schwarzbach MH, Schumacher H, Bockler D, et al. Surgical thrombectomy followed by intraoperative endovascular reconstruction for symptomatic ilio-femoral venous thrombosis. Eur J Vasc Endovasc Surg 2005; 29:58–66.

27. O'Sullivan GJ, Semba CP, Bittner CA, Endovascular management of iliac vein compression (May-Thurner) syndrome. J Vasc Interv Radiol 2000; 11:823–36.

28. Mewissen MW, Seabrook GR, Meissner MH, Cynamon J, Labropoulos N, Haughton SH. Catheter-directed thrombolysis for lower extremity deep venous thrombosis: report of a national multicenter registry. Radiology 1999; 211:39–49.

29. Vedantham S, Vesely TM, Sicard GA, et al. Pharmacomechanical thrombolysis and early stent placement for iliofemoral deep vein thrombosis. J Vasc Interv Radiol 2004; 15:565–574.

30. Blätter W, Heller G, Largiadèr J, Savolainen H, Gloor B, Schmidli J. Combined regional thrombolysis and surgical thrombectomy for treatment of iliofemoral vein thrombosis. J Vas Surg 2004; 40:620–625.

31. Juhan CM, Alimi YS, Barthelemy PJ, Fabre DF, Riviere CS. Late results of iliofemoral venous thrombectomy. J Vasc Surg 1997; 25:417–422.

32. Eklöf B, Neglén P. Venous thrombectomy. In: Raju S, Villavicencio JL, eds. Baltimore, MD, USA: Williams & Wilkins 1997:512–527.

33. Hutschenreiter S, Vollmar J, Loeprecht H, Abendschein A, Rodl W. Reconstructive operations on the venous system: late results with a critical assessment of the functional and vascular morphological criteria. Chirurg 1979; 50:555–563.

34. Greenfield LJ, McCurdy JR, Brown PP, Elkins RC. A new intracaval filter permitting continued flow and resolution of emboli. Surgery 1973; 73:599–606.

35. Participants of the Vena Cava Filter Consensus Conference. Recommended reporting standards for vena cava filter placement and patient follow-up. J Vasc Surg 1999; 30:573–579.

36. Conners M, Becker S, Guzman R, et al. Duplex scan-directed placement of inferior vena cava filters: a five-year institutional experience. J Vasc Surg 2002; 35:286–291.

37. Ebaugh JL, Chiou AC, Morasch MD, Matsumura JS, Pearce WH. Bedside vena cava filter placement guided with intravascular ultrasound. J Vasc Surg 2001; 34:6–21.

38. Athanasoulis CA, Kaufman JA, Halpern EF, Waltman AC, Geller SC, Fan CM. Inferior vena cava filters: review of a 26-year single center clinical experience. Radiology 2000; 216:54–66.

39. Streiff MB. Vena cava filters: a comprehensive review. Blood 2000; 95:3669–3677.

40. Sato DT, Robinson KD, Gregory RT, et al. Duplex directed caval filter insertion in multi-trauma and critically ill patients. Ann Vasc Surg 1999; 13:365–371.

41. Benjamin ME, Sandager GP, Cohn EJ, Jr., et al. Duplex ultrasound insertion of inerior vena cava filters in multitrauma patients. Am J Surg 1999; 178:92–97.

42. PREPIC study group. Eight-year follow-up of patients with permanent vena cava filters in the prevention of pulmonary embolism: the PREPIC (Prevention du Risque d'Embolie Pulmonaire par Interruption Cave) randomized study. Circulation 2005; 112:416–422.

43. Semba CP, Razavi MK, Kee ST, Sze DY, Dake MD. Thrombolysis for lower extremity deep venous thrombosis. Tech Vasc Intervent Radiol 2004; 7:68–78.

44. Cho JS, Martelli E, Mozes G, Miller VM, Gloviczki P. Effects of thrombolysis and venous thrombectomy on valvular competence, thrombogenicity, venous wall morphology, and function. J Vasc Surg 1998; 28:787–799.

45. Rhodes JM, Cho JS, Gloviczki P, Mozes G, Rolle R, Miller VM. Thrombolysis for experimental deep venous thrombosis maintains valvular competence and vasoreactivity. J Vasc Surg 2000; 31:205–1193.

46. Comerota AJ, Aldridge SC. Thrombolytic therapy for deep venous thrombosis: a clinical review. Can J Surg 1993; 36:359–364.

47. Schweizer J, Kirch W, Koch R, et al. Short- and long-term results after thrombolytic treatment of deep venous thrombosis. J Am Coll Cardiol 2000; 36:1336–1343.

48. Laiho MK, Oinonen A, Sugano N, et al. Preservation of venous valve function after catheter-directed and systemic thrombolysis for deep venous thrombosis. Eur J Vasc Endovasc Surg 2004; 28:391–396.

49. Grossman C, McPherson S. Safety and efficacy of catheter-directed thrombolysis for iliofemoral venous thrombosis. Am J Roentgenol 1999; 211:39–49.

50. Comerota AJ, Throm RC, Mathias SD, Haughton S, Mewissen M. Catheter-directed thrombolysis for iliofemoral deep venous thrombosis improves health-related quality of life. J Vasc Surg 2000; 32:130–137.

51. Watson L, Armon M. Thrombolysis for acute deep vein thrombosis. Cochrane Database Syst Rev 2004; 4:CD002783.

52. Uflacker R. Mechanical thrombectomy in acute and subacute thrombosis with use of the Amplatz device: arterial and venous applications. J Vasc Interv Radiol 1997; 8:923–932.

53. Gandini R, Maspes F, Sodani G, Masala S, Assegnati G, Simonetti G. Percutaneous ilio-caval thrombectomy with the Amplatz device: preliminary results. Eur Radiol 1999; 9:951–958.

54. Kasirajan K, Gray B, Ouriel K. Percutaneous AngioJet thrombectomy in the management of extensive deep venous thrombosis. J Vasc Interv Radiol 2001; 12:179–185.

55. Delomez M, Beregi JP, Willoteaux S, et al. Mechanical thrombectomy in patients with deep venous thrombosis. Cardiovasc Intervent Radiol 2001; 24:42–48.

56. Bush RL, Lin PH, Bates JT, Mureebe L, Zhou W, Lumsden AB. Pharmacomechanical thrombectomy for treatment of symptomatic lower extremity deep venous thrombosis: safety and feasibility study. J Vasc Surg 2004; 40:965–970.

17

Inferior Vena Cava Filters

Sumaira Macdonald
*Northern Vascular Centre and the Department of Radiology, Freeman Hospital,
Newcastle upon Tyne, U.K.*

THE SCOPE OF THE CLINICAL PROBLEM

Venous thromboembolism (VTE), defined as including any thromboembolic event occurring within the venous system, encompassing deep venous thrombosis (DVT) and pulmonary embolism (PE), continues to pose a major health problem.

There are no reliable studies of the incidence or prevalence of VTE in the United Kingdom. A prospective Scandinavian study found an annual incidence of 1.6/1000 people in the general population (1). In another longitudinal Scandinavian study, the incidence of DVT was 2 per 100,000 observation-years, with corresponding incidence rates of 98 for nonfatal PE, 107 for fatal PE and 387 for all venous embolic events (2). In the United States, the incidence of VTE exceeds 1 per 1000. Over 200,000 new cases occur annually. Of these, 30% of patients die within 30 days, one-fifth suffering sudden death as a result of PE (3). Of those surviving VTE, 30% will develop recurrent disease within 10 years. Around 28% will develop venous stasis syndrome within 20 years (3). One postmortem study estimated that 600,000 people develop PE each year in the United States, of whom 60,000 die as a result (4).

The calculated prevalence of DVT depends on the extent to which all laboratory records are searched and misclassification of patients represents a major problem for investigators working exclusively from ICD-9-CM coded data. If records of patients who have undergone venous ultrasound or contrast venography are reviewed in addition to discharge summaries, the overall prevalence of DVT in adults over 20 years of age in a general hospital setting in the United States has been found to be 0.78% (271 of 34,567 patients) (5). Twenty-one percent of this population suffer PE. This figure included those patients treated prophylactically with low molecular weight heparin (LMWH).

Anticoagulation remains the treatment standard for venous thromboembolic disease with satisfactory outcomes in 90% of treatment cases. Heparin has been shown to decrease the risk of fatal PE by 75% and to reduce the risk of recurrent PE from 25% to 2% (6). Long-term warfarin therapy reduces the incidence of documented DVT from 47% to 2%. Patients with VTE who receive adequate anticoagulation generally do not die of recurrent disease. However, it should be noted that patients who are treated for PE are almost four times more likely (1.5% versus 0.4%) to die of recurrent VTE in the next year than are

223

patients who are treated for DVT (7), indicating that this population is at the higher-risk end of the spectrum of diseases that characterize VTE.

Recurrence rates however, may be surprisingly high; as many as 33% of patients develop a second PE while receiving adequate anticoagulation therapy. This fact supports an alternative treatment strategy, namely caval filtration.

INFERIOR VENA CAVA INTERRUPTION: AN EVOLUTION

One of the earliest techniques for the prevention of PE in the setting of proximal DVT was pioneered by John Hunter, when he ligated the femoral vein at the level of the thrombus. Homans later addressed the problem by the ligation of both femoral veins. When it became clear that neither of these approaches would reliably prevent recurrent PE, vena caval interruption, involving laparotomy under general anesthesia was performed. These methods were used in parallel with anticoagulation once heparin and warfarin became available in 1935 and 1948 respectively. These procedures were associated with substantial morbidity from lower extremity edema, venous stasis ulceration and the post-thrombotic syndrome. Furthermore, the potential benefits of these early procedures were negated by the fact that retroperitoneal collaterals subsequently developed, exposing the patients to the risk of recurrent PE in upto 15% of cases. Mortality following ligation was also unacceptably high, ranging from 4% in low-risk cases to 39% in those with significant cardiorespiratory co-morbidities (8). Ligation of the inferior vena cava (IVC) was performed initially in patients with clot burden above the level of the superficial femoral veins. Eventually, this replaced lower-level venous ligation. The operative mortality was not significantly different but a lower rate of recurrent PE was reported. The optimal level for ligation was located immediately below the renal veins to prevent thrombosis due to venous stasis between the interrupted IVC and the renal veins. Immediate lower limb swelling occurred in 10–16% of cases.

External caval clips (Moretz clip, Miles clip, Adams-DeWeese clip) and sutures or staple grids were subsequently used in an attempt to provide channels to allow unhindered venous return while preventing PE. These procedures also required laparotomy and general anesthesia. The incidence of limb edema was reduced but the rates of recurrent PE and operative mortality were unchanged. Despite the partial interruption of venous return, caval occlusion rates of 30%–40% were reported.

In the late 1960s, methods were developed that allowed caval interruption devices to be placed directly into the vena cava through the femoral or jugular vein via a small surgical incision under local anesthesia. The first endoluminal filter was devised in 1967, the Mobin-Uddin umbrella (9).

The major complications associated with this device included IVC thrombosis in up to 60% of cases and device migration at a rate of 0.4%. As a result of these complications, this device was withdrawn from the market. The first percutaneous insertion of a Greenfield conical filter was performed in 1984 (10,11). Perhaps as a result of its unique cone geometry, the long-term patency rate has been shown to be over 95% for over three decades (12). Mathematical modeling and in-vitro studies have demonstrated that the unique design allows upto 70% of the cone volume to be filled with thrombus before significant reductions in blood flow occur.

First generation filters were delivered through a 24 French (8 mm) delivery system resulting in a high incidence of insertion site complications. Naturally, this prompted technical refinements and the development of modern low-profile filters delivered through

6 to 10 French introducer systems, which have reduced the incidence of access site complications. Most of the newer generation filters are made of titanium, nitinol or stainless steel alloys that have low ferromagnetic properties, rendering them safe in magnetic resonance imaging (MRI) scanners although imaging may be somewhat degraded by artefact.

FILTER TYPES AND DESIGN

IVC filters are designed for their physical properties, efficacy at trapping clots, ability to preserve flow in the IVC, and ease of placement. Each of the currently available filters achieves some, but not all, of the following ideal properties:

- The filter should maximize clot capture in order to prevent new or recurrent PE.
- The filter should be nonthrombogenic and maintain caval patency
- The filter should be made of a biocompatible material that is durable and noncorrosive
- The shape and structural integrity of the filter should be durable
- The delivery system of the filter should have a low profile and promote easy placement
- Clot trapping should be reasonably effective even if filter deployment is suboptimal, for example, many deployed filters assume a tilted angle in the cava
- Migration after deployment should be minimal
- The filter should not cause caval perforation[a]
- Preferably, the filter should be nonferromagnetic to allow safe subsequent MRI imaging.

The most frequently used filters at the current time are permanent and retrievable models.

Temporary Filters

Temporary filters, which are attached to catheters that protrude from the access site and can be secured in the subcutaneous tissues (much as would an untunneled central venous line), are much less frequently used. Temporary filters include the Tempofilter, (B Braun Medical Inc, Bethlehem, Pensylvania, U.S.A), the Günther temporary filter, (Cook, Leechburg, Pennsylvania, U.S.A.), the Prolyser (Cordis Corporation, Warren, New Jersey, U.S.A.), and the Antheor filters (Boston Scientific, Natick, Massachusetts, U.S.A.). These filters can be left *in situ* for around six weeks. In an *in-vitro* study, temporary filters demonstrated better clot capture efficiency than permanent filters (13) but they are associated with an appreciable risk of migration (fatalities have been reported with the Tempofilter) (14), filter thrombosis and a potential risk of sepsis.

---

[a] Extension of the filter struts beyond the IVC, which is suggestive of perforation, has been noted in high incidence on CT. Recent animal studies evaluated the apparent vena caval penetration following placement of the Greenfield filter (15). All filters appeared to penetrate the IVC on cavography and CT. Laparoscopy failed to demonstrate penetration, and histology revealed remodelling of the intimal surface of the IVC and thinning of the adventitia. The authors further hypothesized that IVC adaptation and remodelling occurred due to the presence of the filter.

Permanent Filters

Currently available permanent filters include; the stainless steel Greenfield, the titanium Greenfield (Boston Scientific), the LGM VenaTech (B. Braun Medical Inc), the Simon Nitinol (CR Bard, Murray Hill, New Jersey, U.S.A.), the Bird's Nest filter (Cook), and the TrapEase (Cordis Corporation). Currently, only the Bird's Nest filter is licensed for use in mega-cava (over 30 mm in diameter), and is sufficient to provide adequate filtration up to 40 mm. The other filters have a working range between 28 mm and 32 mm. The caveat is that the IVC is flattened on an anteroposterior image taken during venography for filter placement and this measurement is likely to represent the largest caval diameter. A measurement taken perpendicularly is likely to be much smaller and this can be readily appreciated on axial computed tomography (CT). All the filters named are United States Food and Drug Administration (FDA) approved and Conformity European (CE) marked.

Currently there are no prospective data comparing the clinical efficacy and complications of these devices. There are a number of retrospective case series for each device but heterogeneity in patient selection, indications for treatment and definitions of technical and clinical success make meaningful comparison difficult (16).

Retrievable Filters

The newer generation of retrievable filters have potential benefits in that they may be utilized to prevent PE during the time when the patient is at increased risk, for example in a multiple trauma setting, thereby harvesting the benefits of shorter-term survival benefit from PE, while avoiding the risks associated with permanent placement (which includes filter thrombosis, caval thrombosis and lower limb edema). Retrievable devices may be retrieved percutaneously after varying periods, without the requirement for an indwelling catheter.

Retrievable filters include:

- Günther Tulip (Cook). This may be retrieved upto 14 days following placement. It must be retrieved via the jugular vein although it may be initially placed via the femoral or jugular routes
- OptEase (Cordis). This may be retrieved up to 14 days post-placement. The Optease can be deployed from either the femoral or the jugular approach using the same system. Currently, it is the only retrievable filter that can be recovered from a femoral approach. One potential benefit of the femoral approach over the jugular approach during retrieval is the avoidance of the heart, thus lessening possible myocardial injury or arrhythmia
- The ALN (Pyramed, Surbiton, Surrey, United Kingdom) can be removed after an indefinite period of time
- The Recovery (Bard) also has no upper limit on time to safe removal. A small prospective analysis of the Recovery filter in 32 patients, indicated a mean implantation period of 53 days (range: 5–134 days) (17).

INDICATIONS FOR USE

It must be appreciated that unlike anticoagulant therapy, vena caval interruption is an incomplete treatment of venous thromboembolic disease. Caval filtration has no beneficial effect on the prevention of DVT, or on the prevention of DVT extension, recurrence, and subsequent postphlebitic syndrome. As anticoagulant therapy effectively prevents PE in the majority of patients with DVT, only absolute contraindications to and documented failures of anticoagulant therapy in patients with acute VTE represent obvious and widely accepted indications for caval interruption (18). It may be considered that controled trials would be unethical in these settings. However, in certain populations, most patients may have neither of the two main indications (19).

Use of filters in a prophylactic sense, in patients at high risk of but with no documented evidence for VTE, or adjuvant caval filtration for patients with VTE who can receive anticoagulant therapy remain a matter of debate (18,20). The prevailing uncertainties in clinical use of caval filters is highlighted spectacularly in the huge variation in practice between countries; from 3 to 140 per million inhabitants per year in Sweden and the United States, respectively (21).

Although categorical indications for filter placement have been given, as recommended by the Vena Cava Filter Consensus Conference (Table 1) (22), various thresholds exist among clinicians, and there is scarce level-1 evidence to support practice.

The rate of prophylactic placement appears to be increasing. Greenfield has reported a summary of 642 placements over 27 years (23). Of note is the increasing use of caval filters in the prophylactic setting (11% of placements in 1977 and 32% in 1999), and the reduction in number of placements for failure of anticoagulation (38% in 1977 and 10% in 1999).

Free-floating iliofemoral thrombus is a relatively rare entity but it comprises a commonly proposed indication for caval filtration (24). A retrospective review of 78 patients with documented iliofemoral DVT treated with anticoagulation concluded that there was an extremely high rate of PE, i.e., 60% among those with free-floating thrombi (25).

Several other retrospective studies have reported similar outcomes but a prospective analysis of 95 patients reported no significant differences in the rates of PE between patients with (3.3%) or without (3.7%) free-floating iliofemoral thrombi treated with anticoagulation (26). Differences in study populations may explain the conflicting conclusions but the use of caval filters in this clinical scenario remains controversial.

Table 1 Categorical Indications for Filter Placement

- Contraindication to anticoagulation (absolute or relative), e.g., thrombocytopenia
- Complication of anticoagulation
  Hemorrhage: major or minor
  Skin necrosis
  Drug reaction
- Failure of anticoagulation, i.e., objectively documented extension of existing DVT or a new
  DVT or PE while therapeutically anticoagulated
- Evidence/probability of poor compliance with anticoagulation therapy
- Prophylaxis: no thromboembolic disease, i.e., multiple trauma
- Prophylaxis in patients with thromboembolism in addition to anticoagulation, e.g., those
  scheduled for major orthopedic or pelvic surgery
- Failure of previous device to prevent PE; central extension of thrombus through an existing filter
  or recurrent PE
- In association with another procedure: thrombectomy, embolectomy, or lytic therapy

Source: From Ref. 22.

There are four main categories of patients who could be at high risk for thromboembolic events and may constitute an indication for prophylactic filter placement. These are:

1. Patients with DVT who are about to undergo surgery (lower-extremity orthopedic surgery, major abdominal surgery, neurosurgery)
2. Patients with chronic pulmonary hypertension and a marginal cardiopulmonary reserve
3. Patients with cancer
4. Trauma patients

The records of 32 cancer patients who were treated with heparin and warfarin for thromboembolic disease were reviewed in a study published in 1981 that concluded that standard techniques for anticoagulation were reported to be neither safe nor effective in this population. Sixteen patients experienced 21 different hemorrhagic complications. Eight patients had major hemorrhages that led to cessation of therapy or death. Six of 32 patients had PE while receiving anticoagulants. It was suggested that venous interruption could be a safer and more effective method of prophylaxis against PE in cancer patients (27). This conclusion was disputed by the American College of Chest Physicians Consensus Committee on Pulmonary Embolism (28), which stated that the case for the routine use of caval filters in patients with cancer and DVT or PE was not supported.

Patients with severe trauma are at risk of VTE. In many such patients, anticoagulation is contraindicated on the basis of an unacceptably high risk of hemorrhage. Other conservative methods, such as foot pumps and compression devices may not adequately prevent DVT. Examples of patients in this category include; patients with severe head injury and prolonged ventilator dependence, major abdominal or pelvic penetrating injury, spinal cord injury with or without paralysis, severe head injury with multiple lower extremity fractures and pelvic fracture with or without lower extremity fracture.

A case-controled study on caval filters in trauma patients was reported in 1996. The results indicated that vena cava filters may have reduced the incidence of PE in multiple trauma patients, that mortality from PE had been reduced as a result of caval filtration and that overall mortality was noted to be reduced. The study was not adjusted for confounding factors and not validated in an independent set of patients. It was set in a tertiary center in the United States. There were 120 patients (mean age 42 years, 63% male). Forty patients were multiply injured and had survived more than 48 hours, with three or more risk factors for PE, compared with 80 retrospective matched controls. Patients were excluded if they were younger than 56 years, or had an injury score of < 16. All patients had VTE prophylaxis (antiembolism—TED stockings, plus or minus heparin). As a non randomized trial, it is likely that the benefits of caval filters may have been overestimated. The PE mortality was high, i.e., around 60% of cases, compared to the more commonly quoted rate of around 2.5%. Also, the filter group in this study were older, had less severe injuries and were immobilized for longer, all of which would comprise important confounding variables.

A review of 4093 titles yielded 73 articles for meta-analysis of prevention of VTE after injury (29). A random-effects model was used for all pooled results. Study quality was evaluated by previously published quality scores. The incidence of DVT and PE reported in the included studies varied widely. The pooled rates were 11.8% for DVT and 1.5% for PE. Only a few randomized controled trials evaluated the methods of VTE prophylaxis among trauma patients, and combining their data was considered difficult because of different designs and differences in the preventive methods used.

The quality of most studies was considered low. Meta-analysis showed no evidence that low-dose heparin, mechanical prophylaxis, or low-molecular-weight heparin were more effective than either no prophylaxis or each other. However, the 95% confidence intervals of many of the comparisons were wide; therefore, a clinically important difference may exist. The review concluded that the trauma literature on VTE prophylaxis provided inconsistent data and highlighted a need for a large high-quality, multicenter trial that could provide definitive answers. In Part II of this two-part review (30), the role of caval filters was analyzed. The same methodology was employed as in Part I of the review. It was noted that spinal fractures and spinal-cord injuries increased the risk of DVT two-fold and three-fold respectively. Patients with DVT were approximately nine years older than those without DVT. No specific cut-off point for increased risk could be established because data could not be combined across studies. Patients with prophylactically placed vena cava filters had a lower incidence of PE (0.2%) compared with concurrently managed patients without caval filtration (1.5%) or historical controls without caval filters (5.8%). The results report on uncontrolled studies with observational design; nevertheless, the authors concluded that placement of a caval filter in selected trauma cases may decrease the incidence of PE. The need for future trials was again emphasized.

THE USE OF CAVAL FILTERS OUTSIDE OF THE TRAUMA SETTING: THE EVIDENCE BASE

Girard and associates performed a systematic review of the literature in an attempt to clarify the indications for filter placement (31). A systematic MEDLINE search produced a total of 568 references with abstracts between 1975 and 2000 inclusively. Each reference was analysed to predetermined criteria. A similar search was undertaken for heparin and thromboembolism.

The annual number of publications ranged from one in 1976 to 42 in 1994 and 1998. Retrospective clinical series ($n=189$) represented exactly one-third (33.3%) of all publications, with only 59 series reporting on ≥ 100 patients, and 90 series reporting on <50 patients. Case reports ($n=180$) represented nearly one-third of the literature (31.7%). Animal studies ($n=38$) and in vitro work ($n=35$) represented 12.9% of the literature. Prospective series accounted for only 7.4% of the literature. Among prospective studies, only 16 series (2.8% of the entire library) included ≥ 100 patients, and there was only one randomized controled trial, representing 0.02% of the library. Among the 16 prospective studies, nine series were partial and/or updated reports from the same authors and/or on the same patients. There were 26 clinical series reporting mainly or exclusively on prophylactic IVC interruption in trauma or major orthopedic surgery patients, all originating from the United States. Only one of these was a prospective series of >100 patients. Sixty of the 568 references (10.6%) reported on temporary filters, with only one prospective series of ≥ 100 patients. The annual number of publications ranged from one article in 1985 to 10 articles in 1995.

By comparison, 531 references concerning heparin therapy in DVT were found, and of those, two-hundred and fifty-two articles (47.7%) reported randomized controled trials.

In 1998, Decousus et al. published the only randomized trial of vena cava filters in the prevention of PE to date (32). This was an unblinded concealed randomized trial without intention-to-treat and took over three and a half years to complete in 44 centers in France. Four-hundred patients were randomized using a 2×2 factorial design to caval filter or no caval filter and a LMWH (enoxaparin) or unfractionated heparin. The mean age was 73 years (range 60–94 years), and 50% were male. Inclusion criteria were an acute proximal deep vein thrombosis, diagnosed by venogram, in a patient considered to be at high risk for PE. Four different types of caval filter were employed. These included the titanium Greenfield, Bird's Nest, LGM Vena Tech and Cardial (CR Bard). All were placed within 48 hours of diagnosis. Ventilation-perfusion scans were performed at baseline and after 8 to 12 days of anticoagulation. Vena cava filters were associated with a significant decrease in the incidence of PE compared with anticoagulation alone (1.1% versus 4.8%, $p=0.03$) at 8 to 12 days of follow-up. After two years, however, this difference was no longer statistically significant, although the trend favoured caval filters (3.4% versus 6.3%, $p=0.16$). Symptomatic PE occurred at a similar frequency in both groups after three months (filter, 4%; no filter, 6%). Fatal emboli were more common among patients treated solely with anticoagulation (0.5% vs. 2.5%). In contrast, vena cava filters were associated with significantly more recurrent DVT than anticoagulation alone (20.8% vs. 11.6%, $p=0.02$). There was no difference in bleeding or overall mortality. Sixteen of the 37 patients (43.2%) with vena cava filters who had recurrent DVT also had IVC thrombosis (8% of the filter population).

The authors concluded that in high-risk patients with proximal DVT, the initial beneficial effect of vena cava filters for the prevention of PE was counterbalanced by an excess of recurrent deep-vein thrombosis, without any difference in mortality.

Clearly, vena cava filters in combination with standard anticoagulation do appear to offer significantly more protection from PE than anticoagulation alone. This additional protection, however, appeared to be short-lived and did not decrease overall mortality. In addition, vena cava filters were associated with a higher incidence of recurrent DVT over two years of follow-up.

Because almost all participants (94%) in this trial received anticoagulants for at least three months, however, the outcomes of these patients cannot be generalized to the typical patient with a filter who does not receive anticoagulation. A further limitation of the trial includes lack of clarity in how high-risk patients were defined. It is also not clear whether patients would have received only positive benefits if filters had been removed after a few weeks, whether patients with thrombophilia would differ in terms of outcomes and whether filters could be an alternative to anticoagulation. Lastly, the data presented at two years reflect the all-cause mortality as the outcome measure of net clinical benefit, with those deaths in the filter group attributable to hemorrhage, myocardial infarction, respiratory failure and renal failure. Arguably, filter efficacy relates specifically to PE mortality. The reduction in symptomatic PE at 2 years with a filter ($p=0.16$) may not have reached statistical significance because of the sample size. The study was originally designed for 800 patients.

The Michigan Filter Registry contains data for a prospective cohort of 2188 patients with a Greenfield filter (33). Data on the percutaneous stainless steel Greenfield were extracted in order to compare outcomes with the titanium Greenfield filter. Since 1995, 600 percutaneous stainless steel Greenfield filters were placed in 599 patients. A one-year mortality rate of 42% left 349 patients available for annual follow-up, and studies were completed for 231 (66%). Periprocedural events occurred in 2.5% of cases with associated morbidity in 1.5%. The rate of new PE was 2.6%, and vena caval patency was 98.3%. The combined rate of new VTE was 12.5%. Left-sided femoral vein placements increased to 20%, and the major indication for filter placement had become for prophylaxis (46%). It was concluded that the ease of use and favorable patient outcomes for the percutaneous stainless steel Greenfield have resulted in more frequent placement for prophylactic indications. This registry provides important data and is notable for its size but is limited in a number of ways. It reflects a heterogeneous population, i.e., prophylactic use has doubled since 1993, follow-up imaging comprised ultrasound in many cases and outcomes were "indeterminate" in 35 cases. Twenty percent of the original retrospective study data which were subsequently incorporated into the registry was missing (34). In common with many registries, it is likely that the results were largely self-audited and this is known to be notoriously unreliable (35).

To a clinician seeking reliable information about the indications for IVC interruption, the overall quality of the abundant literature is disappointing, in contradistinction to the publications pertaining to heparin and VTE. Reliable evidence is still available on the technique and safety profile of IVC interruption, despite the lack of randomized trials, through large retrospective and prospective series. However, regarding indications for use, careful systematic reviews have been unable to provide evidence-based guidelines. Future randomized trials may focus on the trauma setting and on prophylactic use. There are ethical concerns with the randomization of patients who have contraindication to, or failure of, anticoagulant therapy to treatment with anticoagulants. Furthermore there are logistical issues; the only published randomized trial took 3.5 years in 44 centers. However, until results of future randomized trials and subsequent recommendations become available, literature reviews about IVC interruption will remain narrative at best, and many, if not most, indications for filter placement will remain a matter of opinion.

Lastly, there is much industry support for the use of caval filters and a number of clinicians involved in the Vena Cava Filter Consensus Committee have highlighted competitive interests. Even with respect to randomized trials it is known that industry-funded endeavours are more likely to be associated with statistically significant pro-industry findings, both in medical trials and surgical interventions (36).

CLINICAL CONTROVERSIES CONCERNING VENA CAVA FILTERS

Many areas of clinical uncertainty have been highlighted above. The use of caval filtration in free floating iliofemoral thrombus, the use of filters in specific settings such as cancer or trauma and the use of temporary or retrievable filters are all relatively controversial. Many of these areas of uncertainty would be best addressed by means of robust well-designed and preferably randomized trials.

Other specific questions remain unanswered.

The Use of Adjuvant Anticoagulation

It is not clear if anticoagulation is necessary after caval filtration. Many investigators recommend routine anticoagulation after vena cava filter placement (37). However, little data are available to support the utility of this practice. Several case-series have attempted to address this issue. None of these investigators were able to demonstrate any benefit of anticoagulation and the retrospective, unrandomized nature of the studies as well as the limited duration and intensity of anticoagulation used in some of the studies suggest that randomized comparisons will be necessary to resolve this issue.

Comparative Efficacy of Filters and Anticoagulation

The comparative efficacy of caval filters relative to anticoagulation is unclear. The randomized trial of Decousus suggested that filters may provide additional short-term benefit against PE in anticoagulated patients. An unrandomized retrospective series found no significant differences in recurrence rate or lower extremity symptoms between patients treated with anticoagulation and in those in who filters were placed (38). The significant design flaws of this small study mean that larger randomized trials will be necessary to address this issue.

Suprarenal Placement of Caval Filters

The general recommended placement site for caval filters is in the infrarenal portion of the vena cava. This reflects concern about the possibility of caval thrombosis precipitating acute renal failure as a result of renal vein extension of thrombus following suprarenal placement. On occasion, infrarenal placement is impossible. Six studies, including 187 patients in total, highlight this subset of patients (37). All but one study utilized the Greenfield filter exclusively (39–44). Mean follow-up was 70 months. PE occurred in 6% (7 of 112) and venous insufficiency developed in 75% (55 of 73). Although IVC thrombosis was diagnosed in 3.6% (4 of 112), no evidence of significant renal morbidity was noted.

Compared with infrarenal placement, suprarenal filters appear to be associated with a higher rate of PE and venous insufficiency. These differences could reflect differences in study population rather than site of filter placement. Previous PE and malignancy was more common in those studies evaluating suprarenal placement, suggesting that this study population was at particularly high risk of thrombotic events and venous stasis (41). More work will be required to clarify the safety and efficacy of suprarenal deployment.

Superior Vena Cava Filters

Data on superior vena cava filtration (SVC) are scarce and the literature is limited to case reports, a single small case series (45–50) and a report of a retrievable filter placed in the SVC and successfully retrieved (51). To date the reported results are mixed, with some patients remaining asymptomatic and others developing SVC thrombosis. Larger series and longer follow-up will be required before any meaningful comment can be made on the safety and efficacy of SVC filters.

Assessment of Risk and Benefit of Anticoagulation for Venous Thromboembolic Disease

In order to fully appraise the utility of caval filters, an informed decision regarding their use must necessarily include a consideration of the relative risks and benefits of anticoagulation. As highlighted above, there is a wealth of reliable evidence in the form of randomized trials of anticoagulation in VTE which involve thousands of patients worldwide. The rate of symptomatic recurrent thrombosis is 3% over two to four years of surveillance for patients on long-term therapy (52,53). Major hemorrhage may be defined as one resulting in retroperitoneal or intracranial bleeding, requiring blood transfusion or reducing baseline hemoglobin by 2 g/dl. During heparin therapy, 3% of patients (range: 0–7%) will suffer major hemorrhage as will 2% to 5% of patients on subsequent warfarin therapy (54,55). In patients on warfarin therapy, for an indefinite period, major bleeding has been noted in 8.3%

after 4 years of follow-up (53). The risk factors for hemorrhage include duration of therapy, recent surgery or trauma, age over 65 years, concomitant aspirin therapy, renal or hepatic insufficiency, previous gastrointestinal bleeding, alcohol abuse, higher intensity therapy, and, in some studies, malignant disease and female gender (54,55). Clearly these factors would not constitute absolute contraindications, although many clinicians would hesitate to anticoagulate a patient with recent central nervous system trauma or hemorrhage, active hemorrhage, significant thrombocytopenia (less than 50,000/µl), cerebral metastases or a recent large embolic stroke (56–58). The evidence-base for this strategy is limited but anecdotal case reports and series suggest that anticoagulation is probably sufficiently hazardous that vena cava filters should be considered for patients with VTE in these situations.

KEY POINTS

- The evidence base for the use of caval filters is relatively limited.
- There are substantial variations in practice between the United States, the United Kingdom and mainland Europe with respect to numbers of caval filters placed. This may reflect clinical uncertainty, the influence of reimbursement and/or the threat of litigation.
- Caval filters may reduce early PE mortality but there is no reduction in all-cause mortality at two years in a population who also have adjuvant anticoagulation.
- In a population who are also treated with anticoagulation, the use of caval filters may be associated with an increase in recurrent DVT.
- There are no randomized trials to support the use of caval filters for the most widely accepted indications (documented failure of and absolute contra-indication to, anticoagulation) and it is doubtful that an Ethics Committee or Institutional Review Board will support trials in this area.
- The use of caval filters per se in trauma settings is increasing rapidly and the practice would benefit from supporting randomized trial evidence.
- The latest generation of retrievable filters can be retrieved after extended periods and may protect the patient from PE during high-risk periods, e.g., post-operatively, while avoiding the longer-term risks associated with extended placement.
- The practice of retrievable filter placement in trauma or perioperative settings would benefit from evidence from robust trials
- Many controversies exist regarding optimal management of patients with VTE using caval filters including the use of adjuvant anticoagulation therapy (dose and duration of therapy), suprarenal placement and SVC placement and the use of filters for free-floating thrombus.

REFERENCES

1. Nordstrom M, Lindblad B, Bergqvist D, et al. A prospective study of the incidence of deep-vein thrombosis within a defined urban population. J Intern Med 1992; 232:155–160.
2. Hansson PO, Welin L, Tibblin G, et al. Deep vein thrombosis and pulmonary embolism in the general population. The study of men born in 1913. Arch Intern Med 1997; 157:1665–1670.
3. Heit JA. Venous Thromboembolism epidemiology: implications for prevention and management. Semin Thromb Hemost 2002; 28:003–014.

4. Rubenstein I, Murray D, Hoffstein V. Fatal pulmonary emboli in hospitalised patients: an autopsy study. Arch Intern Med 1988; 148:1425–1426.

5. Stein PD, Patel KC, Kalra NK, et al. Deep Venous Thrombosis in a General Hospital. Chest 2002; 122:960–962.

6. Siskin GP, Kwan B. Inferior Vena Cava Filters. E-medicine last updated September 2004.

7. Douketis JD, Kearon C, Bates S, et al. Risk of fatal pulmonary embolism in patients with treated venous thromboembolism. JAMA 1998; 279:458–462.

8. Greenfield LJ, Wakefield T. Prevention of venous thrombosis and pulmonary embolism. In: Tompkins R, Cameron J, Langer B et al., eds. Advances in Surgery. Chicago: Year Book Medical Publishers, 1989:301–323.

9. Mobin-Uddin K, Smith PE, Martines LO, et al. A vena caval filter for the prevention of pulmonary embolus. Surg Forum 1967; 18:209–211.

10. Greenfield LJ, McCrudy JR, Brown PP, et al. A new intracaval filter permitting continued flow and resolution of emboli. Surgery 1973; 73:599–606.

11. Tadarthy SM, Castaneda-Zuniga W, Salomonowitz E, et al. Kimray-Greenfield vena cava filter: percutaneous introduction. Radiology 1984; 151:525–526.

12. Greenfield LJ, Proctor MC. Suprarenal filter placement. J Vasc Surg 1998; 28:432–438.

13. Stoneham GW, Burbridge BE, Millward SF. Temporary inferior vena cava filters: in vitro comparison with permanent IVC filters. J Vasc Interventional Radiol 1995; 5:731–736.

14. Rossi P, Arata FM, Bonaiuti P, et al. Fatal Outcome in Atrial Migration of the Tempofilter. Cardiovasc Interventional Radiol 1999; 22:227–231.

15. Proctor MC, Greenfield LJ, Cho KJ, et al. Assessment of apparent vena caval penetration by the Greenfield filter. J Endovasc Surg 1998; 5:251–258.

16. Kinney TB. Update on Inferior Vena Cava Filters. J Vasc Intervent Radiol 2003; 14:425–440.

17. Asch MR. Initial Experience in Humans with a New Retrievable Inferior Vena Cava Filter. Radiology 2002; 225:835–844.

18. Hyers TM, Agnelli G, Hull RD, et al. Antithrombotic therapy for venous thromboembolic disease. Chest 2001; 119:176S–193S.

19. White RH, Zhou H, Kim J, et al. A population-based study of the effectiveness of inferior vena cava filter use among patients with venous thromboembolism. Arch Intern Med 2000; 160:2033–2041.

20. Geerts WH, Heit JA, Clagett GP, et al. Prevention of venous thromboembolism. Chest 2001; 119:132S–175S.

21. Bergqvist D. The role of vena cava interruption in patients with venous thromboembolism. Prog Cardiovasc Dis 1994; 37:25–37.

22. Recommended reporting standards for vena cava filter placement and patient follow-up: Vena Cava Filter Consensus Conference. J Vasc Surg, 1999; 30:573–579.

23. Greenfield LJ, Proctor MC. Indications and techniques of inferior vena cava interruption. In: Gloviczki P, Yao JST, eds. Handbook of Venous Disorders. 1st ed. London: Chapman and Hall Medical, 1996; 306–320.

24. Jones TK, Barnes RW, Greenfield LJ. Greenfield vena caval filter: rationale and current indications. Ann Thorac Surg 1986; 42:S48–S55.

25. Norris CS, Greenfield LJ, Herrmann JB. Free-floating iliofemoral thrombus. A risk of pulmonary embolism. Arch Surg 1985; 120:806–808.

26. Pacouret G, Alison D, Pottier JM, et al. Free-floating thrombus and embolic risk in patients with angiographically confirmed proximal deep venous thrombosis. A prospective study. Arch Intern Med 1997; 157:305–308.

27. Moore FD, Osteen RT, Karp DD, et al. Anticoagulants, venous thromboembolism, and the cancer patient. Arch Surg 1981; 116:405–407.

28. American College of Chest Physicians. Opinions regarding the diagnosis and management of venous thromboembolic disease. ACCP Consensus Committee on Pulmonary Embolism. American College of Chest Physicians. Chest 1998; 113:499–504.

29. Velmahos GC, Kern J, Chan LS, et al. Prevention of venous thromboembolism after injury: an evidence-based report—part I: analysis of risk factors and evaluation of the role of vena caval filters. J Trauma 2000; 49:132–138 discussion 139.

30. Velmahos GC, Kern J, Chan LS, et al. Prevention of venous thromboembolism after injury: an evidence-based report—part II: analysis of risk factors and evaluation of the role of vena caval filters. J Trauma 2000; 49:140–144.

31. Girard P, Stern J-B, Parent F. Medical Literature and Vena Cava Filters. So Far So Weak. Chest 2002; 122:963–967.

32. Decousus H, Leizorovicz A, Parent F, et al. A Clinical Trial of Vena Cava Filetrs in the Prevention of Pulmonary Embolism in Patients with Proximal Deep-Vein Thrombosis. N J Engl Med 1998; 338:409–416.

33. Greenfield LJ, Proctor M. The Percutaneous Greenfield Filter: Outcomes and practice patterns. J Vasc Surg 2000; 32:888–893.

34. Greenfield LJ, Proctor MC. Twenty-year clinical experience with the Greenfield filter. Cardiovasc Surg 1995; 3:199–205.

35. Rothwell P, Warlow C. Is self-audit reliable? Lancet 1995; 346:1623.

36. Bhandari M, Busse JW, Jackowski D, et al. Association between industry funding and statistically significant pro-industry findings in medical and surgical randomized trials. CMAJ 2004; 170:477–480.

37. Streiff MB. Vena cava filter: a comprehensive review. Blood 2000; 15:3669–3677.

38. Jones BT, Fink JA. A prospective comparison of the status of the deep venous system after treatment with intracaval interruption versus anticoagulation. J Am Coll Surg 1994; 178:220–222.

39. Brenner DW, Brenner CJ, Scott J, et al. Suprarenal Greenfield filter placement to prevent pulmonary embolus in patients with vena caval tumour thrombi. J Urol 1992; 147:19–23.

40. Orsini RA, Jarrell BE. Suprarenal placement of vena cava filters: indications, techniques and result. J Vasc Surg 1984; 1:124–0135.

41. Greenfield LJ, Proctor MC. Suprarenal filter placement. J Vasc Surg 1998; 28:432–438.

42. Greenfield LJ, Cho KJ, Proctor MC, et al. Late results of suprarenal Greenfield vena cava filter placement. Arch Surg 1992; 127:969–973.

43. Stewart JR, Peyton JWR, Crute S, et al. Clinical results of suprarenal placement of the Greenfield vena cava filter. Surgery 1982; 92:1–4.

44. Matchett WJ, Jones MP, McFarland DR, et al. Suprarenal vena cava filter placement:follow-up of four filter types in 22 patients. J Vasc Interv Radiol 1998; 9:588–593.

45. Owen EWJ, Schoettle GPJ, Harrington OB. Placement of a Greenfield filter in the superior vena cava. Ann Thorac Surg 1992; 53:896–897.

46. Ascer E, Gennaro M, Lorenson E, et al. Superior vena caval Greenfield: indications, techniques, and results. J Vasc Surg 1996; 23:498–503.

47. Hoffman MJ, Greenfield LJ. Central venous septic thrombosis managed by superior vena cava Greenfield filter and venous thrombectomy: a case report. J Vasc Surg 1986; 4:606–611.

48. Pais SO, Orchis DF, Mirvis SE. Superior vena caval placement of Kimray-Greenfield filter. Radiology 1987; 165:385–386.

49. Black MD, French GJ, Rasuli P, et al. Upper extremity deep venous thrombosis: underdiagnosed and potentially lethal. Chest 1993; 103:1887–1890.

50. Lidogaster MI, Widman WD, Chevinski AH. Superior vena caval occlusion after filter insertion. J Vasc Surg 1994; 20:158–159.

51. Nadkarni S, Macdonald S, Cleveland TJ, et al. Placement of a retrievable Günther Tulip filter in the superior vena cava for upper extremity deep venous thrombosis. Cardiovasc Intervent Radiol 2002; 25:524–526.

52. Kearon C, Gent M, Hirsh J, et al. A comparison of three months of anticoagulation with extended anticoagulation for a first episode of idiopathic venous thromboembolism. N Engl J Med 1999; 340:901–907.

53. Schulman S, Granqvist S, Holmstrom M, et al. The duration of oral anticoagulant therapy after a second episode of venous thromboembolism. The Duration of Anticoagulation Trial Study Group. N Engl J Med 1997; 336:393–398.

54. Levine M, Gent M, Hirsh J, et al. A comparison of low-molecular-weight heparin administered primarily at home with unfractionated heparin administered in the hospital for proximal deep-vein thrombosis. N Engl J Med 1996; 334:677–681.

55. White RH, White RH, Beyth RJ, et al. Major bleeding after hospitalization for deep-venous thrombosis. Am J Med 1999; 107:414–424.

56. Brathwaite CE, Mure AJ, O'Malley KF, et al. Complications of anticoagulation for pulmonary embolism in low risk trauma patients. Chest 1993; 104:718–720.

57. Olin JW, Young JR, Graor RA, et al. Treatment of deep vein thrombosis and pulmonary emboli in patients with primary and metastatic brain tumors. Anticoagulants or inferior vena cava filter? Arch Intern Med 1987; 147:2177–2179.

58. Cerebral Embolism Study Group. Immediate anticoagulation of embolic stroke: brain hemorrhage and management options. Stroke 1984; 15:779–789.

18

Etiology and Pathophysiology of Varicose Veins

Jonathan Golledge
School of Medicine, James Cook University, Townsville, Queensland, Australia

INTRODUCTION

Review of published studies on varicose veins is hampered by the variety of methods used to assess, define and classify the condition. The definition of varicose veins used in a given study is often not stated or varies, making comparison from one publication to another impossible. The CEAP classification states that "varicose veins are palpable, dilated subcutaneous veins usually larger than 4 mm" (1). Not surprisingly, studies of the prevalence of varicose veins have produced markedly disparate findings, with figures varying from 4.5% to 57% (2). The mechanism(s) responsible for their development are incompletely understood, however, a number of theories of etiology have been suggested with varying degrees of clinical and pathological evidence. The suggested theories have to explain in some form the findings from studies of varicose vein epidemiology, imaging and pathology.

RISK FACTORS FOR VARICOSE VEINS

Most studies suggest that varicose veins are more common in women, older sub-groups and following multiple pregnancies (2). There is little evidence to support other suggested risk factors for varicose veins, including life style factors (3).

DUPLEX FINDINGS IN VARICOSE VEINS

Superficial venous reflux (retrograde flow across a valve of >0.5 sec) is detectable in individuals without prominent superficial lower limb veins (14% in one study) (4). The incidence of reflux is higher in patients with obviously dilated veins (77%) but not invariably present in those with varicose veins (87%) (4). The site of reflux can be anywhere along the great or small saphenous veins and frequently is located at a valve distal to the sapheno–femoral or sapheno–popliteal junctions. For example, Labropoulos and associates studied the site of valvular incompetence in 139 limbs with primary varicose veins and found that in 24% reflux was detected in the main trunk of the long saphenous or a tributary without junctional incompetence (5).

PATHOLOGY OF VARICOSE VEINS

Studies of the pathology of venous disease have been limited. Ono and colleagues examined the great saphenous vein (GSV) from 13 patients undergoing varicose vein surgery in comparison to normal veins removed for coronary artery bypass (6). They found clear valve leaflet shortening in three of seven specimens examined. In addition, they demonstrated monocyte/macrophage infiltration at valve sinuses. These findings were absent in the four specimens of macroscopically normal vein removed from patients undergoing coronary bypass. In a larger study of proximal great saphenous valves Corcos et al. demonstrated dilations of the valve annulus and hypoplasia of valve cusps (7). A variety of other changes in the vein wall have been demonstrated in excised varicose veins, however, whether any of these findings are primary or secondary is unclear (see below).

THEORIES REGARDING VARICOSE VEIN ETIOLOGY

The main discussion regarding the etiology of varicose veins is whether the venous dilatation is secondary to a primary problem in the vein wall or a primary problem in one or more venous valves.

A Primary Valvular Dysfunction in Varicose Veins

In this theory the primary event is valve dysfunction in the great or small saphenous vein or possibly a perforator. Resultant increased venous filling leads to secondary vein wall dilatation.

A Primary Vein Wall Dysfunction in Varicose Veins

In this theory a weakening of the vein wall develops initially as a result of connective tissue problems within the vessel or perhaps loss of venous tone. The other changes typical of varicose veins, including valvular incompetence, are secondary changes due to widening of the valve annulus at the site of vein dilatation.

Arteriovenous Communications as an Etiology for Varicose Veins

Increased inflow to superficial lower limb veins could lead to secondary venous dilatation and valvular incompetence.

Final Common Pathway

Whatever the initiating factor for the venous dilatation, all theories incorporate a common final path of prolonged venous filling, further valvular incompetence and transmitted pressures from the deep to superficial venous systems (Fig. 1).

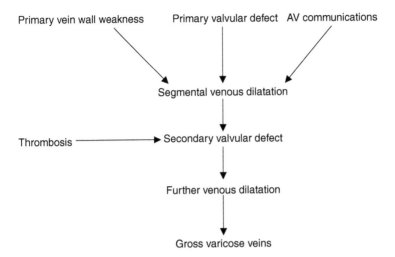

Figure 1 Theories and mechanisms in varicose vein etiology.

VALVE DYSFUNCTION IN VARICOSE VEINS

The original theory regarding varicose veins etiology suggested that valvular failure at the sapheno-femoral junction was the primary event with secondary failure of more distal valves as a result of the increased pressure placed on these sites (descending incompetence) (8). The finding of isolated valvular incompetence at distal sites or tributaries demonstrates that descending incompetence cannot account for all cases of varicose veins (5). However, a primary valvular problem could develop at a distal site with associated increased venous filling and secondary venous dilatation leading to ascending valvular incompetence (9).

Mechanism of Valve Failure

Congenital Valve Abnormalities

There have been remarkably few studies of valve cusp anatomy. In a recent study Yamaki and colleagues correlated the findings on pre-operative duplex imaging with those demonstrated intra-operatively by angioscopy (10). By endoluminal imaging they defined three groups of valve cusp abnormalities in 75% of patients and absent sapheno femoral valves in 25%. While duplex could be used to detect these abnormalities with high sensitivity, the specificity in defining the type of cusp problem was low (10).

Secondary Valvular Failure

It is likely that most valvular abnormalities which can be detected by the time patients come to surgery have developed in response to an episode of thrombophlebitis, prolonged venous stasis or incompetence. An initiating event such as a sub clinical thrombus in the vicinity of a superficial valve could be the initiating factor for valve inflammation, fibrosis and reflux. The role of DVT in the etiology of deep venous incompetence is well established (11–13). Following DVT the incidence of superficial as well as deep reflux appears to be increased. Meissner and colleagues carried out repeat duplex imaging on 69 limbs in which a DVT had occurred (14). Thrombus was demonstrated in the GSV initially in 21%. At eight years the incidence of GSV reflux was 29% in limbs that had developed a DVT, compared to 15% in the contralateral limb (14). The reflux incidence was much higher in limbs in which the initial thrombosis had involved the GSV (77%). Interestingly a recent association has been demonstrated between polymorphism in the gene for the anticoagulant protein thrombomodulin and varicose veins (15).

PRIMARY VEIN WALL WEAKNESS AND VARICOSE VEINS

Structural Weakness of the Vein Wall

A primary weakness in the wall of the vein could result in dilatation of the vein with resultant separation of valve cusps and eventual reflux. Most authors have suggested that this weakness would be a result of structural problems in the wall of the vein (16–20). A number of abnormalities in the structural proteins of the vein have been demonstrated. These include abnormal collagen and elastin content, intimal hyperplasia and changes in matrix controlling enzymes, although the changes demonstrated have varied from one study to another (16–20). Andreotti and colleagues demonstrated a reduction in both collagen and elastin content in varicose compared to macroscopically normal veins (16). They also found alterations in the collagen content of skin taken from patients with varicose veins and suggested a systemic collagen disorder in varicose veins (17). In contrast, most investigators have found an increase in the collagen content of segments of varicose compared to normal veins (18,19). For example, Gandhi et al. demonstrated an increase in the collagen content and a decrease in the elastin concentration, without change in the activity of proteolytic enzymes in the wall of varicose veins (18). Sansilvestri-Morel et al. found an imbalance in the sub types of collagen synthesized by smooth muscle cells derived from varicose veins (19). Collagen type I was increased, while type III was decreased. Badier-Commander and colleagues recently investigated the concentration of enzymes regulating the extracellular matrix in specimens from patients with varicose veins (20). They discovered a relatively high concentration of the tissue inhibitor of metalloproteinase, TIMP-1, and a relatively low concentration of the proteolytic enzyme, metalloproteinase 2 (20). This balance of matrix controlling enzymes would favor the accumulation of matrix within the venous wall and is not reflective of a matrix degrading environment, which might be expected if wall destruction was an important mechanism in varicose vein development. Thus, to date, the matrix changes demonstrated in the wall of varicose veins have not been consistent in different studies. This may relate to the fact that many of the pathological findings are the result rather than the cause of the development of varicose veins.

Impaired Venous Tone

Another possibility is that venous dilatation and secondary reflux results from inability of the vein to contract adequately due to smooth muscle cell or endothelial dysfunction. In support of this theory a number of abnormalities in the contraction and relaxation of varicose vein have been demonstrated compared to normal vein (21–25). Duplex studies suggest reduction in vein wall elasticity in patients with varicose veins (21). Brunner et al. assessed the contraction of a grossly varicosed vein in comparison with a mildly varicosed vein and a competent vein from the same patient (22). They discovered that phenylephrine induced contraction was absent in the overtly varicosed segments. However, of note, the incompetent but macroscopically normal vein contracted normally, suggesting that a primary contractile abnormality, in response to phenylepherine at least, was not an early event in the etiology of valvular incompetence. Mildly varicosed segments had normal endothelial-dependent relaxation but reduced endothelial-independent relaxation to nitroprusside, suggesting a global dysfunction of the smooth muscle in varicose veins. In support of this, in a culture model of varicose veins smooth muscle cells appear to be heparin resistant compared to cells from normal vein (23). Other investigators have demonstrated reduction of endothelin B receptors in varicose veins (24). Other functional abnormalities have also been detected and include reduction in nitric oxide and vascular endothelial growth factor release under conditions of venous hypertension (25).

Endothelial Activation

The endothelium is fundamental in control of vasomotor tone, inflammation and thrombosis. All these processes may play a role in varicose vein development. Loss of venous tone may contribute to venous dilatation and secondary valvular reflux. Sub clinical thrombosis and inflammation could be responsible for valve cusp fibrosis and resultant reflux. There is good evidence of endothelial activation in venous disease. For example, increased expression of the endothelial adhesion molecules ICAM-1 has been demonstrated in varicose veins (26). A study by Biagi and colleagues suggested that varicose veins produced less prostacyclin but more thromboxane A2 and prostaglandin E2 (27). These changes would favor platelet activation and thrombosis. However, Nemcova et al. were unable to confirm these findings in a more recent study (28). In a detailed study by Badier-Commander and associates the concentration of fibroblast growth factor and transforming growth factor beta were found to be increased in atrophic varicose veins segments (29). Thus alteration in endothelial function could play an important role in varicose vein development, however, the changes demonstrated to date could also be explained as secondary phenomenon.

ARTERIOVENOUS COMMUNICATIONS AND VARICOSE VEINS

Arteriovenous communications in patients with varicose veins have been reported in angiographic studies and microsurgical dissections (30,31). Further support for the presence of arteriovenous shunt in varicose veins comes from studies reporting increased oxygen partial pressures in the saphenous vein of varicosed compared to normal veins (32,33). The inability to demonstrate such fistulae during sapheno-femoral ligation to treat varicose veins has led to little promotion of this theory and limited investigation has been carried out to prove or refute the mechanism.

CONCLUSION

The pathogenesis of varicose veins has been relatively underinvestigated. Epidemiological studies have failed to show strong associations between environmental factors and varicose veins. Pathological studies demonstrate abnormalities within the venous wall in endothelial cells, smooth muscle cells and extracellular matrix in patients with varicose veins. However, whether the demonstrated abnormalities are primary or develop secondary to valvular reflux is unclear. Longitudinal studies employing new imaging techniques are likely to provide important new information.

KEY POINTS

- Three principal theories for varicose vein development have been suggested: a primary valvular defect, a primary vein wall defect, and primary arterio-venous communications.
- Irrespective of the initiating stimulus, secondary phenomenon in varicose veins are superficial venous dilatation and valvular incompetence.
- Progressive valve dysfunction can be descending or ascending.
- Numerous vein wall abnormalities have been identified in the connective tissue, smooth muscle cells and endothelium. Whether these changes are primary or secondary is unknown.

REFERENCES

1. Reporting standards in venous disease. Prepared by the Subcommittee on Reporting Standards in Venous Disease, Ad Hoc Committee on Reporting Standards, Society for Vascular Surgery/North American Chapter, International Society for Cardiovascular Surgery. J Vasc Surg 1988; 8:172–181.
2. Callam MJ. Epidemiology of varicose veins. Br J Surg 1994; 81:167–173.
3. Fowkes FG, Lee AJ, Evans CJ, Allan PL, Bradbury AW, Ruckley CV. Lifestyle risk factors for lower limb venous reflux in the general population: Edinburgh Vein Study. Int J Epidemiol 2001; 30:846–852.
4. Labropoulos N, Giannoukas AD, Delis K, et al. Where does venous reflux start? J Vasc Surg 1997; 26:736–742.
5. Labropoulos N, Tassiopoulos AK, Kang SS, Mansour MA, Littooy FN, Baker WH. Prevalence of deep venous reflux in patients with primary superficial vein incompetence. J Vasc Surg 2000; 32:663–668.
6. Ono T, Bergan JJ, Schmid-Schonbein GW, Takase S. Monocyte infiltration into venous valves. J Vasc Surg 1998; 27:158–166.
7. Corcos L, De Anna D, Dini M, Macchi C, Ferrari PA, Dini S. Proximal long saphenous vein valves in primary venous insufficiency. J Mal Vasc 2000; 25:27–36.
8. Moore HD. Deep venous valves in the etiology of varicose veins. Lancet 1951; 2:7–10.
9. Lane RJL, Cuzzilla ML. Aetiology of varicose veins: Haemodynamics. ANZ J Surg 2003; 73:874–876.
10. Yamaki T, Sasaki K, Nozaki M. Preoperative duplex-derived parameters and angioscopic evidence of valvular incompetence associated with superficial venous insufficiency. J Endovasc Ther 2002; 9:229–233.
11. Masuda EM, Kessler DM, Kistner RL, Eklof B, Sato DT. The natural history of calf vein thrombosis: lysis of thrombi and development of reflux. J Vasc Surg 1998; 28:67–74.
12. Haenen JH, Janssen MCH, van Langen H, et al. Duplex ultrasound in the hemodynamic evaluation of the late sequelae of deep venous thrombosis. J Vasc Surg 1998; 27:472–478.
13. van Ramshorst B, van Bemmelen PS, Hoeneveld H, Eikelboom BC. The development of valvular incompetence after deep vein thrombosis: a follow-up study with duplex scanning. J Vasc Surg 1994; 19:1059–1066.
14. Meissner MH, Caps MT, Zierler BK, Bergelin RO, Manzo RA, Strandness DE. Deep venous thrombosis and superficial venous reflux. J Vasc Surg 2000; 32:48–56.
15. Le Flem L, Mennen L, Aubry ML, et al. Thrombomodulin promoter mutations, venous thrombosis and varicose veins. Arterioscler Thromb Vasc Biol 2001; 21:445–451.
16. Andreotti L, Cammelli D. Connective tissue in varicose veins. Angiology 1979; 30:798–805.

17. Andreotti L, Cammelli D, Sampognaro S, et al. Biochemical analysis of dermal connective tissue in subjects affected by primary uncomplicated varicose veins. Angiology 1985; 36:265–270.

18. Gandhi RH, Irizarry E, Nackman GB, Halpern VJ, Mulcare RJ, Tilson MD. Analysis of the connective tissue matrix and proteolytic activity of primary varicose veins. J Vasc Surg 1993; 18:814–820.

19. Sansilvestri-Morel P, Rupin A, Badier-Commander C, et al. Imbalance in the synthesis of collagen type I and collagen type III in smooth muscle cells derived from human varicose veins. J Vasc Res 2001; 38:560–568.

20. Badier-Commander C, Verbeuren T, Lebard C, Michel JB, Jacob MP. Increased TIMP/MMP ratio in varicose veins: Possible explanation for extracellular matrix accumulation. J Pathol 2000; 192:105–112.

21. Clarke GH, Vasdekis SN, Hobbs JT, Nicolaides AN. Venous wall function in the pathogenesis of varicose veins. Surgery 1992; 111:402–408.

22. Brunner F, Hoffman C, Schuller-Petrovic S. Responsiveness of human varicose saphenous vein to vasoactive agents. Br J Clin Pharmacol 2001; 51:219–224.

23. Hollingsworth SJ, Tang CB, Baker SGE. The effects of heparin on cultured explants of varicose long saphenous vein. Phlebology 2001; 16:60–67.

24. Agu O, Hamilton G, Baker DM, Dashwood MR. Endothelin receptors in the etiology and pathophysiology of varicose veins. Eur J Vasc Endovasc Surg 2002; 23:165–171.

25. Hollingsworth SJ, Tang CB, Dialynas M, Barker SG. Varicose veins: loss of release of vascular endothelial growth factor and reduced plasma nitric oxide. Eur J Vasc Endovasc Surg 2001; 22:551–556.

26. Takase S, Bergan JJ, Schmid-Schonbein G. Expression of adhesion molecules and cytokines on saphenous veins in chronic venous insufficiency. Ann Vasc Surg 2000; 14:427–435.

27. Biagi G, Lapilli A, Zendron R, Piccinni L, Coccheri S. Prostanoid production in varicose veins: evidence for decreased prostacyclin with increased thromboxane A2 and prostaglandin E2 formation. Angiology 1988; 39:1036–1042.

28. Nemcova S, Gloviczki P, Rud KS, Miller VM. Cyclic nucleotides and production of prostanoids in human varicose veins. J Vasc Surg 1999; 30:876–884.

29. Badier-Commander C, Couvelard A, Henin D, Verbeuren T, Michel JB, Jacob MP. Smooth muscle cell modulation and cytokine overproduction in varicose veins. An in situ study. J Pathol 2001; 193:398–407.

30. Piulachs P, Vidal-Barraquer F. Pathogenic study of varicose veins. Angiology 1953; 4:59–100.

31. Guis JA. Arteriovenous anastomoses and varicose veins. Observations with the operation microscope. Arch Surg 1960; 81:299–310.

32. Baron HC, Cassaro S. The role of arteriovenous shunts in the pathogenesis of varicose veins. J Vasc Surg 1986; 4:124–128.

33. Scott HJ, Cheatle TR, McMullin GM, Coleridge Smith PD, Scurr JH. Reappraisal of the oxygenation of blood in varicose veins. Brit J Surg 1990; 77:934–936.

19

Indications for Treatments of Varicose Veins

Simon Palfreyman and Jonathan Michaels
Department of Vascular Surgery, University of Sheffield, Sheffield, U.K.

INTRODUCTION

This chapter will examine the physical and nonphysical symptoms ascribed to varicose veins and treatments used to mitigate these. The aim of this chapter is to review the complex interaction between symptoms, complications, and indications for treatment of varicose veins. It will also assess the impact of varicose veins on quality of life, the evidence of effectiveness, and indications for varicose vein treatments.

BACKGROUND

Studies have shown that varicose veins have a prevalence of between 20% and 60%, with up to one quarter of the adult population having at least one varicose vein (1). The resultant impact on health services can be illustrated by the fact that operations for varicose veins are one of the most commonly undertaken surgical procedures, with around 50,000 patients admitted for treatment in the National Health Service annually in the United Kingdom (2), and have a major impact on waiting lists and workload (3). They are also a major reason for patients to seek redress through legal action against clinicians and healthcare providers (4).

Patients report a wide range of symptoms that they attribute to their varicose veins. Some of the symptoms patients associate with their varicose veins may not be directly attributable to the veins themselves (5). A further complication for the clinician is that the extent of the visible veins does not correlate with the severity or number of symptoms experienced (6). There appears to be a complex interaction between cosmetic dislike and perception of symptoms (7).

The reported symptoms for varicose veins include heaviness, aching, itching and concerns about cosmetic appearance. In addition to these are the complications associated with varicose veins that can include varicose eczema, pigmentation, bleeding and varicose ulcers. The patient can experience, to a greater or lesser degree, all of these symptoms and complications or none at all.

The crux of the dilemma for health service providers is to determine whether uncomplicated varicose veins should be treated. The current guidance from the National

Institute for Clinical Excellence (NICE) (8) considers only complications as a clear indication for surgery. However, patients are presenting at General Practitioner (GP) surgeries and outpatients clinics with the expectation that their varicose veins should be treated (9).

Symptoms of Varicose Veins

The most comprehensive study to examine leg symptoms in members of the general public was the Edinburgh Vein Study (5). This study used an age stratified random sample of 1566 people selected from GP practices in Edinburgh, Scotland. Participants were asked to complete a self-administered questionnaire that asked about the presence of symptoms attributed to varicose veins. One surprising finding was that the lower limb symptoms often attributed to varicose veins were present in the general population whether or not varicose veins were present.

The study found that the prevalence of symptoms increased with age and that there was a difference between men and women in terms of the prevalence of symptoms. The most common symptoms for women were aching (53%), cramp (42%), restless legs (35%), heaviness or tension (28.6%), itching (25%) and swelling (23%). While for men, the most common symptoms were cramp (34%), aching (32.5%), restless legs (20%), itching (19%) and swelling (9.2%). But there was no statistical association between symptoms and the presence of varicose veins, except for itching in men.

Another study (9) used qualitative techniques to examine the reasons patients were seeking treatment. The sample was drawn from patients referred to vascular surgeons with varicose veins and so differed from the Edinburgh Vein Study. The patients were therefore a selected group who had been to their GP with the symptoms associated with varicose veins and had been referred on to the vascular surgeon. This could have led to some bias in terms of the patients having an expectation of treatment and the possibility of exaggeration of symptoms to gain treatment. However, the study found that pain and itching were the most common symptoms. For some of the patients in the study the severity of the pain was such that they resorted to taking analgesia—including non steroidal anti-inflammatory drugs (NSAIDs, e.g., ibuprofen, voltarol and naproxen) and codeine (dihyrocodine).

A study by Michaels et al. (10), was a randomized trial examining the cost-effectiveness of treatments for varicose veins. The sample were recruited from secondary care and were patients referred to vascular surgeons. The study compared the self-reported symptoms at baseline and post-treatment (Tables 1 and 2). The most common complaint prior to treatment was of aching in the legs (86.3%). After treatment 45,8% complained of aching and 42,7% stated that the aching was the same as that prior to treatment.

A complicating factor is that there is a subjective element to the perception of the severity, and extent of, the symptoms experienced (7). Varicose veins can be unsightly, cause embarrassment and have a significant impact on people's social activities (9).

Table 1   Symptoms at Initial Assessment of All Patients by Initial Treatment

	Conservative	Sclerotherapy	Surgery	Total
N	387	91	531	1009
Aching	306 (79.1%)	85 (93.4%)	480 (90.4%)	871 (86.3%)
Heaviness	191 (49.4%)	53 (58.2%)	339 (63.8%)	583 (57.8%)
Itching	203 (52.5%)	48 (52.7%)	338 (63.7%)	589 (58.4%)
Swelling	157 (40.6%)	45 (49.5%)	277 (52.2%)	479 (47.5%)
Cosmetic concerns	252 (65.1%)	59 (64.8%)	382 (71.9%)	693 (68.7%)

Table 2 Symptoms at One Year in All Patients, by Initial Treatment

		None	Better	Same	Worse
Aching	Conservative	57 (21.8%)	99 (37.8%)	45 (17.2%)	61 (23.3%)
	Sclerotherapy	20 (32.3%)	17 (27.4%)	21 (33.9%)	4 (6.5%)
	Surgery	159 (45.8%)	28 (8.1%)	148 (42.7%)	12 (3.5%)
Heaviness	Conservative	126 (48.1%)	75 (28.6%)	24 (9.2%)	37 (14.1%)
	Sclerotherapy	36 (58.1%)	14 (22.6%)	12 (19.4%)	(0.0%)
	Surgery	206 (59.4%)	21 (6.1%)	111 (32.0%)	9 (2.6%)
Itching	Conservative	133 (50.8%)	62 (23.7%)	23 (8.8%)	44 (16.8%)
	Sclerotherapy	38 (61.3%)	8 (12.9%)	14 (22.6%)	2 (3.2%)
	Surgery	223 (64.3%)	16 (4.6%)	101 (29.1%)	7 (2.0%)
Swelling	Conservative	155 (59.2%)	61 (23.3%)	20 (7.6%)	26 (9.9%)
	Sclerotherapy	42 (67.7%)	12 (19.4%)	5 (8.1%)	3 (4.8%)
	Surgery	227 (65.4%)	22 (6.3%)	86 (24.8%)	12 (3.5%)
Cosmetic concerns	Conservative	64 (24.4%)	115 (43.9%)	10 (3.8%)	73 (27.9%)
	Sclerotherapy	22 (35.5%)	14 (22.6%)	22 (35.5%)	4 (6.5%)
	Surgery	129 (37.2%)	21 (6.1%)	182 (52.4%)	15 (4.3%)

Underlying problems with the cosmetic appearance may be the motivation for many patients to complain of symptoms and seek treatment for their varicose veins (5,10), even though they may deny that this is their primary motivation (9). However, if patients are approaching clinicians stating that they want relief of symptoms surely it is beholden on the clinician to try and ease the patients burden.

It is the group of patients who are seeking treatment to relieve the symptoms they associate with varicose veins who provide the greatest challenge to both the clinician and health service provider. This is because there is little evidence regarding the cost-effectiveness of treatments currently available.

Complications of Varicose Veins

The complications of varicose veins are thrombophlebitis; bleeding; skin changes, eczema and lipodermatosclerosis; and ulceration.

Superficial thrombophlebitis manifests itself with symptoms of swelling, pain and redness located around a vein. It can occur in the absence of varicose veins and may be associated with malignancy, autoimmune disease and cancer (11), but varicose veins are the commonest underlying cause (12). It is often confused with deep vein thrombosis (DVT) and patients may worry about traveling (particularly flying and the risk of "economy class syndrome") (9). There is also a perceived additional risk of developing a DVT due to having varicose veins, however the evidence for this is equivocal (13).

Bleeding is an uncommon consequence of varicose veins and usually occurs due to minor trauma but can occur spontaneously (14,15). It almost always occurs through an area of obviously compromised skin overlying a varicosity in the lower leg. The bleeding may be minor and internal resulting in a bruise or severe haemorrhage. This can be alarming and poses a potential threat to life (14–16).

Lipodermatosclerosis and ulceration result from the venous hypertension associated with varicose veins and is an important cause of damage to the skin and subcutaneous tissues of the lower leg (17,18). This usually starts with eczema or pigmentation and may then progress through varying severities of lipodermatosclerosis to ulceration. The chance of any individual with varicose veins developing skin damage is both uncertain and small with between 3% and 6% reporting "skin problems" (19,20). Among those who do develop skin changes the risk of ulceration is also unpredictable, but any signs of venous damage to the skin of the leg is usually regarded as an indication to consider preventative measures—either in the form of compression hosiery or treatment of the varicose veins.

Treatments for Varicose Veins

There are currently three established treatment options for varicose veins. These are conservative, sclerotherapy and surgery. There are also a number of newer therapies that are based on Endovascular approaches. However, there is limited published information of sufficient rigor and quality, to determine any of the treatment options relative effectiveness (7). There is also disagreement regarding the indications for treatment (21).

Conservative treatment refers to a range of measures that encompassing life-style advice and compression hosiery. People can develop complex rituals which they use to ease any symptoms they associate with their varicose veins (9). Clinicians tend to concentrate on providing explanations, reassurance, suggesting lifestyle changes and prescribing compression hosiery. There is a need for reassurance and education as there are widespread misconceptions that varicose veins are associated with a likelihood of DVT, heart disease and amputation (9,10). Compression hosiery can be useful in helping the symptoms and treating complications (22). However, many patients find compression hosiery unacceptable and it tends to be used regularly only by those who are extremely motivated (23–25). There are uncertainties about both clinical and cost effectiveness of conservative measures. They are subject to variation in advice given by doctors and their acceptability to patients (10).

Sclerotherapy is usually undertaken on an outpatient basis. It involves the injection of a sclerosant (e.g., sodium tetradecyl sulfate) into the varicosities followed by a period of compression treatment using bandaging or compression hosiery. Sclerotherapy became popular in the 1960s (26) but it has been less widely used in recent decades (27). Sclerotherapy is now generally considered to be most appropriate for varicose veins below the knee (where compression is easier to apply than above the knee) in the absence of saphenous vein reflux (10).

Surgical treatment involves day case or inpatient operation and general anaesthetic. It requires a period of recuperation and time off work. There is also an increased possibility of complications compared to sclerotherapy (4). Recurrence of varicose veins is not uncommon and it has been reported that about 20% of patients seen in secondary care with varicose veins have previously been treated surgically. In terms of surgical technique there is controversy regarding the need for stripping the long saphenous vein (LSV), the level to which it should be stripped, in which direction and with what technique (28). Where the vein strip was extended to the ankle, the direction of the strip had been shown to be important in terms of nerve injury. It has been reported that nerve injury was increased if the vein was stripped in an upward direction (ankle to groin) (28). Additional fears about stripping include the risk of deep vein damage, increased trauma to the tissues and damage to the saphenous nerve, set against the potential benefit in reducing recurrence rates.

Endovascular treatments for varicose veins. Relatively new surgical techniques for ablation of veins are available using radiofrequency (29) or laser (30), as well as a new sclerosant foam; (31–33) however, the effectiveness and costs have not yet been fully assessed.

INDICATIONS FOR TREATMENT OF VARICOSE VEINS

When assessing whether or not varicose veins should be treated, there are a number of questions that need answering.

1. Do varicose vein treatments work? This examines the effectiveness of treatments
2. How much do varicose vein treatments cost? This involves assigning monetary cost to interventions but also include other costs such as complications
3. Do varicose vein treatments make patients happy? This question addresses whether the treatment improves the patients quality of life but also whether patients are satisfied with treatment.

In the real world there is a complex interaction between effectiveness, cost and quality of life. The health service providers use some or all of these when examining the cost-effectiveness of treatments. The treatments for varicose veins, therefore, need to be effective, have reasonable costs and improve the patient's quality of life. However, the priorities of the patient, clinician and health service provider may not be the same and can be diametrically opposed.

Effectiveness

The question of effectiveness should be easy to answer. Do the current treatments for varicose veins work? In order to answer such a question there is a need to examine the evidence for the treatments that are currently available.

Surgery Versus Sclerotherapy

The two most common interventions for varicose veins are surgery and sclerotherapy. However, there is little comparative data regarding their effectiveness (7,13,34).

One source of the comparative effectiveness of surgery compared to sclerotherapy is a Cochrane Collaboration systematic review undertaken by Rigby et al. (34). This systematic review found a total of 63 papers that considered surgery and sclerotherapy but found only seven randomized controlled trials. In these trials there was a wide variation in terms of the outcome measures included to assess the effectiveness of treatments. The trials relied on subjective assessment of the results of the interventions. Subjective measures are always open to bias and no single classification system has been uniformly adopted. This lack of consensus meant that studies developed and used their own classification system and these had not always been piloted or validated. Objective measures such as duplex scanning and foot volumetry can be used but these have not been universally employed and their relationship with clinical benefit is uncertain.

The quality of the included studies was not of the highest standard with the studies being underpowered and being potentially open to bias due to lack of blinding of outcome assessement and unclear randomization procedures.

The review concluded that there was insufficient evidence to preferentially recommend the use of sclerotherapy or surgery. However there was a general trend to better results after surgery than sclerotherapy although this was only consistent when the follow-up period was three years or more. Sclerotherapy had some short term benefit in the first year but these rapidly deteriorated so that by five years, surgery was the most effective intervention due to higher recurrence rates following sclerotherapy.

Surgery Versus Conservative Treatment

There is currently a lack of high quality evidence available comparing surgery and conservative treatment of varicose veins. The only randomized controlled trial currently published is a NHS Health Technology Assessment Programme monograph by Michaels et al. (10).

The study randomized 246 participants with uncomplicated varicose veins between surgery and conservative measures (lifestyle advice and compression hosiery). The study found that those randomized to conservative treatment were dissatisfied and over half (51.6%) chose to withdraw from conservative treatment and undergo surgery. The surgical arm of the trial showed better results in terms of self-reported symptom relief, anatomical extent, quality of life and patient satisfaction at one-year follow up.

Sclerotherapy Versus Conservative Treatment

A Cochrane Collaboration systematic review was undertaken by Tisi and Beverley (35). Their review aimed to examine all randomized controlled trials comparing injection sclerotherapy and conservative treatments (graduated compression stockings and/or observation). They also examined differences in sclerosants and techniques for sclerotherapy. A total of twenty-eight studies were identified for inclusion in their review. Of these 16 were excluded as they did not meet the inclusion criteria or were non-randomized studies.

The review concluded that there was no evidence to support the claims of Fegan (26) regarding the type and duration of compression following sclerotherapy. The review also found no effect of the types and duration of compression on the incidence of superficial thrombophlebitis, obliteration of varicose veins or recurrence rate. In addition they found no difference in results relating to the strength of STD used.

The review concluded that the available evidence on the effectiveness of sclerotherapy was limited and of poor quality. There was a particular lack of evidence comparing sclerotherapy with compression stockings.

Other Treatment for Varicose Veins

There are a number of publications examining less widely used treatments for varicose veins including hydrotherapy and drug treatments.

A randomized controlled trial comparing hydrotherapy and no hydrotherapy (36,37) reported significant reductions in leg volumes and ankle/calf circumference for the hydrotherapy group. However, the study was exploratory in nature, only randomized 61 patients and did not include an a priori sample size calculation. There have been no other studies that have duplicated these findings.

A number of drug treatments have been examined for the treatment of varicose veins including oxerutins (a group of chemicals derived from a naturally occurring bioflavonoid called rutin) (38,39). Both the studies found no statistically significant differences between those randomized to oxerutins and those randomized to placebo. Two other drug studies randomized between heptaminol adenosine phosphate (HAP—a cardiac stimulant and vasodilator) and placebo (40) and calcium dobesilate (a vasoprotectant and capillary dilator) and placebo (41). Although some improvements were seen in venous outflow for HAP it is unclear whether this is of clinical significance.

One study examined a homeopathic preparation (Poikiven) and placebo (42). The study reported significant improvements in objective measures (plesthysmography and leg circumference) but there were significant differences between the groups at baseline and the analysis was not based on intention to treat.

Cost and Effectiveness

Evidence of effectiveness does not necessarily mean that treatments can be or should be adopted because resources for health care interventions are not unlimited and the effect on resources may influence whether health care providers will undertake to provide the treatment (43). Where evidence exists that there is therapeutic equivalence between two or more treatment options, the cheaper option is preferred (44). Cost therefore needs to be included in any evaluation of health care.

Cost-effectiveness is a measure of the cost per unit of effectiveness and is a measure of economic efficiency. The costs are valued in monetary terms and compared with a single primary outcome (45). The outcome that is increasingly being used is the cost per Quality Adjusted Life Year (QALY) gained. The QALY is a measure that combines the length of life and quality of life (valued on an index where one represents perfect health and zero represents death) (46). In the real world with limited resources it allows different treatments to be compared and the most effective care to be obtained for the least cost (47).

There is however limited evidence for the cost-effectiveness of the treatments for varicose veins. The currently published evidence concentrates on clinical effectiveness rather than cost-effectiveness (34). Michaels et al. (10) found that there were some differences in both costs and outcomes between surgery and conservative treatment. Surgical treatment for varicose veins was associated with a modest health benefit for a small additional NHS cost relative to conservative treatment. If £30,000 is taken as the maximum acceptable cost effectiveness ratio, based on the probable threshold set by the United Kingdom NICE (44), then on the basis of the results for patients with severe varicose veins, surgical treatment appeared to be highly cost-effective with a ratio of less than £5000 per QALY.

The results for sclerotherapy for minor varicose veins were insufficient for cost effectiveness analysis and were examined by economic modeling. This found that sclerotherapy had some benefit over conservative treatment but that surgery remained cost-effective when compared to sclerotherapy.

Quality of Life

Quality of life is a concept of which people have an intuitive understanding but it can be difficult to relate this to health (48,49). The potential benefit to patients of including measures of quality of life into evaluations of treatment is that treatment decisions are based on their own priorities and preferences (50).

One aim of treatment is to maximize a person's quality of life by reducing the impact of the disease on the patients. Yet patients with severe disease do not necessarily report having a poor quality of life (51). The relationship between symptoms and quality of life is not linear or necessarily direct. Carr et al. (48) reported problems with measuring health related quality of life. These included differing expectations, which are specific to individuals, assessment may be at different stages of illness and the expectation of "normal" quality of life may change over time.

A number of generic and a disease-specific quality of life tools have been used to examine outcomes from varicose vein treatments. However, there are a limited number of studies that have used validated Quality of Life instruments and these have produced conflicting results. One of the most widely used generic instruments is the SF-36.

It contains 36 questions measuring health across eight dimensions. These are: physical functioning, role limitation due to physical health, social functioning, vitality, pain, mental health, role limitation because of emotional problems and general health. Responses to each question within a dimension are combined to generate a score from 0 to 100, where 100 is "best possible health" and 0 is "worst possible health." It generates a profile of eight dimension scores and two summary scores for physical and mental health (52).

Some studies with the SF-36 have shown that patients with varicose veins have reduced QoL compared to the general population (53), but others have shown no significant difference (54,55). A large international study undertaken in Belgium, France, Canada and Italy (56) found that impairment in quality of life was associated with related venous disease rather than the presence of varicose veins per se.

Michaels et al. used the SF-6D (57) and EQ-5D (58) as primary outcome measures for varicose vein treatments. The SF-6D is a single summary preference-based measure of health derived from the SF-36 and can be regarded as a continuous outcome scored on a 0 to 1.00 scale, with 1.00 indicating "full health" (59). The EQ-5D (commonly referred to as the Euroqol) contains five questions, which measure health across the five dimensions of mobility, self-care, usual activities, pain/discomfort and anxiety depression. It provides a simple descriptive profile and generates a single index value for heath status, based on societal valuations, where full health is assigned a value of 1 and death a value of 0 (58). The scores from the SF-6D and EQ-5D can be used to derive QALYs. Michaels et al. (10) showed that the QALY gain was greater for surgery compared to sclerotherapy at two-years.

A further important issue related to quality of life is that these measures do not necessarily produce a complete picture of the motivations and expectations of treatment (48,49). One method of forming a complete picture from the patients perspective is to directly ask the patient through the qualitative methods of interviews and focus groups.

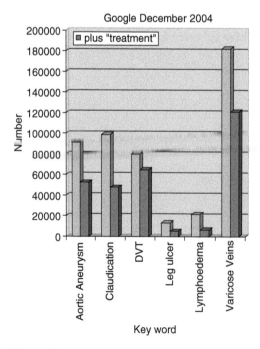

Figure 1 Number of hits on Google.

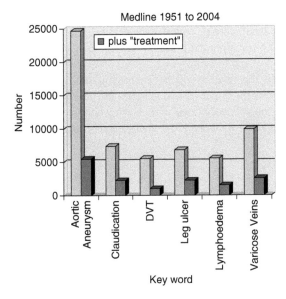

Figure 2 Number of hits on Medline.

Qualitative studies where the patients are asked directly about having varicose veins have shown that it can affect patients social activities, feelings of self-worth, how they dress and interact (9). Palfreyman et al. (9) also showed that patients will actively seek surgery in preference to sclerotherapy and conservative treatment.

Patient, Clinician, or Provider Priorities?

The treatment for varicose veins highlights the dilemma of whose values and priorities should be used to determine treatment. Patients seem to prefer surgery and are seeking treatment from healthcare clinicians (9,10). Varicose veins provide a significant workload for vascular surgeons and the majority of patients see surgery as an appropriate treatment for varicose veins (13). However, some healthcare providers in the United Kingdom are limiting surgery for varicose veins to those with complications (60).

The relative importance of varicose veins to the general public compared to clinicians and healthcare providers can be assessed using a proxy measure comparing the prevalence of literature on the subject on the Internet and in medical publications. This was assessed by recording the relative number of hits on the Internet and Medline for varicose veins.

Undertaking a simple search of common vascular conditions and treatment using Google illustrates that the number of hits for varicose veins is almost twice that of the next highest, claudication (Fig. 1). In comparison, a search of Medline showed that, although varicose veins come second in terms of the number of published journals there are less than half as many fewer articles compared to aortic aneurysm (Fig. 2).

CONCLUSION

The indications for treatment of varicose veins will vary dependent on the perspective considered and is likely to be different in various health care settings. A system that is constructed on the basis of consumer-led demand, such as in the United States, is more likely to respond to the obvious pressure for treatment from patients. However, a system that is funded centrally and is led by healthcare providers will seek to limit varicose vein treatments as they could potentially be spending the limited resources on a condition that has a greater impact on life-expectancy and morbidity.

However, despite doubts about the relationship between symptoms and varicose veins, the best evidence currently available suggests that surgery and sclerotherapy both produce benefits—particularly from the patients perspective. Even when viewed in terms of the health care funders, treatment is still likely to be cost-effective in appropriately selected patients.

KEY POINTS

- Varicose veins are common and have a major impact on health budgets and surgical waiting lists.
- Patients may report a wide range of symptoms, which they attribute to their varicose veins.
- Symptom severity does not correlate with the extent of visible varicose veins.
- In patients referred for surgery, pain and itching are the most common symptoms.
- Symptoms such as aching, heaviness, itching, and swelling may not improve after treatment.
- There is little evidence regarding the cost effectiveness of the currently available treatments.
- Sclerotherapy tends to have short-term benefits but surgical treatments appear more effective when follow-up is 3 years or more.
- Surgery appears to be better than conservative treatments for uncomplicated varicose veins in terms of symptom relief, quality of life, and patient satisfaction.
- Surgery for severe varicose veins is highly cost effective and results in improved quality of life in appropriately selected patients.

REFERENCES

1. Callam MJ. Epidemiology of varicose veins. Br J Surg 1994; 81:167–173.
2. London NJM, Nash R. ABC of arterial and venous disease, Varicose veins. BMJ 2000; 320:1391–1394.
3. O'Leary DP, Chester JF, Jones SM. Management of varicose veins according to reason for presentation. Ann R Coll Surg Engl 1996; 78:214–216.
4. Tennant WG, Ruckley CV. Medicolegal action following treatment for varicose veins. Br J Surg 1996; 83:291–292.
5. Bradbury A, Evans C, Allan P, et al. What are the symptoms of varicose veins? Edinburgh vein study cross sectional population survey BMJ 1999; 318:353–356.
6. Goldman MP, Weiss RA, Bergan JJ. Diagnosis and treatment of varicose-veins—a review. J Am Acad Dermatol 1994; 31:393–413.
7. Robbins MA, Frankel SJ, Nanchal K, Coast J, Williams MH. Varicose vein treatments. In: Stevens A, Raftery J, eds. Health Care Needs Assessment. The Epidemiology Based Needs Assessment. Oxford: Radcliffe Medical Press, 1994:79–133.
8. NICE. Varicose veins—referral practice—version under pilot. NICE website, 2000.
9. Palfreyman SJ, Drewery-Carter K, Rigby KA, Michaels JA, Tod AM. A qualitative study to explore expectations and reasons for seeking treatment for varicose veins. J Clin Nurs 2004; 13:332–340.

10. Michaels JA, Campbell WB, Brazier J, et al. Assessment of Cost-Effectiveness of the Treatment of Varicose Veins (REACTIV Trial)—HTA Project 95/05/06. NHS HTAP. London: Department of Health, in press.

11. Decousus H, Epinat M, Guillot K, et al. Superficial vein thrombosis: risk factors, diagnosis, and treatment. Curr Opin Pulm Med 2003; 9:393–397.

12. Gorty S, Patton AJ, DaLanno M, et al. Superficial venous thrombosis of the lower extremities: analysis of risk factors, and recurrence and role of anticoagulation. Vasc Med 2004; 9:1–6.

13. Lees TA, Beard JD, Ridler BM, Szymanska T. A survey of the current management of varicose veins by members of the Vascular Surgical Society. Ann R Coll Surg Engl 1999; 81:407–417.

14. Evans GA, Evans DM, Seal RM, Craven JL. Spontaneous fatal haemorrhage caused by varicose veins. Lancet 1973; 2:1359–1361.

15. Wigle RL, Anderson GV, Jr. Exsanguinating hemorrhage from peripheral varicosities. Ann Emerg Med 1988; 17:80–82.

16. du Toit DF, Knott-Craig C, Laker L. Bleeding from varicose vein—still potentially fatal. A case report. S Afr Med J 1985; 67:303.

17. Lapropolous N, Delis K, Nicolaides AN, Leon M, Ramaswami G. The role of the distribution and anatomic extent of reflux in the development of signs and symptoms in chronic venous insufficiency. J Vasc Surg 1996; 23:505–510.

18. Shami SK, Sarin S, Cheatle TR, Scurr JH, Smith PD. Venous ulcers and the superficial venous system. J Vasc Surg 1993; 17:487–490.

19. Kurz X, Kahn SR, Abenhaim L, et al. Chronic venous disorders of the leg: epidemiology, outcomes, diagnosis and management—summary of an evidence-based report of the veins task force. Int Angiol 1999; 18:83–102.

20. Coon WW, Willis PW, Keller JB. Venous thromboembolism and other venous disease in the Tecumseh community health study. Circulation 1973; 48:213–217.

21. Tremblay J, Lewis EW, Allen PT. Selecting a treatment for primary varicose veins. CMAJ 1985; 133:20–25 [Review] [50 refs].

22. Chant ADB, Davies LJ, Pike JM, Sparks MJ. Support stockings in practical management of varicose veins. Phlebology 1989; 4:167–169.

23. Kiev J, Noyes LD, Rice JC, Kerstein MD. Patient compliance with fitted compression hosiery monitored by photoplethysmography. Arch Phys Med Rehabil 1990; 71:376–379.

24. Harker J. Influences on patient adherence with compression hosiery. J Wound Care 2000; 9:379–382.

25. Hayes JM, Lehman CA, Castonguay P. Graduated compression stockings: updating practice, improving compliance. Medsurg Nurs 2002; 11:163–166.

26. Fegan WG. Continuous compression technique of injecting varicose veins. Lancet 1963; 2:109–112.

27. Galland RB, Magee TR, Lewis MH. A survey of current attitudes of British and Irish vascular surgeons to venous sclerotherapy. Eur J Vasc Endovasc Surg 1998; 16:43–46.

28. Rigby KA, Palfreyman SJ, Beverley C, Michaels JA. Surgery for varicose veins: use of tourniquet. The Cochrane Database of Systematic Reviews 2002; 4:CD001486.

29. Lurie F, Creton D, Eklof B, et al. Prospective randomized study of endovenous radiofrequency obliteration (closure procedure) versus ligation and stripping in a selected patient population (EVOLVeS Study). J Vasc Surg 2003; 38:207–214.

30. Merchant RF, DePalma RG, Kabnick LS. Endovascular obliteration of saphenous reflux: a multicenter study. J Vasc Surg 2002; 35:1190–1196.

31. Breu FX, Guggenbichler S. European Consensus Meeting on Foam Sclerotherapy April, 4–6, 2003, Tegernsee, Germany. Dermatol Surg 2004; 30:709–717.

32. Barrett JM, Allen B, Ockelford A, Goldman MP. Microfoam ultrasound-guided sclerotherapy of varicose veins in 100 legs. Dermatol Surg 2004; 30:6–12.

33. Hsu TS, Weiss RA. Foam sclerotherapy: a new era. Arch Dermatol 2003; 139:1494–1496.

34. Rigby KA, Palfreyman SJ, Beverley C, Michaels JA. Surgery versus sclerotherapy for the treatment of varicose veins. The Cochrane Database of Systematic Reviews 2004, Issue 4. Art. No.: CD004980. DOI: 10.1002/14651858. CD004980.

35. Tisi PV, Beverley CA. Injection sclerotherapy for varicose veins. The Cochrane Database of Systematic Reviews 2002, Issue 1. Art. No.: CD001732. DOI: 10.1002/14651858. CD001732.
36. Ernst E, Saradeth T, Resch KL. Hydrotherapy for varicose-veins—a randomized, controlled trial. Phlebology 1992; 7:154–157.
37. Ernst E, Saradeth T, Resch KL. A single blind randomized, controlled trial of hydrotherapy for varicose-veins. VASA—J Vasc Dis 1991; 20:147–152.
38. Anderson JH, Geraghty JG, Wilson YT, et al. Paroven and graduated compression hosiery for superficial venous insufficiency. Phlebology 1990; 5:271–276.
39. Schuller-Petrovic S, Wolzt M, Bohler K, Jima B, Eichler HG. Studies on the effect of short-term oral dihydroergotamine a dn troxerutin in patients with varicose veins. Clin Pharmacol Ther 1994; 56:452–459.
40. Schmidt CGR, Perez P, Schmitt J. Double blind plethysmographic study of venos effects of heptaminol adenosine phosphate (HAP) in patients with primary varicose veins. Eur J Clin Pharmacol 1989; 37:37–40.
41. Androulakis GPP. Plethysmographic confirmation of the beneficial effects of calcium dobesilate in primary varicose veins. Angiology 1989; 40:1–4.
42. Ernst E, Saradeth T, Resch KL. Complementary treatment of varicose veins—a randomized, placebo-controlled, double-blind trial. Phlebology 1990; 5:157–163.
43. Sculpher M, Drummond M, O'Brien B. Effectiveness, efficiency, and NICE. BMJ 2001; 322:943–944.
44. Rawlins MD, Culyer AJ. National Institute for Clinical Excellence and its value judgments. BMJ 2004; 329:224–227.
45. Coast J. Is economic evaluation in touch with society's health values? BMJ 2004; 329:1233–1236.
46. Raftery J. Economics notes: economic evaluation: an introduction. BMJ 1998; 316:1013–1014.
47. Jefferson T, Demicheli V. Quality of economic evaluations in health care. BMJ 2002; 324:313–314.
48. Carr AJ, Gibson B, Robinson PG. Measuring quality of life: is quality of life determined by expectations or experience? BMJ 2001; 322:1240–1243.
49. Addington-Hall J, Kalra L. Measuring quality of life: who should measure quality of life? BMJ 2001; 322:1417–1420.
50. Higginson IJ, Carr AJ. Measuring quality of life: using quality of life measures in the clinical setting. BMJ 2001; 322:1297–1300.
51. Evans RW. Quality of life. Lancet 1991; 338:363.
52. Resnick B, Parker R. Simplified scoring and psychometrics of the revised 12-item short-form health survey. Outcomes Manag Nurs Pract 2001; 5:161–166.
53. Garratt AM, Macdonald LM, Ruta DA, et al. Towards measurement of outcome for patients with varicose veins. Qual Health Care 1993; 2:5–10.
54. Baker DM, Turnbull NB, Pearson JC, Makin GS How successful is varicose vein surgery? A patient outcome study following varicose vein surgery using the SF-36 health assessment questionnaire Eur J Vasc Endovas Surg 1995; 9:299–304.
55. Smith JJ, Garratt AM, Guest M, Greenhalgh RM, Davies AH. Evaluating and improving health-related quality of life in patients with varicose veins. J Vasc Surg 1999; 30:709–710.
56. Kurz X, Lamping DL, Kahn SR, et al. Do varicose veins affect quality of life? Results of an international population-based study J Vasc Surg 2001; 34:641–648.
57. Brazier J, Roberts JF, Deverill MD. The estimation of a preference based measure of health from the SF-36. Health Econ 2002; 21:92.
58. The EuroQol Group. EuroQol—a new facility for the measurement of health related quality of life. Health Policy 1990; 16:199–208.
59. Walters S, Brazier J. What is the relationship between the minimally important difference and health state utility values? The case of the SF-6D Health Qual Life Outcomes 2003; 1:4.
60. Tiwari A, Douek M, Ackroyd JS. Rationing of surgery for varicose veins based on the presence or absence of cosmetic symptoms. J Eval Clin Prac 2002; 8:425.

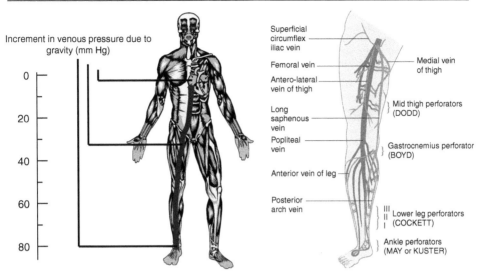

Increment in venous pressure due to gravity (mm Hg)

Superficial circumflex iliac vein
Femoral vein
Antero-lateral vein of thigh
Long saphenous vein
Popliteal vein
Anterior vein of leg
Posterior arch vein

Medial vein of thigh
Mid thigh perforators (DODD)
Gastrocnemius perforator (BOYD)
III
II Lower leg perforators
I   (COCKETT)
Ankle perforators (MAY or KUSTER)

Figure 3.2 *See p. 25.*

Figure 3.3 *See p. 27.*

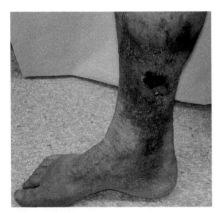

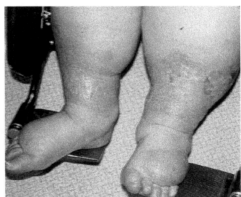

Figure 7.3 *See p. 84.*

Figure 14.1 *See p. 175.*

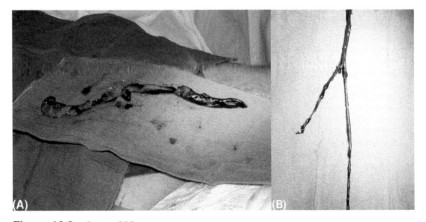

(A) (B)

Figure 16.3 *See p. 208.*

1

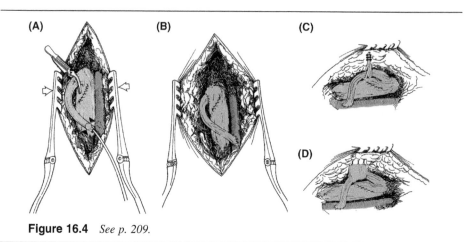

Figure 16.4 *See p. 209.*

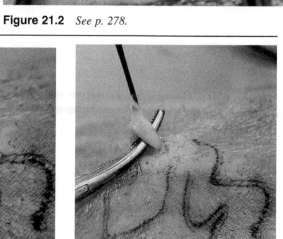

Figure 21.1 *See p. 278.* **Figure 21.2** *See p. 278.*

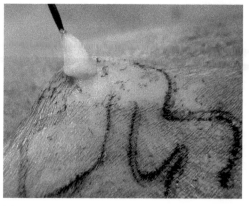

Figure 21.3 *See p. 280.* **Figure 21.4** *See p. 280.*

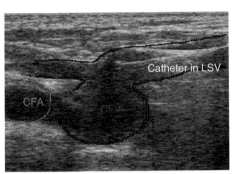

Catheter in LSV

CFA

Figure 23.2 *See p. 301.*

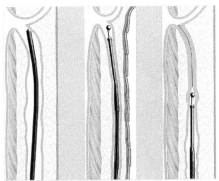

Figure 23.3 *See p. 301.*

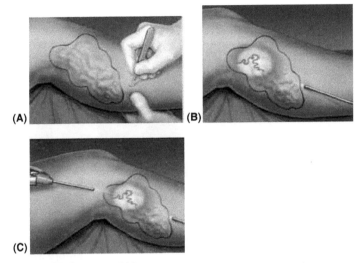

(A)

(B)

(C)

Figure 23.4 *See p. 305.*

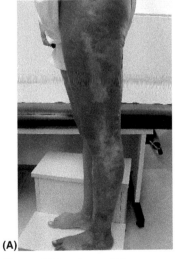

(A)

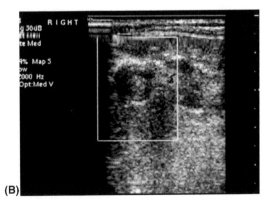

RIGHT

(B)

Figure 35.2 *See p. 476.*

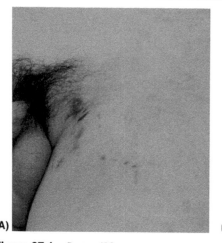

(A)

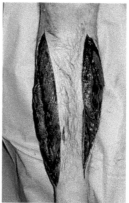

(B)

Figure 37.1 *See p. 498.*

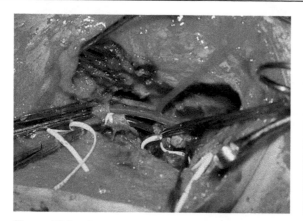

Figure 37.2 *See p. 499.*

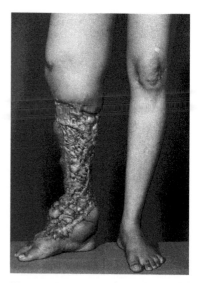

Figure 37.3 *See p. 500.*

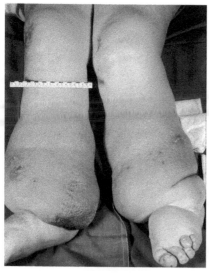

Figure 38.1 *See p. 515.*

Figure 39.1 *See p. 532.*

20

Conservative Treatments: Medical/Drug Therapies

Stavros K. Kakkos
Vascular Unit, Ealing Hospital, Southall, U.K.

Michel Perrin
University of Lyon, Lyon, France

Keith F. Cutting
Vascular Unit, Ealing Hospital, Southall, U.K.

George Geroulakos
*Vascular Unit, Ealing Hospital, Southall, and Department
of Vascular Surgery, Imperial College, London, U.K.*

COMPRESSION

Historical Aspects

Leg compression has been used to treat varicose veins and leg ulcers since ancient times, probably before Hippocrates' era. Leg wrapping with bandages was used by Hippocrates, Celsus, Ambrose Paré, and others, but it was Wiseman in 1676 who introduced a laced stocking made of a number of different materials but primarily of soft leather (1). The dermatologist Unna in 1893 used zinc and lanolin impregnated bandages to treat leg ulcers, offering compression with antimicrobial properties. Elastic compression in the form of bandages or stockings was developed during the nineteenth century. Elastic stockings initially exerted uniform compression, but in the 1940s Jobst introduced graded elastic stockings, which are widely used nowadays (1).

Types of Compression

Table 1 shows the different types of compression with particular emphasis to their characteristics. Elastic stockings are the most widely used form of compression, perhaps because they are generally easy to apply and comfortable to wear. This advantage renders them practical, but they are also cost-effective because they do not lose their elastic properties for several weeks. Thigh or knee length types are available, the former useful in varicose veins with thigh involvement or post-thrombotic leg. Various compression

Table 1 Different Types of Compression

Types of compression	Characteristics	Indications
Elastic compression	Stockings or bandages (short or long-stretch) made from woven textile with elastic properties	Varicose veins, varicose vein surgery Sclerotherapy
Inelastic compression	Rigid compression garments or bandages with no elastic properties	Varicose veins, venous ulcers
Compression systems	Multiple layers of bandages able to sustain a high compression profile for several days	Venous ulcers
Intermittent pneumatic compression	Pneumatic sleeves, periodically inflated	Venous ulcers

classes are available applying variable level of compression, but unfortunately there is no uniform agreement on the nomenclature of compression classes.

Pathophysiology and Mechanism of Compression

Several mechanisms are responsible for the improvement of symptoms of varicose veins and healing of venous ulcers by leg compression. Leg compression reduces the volume of blood pooled inside the varicose veins and restores the valvular function of the long or short saphenous vein or even occludes them; this prevents venous over-distension and minimises venous wall tension, which is responsible for local symptoms like ache, pain, itching, etc. Similarly, high-grade compression reduces popliteal vein reflux in post-thrombotic patients (2).

Elastic compression has been shown to reduce the venous filling index (VFI); (3–5) it is not known if this is the result of reducing the rate of venous wall expansion or because the reduction of the diameter of superficial venous segments abolishes reflux. VFI improvement has been shown to be greater with inelastic compression (4,6). It is also thought that compression diverts blood toward the deep veins via the perforating veins, or in cases where the latter are incompetent, that compression prevents the outward surge of blood during walking. This could be responsible for the improvement in muscle pump function expressed as reduction in residual volume fraction observed both during resting (3,5) and walking (7). The combination of inelastic (Unna boot) and elastic compression is probably more effective in normalizing venous hemodynamics, and one study has demonstrated further increases in venous refill time (8). Higher grades of compression could also improve deep vein hemodynamics, a significant problem in post-thrombotic legs. As a result of improving venous hemodynamics, elastic stockings reduce ambulatory venous pressure (9,10). Partsch has shown that thigh compression at the pressure range of 40 to 60 mm Hg with strongly applied short-stretch bandages on the thigh, but not class II thigh-length compression stockings, is able to significantly reduce venous diameter or venous reflux (11).

Compression increases interstitial pressure in the skin and subcutaneous tissues, preventing their expansion and reducing edema formation; (12–14) this is probably accomplished by improvement in lymphatic drainage resulting in improvement of patient symptoms, including leg heaviness and promotes ulcer healing. A result of direct skin compression is the improvement of venous hypertensive microangiopathy (15). Long-term use of elastic compression has been shown to improve venous elasticity (16), and prevent anatomical deterioration of the disease pattern (12). Labropoulos reported that the beneficial effect of elastic stockings on the venous hemodynamics is present mainly when the stockings are worn and completely abolished within a day after their removal (17).

Limbs with chronic venous insufficiency (CVI) have a reduced ankle range of movement (ROM), which may contribute to poor calf pump function (18). ROM is worse in advanced venous disease (18), and is a predictor of poor healing of venous ulcers by compression (19).

Level of Compression Applied According to Disease Severity

Advanced venous disease, especially if complicated with edema or ulcers, typically necessitates stronger compression, as shown in Table 2. This is to compensate the higher ambulatory pressure observed especially in post-thrombotic syndrome. In the latter case, compression pressure at the ankle level should be as strong as the four-layer compression system (40 mmHg) (20). High compression is more effective than low compression (21), but limitations of this are patient concordance. Occasionally, and mainly in cases of phlebolymphedema compression, should be even higher, above 45 mmHg.

Effectiveness of Compression

Compression therapy has shown variable success in treating varicose veins and its complications. Graded elastic stockings reduce leg symptoms, including edema and pain (22–24), and improve quality of life (24). In a recent study, severity score reduction for lower extremity swelling, pain, skin discoloration, activity tolerance, depression and sleeping problems after 1 and 16 months of treatment with compression stockings varied from 25% to 54% (25). In mesomorphic patients, noncustom graded compression stockings are equally effective with custom stockings (26).

A recent Cochrane review confirmed that compression increases ulcer healing rates compared with no compression (21). Compression significantly improves quality of life in patients with venous ulcers as estimated with the SF-36 (27), and EuroQol questionnaires (28), comparable with surgery (28). Similarly elastic stockings, compared to placebo stockings, improve quality of life in patients with symptomatic varicose veins as estimated by the CIVIC questionnaire (24).

In patients with venous ulcers, healing rate with the four-layer bandaging has been reported to be about 65%–80% at 6 to 12 months (19,29,30), significantly better (19),

Table 2 Severity of Venous Disease and Recommended Compression

Compression level (mmHg)	Indication
15–20 mmHg	Mild varicose veins, including those which appear during pregnancy Post-surgery
21–30 mmHg	Symptomatic varicose veins Post-sclerotherapy
31–45 mmHg	Post-thrombotic syndrome Healed venous ulcer to prevent recurrence
>45 mmHg	Phlebolymphedema

and faster compared to inelastic compression (19,31), or usual practice (32). A recent Cochrane review concluded that multi-layered systems are more effective than single-layered systems (21).

Compression effectiveness is affected by proper use. Bad or no usage due to compliance problems was associated with 97% of recurrent ulcerations in one study (33).

Two studies have shown that although compression is equally effective with superficial venous surgery in healing leg ulcers (29,34), recurrence rate is higher with compression when this is stopped. Recurrence varied from 28% to 36% at one to three years (29,34). Based on these results, surgical correction should be offered, ideally when all ulcers have healed and edema is minimal. Similarly, treatment failures of compression should be managed with superficial or deep venous surgery in fit patients. Although improved diagnostic and operative techniques make possible more active approaches to venous ulceration (35), unfortunately, some patients with post-thrombotic syndrome will need to use compression indefinitely; this is because surgery is not feasible or because it is partially or not effective whatsoever.

Special Indications of Compression (Post-Surgery, Sclerotherapy)

Elastic stockings are routinely used after sclerotherapy is performed; this has been shown to increase efficacy from 80% to 92% and reduce the incidence of superficial thrombophlebitis (36). Provided that high compression stockings are worn, the additional use of elastic compression is not necessary (37).

Adequate compression bandaging can decrease subcutaneous haematoma formation after varicose vein stripping (38). This is replaced after a variable period of time with elastic stockings. Low compression stockings (15–20 mmHg) are preferred because they are more comfortable and equally effective in controlling bruising and thrombophlebitis compared to high compression stockings (40 mmHg) (37).

Compliance, Cost-Effectiveness, and Complications of Leg Compression

In some 20–25% of patients, compliance or concordance with elastic stockings is moderate or poor (24). Socio-economic and cost issues are a major reason for non-compliance (33,39). Non-compliance with elastic compression stockings significantly decreases ulcer healing and increases recurrence. One study has shown that all patients who were noncompliant had recurrent ulceration by 36 months (40).

Cost-effectiveness analysis has shown that elastic stockings in patients with prior venous ulceration are cost saving, even with the most conservative of assumptions (41). Similarly, four-layer bandaging is associated with lower treatment cost compared to two-layer compression and short-stretch bandaging (42,43).

The four-layer bandage offers advantages over the two-layer bandage in terms of fewer adverse events and withdrawals from treatment (42,44). Skin maceration, excoriation, dryness or other damage, ulcer deterioration or infection or bandage failure have been reported (19). Ischemic complications associated with the use of these stockings also appears to be more common than previously thought (45). Toe ulceration associated with compression bandaging has been also reported (46). In order to prevent these ischemic complications, an ankle/arm index <0.6 is a contraindication for compression hosiery therapy (47). Other contraindications include peripheral neuropathy and allergy to the elastic material used.

Durability of Compression

Elastic compression material loses its elasticity over time. Three new stockings each year have been recommended to ensure an effective function (48). Similarly, compression systems maintain their compression profile up to a week; this is significantly better than single layer compression (20).

INTERMITTENT PNEUMATIC COMPRESSION

It has been shown that intermittent pneumatic leg compression (IPC) plus compression increased ulcer healing more than compression alone, the relative risk for healing being 11.4 (49). However, in view of the small size of this study, a Cochrane Review suggested that further trials are required to determine whether IPC increases the healing of venous leg ulcers (50). Since compression alone frequently fails, the additional use of IPC by these difficult-to-heal ulcer patients is probably helpful, as indicated by Rowland, who found that a crossover policy (compression to IPC and vice-versa) is more effective in healing ulcers (51). Home use of impulse compression of the foot and compression stockings has also been proposed for patients with CVI, with patients reporting significant improvement of swelling and pain (52). Awaiting methodologically rigorous research designed to identify the optimal choice of compression therapy or optimal protocol for patients with CVI or venous ulcers, Medicare USA has issued a decision that pneumatic compression will only be covered for patients with refractory edema with significant ulceration of the lower extremities after a six-month trial of standard therapies, such as compression stockings, has failed (53).

SUPERVISED EXERCISE

CVI is associated with impaired calf muscle pump function (3). Structured exercise has been shown not only to improve not only dynamic calf muscle strength but also calf muscle pump function (54,55). It remains unclear if exercise will improve leg ulcer healing rate and further research is warranted.

SKIN SUBSTITUTES

Acceleration of wound closure particularly in wounds that are slow to heal may be achieved through the application of skin substitutes. Commercially available skin substitutes hold a number of advantages over autologous skin grafts; they do not generate a donor site or cause associated acute wound pain, they therefore avoid the not need for the administration of an anaesthetic and they avoid the risk of scarring at the donor site (56). Additionally it has been found that the donation of connective tissue to the wound may enhance the strength of the wound and reduce scarring (57–59).

Bio-engineered skin substitutes applied to a wound can donate both epidermal and dermal components. Fibroblasts found in the dermis are important contributors to healing through the synthesis of collagen, the expression of cytokines and the formation of myofibroblasts.

Fibroblasts may be applied to the wound in the form of an allograft (sometimes called homograft) or as an autograft. In either case fibroblasts are harvested from dermal cells and then cultured in the laboratory in a suitable growth medium. It can take up to four weeks to "grow" the graft ready for application to the wound. Wounds should be free of infection and patients should be checked for any known hypersensitivities to agents (e.g., bovine proteins) that may have been used during the manufacturing process or in storage solutions.

Cultured fibroblast may be used on a variety of wounds and provide a "high tech" off-the-shelf approach to achieving wound closure (60).

Views on cost effectiveness vary. When considering skin substitutes and ulcer healing, Sibbald et al. (61) and Harding et al. (62) remain sceptical, although Sibbald et al. (61) indicated that greater gains were evident when the ulcers were of longer duration. Others have found a positive cost benefit. Kirsner et al. found reduced healing time and fewer complications together with a cost benefit (63). Positive findings have also been recorded by Nunez-Gutierrez with burns (64) and Redekop in diabetic foot patients (65).

Although undoubtedly expensive when compared on a unit cost basis with wound dressings, skin substitutes would appear to offer a useful therapeutic alternative. Their advantage would appear to currently lie in the treatment of those wounds that are resistant to "traditional" approaches (60). Brief details are provided of two commercial products that are widely available.

Apligraf® consists of living cells and proteins and is the only bi-layered skin substitute available. Apligraf does not contain all of the cells and structures normally found in skin and in common with other substitutes is limited to providing a stimulus to healing through the donation of growth factors and matrix components while at the same time affording a degree of protection to the wound bed. Keratinocytes are found in the upper (epidermal) layer of Apligraf and type one collagen and fibroblasts in the lower dermal layer.

Dermagraft® is also composed of human fibroblasts that are derived, like Apligraf, from neonatal foreskin. The graft is presented as a cryo-preserved sheet where the fibroblasts are seeded onto a bio-absorbable mesh scaffold.

Apligraf and Dermagraft do not contain melanocytes, Langerhans' cells, macrophages, or lymphocytes.

Lindgren et al. reported on a randomized controlled trial where 27 venous leg ulcers were treated with cryopreserved cultured allogenic keratinocytes and compression or compression only (66). Their results are inconclusive and inferred that the cryopreserved nature of the skin substitute adversely affected the capacity of the keratinocytes to produce cytokines and growth factors.

Encouraging results with a bilayed product were, however, reported by Falanga and Sabolinski (67). In this randomized controlled trial ($n = 120$), patients with venous leg ulcers of at least one year's duration were treated with compression only or with compression and the bilayered skin substitute. The results showed that the bilayered product was able to significantly accelerate healing in long-standing venous leg ulcers.

Hjerppe et al. have presented data of a noncomparative series of case studies of 114 patients with 151 difficult-to-heal chronic ulcers of various etiologies (68). The chronic leg ulcers were treated with human fibroblast-derived dermal substitute and showed the benefits obtained with an overall reduction in size of the ulcers being 63%.

Irrespective of the encouraging results demonstrated by a variety of clinical studies, it is important to remember that whatever improvement in healing rates are demonstrated with whatever product is used, the underlying cause of the ulcer is not being addressed with the application of bio-materials, and consequently there is a high risk of recurrence if maintenance therapy is not strictly adhered to.

PHARMACOLOGICAL TREATMENT OF CHRONIC VENOUS DISORDERS

The term chronic venous disorders (CVD) is used to denote all abnormal clinical changes that result from venous disease of the lower extremities and that have a chronic course (69). According to this definition, CVD includes patients who present with so-called symptoms and/or signs of venous disease which characterize each class of CVD in the CEAP classification (70), from class C0s to class C6.

A review of the literature (71) shows that CVD is most commonly manifest by the following symptoms: heaviness in the legs, pain, a sensation of swelling, restless legs, paresthesias, nighttime cramps, tiredness, and itching.

It must be stated that none of these symptoms is specific for CVD and is even less so pathognomonic. Since it is not possible to confirm whether such symptoms are related to venous disease, it appears important to try to characterize these symptoms based on the following secondary criteria:

- *Variability with position or physical activity*: Symptoms generally occur after prolonged standing, at the end of the day and do not exist or are diminished in the morning, by supine position or with the legs elevated
- *Variability with temperature*: Symptoms occur or are exacerbated by warmth, the summertime season, hot baths, hot waxing to remove body hair, floor-based heating systems, and regress; symptoms are diminished in winter and with cold temperatures
- *Variability with levels of circulating sex hormones*: Symptoms fluctuate with the menstrual cycle; they can occur with hormonal therapy (estrogens or estrogen-progestin) and disappear with discontinuation of such treatment.

The existence of at least two secondary criteria is necessary to confirm that symptoms are related to CVD, but the absence of such criteria does not rule out the possible venous-related origin of the symptoms.

Whatever the therapy used, the effect of treatment on symptoms is difficult to quantify because these symptoms are subjective variables.

Therapeutic efficacy can be assessed more readily based on a certain number of signs such as edema or venous ulcers.

Classification of Phlebotropic Drugs

Phlebotropic drugs belong to several different chemical families. The majority of them are plant-derived compounds. Some have been produced by chemical synthesis. The main phlebotropic drugs (72) are summarized in Table 3.

Pathophysiological Targets of Phlebotropic Drugs

It is important to specifically identify the mode of action of phlebotropic drugs depending on the pathophysiological mechanisms that they aim to treat. Among such mechanisms, we can differentiate the following:

- Those that are identified before microcirculatory disorders occur, consisting mainly of alterations in the venous wall; and
- Those consisting of microcirculatory disorders.

Pharmacological Targets Before the Occurrence of Abnormal Changes in the Microcirculation

Two major mechanisms may be responsible for pain in the absence of trophic changes:

- First, venous wall tension, which results from dilatation of the vein in a normal subject in erect position and valvular incompetence during dynamic movement in erect position in a subject with valvular insufficiency; and
- Second, hypoxia of the tunica media of the venous wall due to alteration of the vasa vasorum.

    Pain seems more related to hypoxia; indeed, in the early stages of CVD, superficial venous distensibility is slight, while pain is more severe than in the advanced stages of CVD where venous pressure is elevated and therefore high venous wall pressure exists (73). However, the venous remodeling phase that precedes the development of varicose veins, which is accompanied by the process of venous distention, hemorrheological disturbances, and conditions of hypoxia can be painful.

   Pain and Heaviness in the Legs.   Two specific targets for phlebotropic drugs exist that aim to decrease the sensation of heaviness in the legs, pain, and ankle edema at the end of the day. The first target of such therapy is increased venous wall pressure: indeed, it is known that distensibility is increased by 10–50% in patients (74) according to different studies and that this is due to a decrease in venous tone. The second target is hypoxia of the tunica media related to disease of the vasa vasorum (73).

Table 3   Classification of the Main Phlebotropic Drugs

---
1. Benzopyrones
    a) Alpha-benzopyrones
       Coumarin (1,2-benzopyrone; 5,6-alpha-benzopyrone)
       Dicoumarols (dimers of 4 hydroxycourmarins): oral anticoagulants
    b) Chromenones (flavonoids)
       Micronized purified flavonoid fraction (MPFF)
       Diosmin, kacinprerol, diosmethin, quercetin, rutin and derivatives, *O*-(β-hydroxyethyl) rutosides (HR or oxerutins)
2. Saponins
       Escin, horse-chestnut extracts
       Extracts of ruscus, centella asiatica
3. Other plant extracts
       Anthocyanosides: blueberry extract (protoescigenin, barringtogenol, α- and β-escin, cryptoescin)
       Proanthocyanidols: grape seed extracts
       Ginkgo biloba
4. Synthetic products
       Calcium dobesilate
       Benzarone, naftazone

Source: Adapted from Ref. 72.

Table 4 Possible Links Between Pathophysiological Variables, Symptoms, and Signs of Chronic
Venous Disorders

Pathophysiology	Symptom	Sign
Leukocyte adhesion in subvalvular areas/areas of inflammation	Pain	Early valvular reflux
Valvular incompetence		Reflux
Venous hypertension and venous wall tension	Pain	Edema
Venous wall hypoxia	Pain	
Increased capillary pressure	Sensation of heavy legs and swelling	Edema
Hemorrheological disorders and platelet hyperaggregability	Nighttime cramps Restless legs	

Source: Adapted from Ref. 73.

Restless Legs, Nighttime Cramps.   These symptoms most often occur during the
latter half of the night, but also can occur during prolonged seated position. They can also
be related to hypoxia of the tunica media, but more specifically may be associated with
hemorheological disorders (73). In fact, red blood cell hyperviscosity and hyperaggregation are constant findings in venous disease (75,76). It appears likely that hemorheological
disorders worsen the circulation in the vasa vasorum. Hypoxia in the tunica media, in turn,
induces deterioration of the venous wall. Indeed, hypoxia has a potent effect in inducing
metabolic disorders: triggering of enzymatic activities, such as those of matrix metollo-
proteinases (MMP), and dedifferenciation and migration of smooth muscle cells which
secrete growth factors. Fibrosis of the venous wall governs the development of the
varicose vein. The diseased venous wall generates several metabolic disorders, including
hypofibrinolysis due to elevated levels of plasminogen activating inhibitor (PAI-1).
The links between pathophysiology, symptoms and clinical signs of CVD are
summarized in Table 4.

Pharmacological Targets Related to Microcirculatory Disorders
The process of edema manifestly is due to increased capillary permeability related to
permanent venous hypertension (73), whose mechanisms vary: reflux or obstruction.
     Two stages should be distinguished in the progression of capillary disorders as
venous disease becomes progressively worse: first, the existence of a functional disorder
followed by development of a lesional disorder, which characterizes chronic
venous insufficiency.
     Capillary Functional Disorder.   At a relatively early stage, the existence of a
reduction in capillary permeability is observed in patients, as assessed by ankle
plethysmography following proximal venous hypertension with fluorescein capillary
angioscopy and the Gibbon-Landis radioisotope test. A second aspect is capillary fragility
demonstrated by the suction cup test.
     Traditionally, such disorders are taken as targets for studying the effects of
phlebotropic drugs (Table 5). However, it is not known whether they play a part in the
development of lesional disorders. An argument in support of a possible action is that they
are accompanied by micro-edema and hemorrheological disorders, which exist at an early
stage of venous disease. And yet, it is known that red blood cell hyperaggregation
promotes microcirculatory disorders.

Table 5 Pharmacological Targets of Phlebotropic Drugs

1. Analgesic, anti-edema and capillary protection effects: *all products*
2. Effect on venous tone: *all products*
   Ruscus: partial agonist action on venular alpha-1 adrenergic receptors (neutralized by NO on the arterial side)
3. Lymphotrophic effects: *Ruscus, coumarin, micronized purified flavonoid fraction*
4. Improvement of red blood cell rheology: *micronized purified flavonoid fraction, troxerutin, rutin*
5. Profibrinolytic action: *micronized purified flavonoid fraction, troxerutin, diosmins*
6. Anti-inflammatory action: *micronized purified flavonoid fraction, Gingko biloba, diosmins*
7. Decreased adhesive properties of neutrophils and monocytes: *micronized purified flavonoid fraction*
8. Protective effect on the venous valve: *micronized purified flavonoid fraction*
9. Protective effect on the venous wall
   9.1: inhibition of lysosomial enzymes: *melitot extract, rutins, pycnogenols*
   9.2: protection of fibrous proteins (collagen): *procyanidolic oligomers*
   9.3: anti-free radical properties: *micronized purified flavonoid fraction, Gingko biloba*
   9.4: normalization of the synthesis of prostaglandine E2 : *micronized purified flavonoid fraction*
   9.5: improvement of circulation in the vasa vasorum: *troxerutin*

Source: Adapted from Ref. 73.

Microvascular Lesional Disease. Alteration of the cutaneous microcirculation in the lower extremities is the long-term result of permanent venous hypertension, as the distal venous valves gradually become incompetent. The result is trophic changes whose incidence is proportional to the increase in ambulatory venous pressure.

Over the last few years, advances have been made in understanding the pathophysiology of events, allowing better identification of the structures targeted by phlebotropic drugs:

- Doppler-laser investigation has shown an increase in cutaneous blood flow at rest, related to increased concentrations of circulating red blood cells. This involves impairment of blood distribution affecting the most superficial areas where hypoxia develops, while intra- and subcutaneous PO2 concentrations are normal (77);
- Hypofibrinolysis increases concomitantly with increasing severity of trophic changes, usually with very high levels of PAI-1 (78);
- The hemorheological disorder, in particular, red blood cell hyperaggregation, is exacerbated and correlated with the clinical severity of the disease;
- Hypoxia and excess delivery of oxygenated free radicals in the most superficial capillaries promote endothelial and leukocyte activation (79);
- Therefore, leukocyte accumulation and activation in dilated capillary loops appears as a factor which worsens the condition, extensively involved in the pathogenesis of venous ulcer (79).

In summary, microcirculatory disorders progressively worsen with hemo-dynamic alterations. During this process, leukocyte adhesion to the vascular endothelium produces endothelial activation with release of proteolytic enzymes and free radicals in the tissues (80). In addition, *in vitro* studies have demonstrated the release of prostaglandin (especially PGF2α) and basic fibroblast growth factor (bFGF) which may be directly involved in venous wall remodeling (81). These mediators are found in an abnormal quantity in varicose veins (82). During this process, venous valves may be the first to be damaged (83).

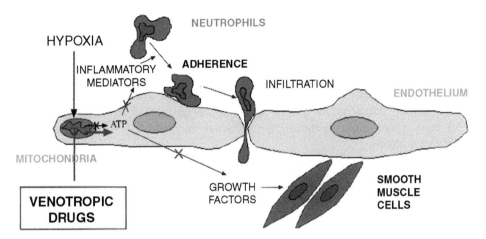

Figure 1 Representation of the possible protective mechanism of phlebotropic drugs on the endothelial cells. *Source*: Adapted from Ref. 85.

The interaction between leukocyte and endothelium may be the key component in the pathogenesis of CVD and its complications, and may be an essential entity targeted by phlebotropic drugs.

Pharmacological Action of Phlebotropic Drugs on These Different Targets

Remacle's team has demonstrated the ability of phlebotropic drugs to inhibit the release of mediators of inflammation in endothelial cells placed under conditions of hypoxia (Fig. 1) (84,85).

A recent pharmacological study has demonstrated the ability of the micronized purified flavonoid fraction (MPFF) to protect venous valves from destruction caused by venous hypertension (86). It is by inhibiting the expression of adhesion molecules on the surface of leucocytes and the endothelium that this phlebotropic drug would limit leukocyte adhesion and subsequently leukocyte infiltration into the valvular subendothelium, limiting inflammatory events (86). This effect had been demonstrated previously with the same preparation in the microcirculation (87).

Clinical Trials of Phlebotropic Drugs

Action on Symptoms

Pain and heaviness in the legs are the two symptoms most commonly identified in studies on symptoms of venous disease (71).

Symptoms, and in particular, pain, can be evaluated with self-evaluation rating scales. Three types of scales have been validated: (88) the simple verbal scale, the numerical scale and the visual analog scale. All these scales evaluate pain intensity but do not provide information on the nature of the pain complaint. They make it possible to compare intra-individual variations between groups of patients in evaluation studies or longitudinal observational surveys.

Symptoms have an effect on the quality of life of patients with CVD. Overall assessment of quality of life allows quantification of the impact of symptoms on functional ability. Several quality of life questionnaires have been specifically adapted to CVD (89–91).

Evaluation of symptoms associated with venous disease and the expected benefit of therapy with phlebotropic drugs is not easy because many intercurrent factors exist. However, many double-blind, placebo-controlled studies with a washout period have been conducted using measurable criteria for evaluation of pain and heaviness in the legs.

We will briefly summarize the studies conducted on calcium dobesilate (92–96), Horse chestnut extract (97,98), hydroxyrutin (99–101), and micronized purified flavonoid fraction (102–105), and to which a few meta-analyses and reviews may be added (106–115). All these studies have confirmed the reduction in symptoms with all the different therapeutic agents.

Measurement of quality of life was assessed during treatment with a phlebotropic drug. It markedly improved after 6 months of treatment, in particular in symptomatic patients, and was greater in patients in whom a reflux had not been identified (116).

Action on Edema

Several methods have been used to measure edema and study the efficacy of phlebotropic drugs on this sign.

The simplest method is measurement of ankle circumference, as done most often with a Leg-O-Meter®. This instrument, which has been validated (117), takes into account the height at which the measurement is made. However, changes observed in ankle circumference are not always correlated with changes in volume of the lower limb. This is why methods to measure differences in leg volume are preferable. The most well-known is the volumetric method of fluid displacement (118–119), which has been validated.

Volumetric measurement has been used to show that the most painful legs are those in which edema exists. Furthermore, volumetric method has demonstrated that the standing position, or even prolonged sitting with no activity of the calf muscle pump system, produces an increase in leg volume. Moreover, such edema is correlated with the degree of venous insufficiency (120). Thus, this accounts for the existence of leg edema during long-distance airline travel.

Other methods have been used to assess edema in CVD: the optoelectronic method (121), the tomographic method (122), high-resolution magnetic resonance imaging, and X-ray absorptiometry (122).

In the literature, a certain number of randomized, controlled studies have demonstrated the efficacy of phlebotropic drugs on edema. Let us mention studies by Jaeger et al. (93), and Casley–Smith (94) on calcium dobesilate, Vayssairat's study on naphtazone (123), Diehm's study on horsechestnut extract (124), that of Blume on micronized purified flavonoid fraction (125), and a study by Cesarone on the effect of hydroxyrutin (126,127) on edema associated with long-distance airline travel. They have demonstrated a significant decrease in edema.

In Chronic Venous Insufficiency: Classes C4–C6

Few phlebotropic drugs have been studied in the treatment of chronic venous insufficiency. The phlebotropic drug most widely studied by far in venous ulcer and its complications is mircronized purified flavonoid fraction (128–131). A recent meta-analysis of five clinical trials conducted with this drug on venous ulcer revealed its beneficial action on reduction of time needed for healing of the ulcer (132).

Among phlebotropic drugs, the use of horse chestnut seed extract (123,133), and hydroxyrutosides (134) have resulted in a reduction in both edema and symptoms of chronic venous insufficiency, but have failed to demonstrate superiority over compression in advanced chronic venous insufficiency (133) or in preventing venous ulcer recurrence

(134). This may be because reduction in edema alone is insufficient to treat leg ulceration. Additional factors must be influenced in order to speed ulcer healing, which the micronized purified flavonoid fraction might be able to address. Recently much attention has been focused on the involvement of growth factors (135), and leukocytes in the development of venous ulceration (87). This has opened up new areas of investigation.

By reducing the likelihood of leukocyte adhesion, micronized purified flavonoid fraction presumably acts through an anti-inflammatory mechanism (87). Thus, among the many mechanisms at work in the pathogenesis of venous ulceration, the mechanism involving leukocyte activation and interaction with the endothelium seems to be the one most responsive to pharmacological treatment up to now.

Place of Phlebotropic Drugs in the Treatment of Chronic Venous Disorders

Phlebotropic drugs have a well-established effect on edema. They also effectively decrease the so-called symptoms of venous disease such as heaviness of the legs, pain, sensation of swelling and nighttime cramps.

In both patients classified as having stage C0 disease and in those classified as C1s and C2s for whom invasive therapy (sclerotherapy, surgery) does not appear warranted, phlebotonic drugs appear to represent good first-line treatment of chronic venous disorder, possibly in conjunction with compression therapy.

In more advanced disease stages, phlebotropic drugs have not demonstrated any additional benefit over compression on improvement of skin changes or in ulcer healing, except for micronized purified flavonoid fraction that may be used in conjunction with sclerotherapy, surgery and/or compression therapy, or as an alternative treatment when surgery is not indicated or is not feasible (114).

KEY POINTS

- Compression increases ulcer healing rates and is cost effective.
- Compression reduces the venous volume and may restore venous valve function.
- Elastic stockings are the most widely used form of compression but lose elasticity with time and should be replaced regularly.
- Various forms of bandaging are available but multi-layer systems are the most effective.
- To prevent ischemic complications, an ankle/arm index <0.6 is a contra-indication for compression hosiery therapy.
- Intermittent pneumatic compression may increase the healing rate of venous ulcers but the evidence for this is currently small.
- Exercise may improve calf muscle pump function but it is not clear if this increases ulcer healing rates. Skin substitutes may increase healing rates but are relatively expensive.
- Few phlebotropic drugs have been studied in the treatment of chronic venous insufficiency and their role remains controversial.
- Phlebotropic drugs have a well-established effect on edema. They may also effectively decrease the so-called symptoms of venous disease such as heaviness of the legs, pain, sensation of swelling, and night-time cramps.

REFERENCES

1. Laufmann H, Clio Chirurgica. The Veins. Austin, TX: Silvergirl, Inc., 1986.
2. Evers EJ, Wuppermann T. Effect of different compression therapies on the reflux in deep veins with a post-thrombotic syndrome. Vasa 1999; 28:19–23.
3. Christopoulos DG, Nicolaides AN, Szendro G, Irvine AT, Bull ML, Eastcott HHG. Air-plethysmography and the effect of elastic compression on venous hemodynamics of the leg. J Vasc Surg 1987; 5:148–159.
4. Partsch H, Menzinger G, Mostbeck A. Inelastic leg compression is more effective to reduce deep venous refluxes than elastic bandages. Dermatol Surg 1999; 25:695–700.
5. Ibegbuna V, Delis K, Nicolaides AN. Effect of lightweight compression stockings on venous haemodynamics. Int Angiol 1997; 16:185–188.
6. Spence RK, Cahall E. Inelastic versus elastic leg compression in chronic venous insufficiency: a comparison of limb size and venous hemodynamics. J Vasc Surg 1996; 24:783–787.
7. Ibegbuna V, Delis KT, Nicolaides AN, Aina O. Effect of elastic compression stockings on venous hemodynamics during walking. J Vasc Surg 2003; 37:420–425.
8. Samson RH, Scher LH, Veith FJ, Gupta SK, Ascer E. Photoplethysmographic evaluation of external compressive therapy for chronic venous ulceration. J Cardiovasc Surg (Torino) 1986; 27:24–26.
9. Horner J, Fernandes J, Fernandes E, Nicolaides AN. Value of graduated compression stockings in deep venous insufficiency. Br Med J 1980; 280:820–821.
10. O'Donnell TF, Jr., Rosenthal DA, Callow AD, Ledig BL. Effect of elastic compression on venous hemodynamics in postphlebitic limbs. JAMA 1979; 242:2766–2768.
11. Partsch H, Menzinger G, Borst-Krafek B, Groiss E. Does thigh compression improve venous hemodynamics in chronic venous insufficiency? J Vasc Surg 2002; 36:948–952.
12. Buhs CL, Bendick PJ, Glover JL. The effect of graded compression elastic stockings on the lower leg venous system during daily activity. J Vasc Surg 1999; 30:830–834.
13. Hirai M, Iwata H, Hayakawa N. Effect of elastic compression stockings in patients with varicose veins and healthy controls measured by strain gauge plethysmography. Skin Res Technol 2002; 8:236–239.
14. Nehler MR, Moneta GL, Woodard DM, et al. Perimalleolar subcutaneous tissue pressure effects of elastic compression stockings. Vasc Surg 1993; 18:783–788.
15. Christopoulos DC, Nicolaides AN, Belcaro G, Kalodiki E. Venous hypertensive microangiopathy in relation to clinical severity and effect of elastic compression. J Dermatol Surg Oncol 1991; 17:809–813.
16. Leon M, Volteas N, Labropoulos N, et al. The effect of elastic stockings on the elasticity of varicose veins. Int Angiol 1993; 12:173–177.
17. Labropoulos N, Leon M, Volteas N, Nicolaides AN. Acute and long term effect of elastic stockings in patients with varicose veins. Int Angiol 1994; 13:119–123.
18. Back TL, Padberg FT, Jr., Araki CT, Thompson PN, Hobson RWII. Limited range of motion is a significant factor in venous ulceration. J Vasc Surg 1995; 22:519–523.
19. Nelson EA, Iglesias CP, Cullum N, Torgerson DJ. VenUS I collaborators. Randomized clinical trial of four-layer and short-stretch compression bandages for venous leg ulcers (VenUS I). Br J Surg 2004; 91:1292–1299.
20. Blair SD, Wright DD, Backhouse CM, Riddle E, McCollum CN. Sustained compression and healing of chronic venous ulcers. BMJ 1988; 297:1159–1161.
21. Cullum N, Nelson EA, Fletcher AW, Sheldon TA. Compression for venous leg ulcers. Cochrane Database Syst Rev 2001;CD000265.
22. Pierson S, Pierson D, Swallow R, Johnson G, Jr. Efficacy of graded elastic compression in the lower leg. JAMA 1983; 249:242–243.
23. Buchtemann AS, Steins A, Volkert B, Hahn M, Klyscz T, Junger M. The effect of compression therapy on venous haemodynamics in pregnant women. Br J Obstet Gynaecol 1999; 106:563–569.

24. Vayssairat M, Ziani E, Houot B. Efficacité versus placebo de la contention classe 1 dans l'insuffisance veineuse chronique des membres inférieurs. J Mal Vasc 2000; 25:256–262.

25. Motykie GD, Caprini JA, Arcelus JI, Reyna JJ, Overom E, Mokhtee D. Evaluation of therapeutic compression stockings in the treatment of chronic venous insufficiency. Dermatol Surg 1999; 25:116–120.

26. Johnson G, Jr., Kupper C, Farrar DJ, Swallow RT. Graded compression stockings: custom vs noncustom. Arch Surg 1982; 117:69–72.

27. Charles H. Does leg ulcer treatment improve patients' quality of life? J Wound Care 2004; 13:209–213.

28. Loftus S. A longitudinal, quality of life study comparing four layer bandaging and superficial venous surgery for the treatment of venous leg ulcers. J Tissue Viability 2001; 11:14–19.

29. Barwell JR, Davies CE, Deacon J, et al. Comparison of surgery and compression with compression alone in chronic venous ulceration (ESCHAR study): randomized controlled trial. Lancet 2004; 363:1854–1859.

30. Meyer FJ, McGuinness CL, Lagattolla NR, Eastham D, Burnand KG. Randomized clinical trial of three-layer paste and four-layer bandages for venous leg ulcers. Br J Surg 2003; 90:934–940.

31. Ukat A, Konig M, Vanscheidt W, Munter KC. Short-stretch versus multilayer compression for venous leg ulcers: a comparison of healing rates. J Wound Care 2003; 12:139–143.

32. O'Brien JF, Grace PA, Perry IJ, Hannigan A, Clarke Moloney M, Burke PE. Randomized clinical trial and economic analysis of four-layer compression bandaging for venous ulcers. Br J Surg 2003; 90:794–798.

33. Samson RH, Showalter DP. Stockings and the prevention of recurrent venous ulcers. Dermatol Surg 1996; 22:373–376.

34. Zamboni P, Cisno C, Marchetti F, et al. Minimally invasive surgical management of primary venous ulcers vs compression treatment: a randomized clinical trial. Eur J Vasc Endovasc Surg 2003; 25:313–318.

35. DePalma RG, Kowallek DL. Venous ulceration: a cross-over study from nonoperative to operative treatment. J Vasc Surg 1996; 24:788–792.

36. Scurr JH, Coleridge-Smith P, Cutting P. Varicose veins: optimum compression following sclerotherapy. Ann R Coll Surg Engl 1985; 67:109–111.

37. Shouler PJ, Runchman PC. Varicose veins: optimum compression after surgery and sclerotherapy. Ann R Coll Surg Engl 1989; 71:402–404.

38. Travers JP, Rhodes JE, Hardy JG, Makin GS. Postoperative limb compression in reduction of haemorrhage after varicose vein surgery. Ann R Coll Surg Engl 1993; 75:119–122.

39. Kiev J, Noyes LD, Rice JC, Kerstein MD. Patient compliance with fitted compression hosiery monitored by photoplethysmography. Arch Phys Med Rehabil 1990; 71:376–379.

40. Mayberry JC, Moneta GL, Taylor LM, Jr,, Porter JM. Fifteen-year results of ambulatory compression therapy for chronic venous ulcers. Surgery 1991; 109:575–581.

41. Korn P, Patel ST, Heller JA, et al. Why insurers should reimburse for compression stockings in patients with chronic venous stasis. J Vasc Surg 2002; 35:950–957.

42. Moffatt CJ, McCullagh L, O'Connor T, et al. Randomized trial of four-layer and two-layer bandage systems in the management of chronic venous ulceration. Wound Repair Regen 2003; 11:166–171.

43. Iglesias CP, Nelson EA, Cullum N, Torgerson DJ. On behalf of the VenUS I collaborators. Economic analysis of VenUS I, a randomized trial of two bandages for treating venous leg ulcers. Br J Surg 2004; 91:1300–1306.

44. Scriven JM, Taylor LE, Wood AJ, Bell PR, Naylor AR, London NJ. A prospective randomised trial of four-layer versus short stretch compression bandages for the treatment of venous leg ulcers. Ann R Coll Surg Engl 1998; 80:215–220.

45. Merrett ND, Hanel KC. Ischaemic complications of graduated compression stockings in the treatment of deep venous thrombosis. Postgrad Med J 1993; 69:232–234.

46. Chan CLH, Meyer FJ, Hay RJ, Burnand KG. Toe ulceration associated with compression bandaging: observational study. BMJ 2001; 323:1099.

47. Neumann HA. Compression therapy with medical elastic stockings for venous diseases. Dermatol Surg 1998; 24:765–770.

48. Veraart JC, Daamen E, de Vet HC, Neumann HA. Elastic compression stockings: durability of pressure in daily practice. Vasa 1997; 26:282–286.

49. Coleridge-Smith P, Sarin S, Hasty J, Scurr JH. Sequential gradient pneumatic compression enhances venous ulcer healing: a randomized trial. Surgery 1990; 108:871–875.

50. Mani R, Vowden K, Nelson EA. Intermittent pneumatic compression for treating venous leg ulcers. Cochrane Database Syst Rev 2001;CD001899.

51. Rowland J. Intermittent pneumatic compression versus compression bandages in the treatment of venous leg ulcers. Aust NZ J Surg 2000; 70:110–113.

52. Arcelus JI, Caprini JA, Sehgal LR, Reyna JJ. Home use of impulse compression of the foot and compression stockings in the treatment of chronic venous insufficiency. J Vasc Surg 2001; 34:805–811.

53. Berliner E, Ozbilgin B, Zarin DA. A systematic review of pneumatic compression for treatment of chronic venous insufficiency and venous ulcers. J Vasc Surg 2003; 37:539–544.

54. Padberg FT, Jr., Johnston MV, Sisto SA. Structured exercise improves calf muscle pump function in chronic venous insufficiency: a randomized trial. J Vasc Surg 2004; 39:79–87.

55. Kan YM, Delis KT. Hemodynamic effects of supervised calf muscle exercise in patients with venous leg ulceration: a prospective controlled study. Arch Surg 2001; 136:1364–1369.

56. Valencia IC, Falabella AF, Eaglstein WH. Skin grafting. Dermatol Clin 2000; 18:521–532.

57. Cuono CB, Langdon R, Birchall N, Barttelbort S, McGuire J. Composite autologous-allogeneic skin replacement: Development and clinical application. Plast Reconstr Surg 1987; 80:626–637.

58. Desai MH, Mlakar JM, McCauley RL, et al. Lack of long-term durability of cultured keratinocyte burn-wound coverage: a case report. Burn Care Rehabil 1991; 12:540–545.

59. Gallico GG, III. Biologic skin substitutes. Clin Plast Surg 1990; 17:519–526.

60. Eisenbud D, Huang NF, Luke S, Silberklang M. Skin Substitutes and Wound Healing: Current Status and Challenges. Wounds 2004; 16:2–17.

61. Sibbald RG, Torrance GW, Walker V, et al. Cost-effectiveness of Apligraf in the treatment of venous leg ulcers. Ost Wound Manage 2001; 47:36–46.

62. Harding K, Cutting K, Price P. The cost-effectiveness of wound management protocols of care. Br J Nurs 2000; 9:S6,S8,S10.

63. Kirsner RS, Fastenau J, Falabella A, et al. Clinical and economic outcomes with graftskin for hard-to-heal venous leg ulcers: A single-center experience. Dermatol Surg 2002; 28:81–82.

64. Nunez-Gutierrez H, Castro-Munozledo F, Kuri-Harcuch W. Combined use of allograft and autograft epidermal cultures in therapy of burns. Plast Reconstr Surg 1996, 98:929–939.

65. Redekop WK, McDonnell J, Verboom P, et al. The cost effectiveness of Apligraf® treatment of diabetic foot ulcers. Pharmacoeconomics 2003; 21:1171–1183.

66. Lindgren C, Marousson JA, Toftgard R. Treatment of venous leg ulcers with cryopreserved cultured allogeneic keratinocytes: a prospective open controlled study. Br J Dermatol 1998; 139:271–275.

67. Falanga V, Sabolinski M. A bilayered living skin construct (APLIGRAF®) accelerates complete closure of hard to heal venous leg ulcers. Wound Rep Reg 1999; 7:201–207.

68. Hjerppe A, Hjerppe M, Autio V, Raudasoja R, Vaalasti A. Treatment of chronic leg ulcers with a human fibroblast-derived dermal substitute: a case series of 114 patients wounds. Wounds 2004; 16:97–104.

69. Ramelet AA, Kern P, Perrin M, eds. Varicose veins and telangiectasias. Paris: Masson, 2003. Chapter 1 (definitions), pp. 7–16.

70. Porter JM, Moneta GL. International Consensus Committee on chronic venous disease. Reporting standards in venous disease: an update. J Vasc Surg 1995; 21:635–645.

71. Garde C, Perrin M, Chleir F, Henriet JP, et al. First meeting of review and consensus on venoactive agents on the symptoms of chronic venous disease (in French). Phlébologie 2003; 56:103–109.

72. Ramelet AA, Kern P, Perrin M, eds. Varicose veins and telangiectasias. Paris: Masson, 2003. Chapter 13 (Drug therapy) pp. 166–168.

73. Boisseau MR. Pharmacologie des médicaments veinotoniques: données actuelles sur leur mode d'action et les cibles thérapeutiques.(in French). Angéiologie 2000; 52:71–77.

74. Clarke GH, Vasdekis SN, Hobbs JT, Nicolaides AN. Venous wall function in the pathogenesis of varicose veins. Surgery 1992; 111:402–408.

75. Boisseau M, Freyburger G, Busquet M, et al. Hemorheological disturbances in venous insufficiency after induced stasis. Clin Hemorheol 1989; 9:161–163.

76. Le Devehat C, Boisseau MR, Vimeux M, et al. Hemorheological factors in the pathophysiology of venous disease. Clin Hemorheol 1989; 9:861–870.

77. Taccoen A, Belcaro G, Lebard C, Zuccarelli F. Etiologies et mécanismes des varices: réalités et perspectives. STV 1997; 9:354–363.

78. Boisseau MR, Taccoen A, Garreau C, et al. Fibrinolysis and hemorheology in chronic venous insufficiency: a double blind study of troxerutin efficiency. J Cardiovasc Surg 1995; 36:369–374.

79. Saharay M, Shields DA, Georgiannos SN, et al. Endothelial activation in patients with chronic venous disease. Eur J Vasc Endovasc Surg 1998; 15:342–349.

80. Michiels C, Arnould T, Thibaut-Vercruyssen R, Bouaziz N, Janssens D, Remacle J. Perfused human saphenous veins for the study of the origin of varicose veins: role of the endothelium and of hypoxia. Int Angiol 1997; 16:135–141.

81. Michiels C, De Leener F, Arnould T, Dieu M, Remacle J. Hypoxia stimulates human endothelial cells to release smooth muscle cell mitogens: role of prostaglandins and bFGF. Exp Cell Res 1994; 213:43–54.

82. Badier-Commander C, Couvelard A, Henin D, Verbeuren T, Michel JB, Jacob MP. Smooth muscle cell modulation and cytokine overproduction in varicose veins. An in situ study. J Pathol 2001; 193:398–407.

83. Takase S, Pascarella L, Bergan J, Schmid-Schönbein GW. Hypertension-induced valve remodeling. J Vasc Surg 2004; 39:1329–1334.

84. Janssens D, Delaive E, Houbion A, Eliaers F, Remacle J, Michiels C. Effect of venotropic drugs on the respiratory activity of isolated mitochondria and in endothelial cells. Br J Pharmacol 2000; 130:1513–1524.

85. Michiels C, Bouaziz N, Remacle J. Role of the endothelium and blood stasis in the appearance of varicose veins. Int Angiol 2002; 21:1–8.

86. Takase S, Pascarella L, Lerond L, Bergan J, Schmid-Schönbein GW. Venous Hypertension. Inflammation and Valve Remodeling. Eur J Vasc Endovasc Surg 2004; 28:484–493.

87. Shoab SS, Porter JB, Coleridge-Smith PD. Effect of oral micronised flavonoid fraction treatment on leukocyte adhesion molecule expression in patients with chronic venous disease: a pilot study. J Vasc Surg 2000; 31:456–461.

88. Agence Nationale d'Accréditation et d'Evaluation de la Santé (in French). Evaluation et suivi de la douleur chronique chez l'adulte en médecine ambulatoire (in French). www.anaes.fr.

89. Launois R, Reboul-Marty J, Henry B. Construction and validation of a quality of life questionnaire in chronic lower limb venous insufficiency (CIVIQ). Qual Life Res 1996; 5:539–550.

90. Lamping DL, Abenhaim L, Kurz X, et al. Measuring quality of life and symptoms in chronic venous disorders of the leg: development and psychometric evaluation of the VEINES-Qol/SYM questionnaire. Qual Life Res 1998; 7:621–622.

91. Klyscz T, Junder M, Schanz S, Janz M, Rassner G, Kohnen R. Quality of Life in chronic venous insufficiency (CVI). Results of a study with the newly developed Tubingen questionnaire for measuring quality of life with CVI. Hautartz 1998; 49:372–381.

92. Hachen HJ, Lorenz P. Double-blind clinical and plethysmographic study of calcium dobesilate in patients with peripheral microvascular disorders. Angiology 1982; 33:480–487.

93. Labs KH, Degischer S, Gamba G, Jaeger KA. Effectiveness and safety of calcium dobesilate in treating chronic venous insufficiency: randomized, double-blind, placebo-controlled trial. Phlebology 2004; 19:123–130.

94. Casley-Smith JR. A double blind trial of calcium dobesilate in chronic venous insufficiency. Angiology 1988; 39:853–857.

95. Pecchi S, De Franco V, Damiani P, et al. Calcium dobesilate in the treatment of primary venous insufficiency of the lower limbs. A controlled clinical study. Clin Ter 1990; 32:409–417.

96. Widmer L, Biland L, Barras JP. Doxium 500 in chronic venous insufficiency: a double-blind placebo-controlled multicentre study. Int Angiol 1990; 9:105–110.

97. Le Devehat C, Lemoine A, Roux E, et al. Aspects clinique et hemodynamique de Cyclo 3 dans l'insuffisance veineuse. (in French). Angeiologie 1984; 36:119–122.

98. Sentou Y, Bernard-Fernier MF, Demarez JP, et al. Symptomatologie et plethysmographie: parallelisme des resultats obtenus lors d'un traitment par Cyclo 3 de patients porteuses d'une insuffisance veineuse chronique (etude en double insu contre placebo). Gaz Med 1985; 92:73–77.

99. Petruzzellis V, Troccoli T, Candiani C, et al. Oxerutins (Venoruton): efficacy in chronic venous insufficiency–a double-blind, randomized, controlled study. Angiology 2002; 53:257–263.

100. Balmer A, Limoni C. Adouble blind placebo controlled clinical trial of Venoruton on the symptoms and signs of chronic venous insufficiency. The importance of patient selection. VASA 1980; 9:1–7.

101. MacLennan WJ, Wilson J, Rattenhuber V, et al. Hydroxyethylrutosides in elderly patients with chronic venous insufficiency: its efficacy and tolerability. Gerontology 1994; 40:45–52.

102. Chassignolle J-F, Amiel M, Lanfranchi G, et al. Activité thérapeutique de Daflon 500 mg dans l'insuffisance veineuse fonctionnelle [in French]. J Int Med 1987; 99:32–37.

103. Gilly R, Pillion G, Frileux C. Evaluation of a new venoactive micronized flavonoid fraction (S 5682) in symptomatic disturbances of the veinolymphatic circulation of the lower limb: a double-blind, placebo-controlled study. Phlebology 1994; 9:67–70.

104. Cospite M, Dominici A. Double blind study of the pharmacodynamic and clinical activities of 5682 SE in venous insufficiency. Advantages of the new micronized form. Int Angiol 1989; 8:61–65.

105. Tsouderos Y. Are the phlebotonic properties shown in clinical pharmacology predictive of a therapeutic benefit in chronic venous insufficiency? Our experience with Daflon 500 mg Int Angiol 1989; 8:53–59.

106. Ciapponi A, Laffaire E, Roque M. Calcium dobesilate for chronic venous insufficiency: a systermatic review. Angiology 2004; 55:147–154.

107. Arceo A, Berber A, Trevino C. Clinical evaluation of the efficacy and safety of calcium dobesilate in patients with chronic venous insufficiency of the lower limbs. Angiology 2002; 53:539–544.

108. Poynard T, Valterio C. Meta-analysis of hydroxyethylrutosides in the treatment of chronic venous insufficiency. VASA 1994; 23:244–250.

109. Wadworth AV, Faulds D. Hydroxyethylrutosides: a review of its pharmacology, and therapeutic efficacy in venous insufficiency and related disorders. Drugs 1992; 44:1013–1032.

110. Boyle P, Diehm C, Robertson C. Meta-analysis of clinical trials of Cyclo 3 Fort in the treatment of chronic venous insufficiency. Int Angiol 2003; 22:250–262.

111. Siebert U, Brach M, Sroczynski G, et al. Efficacy, routine effectiveness, and safety of horsechestnut seed extract in the treatment of chronic venous insufficiency. A meta-analysis of randomized controlled trials and large observational studies. Int Angiol 2002; 21:305–315.

112. Pittler MH, Ernst E. Horse-chestnut seed extract for chronic venous insufficiency. A criteria-based systematic review. Arch Dermatol 1998; 134:1356–1360.

113. Geroulakos G, Nicolaides AN. Controlled studies of Daflon 500 mg in chronic venous insufficiency. Angiology 1994; 45:549–553.

114. Lyseng-Williamson KA, Perry CM. Micronised Purified Flavonoid Fraction. A review of its use in chronic venous insufficiency, venous ulcers and haemorrhoids. Drugs 2003; 63:71–100.

115. Boada JN. Therapeutic effect of venotonics in chronic venous insufficiency. Clin Drug Invest 1999; 18:413–432.

116. Jantet G, the RELIEF Study Group. Chronic venous insufficiency: worldwide results of the RELIEF study. Reflux assEssment and quaLity of life improvEment with micronized Flavonoids. Angiology 2002; 53:245–256.

117. Bérard A, Kurz X, Zuccarelli F, et al. Reliability study of Leg-O-Meter, an improved tape measure device in patients with chronic venous insufficiency of the leg. Angiology 1998; 49:169–173.

118. Brijker F, Heijdra YF, Van den Elshout FJJ, et al. Volumetric measurements of peripheral oedema in clinical conditions. Clin Physio 2000; 20:56–61.

119. Vayssairat M, Maurel A, Gouny, et al. La volumétrie: une méthode précise de quantification en phlébologie (in French). J Mal Vasc 1994; 19:108–110.

120. Garde C, Nicolaides A, Guex JJ, Grondin L, et al. Consensus meeting on the action of phlebotropic drugs on chronic venous disease-related edema (in French). Phlébologie 2004; 57:7–13.

121. Stanton AWB, Northfield JW, Holroyd B, et al. Validation of an optoelectronic limb volumeter (Perometer®). Lymphology 1997; 30:77–97.

122. Perrin M, Guex JJ. Edema and leg volume: methods of assessment. Angiology 2000; 51:9–12.

123. Vayssairat M. and the French Venous Naphtazone Trial Group. Placebo-controlled trial of naphtazone in women with primary uncomplicated symptomatic varicose veins. Phlebology 1997; 12:17–20.

124. Diehm C, Trampish HJ, Lange S, Schmidt C. Comparison of leg compression stocking and oral horse-chestnut extract therapy in patients with chronic venous insufficiency. Lancet 1996; 347:292–294.

125. Blume J, Langenbahn H, de Champvallins M. Quantification of edema using the volometer technique; therapeutic application of Daflon 500 mg in chronic venous insufficiency. Phlebology 1992; 7:S37–S40.

126. Cesarone MR, Belcaro G, Brandolini R, et al. The LONFLIT4-Venoruton Study: a randomized trial–prophylaxis of flight-edema in venous patients. Angiology 2003; 54:137–142.

127. Cesarone MR, Belcaro G, Geroulakos G, et al. Flight microangiopathy on long-haul flights: prevention of edema and microcirculation alterations with Venoruton. Clin Appl Thromb Hemost 2003; 9:109–114.

128. Guilhou J-J, Dereure O, Marzin L, et al. Efficacy of Daflon 500 mg in venous leg ulcer healing: a double-blind, randomized, controlled versus placebo trial in 107 patients. Angiology 1997; 48:77–85.

129. Gliński W, Chodynicka B, Roszkiewicz J, et al. The beneficial augmentative effect of micronised purified flavonoid fraction (MPFF) on the healing of leg ulcers: an open, multicentre, controlled, randomised study. Phlebology 1999; 14:151–157.

130. Roztocil K, Sterinova V, Strejcek J. Efficacy of a 6-month treatment with Daflon 500 mg in patients with venous leg ulcers associated with chronic venous insufficiency. Int Angiol 2003; 22:24–31.

131. Ramelet AA. Clinical benefits of Daflon 500 mg in the most severe stages of chronic venous insufficiency. Angiology 2001; 52:S49–S56.

132. Ramelet AA, Coleridge-Smith PD, Gloviczki P. A meta-analysis of venous leg ulcer healing in prospective randomised studies using Micronized Purified Flavonoid Fraction. J Mal Vasc 2004; 29:1S43.

133. Ottillinger B, Greeske K. Rational therapy of chronic venous insufficiency—chances and limits of the therapeutic use of horse-chestnut seeds extract. BMC Cardiovasc Disord 2001; 1:5.

134. Wright DD, Franks PJ, Blair SD, Backhouse CM, Moffatt C, McCollum CN. Oxerutins in the prevention of recurrence in chronic venous ulceration: randomized controlled trial. Br J Surg 1991; 78:1269–1270.

135. Jull A, Waters J, Arroll B. Pentoxifylline for treatment of venous leg ulcers: a systematic review. Lancet 2002; 359:1550.

21

Surgical Treatment of Varicose Veins

Steven S. Kang
South Miami Heart Center, Miami, Florida, U.S.A.

The surgical treatment of varicose veins most commonly consists of ligation and stripping the great saphenous vein, which eliminates or reduces venous hypertension from truncal reflux, and avulsion of subcutaneous varicose veins. The small saphenous is less frequently treated. The following is a description of these procedures, which are effective and cosmetic.

GREAT SAPHENOUS VEIN LIGATION AND STRIPPING

Before being taken to the operating room, I have the patient stand to distend the veins and use an indelible marker to draw the outlines of varicose veins (Fig. 1). I draw lines on either side of the varicose vein so that I know the relative size. Often the saphenous vein itself is visible or palpable about the knee and this should be marked as well.

Light general or spinal anesthesia is used although the procedure can be done with local anesthesia in the groin with a femoral nerve block. The patient is placed supine. Some surgeons use a tourniquet but I do not think it is necessary. The incision to expose the saphenofemoral junction is made directly in the groin skin crease just medial to the femoral pulse. This is more cosmetic than below the skin crease. In thin patients, it need not be longer than two or three cm.

After dividing the saphenous fascia, blunt finger dissection will readily reveal the saphenous vein or one of it proximal branches. A small self-retaining retractor or Army–Navy retractors can be used. Branches are exposed sufficiently to ligate and divide them. This allows dissection and mobilization of the saphenous vein proximally to the fossa ovalis (Fig. 2). The junction of the saphenous and femoral veins should be clearly visualized. A right-angled clamp then is placed across the saphenous vein a couple of centimeters distal to the saphenofemoral junction and another clamp placed further down. The vein is divided between the clamps. The origin of the saphenous vein then is simply ligated with a 2–0 silk; any complicated suturing is not necessary. The clamp is removed before cutting the suture to visualize that the ligature is flush with the femoral vein.

The remaining distal end of the saphenous vein is addressed next. It is worthwhile to place the Army–Navy retractor in the inferior aspect of the incision to see if the

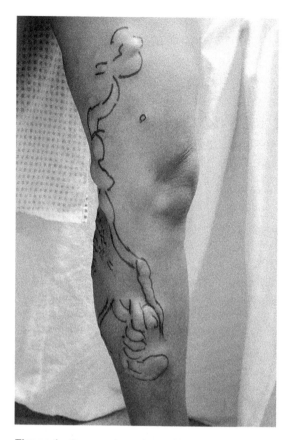

Figure 1 Preoperative vein marking. (*See color insert.*)

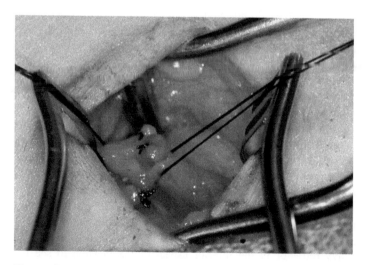

Figure 2 Groin incision. The foot is to the left. The silk loop on the right is just distal to the saphenofemoral junction. (*See color insert.*)

anterior or posterior branches are visible. Clipping and dividing the branches will reduce bleeding in the upper thigh. A disposable plastic Codman stripper is then passed into the open end of the saphenous vein down to below the knee. The tip of the stripper then can be palpated posterior to the medial edge of the proximal tibia. Sometimes the tip will be felt a short distance into the posterior or anterior arch vein. A 4 or 5 mm incision is then made on the skin directly over the tip of the stripper, and with blunt dissection the vein containing the tip can be exposed. The vein is incised and the stripper pushed or pulled out above the skin.

Sometimes the stripper will enter a branch and end up near the skin of the medial or anterior thigh. The stripper can be retracted and by twisting it, can be reoriented in the main trunk. Occasionally, the saphenous itself is tortuous enough to prevent passage down to the knee. In those cases, the saphenous vein can be exposed in the thigh where the tip is held up, and a second stripper can be passed from there to the proximal calf. Another option, when the location of the saphenous vein below the knee has been marked, is to bluntly deliver the saphenous vein through a small incision there and pass the stripper to the groin.

Once the distal end of the stripper has been delivered through the skin incision, a long #1 silk suture is tied securely around the proximal end of the vein. The acorn head that comes with the stripper is not used. The bed is placed in slight Trendelenberg to reduce bleeding. The distal end of the stripper is pulled toward the foot causing the bulbous end of the stripper to invaginate into the lumen of the saphenous vein. Continued traction causes the proximal end of the vein to follow the stripper into the vein, with tearing of branches, and inversion of the vein. As the stripper exits the distal incision, the inverted vein follows it and the entire segment cannulated by the stripper can be removed. If the vein breaks before the distal end is delivered, the silk suture can be used as a guide to allow retrieval of the retained segment through limited incisions on the thigh. After the vein is delivered, manual compression is applied for a few minutes along the course of the vein to stop bleeding from the avulsed branches. The groin incision is closed with absorbable suture and skin approximated with subcuticular suture and steristrip. The distal incision may use a single subcuticular stitch or just a steristrip.

SMALL SAPHENOUS LIGATION AND STRIPPING

The small saphenous vein may require ligation alone or ligation and stripping. Since the termination of the small saphenous vein is quite variable, its location should be marked on the skin with duplex ultrasound evaluation prior to surgery. After anesthesia is administered, the patient is placed prone. A skin crease incision is made at the popliteal fossa or more proximally where the saphenopopliteal junction has been marked. After incision of the fascia, the saphenous vein is identified and dissected proximally to the popliteal vein. The gastrocnemial and Giacomini veins are often encountered and may be confused with the saphenopopliteal junction. The true saphenopopliteal junction is clear when the popliteal artery and common peroneal nerve are identified. Ligation and division of the saphenopopliteal junction is performed as for the saphenofemoral junction. Stripping of the small saphenous vein is not considered necessary by many surgeons and often only a few centimeters within reach of the incision are avulsed. A stripper may be passed distally and various lengths may be stripped with the inversion technique as described above. The incision is closed in similar fashion to the groin expect that a heavier suture (0 or 2–0) is used for the fascia.

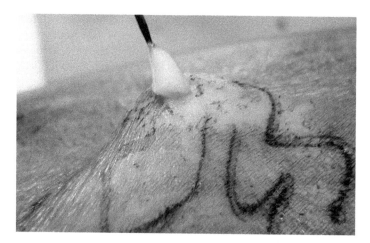

Figure 3   A crochet hook delivers the varicose vein out of the stab incision. (*See color insert.*)

STAB AVULSIONS

The previously marked varicose veins are removed piecemeal. A 3 or 4 mm incision is made by stabbing the skin with an 11 scalpel blade deep enough to penetrate the subcutaneous fat. These incisions are oriented vertically except in the groin, knee, and ankle creases, where Langer's line are followed. Various crochet-type hooks are available to fish out the vein. The hook is inserted into the incision and bluntly moved back and forth across the course of the varicose vein to isolate it from the surrounding tissues. The adventitia of the vein is then caught with the hook and the vein is drawn out above the skin (Fig 3). Instead of hooks, a very fine-tipped mosquito clamp may be used to dissect and pull up the vein. Once the vein is exposed outside of the incision, it is grasped with a heavier mosquito clamp or the loop of the vein controlled (Fig. 4). Additional clamps are placed on either end of the loop and each end is pulled. As more length of vein is exposed,

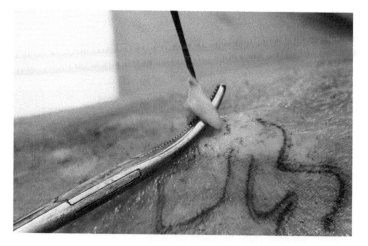

Figure 4   A clamp is placed through the loop of vein prior to clamping the vein on either end. (*See color insert.*)

the clamps are moved closer to the incision so that when the vein breaks, it will not retract so much. After both ends have broken off, another stab incision is made far enough away from the previous incision to find another segment of vein. Bleeding points are controlled with manual compression. Incisions are approximated with steristrips only.

POSTOPERATIVE CARE

The foot and leg are wrapped with gauze rolls and compression bandages. Patients are discharged after a short recovery. They are instructed to walk at least several minutes every waking hour and to elevate their legs when not walking. The bandages are removed after four or five days. Compression stockings are worn daily for at least one month.

KEY POINTS

- Preoperatively the varicosities should be marked on the skin with the patient standing
- The sapheno-femoral junction should be clearly identified before division
- The great saphenous vein should be stripped from groin to below knee using an invaginating technique
- The sapheno-politeal junction should be marked on the skin with Duplex preoperatively
- Stripping of the short saphenous vein is not always needed
- Small "stab" incisions are used to avulse varicosities as marked using hooks or fine clips.

22

Assessment and Surgical Treatment of Recurrent Varicose Veins

James E. McCaslin and Ronald K. G. Eifell
Department of Vascular and General Surgery, Queen Elizabeth Hospital, Gateshead, U.K.

Gerard Stansby
University of Newcastle upon Tyne, Newcastle upon Tyne, U.K.

INTRODUCTION

Recurrent varicose veins are relatively common and pose a particular problem to the surgeon. Prevention is better than cure and the rates of recurrence can be minimized by preoperative color duplex scanning and meticulous technique at primary surgery such as ensuring the ligation of the long saphenous vein is flush with the femoral vein and stripping the long-saphenous vein (1). Before any surgical intervention can be planned, a careful assessment of the sites of recurrence has to be rigorously performed. Re-do surgery is altogether more complex and should be dealt with in a different manner to primary surgery. The patient's expectations must be carefully managed and the surgery should be carried out only by an experienced surgeon.

ASSESSMENT

First, a thorough history of the patients symptoms and expectations should be taken. In some cases all that is required is reassurance rather than further intervention. In other cases sclerotherapy may be appropriate—but usually this will not provide long-term benefit if there are major sites of deep to superficial reflux. This should be carefully discussed with the patient. During the taking of the history the patients should be specifically asked about previous surgery and sclerotherapy including dates and an enquiry as to whether groins or popliteal fossae were operated on. Secondly the limb should be carefully examined to assess the pattern of the varicose veins and the sites of any previous surgical scars. Groin scars particularly can be very hard to identify and patients frequently fail to remember that a groin exploration had previously been performed.

The main investigation in most centers will be duplex scanning which has now largely replaced venography. This can define the anatomical pattern of recurrence and aid planning of surgical intervention. In most reports of recurrent varicose veins the majority

283

of recurrences are from the groin, with other major sites being thigh or calf perforators and short saphenous disease (2–5). There may also be multiple sites in a significant number of patients. Duplex scanning will also help assess deep venous disease which may be contributory in some cases.

The main causes of groin recurrence are either inadequate original surgery or neovascularization (6–8). In inadequate original surgery the sapheno-femoral junction will not have been ligated at it origin. In neovascularization thin-walled, new veins have developed to reconnect to the saphenous stump. Another important issue is whether the recurrence is feeding into a residual long saphenous trunk or accessory saphenous vein. It is important that these are identified, as surgery should aim to remove this to make clinical recurrence less likely if further groin neovascularization occurs. There is good evidence that neovascularization often occurs without leading to clinically relevant varicosities. Duplex scanning is good at classifying the nature of groin recurrences and residual or accessory trunks can be marked preoperatively to ensure complete removal. Likewise saphenopopliteal reflux and recurrence due to perforators can be identified and marked. In our view all patients with recurrent varicose veins require color duplex scanning preoperatively and failure to do so should be regarded as negligent.

Several studies have investigated the technique of interposing a barrier to neovascularization around the saphenofemoral junction. Material used include a reflected flap of pectineus fascia (9) and artificial materials such as PTFE, silicone and polyester mesh (10–12). Although there are some promising results more data would be needed before these could be recommended for routine practice in recurrent varicose vein surgery.

SURGICAL MANAGEMENT

Once the pattern of the recurrence has been defined, appropriate surgical management can be planned. In some cases, where inadequate surgery has left an intact saphenofemoral junction, surgery will essentially be the same as a primary procedure with the additional feature of difficulty in the groin due to scar tissue. This difficulty will be increased if neovascularization is present. Surgery in these cases is fraught with hazards, as thin-walled neovessels surround the sapheno-femoral junction encapsulated in scar tissue from the previous surgery (13). The surgical maxim of dissecting from normal to abnormal should be used. We favour the approach of Li (14–16). The incision is made either through the previous scar, or else just above the groin skin crease. The previous wound should be assessed in relation to the anatomical landmarks as often, in the case of a missed junction, it will be found to have been placed too low. It is usually sensible to make the wound somewhat longer than would normally be necessary for primary procedures, to allow better access and to approach the junction from a lateral direction. Li describes first dissecting down to the femoral artery, with care taken not to damage the femoral nerve. The femoral sheath is then opened, and the femoral vein carefully identified. The gives a safe guide to the level of the sapheno femoral junction and reduces the risk of damage to the femoral vein. Progress is made inferiorly, until the residual stump of the long saphenous vein is found, dissected, surrounded and clamped. Another approach which is sometimes useful is to identify the inguinal ligament and use this to identify the femoral vein superiorly and then dissect downwards to the saphenofemoral junction.

Any residual saphenous trunk should be removed and should have been marked preoperatively. Stripping or multiple avulsions can be performed, but stripping is to be preferred, and this may be done in an anterograde fashion. If this is not possible, retrograde stripping has been described (17). Preoperative duplex marking of the vein as it traverses the medial condyle of the femur allows a stripper to be passed superiorly along its course via a small transverse incision. This technique can also be used in the patient who does not require groin exploration, but has a significant portion of residual long-saphenous vein on duplex scanning. Care must be taken when employing this method not to pass the stripper into the deep venous system by way of a large mid-thigh perforator.

The recurrence rate following short saphenous surgery is higher than after saphenofemoral disconnection (18–20). Reported recurrence rates range from 40% to 61% following saphenopopliteal junction disconnection, despite the use of preoperative duplex marking (21–23). Saphenopoliteal re-exploration needs careful identification and avoidance of damage to the popliteal and sural nerves and the patient needs to be carefully counselled about the risks of nerve injury beforehand. Duplex marking or varicography to identify the junction is absolutely essential. If a Giacomini vein is present it should also be marked preoperatively.

COMPLICATIONS

Complications are more likely after redo than primary surgery. One of the more common complications seen in redo surgery for recurrent veins is the formation of a lymphocoele or lymphatic fistula (15). It is important to minimize disturbance to lymphatic channels in the groin if possible and ligation should be performed rather than relying on diathermy. Lymphocoele and lymphatic fistulae usually resolve spontaneously (24), although it may take many months and occasionally they have to be aspirated or excised (15). With the increased incidence of lymphatic leakage and consequent infection following redo groin dissection for recurrence (24), there may be a role for routine antibiotic prophylaxis in patients undergoing redo groin dissection, although no direct evidence exists to support or refute this. Certainly if there is pre-existing intertrigo then we recommend their use. Careful attention should be paid to closure of the wound to eliminate dead space and we advocate the use of interrupted (not continuous) absorbable sutures. We do not routinely use any wound drains although careful attention should be paid to hemostasis. Interestingly, advocates of endovenous ablation have postulated that haematoma formation after surgery may be a stimulus for new vessel formation after open surgery (25). We also routinely use subcutaneous low-molecular weight heparin as prophylaxis against DVT in these patients and have not noticed any major problem with bleeding or wound haematoma.

CONCLUSION

Recurrent varicose veins need careful assessment and an experienced surgeon. The use of color duplex scanning to plan intervention is now widely accepted as standard practice. The advent of new treatment modalities such as endovenous ablation may further improve the results of surgery for recurrence in the future.

KEY POINTS

- Recurrent varicose veins are relatively common.
- Patients should undergo color duplex scanning preoperatively.
- Common reasons for recurrence include inadequate previous surgery, neovascularization and missed perforators.

- Surgery for long saphenous recurrence may require re-exploration of the groin, local avulsion of varicosities or a combination of both.
- Residual long saphenous segments should be stripped or avulsed.
- Complications are more common than with primary surgery and patients should be warned of this.
- Newer modalities may improve long-term results in both primary and redo surgery.

REFERENCES

1. Winterborn RJ, Foy C, Earnshaw JJ. Causes of varicose vein recurrence: late results of a randomized controlled trial of stripping the long saphenous vein. J Vasc Surg 2004;634–639.
2. Garner JP, Heppell PSJ, Leopold PW. The lateral accessory saphenous vein—a common cause of recurrent varicose veins. An R Coll Surg Engl 2003;389–392.
3. Darke SG. The morphology of recurrent varicose veins. see comment Eur J Vasc Surg 1992;512–517.
4. Tong Y, Royle J. Recurrent varicose veins following high ligation of long saphenous vein: a duplex ultrasound study. Cardiovasc Surg 1995;485–487.
5. Jiang P, van Rij AM, Christie R, Hill G, Solomon C, Thomson I. Recurrent varicose veins: patterns of reflux and clinical severity. Cardiovasc Surg 1999;332–339.
6. Fischer R, Chandler JG, De Maeseneer MG, et al. The unresolved problem of recurrent saphenofemoral reflux. J Am Coll Surg 2002;80–94.
7. Van Rij AM, Jones GT, Hill GB, Jiang P. Neovascularization and recurrent varicose veins: more histologic and ultrasound evidence. J Vasc Surg 2004; 40:296–302.
8. Winterborn RJ, Foy C, Earnshaw JJ. Causes of varicose vein recurrence: late results of a randomised controlled trial of stripping the long saphenous vein. J Vasc Surg 2004;634–639.
9. Gibbs PJ, Foy DM, Darke SG. Reoperation for recurrent saphenofemoral incompetence: a prospective randomised trial using a reflected flap of pectineus fascia. Eur J Vasc Endovasc Surg 1999;494–498.
10. Bhatti TS, Whitman B, Harradine K, Cooke SG, Heather BP, Earnshaw JJ. Causes of re-recurrence after polytetrafluoroethylene patch saphenoplasty for recurrent varicose veins. see comment Br J Surg 2000;1356–1360.
11. De Maeseneer MG, Vandenbroeck CP, Van Schil PE. Silicone patch saphenoplasty to prevent repeat recurrence after surgery to treat recurrent saphenofemoral incompetence: long-term follow-up study. J Vasc Surg 2004;98–105.
12. Glass GM. Prevention of sapheno-femoral and sapheno-popliteal recurrence of varicose veins by forming a partition to contain neovascularization. Phlebology 1990;3 9.
13. Tibbs DJ. Superficial vein incompetence. 1st ed. Varicose Veins and Related Disorders. Oxford: Butterworth-Heinemann Ltd, 1995 pp. 86–126.
14. Li AK. A technique for re-exploration of the saphenofemoral junction for recurrent varicose veins. Br J Surg 1975;745–746.
15. Browse NL, Burnand KG, Irvine AT, Wilson NM. Recurrent varicose veins. 2nd ed. Diseases of the Veins. London: Arnold, 1999 pp. 225–230.
16. Bergan JJ. Surgical management of primary and recurrent varicose veins. In: Yao JST, ed. Handbook of Venous Disorders. 2nd ed. London: Arnold, 2001:289–302.
17. Mitton D, Thornton M, Beard J. Retrograde stripping of recurrent varicose veins. Eur J Vasc Endovasc Surg 2001;90–91.
18. Hobbs JT, Surgery and sclerotherapy in the treatment of varicose veins. A random trial. Arch Surg 1974; 109:793–796.
19. Doran FS, Barkat S, The management of recurrent varicose veins. Ann R Coll Surg Eng 1981; 63:432–436.

20. Mitchell DC, Darke SG, The assessment of primary varicose veins by Doppler ultrasound—the role of sapheno-popliteal incompetence and the short saphenous systems in calf varicosities. Eur J Vasc Surg 1987; 1:113-115.

21. Rashid HI, Ajeel A, Tyrrell MR. Persistent popliteal fossa reflux following saphenopopliteal disconnection. Br J Surg 2002;748–751.

22. Spronk S, B R, Veen HF. Subfascial ligation of the incompetent short saphenous vein:technical success measured by duple sonography. J Vasc Nursing 2003;92–95.

23. Sheppard M. The incidence, diagnosis and management of saphenopopliteal incompetence. Phlebology 1986;23–32.

24. Hayden A, Holdsworth J. Complications following re-exploration of the groin for recurrent varicose veins. Ann R Coll Surg Engl 2001;272–273.

25. Pichot O, Kabnick LS, Creton D, et al. Duplex ultrasound scan findings two years after great saphenous vein radiofrequency endovenous ablation. J Vasc Surg 2004;189–195.

23
Surgical Treatments and New Technologies/Day Care Strategies

Ronald K. G. Eifell
Department of Vascular and General Surgery, Queen Elizabeth Hospital, Gateshead, U.K.

Tim A. Lees
Department of Vascular Surgery, Freeman Hospital, Newcastle upon Tyne, U.K.

INTRODUCTION

Historical Perspective

Venous ulceration had been documented as a medical problem since the fourth century B.C., and the association between venous disease and lower limb ulcers was most likely made by Hippocrates (1) who was also the first to propose the treatment of venous ulcers using compression bandaging. Open surgery and elastic compression therapy have long been the mainstay of treatment of varicose veins and chronic venous insufficiency (CVI); however, relatively high recurrence rates and postoperative complications have led to the search for more efficient and less invasive treatments. As a result, the treatment of varicose veins has started to undergo a transformation.

Injection sclerotherapy has been used for many years with interest in foam sclerotherapy initially developing in the 1950s, although the technique never really became popular due to complications. Over the last 10 years there has been renewed interest in foam sclerotherapy with the development of techniques that have improved the quality of the foam sclerosants, enabling the treatment of varices that cannot be successfully treated with liquid sclerosants.

Subfascial endoscopic perforator surgery was described in the mid 1980s, but its role in the treatment of CVI remains uncertain and controversial, and as a result the technique has been losing popularity. Other less invasive methods of treating varicose veins such as endovenous ablation were pioneered over 40 years ago, but the techniques have only recently been developed using radiofrequency and laser energy to produce promising results. Other techniques such as transilluminated powered phlebectomy (TIPP) and external valvular stenting (EVS) have been reported in Belgium and Australia, respectively, over the past 2 years, but their benefits have not yet been proven over other techniques.

With the advent of less invasive, shorter duration procedures that do not necessarily require an operating theater environment, more healthcare professionals such as specialist nurses and radiologists have become involved in the treatment of varicose veins and CVI.

Indications for Treatment

The presence of varicose veins is not in itself an indication for surgery, but patients with symptoms and complications secondary to varicose veins should be considered for treatment (2). Signs and symptoms of varicose veins and chronic venous insufficiency are listed below:

- Venous ulcer
- Atrophie blanche
- Lipodermatosclerosis
- External bleeding
- Cosmetic appearance
- Aching
- Leg heaviness and leg fatigue
- Superficial thrombophlebitis

Treatment Options for Varicose Veins

These can be divided into surgical and non-surgical methods.

Conventional surgical options for varicose vein surgery include:

1. Saphenofemoral disconnection and groin-to-knee long saphenous stripping
2. Saphenopopliteal disconnection ± short saphenous stripping
3. Multiple phlebectomies

Non-surgical options include:

1. Reassurance
2. Elastic compression therapy
3. Sclerotherapy

New treatments include:

1. Subfascial endoscopic perforator surgery (SEPS)
2. Radiofrequency endovenous ablation (RFA)
3. Laser endovenous ablation (EVLT)
4. Powered phlebectomy (TIPP)
5. Venous cuffs/external valvular stenting (EVS)
6. Foam sclerotherapy

SURGICAL TREATMENTS

The objectives behind open surgery on incompetent superficial veins are the correction of the hydrostatic forces of saphenous vein reflux and removal of hemodynamic forces of perforating vein reflux, along with improved cosmesis. These can be achieved by the following methods:

- Ligation and disconnection of the long saphenous vein (LSV) and short saphenous vein (SSV) at the saphenofemoral and saphenopopliteal junctions, respectively
- Stripping of the LSV and SSV
- Avulsion of varices by performing multiple phlebectomies
- Ligation and division of incompetent perforators

SAPHENOFEMORAL DISCONNECTION (SFD) COMBINED WITH LSV STRIPPING

Technique

In stripping the LSV, a 2–3 cm oblique incision is made in or 1 cm above the inguinal skin crease, the lateral one-third of the incision being over the femoral pulse. All tributaries at the saphenofemoral junction are ligated and divided and the junction is flush ligated, taking special care not to narrow the lumen of the common femoral vein. A disposable, flexible vein stripper, such as a Codman® Disposable Vein Stripper (Johnson & Johnson, Raynham, MA, U.S.A.) or a rigid stripper such as the perforate-invaginate PIN® stripper (Credenhill Ltd, Derbyshire, U.K.) is then introduced into the cut end of the vein at the groin and passed distally along the LSV in the thigh. It is exposed distally through a short incision made close to the knee. The stripper is pulled through the wound and the distal end of the vein is ligated or avulsed. The proximal end is ligated around the stripper with a strong suture, which is left long. The stripper is then pulled distally, inverting the LSV, which is then removed through the lower incision. The groin wound is closed with absorbable sutures and the distal wound for stripping can be closed with Steri-Strips®. If concomitant multiple phlebectomies are required (see below), these are performed following stripping and the avulsion wounds closed with Steri-Strips®.

Results

The recurrence rate following SFD and LSV stripping is reported to be between 20% and 28% at five years (3,4) and Fischer et al. found that the prevalence of recurrent varicose veins following SFD approached 60% in patients surviving 30 years or more (3). In comparison, SFD alone has a five-year recurrence rate that is double that of disconnection and stripping (3,5).

Complications following SFD depend on whether surgery is done for primary or recurrent disease. The overall rate of minor complications (wound hematomas, wound abscess, cellulitis and minor neurological symptoms) is about 17% (6), whereas major complications such as deep femoral vein or arterial injuries occur in 0.05% to 0.8% of patients who have undergone primary surgery (Table 1) (6,7). The overall complication rate for primary SFD and LSV stripping is between 17% to 20% (6), while that reported for recurrent groin exploration is 40% (8). Lymphatic complications and infection are more common following surgery for recurrent varicose veins, where the incidence of each complication is 26% and 16% respectively (8). The reported prevalence of symptoms related to the saphenous nerve following surgery ranges from 6% to 40% immediately postoperatively (6,9,10), but in the long term, the patient's quality of life is

Table 1 Complications of saphenofemoral Disconnection and Stripping with Stab Avulsions

	Complication	Overall incidence
Minor	Wound hematoma/infection	2.8%
	Nerve injury (numbness/tingling/pain)	6.6%
	Lymphatic leakage	<1%
Major	CFV or CFA injury	0.05% to 0.8%

Abbreviations: CFV, common femoral vein; CFA, common femoral artery.

only affected by saphenous nerve injury, which occurs in approximately 6.7% of operations (9).

Discomfort and skin pigmentation can result from extravasation of blood subcutaneously during and after stripping. Methods employed to try to minimize this include leg elevation before and during stripping, use of a thigh tourniquet, and injection along the vein tract prior to stripping with a solution of lignocaine and adrenaline (2). There is no clear difference in the outcome whether the PIN® or the Codman® stripper is used, but the exit wound with the PIN stripper has been shown to be smaller (11,12). The risk of saphenous nerve injury is higher with full length stripping of the LSV to the ankle (13) and is reduced if stripping is performed from groin to the knee. In addition, the most significant calf perforators, known as Cockett's perforators, do not originate from the LSV but rather from the posterior arch vein of the calf. Therefore, stripping the LSV below the knee will not treat perforator reflux (14).

SFD ONLY

Saphenofemoral junction disconnection has been practiced with the objectives of controlling gravitational reflux while preserving the vein so that it may be used for arterial bypass in the future. Hydrostatic forces, however, are not controlled along the vein distal to the disconnection and reflux continues (15). Stripping of the LSV results in greater diminution of the hydrostatic forces that result from venous reflux than that achieved following high ligation and disconnection alone. As a result, recurrence of varicose veins is more common when compared with disconnection and LSV stripping with or without concomitant multiple phlebectomies or sclerotherapy (16,17).

SAPHENOPOPLITEAL JUNCTION DISCONNECTION (SPJ)

Saphenopopliteal and SSV incompetence occurs in approximately 15% of patients with primary varicose veins. It is well known that the anatomy of the saphenopopliteal junction (SPJ) is highly variable, as 60% of cases lie between 2 cm and 7 cm above the level of the knee joint (18). The SSV joins the deep venous system in the thigh or joins the LSV in 30% of individuals, and in 10% it joins the gastrocnaemius vein or LSV in the calf (18). It is for this reason that pre-operative duplex mapping and marking of an incompetent SPJ is essential. Ideally, both the junction and the point at which the vein penetrates the deep fascia of the leg, as well as the course of the proximal segment of the vein, should be marked.

Technique

With the patient in the prone position, a 2 to 3 cm transverse skin incision is made between the pre-marked sites of the junction and point at which the vein pierces the fascia. The fascia is opened transversely or vertically and the vein is ligated deep to the fascia. Any tributaries connected to the SSV are also ligated and as long a segment of the SSV as possible should be removed (2). Some surgeons advocate stripping of the SSV to the mid or distal third of the calf. Stripping the full length of the vein is unnecessary as reflux in the SSV is usually segmental (19) and the sural nerve is in close proximity to the SSV in the lower two-thirds of the calf. During stripping, the stripper and vein are brought through the skin distally through a small transverse skin incision and the vein is carefully separated from the sural nerve prior to stripping to avoid damage to the nerve.

Results

Relatively high reflux recurrence rates (40%–61%) have been reported following SPJ disconnection (20,21), despite the use of preoperative duplex marking. This has been attributed to poor operative technique (missed SPJ or suprafascial SSV disconnection), inadequate preoperative duplex mapping (poor identification of SPJ anatomy or perforators) or neovascularization reconnecting the popliteal vein to the SSV.

These recurrence rates might reflect a wide variation in practice by vascular surgeons performing saphenopopliteal disconnections. In a large survey of over 370 vascular surgeons in the United Kingdom, there was much diversity in the management of saphenopopliteal reflux (22). Duplex scanning was arranged for all patients by 89% of surgeons, while preoperative duplex marking of the SPJ was practiced by only 59% of surgeons (22). The low usage of preoperative duplex marking may contribute significantly to the recurrence rate, as failure to identify the junction is known to be a major cause of recurrence (23).

Complications include hematoma formation, bruising, popliteal DVT, sural and/or cutaneous nerve injury, and herniation through a residual defect in the fascia of the popliteal fossa, with an overall complication rate (excluding recurrence) reported in the region of 5% of cases (21).

SAPHENOFEMORAL JUNCTION (SFJ) RECURRENCE AND REDO SURGERY

It is estimated that up to 20% of all varicose vein operations are done for recurrent varicose veins (24) and the recurrence rate following SFD has been reported to be between 20% to 28% at five years (3,4). Stonebridge et al. found that the majority of SFJ recurrences appear to be due to inadequate groin surgery resulting from failure to ligate the saphenous vein flush with the common femoral vein or failure to strip the LSV (25). This is thought to result in dilatation of small venous channels due to altered venous hemodynamics and is one theory on the development of groin reflux. Later ultrasound and histological studies have found that neovascularization (serpentine, irregular tributaries) appears to be a principle cause of recurrence at the saphenofemoral junction, but only in the presence of a persistent LSV or major thigh vein (26–28). These findings support the discovery that using interposition silicon or PTFE (polytetrafluoroethelyne) implants may lower the incidence of neovascularization after SFD and LSV stripping (29,30). Only one recently published histological study failed to demonstrate that neovascularization occurs, favoring the argument that new vessels at the site of groin recurrence represent adaptive dilatation of pre-existing venous channels due to the change in venous hemodynamics (31). This finding, however, has not been reported by other researchers.

The commonly held practical principle in performing redo varicose vein surgery in the groin is to approach the SFJ laterally, by first exposing the artery, then continuing the dissection medially, as described by Li (32). Ideally the recurrent SFJ should be ligated and divided before more superficial dissection is performed. This approach is preferred to direct dissection to the SFJ through the previous scar, which is often associated with significant bleeding from irregular friable neovascularization around the wound, damage to the common femoral vein, and consequently inadequate surgery. Hayden et al. reported that this approach is associated with an increased incidence of lymphatic leakage resulting from disruption of lymphatic channels around the femoral artery (8). Such leakage, however, tends to settle with conservative management but can last for several weeks. The LSV should be stripped if still present. Occasionally a residual LSV may not be accessible from the groin if the upper portion of the vein has been stripped. This should be documented by preoperative ultrasound scanning and the course of the LSV marked on the skin before operation. The vein can then be accessed at the knee and a stripper passed from knee to groin allowing retrograde stripping of the vein. As mentioned, there is an increased incidence of lymphatic leakage and infection following redo groin dissection for recurrence (8), indicating that there may be a role for routine antibiotic prophylaxis in patients undergoing redo groin dissection.

MULTIPLE PHLEBECTOMIES (STAB AVULSIONS)

These are performed using a small blade and a special hook to deliver the vein through the incision, such as a Müller hook. Incisions are made over visible varicosities and are usually 2 to 3 mm in length. The risk of saphenous nerve injury is low compared to stripping the LSV below the knee. There is also a theoretical risk of injury to the common peroneal nerve during avulsions performed in the region of the neck of the fibula where the nerve is relatively superficial, however the authors have never seen this complication. Hemostasis is maintained with leg elevation, direct pressure, and venospasm.

PERFORATOR SURGERY

Incompetent calf perforators in the presence of significant skin changes of CVI are possible indications for perforator surgery. The most significant of the medial calf perforators (named Cockett perforators) connect the paired posterior tibial veins to the posterior arch vein rather than the LSV. There are three groups of Cockett perforators, called Cockett I to III. Cockett I perforators lie just posterior to the medial malleolus, while Cockett II and III perforators lie 7–9 cm and 10–12 cm proximal to the lower border of the medial malleolus respectively (14,33). These three groups of perforators lie 2–4 cm posterior to the medial border of the tibia (Linton's line or lane). Three other medial perforator groups known as the paratibials are located at 18–22 cm, 23–27 cm, and 28–32 cm from the lower border of the medial malleolus, respectively (14,33). They lie in a column about 1–2 cm posterior to the medial border of the tibia. Just distal to the knee is Boyd's perforator, which is the most proximal calf perforator that connects the LSV to the popliteal vein.

In the presence of a post-thrombotic syndrome, perforator surgery has been shown to be ineffective, with 100% ulcer recurrence compared with a 6% recurrence in the absence of post-thrombotic syndrome (34). This may be because the perforators are acting as collaterals for venous outflow obstruction.

OPEN PERFORATOR SURGERY

Technique

Most surgeons will only perform open perforator surgery after any existing ulcers have healed. Linton's procedure and subsequent modifications of this operation sought to eliminate perforator incompetence, so improving ulcer healing, but high morbidity resulting from wound complications has led many surgeons to abandon this operation (35). If the overlying skin is not in an acceptable state for open operation or in the presence of a clean, granulating ulcer, the SEPS procedure is preferable. Incompetent calf perforators should be confirmed and marked pre-operatively with duplex sonography. A longitudinal incision made directly over the incompetent perforator allows targeted dissection down to the incompetent vein. Sherman highlighted the importance of ligating perforating veins deep to the deep fascia (36), because perforating veins branch as they pierce the fascia from the deep compartment. This, however, is not proven necessary once the incompetent perforators are identified pre-operatively with ultrasound. The Cockett I perforator is inaccessible via endoscopic perforator surgery, so open ligation is indicated if this perforator must be ligated.

HEPARIN PROPHYLAXIS

There is no general consensus on the use of heparin prophylaxis in varicose vein surgery. There was notable variation in the use of prophylactic heparin reported in a survey of the members of the Vascular Surgical Society of Great Britain and Ireland, with just 12% of members using heparin routinely and 71% using it on a selective basis (37). Patients with obvious risk factors such as poor mobility, obesity, and advanced age should receive heparin prophylaxis (38).

NON-SURGICAL PROCEDURES

Liquid Sclerotherapy

Sclerotherapy involves the use of a sclerosing agent and has its greatest effect in the smallest incompetent veins, usually non-truncal varices below the knee (macrosclerotherapy) and telangiectasias (microsclerotherapy). The technique is not useful, however, if proximal venous hypertension exists and any proximal venous reflux should be corrected first. (With the new foam sclerotherapy techniques it is possible to treat truncal incompetence).

Sclerotherapy relies on the basic principle of inducing fibrosis of the vein and obliteration of the lumen by causing inflammation in the endothelial and subendothelial layers of the vein wall, produced by introduction of an irritant followed by external compression of the vein so that the walls lie in apposition. Following a consensus conference on sclerotherapy of varicose veins of the lower limbs in 1996 (39), it was unanimously decided that sclerotherapy is the preferred treatment of small varicose veins. These include telangiectasias, reticular veins, and venulectases. The definitions of these veins are given below, and the contraindications to sclerotherapy (40) are listed in Table 2.

- *Telangiectasias*: Flat red vessels between 0.1 mm and 1 mm in diameter
- *Reticular veins*: Dilated subcuticular veins, not connected to truncal veins or their capillaries
- *Intradermal venulectases*: These are visible bluish intradermal vessels that are sometimes visible above the skin surface, which measure from 0.1 mm to 2 mm in diameter

Sclerosing Agents

Following the consensus conference on sclerotherapy in 1996, the recommended agents for use in sclerotherapy (39) include:

- Sodium tetradecyl sulphate 0.2%–3%
- Chromated glycerine 25%–100%
- Polidocanol 0.2%–1%
- Sodium salicylate 6%–12%
- Hypertonic glucose

Other agents used include:

- Polyiodinated iodine 0.1%–2%
- Ethanolamine oleate
- Sodium morrhuate 1%–5%

Techniques

The veins should be distended before treatment begins, so the patient should be asked to stand or sit up for at least five min to ensure adequate venous filling. An alternative is

Table 2 Contraindications to Sclerotherapy

Absolute contraindications	Relative contraindications
Known allergy to the sclerosants	Leg edema
Severe systemic disease	Late complications in diabetes (e.g., polyneuropathy)
Acute superficial or deep vein thrombosis	Mild peripheral arterial occlusive disease
Local infection in the area of sclerotherapy or severe generalized infection	Poor general health
Immobility	
Confinement to bed	Bronchial asthma
Severe peripheral arterial occlusive disease	Marked allergic diathesis
Hyperthyroidism (in the case of sclerosants containing iodine)	Known hypercoagulability
Pregnancy in the first trimester and after the 36th week of gestation	Thrombophilia with history of deep vein thrombosis

to use a blood pressure cuff placed proximal to the veins to be treated and inflated to 40 mmHg. With the patient then lying supine or sitting with the legs horizontal, the skin over the veins to be treated is prepared with either alcohol or acetic acid wipes. A small caliber needle, usually between 25 and 30 gauge, is inserted into the lumen of the vessel to be treated and blood should be aspirated back into the syringe to ensure accurate placement of the needle prior to injection of the sclerosing agent (this, however, may not be possible with telangiectasias). If there is any evidence of extravasation, injection should be stopped immediately. The strength of the sclerosant used depends on the size of the veins to be treated. The manufacturer's recommendation of the maximum dose of sclerosants should be noted before treatment, as this will vary with the concentration of sclerosants. For example, a maximum dose of 4 ml of sodium tetradecyl sulphate–3% (Fibro-Vein™, STD Pharmaceuticals Ltd, Hereford, U.K.) can be injected per session. The volume of sclerosant used can be maximized if an "air block" is used by injecting the vein with air prior to injection of the sclerosant to empty it of blood and reduce dilution of the sclerosants (41). Compression is applied post injection with the use of a foam pad or cotton roll, a crepe bandage, and a TED stocking over the crepe bandage. Repeat sessions are usually required, but the interval between sessions should not be less than one week. Should further treatment be required in the same area, this should be done after three weeks. Compression should be applied immediately and remain uninterrupted for six weeks. After injection the segment of injected vein should have become a palpable firm fibrous cord and there should be no surrounding tenderness. Compression is best maintained with the use of cotton crepe bandages and firm cotton or rubber pads over the sites of injection. Applying class 1 elastic stockings over the bandage helps with compression and keeps the bandage in position.

Patients are encouraged to mobilize immediately after injections and should be advised to avoid prolonged periods of inactive standing until the compression bandages are removed.

Results

Recurrence of varicosities smaller than 4 mm in diameter is reported to be low. The permanent closure rate is approximately 90% to 95% (39,42,43). In larger diameter vessels (>4 mm), the recurrence rate is approximately 10% to 25%. Complications of liquid sclerotherapy include allergic reaction, skin necroses, excessive sclerosing reaction (thrombophlebitis), pigmentation, matting, nerve damage, scotomata orthostatic collapse, and thromboembolism.

NEW TECHNOLOGIES

New treatment modalities have been developed to minimize surgical trauma, reduce post-operative discomfort and shorten post-operative recovery.

Subfascial Endoscopic Perforator Surgery

The advantage of subfascial endoscopic perforator surgery (SEPS) is that it offers the opportunity to treat perforating veins using an incision away from the diseased area of skin, thereby avoiding many of the complications associated with open surgery. Hauer first introduced the technique in 1985 (44) and since then two techniques for SEPS have been developed. The "single port" technique (45,46), employs the use of a single scope with channels for the camera and instruments. Newer scopes allow carbon dioxide insufflation into the subfascial plane. The "two-port" technique uses one port for the camera and a separate port for instruments, providing improved visualization of subfascial perforators. The authors use a balloon technique using the Spacemaker® surgical balloon dissector (General Surgical Innovations, Cupertino, CA, U.S.A.) described below.

Technique

With a thigh tourniquet inflated, a 10 mm endoscopic port is inserted into the subfascial medial compartment of the calf 10 cm distal to the tibial tuberosity, but away from any diseased skin. Balloon dissection is used to separate the subfascial space, which facilitates port placement. CO_2 insufflation is used to enhance visibility and a second 5 mm operator port is then inserted under direct vision, distal and posterior to the camera port. Medial perforators encountered are divided using clips and sharp dissection, a harmonic scalpel, or electrocautery. Cockett II and III perforators and the paratibial perforators are accessed via a separate paratibial fasciotomy and are usually found within an intermuscular septum, which must be incised before the perforators can be divided. In order to visualize proximal paratibial perforators, the medial insertion of the soleus on the tibial may have to be exposed.

After all incompetent perforators have been treated, the ports are removed, the subfascial space is manually deflated, and the tourniquet is released. Any additional treatment, such as stab avulsions or high ligation and stripping, is then carried out and the subfascial compartment can be instilled with local anesthetic to reduce post-operative pain. The wounds are closed and the limb is wrapped with an elastic compression bandage.

Comparison of SEPS and Open Perforator Surgery

The main advantage of SEPS over the traditional open surgical techniques is a lower wound complication rate (45,47). In a review by the North American SEPS registry (NASEPS) of 155 SEPS procedures with concomitant venous procedures in 72% of patients, the one-year cumulative ulcer-healing rate was 88% following SEPS and superficial venous surgery with a median time to healing of 54 days (47,48). The cumulative rate of ulcer recurrence was 16% at one year and 28% at two years.

In a systematic review of the outcomes after surgical management including SEPS for perforator reflux (49,50), 20 studies comprising 19 case series and one randomized trial were identified. One thousand thirty-one patients with 1140 treated limbs were reviewed, and of those limbs that underwent SEPS, the ulcer-healing rate ranged from 56% to 100%, with a combined healing rate in 88% of limbs at a mean follow-up of 10 months. The reported median time to healing was 30 to 60 days and significant risk factors for non-healing and ulcer recurrence, as well as the early complication rates, are shown in Table 3. The overall probability of ulcer recurrence during follow-up is 16%.

Sybrandy et al. compared SEPS to open perforator surgery in a randomized study of 39 patients with perforator vein incompetence using duplex sonography (50), which revealed that both the ulcer healing rates and the recurrence rates were similar following both procedures. It was also found that deep venous incompetence, superficial venous incompetence, and the number of perforating veins had no influence on recurrence rates in either group. The complication rates were, however, significantly different. In the Linton group, 53% of patients developed wound infections while there were no reported complications in the SEPS group.

Table 3 Risk Factors and Early Complications of SEPS

Significant risk factors for non-healing	Persistent postoperative incompetent perforators
	Ulcer diameter > 2 cm
	Secondary etiology
Significant risk factors for ulcer recurrence	Obstructive pathophysiology
	Secondary etiology
	Postoperative incompetent perforators
Early complications ($<$30 days)	Infection (6%)
	Hematoma (9%)
	Neuralgia (7%)
	DVT (1%)

Abbreviation: DVT, deep vein thrombosis.

Ablation of the LSV

There has been a resurgence of interest in endovenous closure of the LSV since the concept was first explored over 40 years ago. Two techniques that are presently in use are radiofrequency and laser ablation.

Radiofrequency Ablation (RFA)

RFA uses radiofrequency energy supplied via a catheter electrode inserted into to the LSV. This is coupled with compression of the vein around the catheter. The result is resistive heating of the vein wall, which is maintained at a constant temperature by a thermocouple, inducing vein wall thickening, contraction of the lumen, and formation of a fibrotic seal of the vein's lumen. The Closure® radiofrequency catheter (VNUS Medical Technologies Inc, Sunnyvale, CA, U.S.A.) was first introduced in Europe in 1998 and was granted Australian and U.S. FDA approval in March 1999 (51). The system consists of a microprocessor-controlled bipolar generator and sheathable electrode catheters that are introduced intravenously. Two catheters measuring 1.7 mm (6F) and 2.7 mm (8F) are available (Fig. 1) and allow radiofrequency obliteration of veins measuring between 2 and 12 mm in diameter. Direct heating of the vein to a depth of 1 mm occurs in rings 6 to 8 mm in length during withdrawal of the catheter along the vein.

Patients with confirmed primary or secondary SFJ and LSV incompetence on duplex sonography are suitable for the procedure. The authors consider the following conditions unsuitable for RFA:

1. Vein diameter <2 mm or >12 mm. If less than 2 mm the vein is too small to cannulate, while vein diameters >12 mm give poor impedance when the patient is supine.
2. Very tortuous veins above the knee (curves $>90°$). This makes advancement of the catheter very difficult.
3. Thrombus in the LSV.
4. Any patient with a pacemaker or internal defibrillator.

The treatment of the SSV by ablation is not advocated by the authors due to the potential risk of sural nerve injury. The National Institute for Clinical Excellence

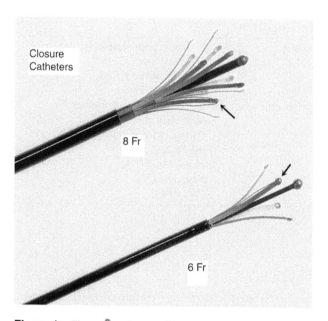

Figure 1 Closure® catheters with unsheathed electrodes. Arrows indicate the microthermocouple that continuously measures vein wall temperature and provides feedback to the radiofrequency generator. *Source*: VNUS® Medical Technologies, Inc.

(NICE) published guidelines for the procedure in September 2003 and they can be found at www.nice.org.uk/pdf/ip/ipg008guidance.pdf.

Technique

Ablation can be performed under general, regional or local (tumescent) anesthetic, with or without sedation (52,53). After adequate skin preparation, duplex ultrasound is used to map the course of the LSV from the SFJ to the knee, where it is accessed either percutaneously or via a cut-down procedure. Access can be achieved at the ankle, however passage of the catheter from this level can sometimes be difficult and the authors now favor access at the knee level (54). Access to the lumen of the LSV is established using ultrasound control and a seven or nine French sheath (dependent on the size of the catheter to be used) is inserted. The ablation catheter is then fed through the sheath and passed along the LSV into the common femoral vein under ultrasound control. Infiltration of the tissue surrounding the LSV with 0.9% saline and local anesthetic helps to achieve vein wall compression and reduces the risks of skin burns and paraesthesia from saphenous nerve injury. Following infiltration, the leg is exsanguinated by tilting the patient to 30° Trendelenberg position, elevating the limb to be treated and wrapping the thigh with an Esmark® bandage to compress the vein around the catheter. Manual compression is applied between the upper limit of the bandage and the SFJ. The catheter is withdrawn to a position just below the SFJ (usually below the inferior epigastric vein) (Fig. 2), and the catheter electrodes are unsheathed. At this stage, wall contact is assessed by measuring the impedance and the power level, and maximum temperature and duration of treatment are also recorded. With the target temperature set at 85°C, ablation is performed from just below the SFJ

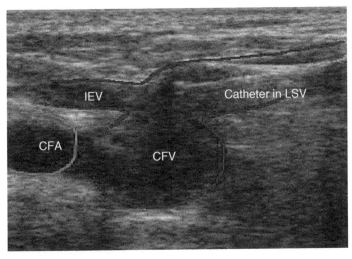

Figure 2 Positioning the Closure® catheter under ultrasound guidance. The electrodes are sheathed as the catheter is positioned in the long saphenous vein just below the saphenofemoral junction. *Abbrevations:* CFV, common femoral vein; CFA, common femoral artery; IEV, inferior epigastric vein. *Source:* Courtesy of Olivier Pichot, MD. (*See color insert.*)

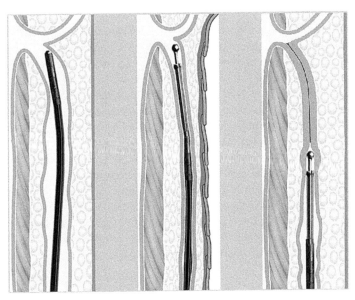

Figure 3 Schematic diagram of long saphenous endovenous ablation with Closure® catheter. The catheter is inserted up to the saphenofemoral junction with the electrodes sheathed. The electrodes are unsheathed with the catheter withdrawn to just below the saphenofemoral junction and the vein is compressed. The electrodes are then activated and the temperature allowed to reach 85°C. The catheter is gradually withdrawn as radiofrequency energy heats and contracts the vein wall. (*See color insert.*)

to the knee, by withdrawing the catheter at a rate of 2.5 to 3 cm/min and maintaining the temperature at $85°C \pm 3°C$ (Fig. 3). Heparinized saline is infused continuously into the catheter via a central lumen to avoid thrombus formation on the electrodes. Following completion, there will be minimal flow in the vein lumen before complete occlusion occurs. A duplex scan is performed to assess adequacy of the procedure and any residual patent segments are re-treated until satisfactory vein treatment is achieved. Local varicosities can be treated either by avulsions at the same operation or by subsequent sclerotherapy.

Results Following RFA

The vein occlusion rate following RFA is between 88% to 100% at one week and 85% to 90% remain occluded at two years (54). To date, two randomized controlled trials comparing the outcome of radiofrequency ablation with conventional surgery have been reported (55,56). Both trials have shown that endovenous obliteration resulted in less postoperative pain, shorter sick leaves, and faster recovery of physical function than following conventional surgery; however, both VNUS and conventional surgery have been shown to be equally effective in elimination of reflux in the treated LSV segments.

Complication rates were similar after both procedures, though the types of complications differed, with hematoma formation more likely in the conventional group, while thrombophlebitis and thermal skin injury occurred in the RFA group. In one case series only, a high incidence of DVT following RFA was reported (16%) requiring anticoagulation therapy and, in some cases, insertion of an IVC filter (57).

Overall operating times were longer in the RFA groups, but this was thought to reflect the associated learning curve as the studies were performed soon after the introduction of the technique.

Neither RCT assessed the long-term recurrence rate of varicose veins, but other follow-up studies have reported 10% persistent reflux and 5–13% recurrence at two years (55,56). There was no neovascularization reported after two years in limbs that underwent RFA (58), whereas neovascularization following conventional surgery at two years postprocedure has been reported to be as high as 52% (26). This is thought to be due to the lack of hematoma formation in the groin with RFA and preservation of the superficial epigastric and superficial pudendal venous drainage via the SFJ tributaries.

The treatment cost of RFA is higher than conventional surgery due to the cost of the generator, the radiofrequency catheter, use of intraoperative duplex, and possibly longer operating time. One RCT compared the cost of RFA to that of conventional surgery (56). Though the direct operative cost of RFA is greater than conventional surgery, the earlier return to work following RFA in employed patients influences the overall cost to society. The sensitivity analysis in one RCT showed that if 60% to 75% of patients are employed, RFA could be economically cost minimizing due to the earlier return to work following the procedure compared with that following conventional surgery.

Endovenous Laser Treatment (EVLT™)

The use of laser energy delivered endovenously via fiberoptic laser fibers was first reported in 1999 in Spain and soon after in New York (59). Laser ablation involves insertion of an optical fiber with a bare tip into the LSV. Partial compression is applied to the vein with a modified tumescent anesthesia technique. Some intravascular blood is necessary for heating of the vein as the chromophore for 810 nm laser is hemoglobin. Pulses of energy are delivered in 0.5–1 sec bursts, with a total power of 8–12 W for each pulse. Intravascular coagulation therefore occurs with this method.

Patients with confirmed primary or secondary SFJ and LSV incompetence on duplex sonography are suitable for the procedure. Based on preliminary reports on the technique from New York and Spain (59), there are no limitations based on the vein diameter. Contraindications for the procedure are as follows:

1. History of deep venous thrombosis
2. Hypercoagulability
3. Arterial occlusive disease
4. Poor general health
5. Pregnancy

NICE published guidelines on this procedure in March 2004. These guidelines can be found at www.nice.org.uk/pdf/ipg052uidance.pdf.

Technique

The following technique is a summary of that described by Navarro, Min, and Boné (59). Using duplex ultrasound, the site of the SFJ and the course of the LSV and varicose branches in the thigh are marked in the upright position. These markings are verified with the patient in the supine position and the skin is prepared for surgery with appropriate solution. The procedure can be performed under general anesthetic or local anesthetic, with or without sedation. Under ultrasound control, the LSV is entered on the lower thigh or at the knee, either via percutaneous needle puncture with a 7 cm, 19-gauge needle or a stab wound using a Müeller hook approach. A 0.035 inch J-tip guide wire is fed into the LSV through the needle and the needle removed. A 45 cm, 5 or 5.5 French catheter is placed over the guidewire and advanced to the SFJ. The position is confirmed by visualization on ultrasound and aspiration of non-pulsatile venous blood.

A bare-tipped laser fiber measuring 400–750 µm in diameter is introduced into the vein via the catheter and advanced to the SFJ. The patient and all staff in the treatment room must wear 810 nm laser safety glasses. The sheath is withdrawn by 3 cm leaving the distal tip of the laser fiber positioned 1–2 cm below the SFJ. The position can be confirmed in three ways: (1) by direct visualization of the red aiming beam of the laser fiber through the skin, (2) by ultrasound imaging, (3) and by previous marking of the distance from the point of entry to the SFJ on the catheter and fiber with Steri-strips. By observing the aiming beam, any inadvertent slippage of the laser fiber into the common femoral vein or the sheath can be immediately detected, as the beam would suddenly disappear. The fiber and catheter should be taped to reduce the risk of them moving independently. Tumescent anesthesia is provided with local anesthetic (lignocaine 0.5%–1% ± adrenaline) infiltrated to form a cuff along the LSV under direct ultrasound guidance and vein emptying is facilitated by Trendelenberg position. Manual finger pressure is applied to oppose the vein walls around the tip of the laser fiber. A wavelength of 810 nm diode laser energy is then delivered to the LSV 1–2 cm below the SFJ and along the course of the LSV as the fiber and catheter are withdrawn in increments of 1–2 mm. The parameters used depend on the operating surgeon and vary from 3–12 W in continuous mode with 0.8–2.0 sec pulse duration of 15–20 J of energy with an interval of 1 sec. The fiber is slowly withdrawn between pulses at a rate of 2–3 mm per pulse of laser energy delivered. A duplex scan is performed after completion of the procedure to assess the adequacy of treatment. If warranted additional treatments such as stab avulsions or sclerotherapy are carried out.

Class II graduated compression stockings are applied and worn for one week after surgery and patients are encouraged to start walking immediately after the procedure.

Results Following EVLT

There are currently no randomized controlled trials of laser treatment compared to conventional surgery in the treatment of varicose veins. Case studies report that the vein occlusion rate following EVLT was between 97%–100% at 1 week in two clinical studies totaling 130 treated limbs (59,60). Those that were not successfully treated at 1-week follow-up were re-treated with 100% of treated LSV remaining closed at nine months. The recurrence rate after two year follow-up is 7%, with the majority of recurrences occurring within the first three months (61).

Complication rates following EVLT are low. In reported series, there were no complications related to cannulation of the LSV such as hematoma or infection. Ecchymoses and induration around the site of local anesthetic infiltration have been reported. In addition, the procedure has been associated with no heat-related complications such as thermal skin injury and paraesthesia. There are also no reported cases of superficial phlebitis or deep vein thrombosis.

The equipment required for EVLT is expensive. The set-up cost amounts to approximately UK$27000 plus the cost of the ultrasound equipment, with a consumable cost of UK$250 per treatment. No published studies have compared the overall operative cost of EVLT with that of any other treatment for varicose veins. However, as with RFA, the overall comparative cost may be lower that expected as the procedure can be undertaken under local anesthetic, recovery and return to work is quick, and the consumable cost is relatively low.

One possible advantage of EVLT over RFA is larger vessels can be treated, as the largest diameter vein successfully treated with EVLT was 32 mm although long-term results still need to be assessed.

Transilluminated Powered Phlebectomy (TIPP)

This has been advocated as a minimally invasive treatment of non-truncal superficial varices. The TriVex™ system (Smith & Nephew, Andover, MA, U.S.A.) consists of an illuminator device, a powered vein resector, a system control unit, and a light source (62). The TriVex™ illuminator combines an irrigator device connected to a tumescent solution that is placed in a pressure cuff at 400 mmHg. Tumescent irrigation hydrodissects the tissue surrounding the vein clusters, which assists in their resection. The resector consists of a rotating inner blade with a speed ranging from 700 to 3000 rpm (forward and reverse).

Technique

The procedure is performed with the patient in the Trendelenberg position. After LSV stripping is completed, the irrigated illuminator and resector devices are inserted via two separate 2–3 mm incisions made just around the previously marked varicose cluster to be treated. Hydrodissection of the venous cluster is performed with a

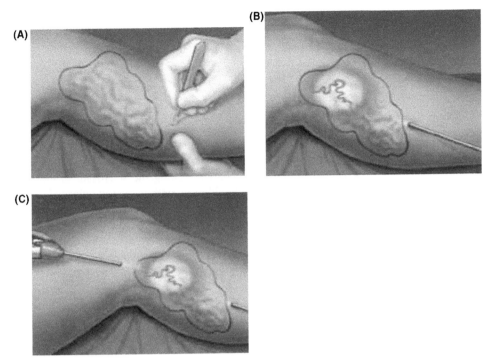

Figure 4 TriVex® system. (**A**) The surgeon makes incisions—as few as 2 per cluster. (**B**) The illumination device is inserted through one incision, allowing surgeon to highlight the veins. (**C**) The resection device is inserted through the other incision to remove the vein. *Source*: Courtesy of Smith & Nephew. (*See color insert.*)

solution of 1000 ml of 0.9% normal saline with 50 ml of lignocaine 1% with adrenaline 1:200,000, which helps to reduce postoperative pain and hematoma. With the veins transilluminated, the resector is inserted via the second incision and the veins avulsed and aspirated with this device (Fig. 4). Once the procedure is completed, the devices are removed and the wounds closed with Steri-Strips™.

Results Following TIPP

One reported case series of 15 patients with varicose vein classification CEAP C2 to C4 (chap. 6), found that postoperative pain is limited as the number of skin incisions is less than with conventional phlebectomies. All patients reported significantly improved symptoms with very good cosmetic results (62). There was one report of paraesthesia, which was thought to result from concomitant ankle to groin LSV stripping. These findings were not supported, however, in a randomized controlled study by Aremu et al. (63), who found that although there are fewer incisions in the TIPP procedure compared with hook phlebectomy (ratio: 1:7), overall cosmesis was similar in both groups. They also found no significant difference in postoperative pain, cutaneous nerve injury, or operating time. Other authors, however, noted significantly greater incidences of postoperative hematoma (64) but this was not evident in the RCT. NICE guidelines were published in January 2004 and can be found at www.nice.org.uk/pdf/ip/IPG037guidance.pdf. These guidelines have high-lighted that current evidence on the efficacy and safety of the procedure is of limited value due to the small number of patients and limited quality of reported data. It is recommended that clinicians wishing to undertake the procedure in the UK should have appropriate systems in place to cover adequate patient consent and to perform surgical audit.

Foam Sclerotherapy

Orbach first described the use of a foam sclerosant in 1950 (65). He suggested that vigorously shaking a 3% sodium tetradecyl sulphate solution improved the thrombogenic effect. Initial sclerosant foams were produced by shaking the sclerosant in the vial or syringe, producing bubbles with a high air:liquid ratio, with increased efficacy in smaller veins only. With larger veins, the air would position itself along the upper side of the vein, impeding contact with endothelium. Several surgeons have since proposed different methods of producing sclerosing foam for the treatment of varicose veins with the aim of increasing the efficacy and safety of the treatment (Table 4). By definition "sclerosing foam (SF) is a mixture of gas and liquid sclerosing solution with tensio-active properties (66)." The gas should be well tolerated or physiologic and the bubble sizes less than 100 μ.

Table 4 Techniques Employed to Produce Foam

Name/year described	Method	Foam quality	Duration
Orbach 1950 (65)	Shaking syringe/vial manually	Poor; of use only in small veins	Short lasting
Monfreux 1995 (78)[a]	Spigotted glass syringe with 0.3–0.5 ml liquid; piston effect of plunger to create 2–3 ml foam	Poor; low consistency, large bubbles	Long lasting (3 h in vivo, 20 min in vitro)
Cabrera 1997 (79)	CO_2 used in place of air	Medium quality	Unknown
Benigni–Sadoun 1999 (80,81)	Plastic syringes with fast pulling and release of piston	Medium quality	Short lasting
Mingo–Garcia 1999 (82) (minimal data available)	Device producing compressed air	Low to medium quality	Unknown
Tessari 1999 (83)	Two disposable syringes and a 3–way tap (sterile, dedicated kit)	High quality using STS	Reconstitution possible[b]
Frullini 2000 (84)	Similar to Tessari; different quantities of sclerosant and air used	High quality	Reconstitution possible[b]

[a] Dizziness and confusion are recognized self-limited side effects of treatment.
[b] System allows reconstitution of foam if treatment takes a long time.
Abbreviation:STS, sodium tetradecylsulfate.

Table 5 Recommendations on Safe Volumes of Foam

Vein Caliber	Volume of foam per single injection	Volume of foam per session
Telangiectasia and reticular veins	<0.5 mL with the Tessari and Monfreux techniques	Tessari technique: 6–8 mL Monfreux technique: 4 mL
CEAP C2–C6	No consensus reached	Tessari technique: 6–8 mL Monfreux technique: 4 mL
Small caliber saphenous veins	No consensus reached	Less than 3mL

Source: European Consensus Meeting on Foam Sclerotherapy, 2003.

Sclerosing foam displaces the blood in the vein, which enhances the sclerosant power of the agent. By using the foam technique it is possible to reduce the volume of the necessary sclerosing liquid and its concentration.

The authors advocate the use of the Tessari method, which produces a high-quality foam that is very compact with a small bubble diameter in a kit that includes two syringes and three-way tap. One syringe is pre-filled with air, which avoids the problem of using "nonsterile air" for injections. The foam lasts for at least two min and if injections take longer, new foam can be reconstituted easily. Following the European Consensus Meeting on Foam Sclerotherapy in 2003 (67), the following recommendations (Table 5) on the maximum safe volumes for use in foam sclerotherapy were prepared for different vein calibers taking into consideration the CEAP classification (chap. 6).

Results Following Foam Sclerotherapy

Foam sclerotherapy allows treatment of large truncal varices, which would otherwise not be amenable to treatment with conventional sclerotherapy. The success rate varies from 88.1% with the Monfreux technique to 93.3% with the Tessari technique at six months follow-up (66). Frullini et al. found that air sclerosing foam is as safe as liquid solution in terms of major complications such as DVT's pulmonary embolism, allergies and skin necrosis. The types of complications are similar to those occurring with conventional sclerotherapy (Table 6).

Table 6 Advantages and Complications of Foam Sclerotherapy

Advantages	Complications
There is no need for general anesthetic	Superficial thrombophlebitis
Can be performed as an out-patient procedure	Skin staining
The procedure can be easily repeated	Skin ulceration
Normal activity can be resumed almost immediately	DVT
	Scotoma (temporary)

Abbreviation: DVT, deep vein thrombosis.

External Valvular Stenting (EVS)

The principle behind external valvular stenting in the treatment of long saphenous varicose veins is correction of valvular incompetence at the SFJ with preservation of venous return via the LSV. This has been proposed to be beneficial as stripping or ablation of the LSV results in a functional obstruction to the movement of blood upward from the limb, possibly resulting in valveless collateral proliferation, which manifests as recurrent varices. The Venocuff™ and Venocuff II™ (Imthage Pty. Ltd, St. Leonards, NSW, Australia) has been tested both in animal and human trials (68–70) and for the procedure to be successful, functionally normal terminal and sub-terminal LSV valves within a dilated LSV must be present.

Technique

The Venocuff II™ Kit consists of designated "L," "R," and "D" stents for repairing the left and right SFJ, and deep venous valve or subterminal LSV valves, respectively. Cuffs have three holes on the belt to allow variation of the cuff diameter. The approach to the SFJ is via a standard groin incision. The Venocuff™ is introduced around the terminal valve of the LSV and the end of the Venocuff™ belt is introduced into its buckle and tightened to an internal diameter that is determined preoperatively by ultrasound assessment of the LSV internal diameter. The cuff should be positioned as high as possible on the LSV or CFV using the notch on the belt to ensure that it covers the valve ring. The valve repair can be tested by inducing a Valsalva maneuvre, and if no reflux is demonstrated using intraoperative ultrasound, the diameter of the Venocuff™ is fixed with a Prolene® suture through the buckle, the belt, and the common femoral vein.

As reported by Lane et al. (71), occasions where the SFJ valve cannot be made competent warrant EVS of the sub-terminal valve as well. If both the terminal and sub-terminal valves cannot be made competent, standard ligation and stripping should be performed.

Postoperative compression is important to reduce the incidence of SFJ thrombo-phlebitis, which is thought to be related to the rapid change in diameter of the SFJ. Compression is applied with a wool and crepe bandage immediately postoperatively and remains for three days. Thereafter further compression with single layer elastic bandaging is continued for a further four days. Based on work by the pioneers of the technique (70), the following situations are considered contraindications to the procedure:

1. Thrombophlebitis affecting the LSV or its tributaries
2. Greatly dilated LSV, >11 mm in male and >10 mm in females
3. Gross tortuosity and aneurysmal dilatation along the course of the vein

Results Following EVS

There are no reported randomized controlled trials comparing the results of EVS to conventional ligation and stripping. The largest reported case series assessed over 1500 Venocuff™ stents inserted over 15 years (71) and the same authors compared EVS with conventional surgery in contralateral limbs in the same patients. Studies have shown that 25% of terminal and sub-terminal valves are destroyed, stunted, perforated, split or in some other way damaged in patients with varicose veins. As a result the procedure is only successful in 50% of patients presenting with varicose veins (71). The technique has been found to be very useful in patients with varicose veins in pregnancy, however.

Recurrence in the long term has been reported at 8% in patients suitable for the procedure and the main complications include wound infections, which necessitate removal of the cuff (0.3%) and thrombophlebitis, which may or may not warrant removing the LSV. DVT requiring anticoagulation therapy has not been reported. Treatment of EVS failure as recommended by the advocates of this technique is by one of three methods: external stenting of the sub-terminal valve, removal of the stent with LSV disconnection, and stripping or preservation of the stent in situ with stripping of the LSV distal to the stent. Preservation of the stent is thought to prevent the formation of neovascularization. There are no trials assessing the efficacy and safety of this procedure, therefore more research and evaluation is required before this technique can be recommended.

DAY CARE STRATEGIES

The Royal College of Surgeons of England published *Guidelines for Day Case Surgery* in 1985, later republished in 1992 (72), which set the College's views on the scope of day case surgery and the facilities required. Since then reports by the Audit Commission for the National Health Service (73) endorsed the College's views and encouraged an increased provision of day surgery. Similar recommendations have also been made by the Department of Health Value for Money Unit (74) and the Bevan Report (75) on the management and utilization of operating departments. Since then the Department of Health launched the Day Surgery Strategy in January 2002 with the aim of improving day surgery strategies in the NHS. It was recognized that there is a need to increase the capacity within the NHS to meet current surgical demands, and day surgery has an important role to play in achieving this (76).

Day surgery is defined by the department of health as "the admission of selected patients to the hospital for a planned surgical procedure, returning home on the same day". Day case patients require operating theater facilities including general anesthetic and recovery facilities. This excludes minor operative procedures undertaken in outpatient or Accident and Emergency departments.

Selection Criteria

Suitability for day case surgery is determined by the type of operation performed, and the patient's health and social circumstances. The anesthetic and social criteria for day case surgery can be found in the Royal College of Surgeons of England *Guidelines for Day Case Surgery* (72) and is summarized in Table 7. These criteria should serve as guidelines for the surgical team and not restrict clinical judgment of the surgeon for individual patients.

The Audit Commission published an updated "basket" of procedures in 2001 that lists 25 operations that can frequently be performed as day cases. "Varicose vein stripping or ligation" is included in this list and "varicose veins, ligation and avulsions" is included in the list of appropriate operations for day case surgery provided by the Royal College of Surgeons. This includes saphenofemoral and saphenopopliteal disconnection and perforator surgery. SEPS, RFA, and EVLT should meet the anesthetic and social criteria set out for day case surgery (72,77) and based on these criteria they are suitable for day case surgery in the U.K. Redo and bilateral

Table 7 Criteria for Day Case Surgery

	Criteria
Patient information	Patients must be fully informed of the procedure to be undertaken and their likely postoperative course
Anesthetic	Age <65 years (Dependent on the individuals state of health)
	Patients requiring general anesthesia should be of physical status ASA I or II
	General anesthetic should last no longer than 1 hour
	The procedure should have a low postoperative complication risk
Social	Housing conditions must be sufficient to allow comfortable recovery and have an inside lavatory
	A responsible adult must be with the patient for 24–48 hr post surgery
	An escort must be available to take the patient home by car (not public transport)
	The patient/guardian must have access to a private telephone
	The journey home should take no longer than 1 hr by car

varicose vein surgery are associated with prolonged general anesthetic times and redo surgery also has an increased risk of postoperative bleeding and hematoma. There are no set guidelines with regard to redo or bilateral surgery; however, these factors should be taken into consideration when planning day surgery for such patients.

More experience and published data on TIPP and EVS are needed, however, in order to fully inform patients as to the risks and possible outcomes of the procedures before they can be widely accepted as day case strategies in the United Kingdom.

Liquid and foam sclerotherapy are performed in out-patient departments as they do not require an anesthetic or any supervision post-procedure. The suitability of various procedures for day case, in-patient, and out-patient surgery is summarized in Table 8.

Table 8 Suitability of Techniques of Day Surgery, In-Patient, and Out-Patient Procedures

Procedure	Suitable for		
	Day case	In-Patient	Out-Patient
SFD, LSV stripping and MSA	✓	✓	X
SPD and MSA	✓	✓	X
Redo surgery	✓[a]	✓	X
Bilateral surgery	✓[a]	✓	X
RFA	✓	✓	X
EVLT	✓	✓	X
TIPP	✓	✓	X
EVS	✓	✓	X
SEPS	✓	✓	X
Liquid sclerotherapy	X	X	✓
Foam sclerotherapy	X	X	✓

[a] The decision for day case surgery should be made on an individual basis.
Abbreviations: SFD, saphenofemoral disconnection; MSA, multiple stab avulsions.

APPENDIX I

CEAP Classification of Venous Disorders
American College of Phlebology (Revised Version 2004)

The letter "C" is based on the clinical findings, usually easily seen on physical examination.

- C0 = no visible venous disease
- C1 = telangiectasies or reticular veins
- C2 = varicose veins; distinguished from reticular veins by a diameter of 3 mm or more
- C3 = edema
- C4 = skin changes without ulceration
  - (i) C4a = pigmentation or eczema
  - (ii) C4b = lipodermatosclerosis or atrophie blanche
- C5 = skin changes with healed ulceration
- C6 = skin changes with active ulceration

After this number, the letter "a" is assigned if the patient is asymptomatic, and the letter "s" is assigned if the patient experiences symptoms. An additional number may follow the "s" to denote the severity of the symptom. More than one number may be assigned if the patient has several findings on clinical examination.

The "E" stands for etiology, and the options are "c" for congenital disease, "p" for primary disease (not due to another cause), "s" for secondary venous disease, usually due to prior deep venous thrombosis and "n" if no venous cause is identified.

The "A" refers to anatomic findings, and is usually based on duplex ultrasound examination. The options are as follows:

Superficial Veins (As)

1. Telangiectasias or reticular veins
2. Greater saphenous vein—above the knee
3. Greater saphenous vein—below the knee
4. Lesser (short) saphenous vein
5. Nonsaphenous

Deep Veins (Ad)

6. Inferior vena cava
7. Common iliac
8. Internal iliac
9. External iliac
10. Pelvic: gonadal, broad ligament, etc.
11. Common femoral
12. Deep femoral
13. Superficial femoral
14. Popliteal
15. Crural: anterior tibial, posterior tibial, peroneal
16. Muscular: gastrocnemius, soleus, etc.

Perforating Veins (Ap)

    17. Thigh
    18. Calf

    The "p" refers to the pathophysiologic component, and the notations "r" for reflux, "o" for obstruction, or "r,o" for both reflux and obstruction may be used.

    In addition, a disability score for chronic venous insufficiency may be used, with:

- "0" denoting a patient who is asymptomatic, and thus has no disability
- "1" denoting a patient who is symptomatic but can function without a support device
- "2" denoting a patient who can work an 8 hour day *only* with a support device
- "3" denoting a patient who is unable to work even with a support device

APPENDIX II

American Society of Anesthesiology (ASA) Classification of Patient Status

Class 1	Healthy patient, no medical problems
Class 2	Mild systemic disease
Class 3	Severe systemic disease, but not incapacitating
Class 4	Severe systemic disease that is a constant threat to life
Class 5	Moribund patient

KEY POINTS

Saphenofemoral Disconnection (SFD), Stripping to Knee and Multiple Phlebectomies:

- Widely accepted practice for the conventional treatment of SFJ and LSV reflux.
- The recurrence rate following SFD is between 20% and 28% after 5 years.

Saphenopopliteal Disconnection

- Preoperative ultrasound guided marking of the SPJ is essential.
- The recurrence rate is between 40% and 61% after 2 years.

Saphenofemoral Junction Recurrence and Redo Surgery

- Neovascularization appears to be the major cause of groin recurrence.
- Complication rate is twice that of primary surgery.

Scierotherapy

- Liquid sclerotherapy is useful in treating small varicose veins without truncal saphenous incompetence.
- Foam sclerotherapy allows treatment of truncal varices.
- The recurrence rate following foam sclerotherapy is less than 7% with the Tessari Technique.

Subfascial Endoscopic Perforator Surgery

- The ulcer healing rates are comparable to open surgery with fewer complications.

Endovenous Ablation

- Overall complication risks are low with no evidence of groin neovascularization.
- The procedures can be performed safely under local (tumescent) anesthesia.
- Radiofrequency ablation achieves 85–90% vein occlusion rate after 2 years.
- Laser ablation achieves 97–100% vein occlusion after 9 months.
- Larger vessels can be treated with endovenous laser rather than with radiofrequency ablation.

REFERENCES

1. Adams E. The Genuine Works of Hippocrates. London: Sydenham Press, 1849.
2. Bergan JJ. Varicoase veins: treatment by surgery and sclerotherapy. In: Rutherford RB, ed. Vascular Surgery. Philadelphia: WB Saunders, 2000:2007–2021.
3. Fischer R, Chandler JG, Earnshaw JJ, et al. The unresolved problem of recurrent saphenofemoral reflux. J Am Coll Surg 2002; 195:80–94.
4. Darke SG. The morphology of recurrent varicose veins. J Vasc Surg 1992; 6:512–517.
5. Sarin S, Scurr JH, Coleridge Smith PD. Assessment of stripping the long saphenous vein in treatment of primary varicose veins. Br J Surg 1992; 79:889–893.
6. Critchley G, Handa A, Maw A, Harvey A, Harvey MR, Corbett CR. Complications of varicose vein surgery. Ann R Coll Surg Eng 1997; 79.105–110.
7. Wigger P. Surgical therapy of primary varicose veins. J Suisse de Medecine 1998, 128:1781–1788.
8. Hayden A, Holdsworth J. Complications following re-exploration of the groin for recurrent varicose veins. Ann R Coll Surg Eng 2001; 83:272–273.
9. Morrison C, Dalsing MC. Signs and symptoms of saphenous nerve injury after greater saphenous vein stripping: prevalence, severity and relevance for modern practice. J Vasc Surg 2003; 38:886–890.
10. Holme JB, Skajaa K, Holme K. Incidence of lesions of the saphenous nerve after partial or complete stripping of the long saphenous vein. Acta Chir Scan 1990; 156:145–148.
11. Durkin MT, Turton EPL, Scott DJA, Berridge DC. A prospective randomised trial of PIN versus conventional stripping in varicose vein surgery. Ann R Coll Surg Engl 1999; 81:171–174.
12. Lacroix H, Nevelsteen A, Suy R. Invaginating versus classic stripping of the long saphenous vein: a randomised prospective study. Acta Chir Belg 1999; 99:22–25.
13. Bergan JJ. Surgery of the Veins of the Lower Extremity. Philadelphia: WB Saunders, 1985.

14. Mozes G, Gloviczki P, Menawat SS, Fisher DR, Carmichael SW, Kadar A. Surgical anatomy for endoscopic subfascial division of perforating veins. J Vasc Surg 1996; 24:800–808.

15. McMullin GM, Coleridge Smith P, Scurr JH. Objective assessment of high ligation without stripping the long saphenous vein. Br J Surg 1991; 78:1139–1142.

16. Munn SR, Morton JB, MacBeth WAAG, McLeish AR. To strip or not to strip the long saphenous vein? A caricose veins trial. Br J Surg 1981; 68:426–428.

17. Neglen P. Treatment of varicosities of saphenous origin. In: Bergan MGJJ, ed. Varicose Veins and Telangiectasias. St Louis: Quality Medical Publishing, 1993.

18. Vasdekis SN, Clarke GH, Hobbs JT, Nicolaides AN. Evaluation of non-invasive and invasive methods in the assessment of short saphenous vein termination. B J Surg 1989; 76:929.

19. van Bemmelen PS, Bedford G, Beach K, Strandness DEJ. Quantitative segmental evaluation of venous valvular reflux with ultrasound scanning. J Vasc Surg 1989; 10:425–431.

20. Rashid HI, Ajeel A, Tyrrell MR. Persistent popliteal fossa reflux following saphenopopliteal disconnection. B J Surg 2002; 89:748–751.

21. Spronk S, Boelhouwer RU, Veen HF, den Hoed PT. Subfascial ligation of the incompetent short saphenous vein: technical success measured by duplex sonography. Vascular Nursing 2003; 21:92–95, quiz 96–7.

22. Winterborn RJ, Campbell WB, Heather BP, Earnshaw JJ. The management of short saphenous varicose veins: a survey of the members of the vascular surgical society of Great Britain and Ireland. Eur J Endovasc Surg 2004; 28:400–403.

23. Doran FS, Barkat S. The management of recurrent varicose veins. Ann R Coll Surg Eng 1981; 63:432–436.

24. Bradbury AW, Stonebridge PA, Ruckley CV, Beggs I. Recurrent varicose veins: correlation between preoperative clinical and hand held doppler ultrasonographic examination and anatomical findings at surgery. B J Surg 1993; 80:849–851.

25. Stonebridge PA, Chalmers N, Beggs I, Bradbury AW, Ruckley CV. Recurrent varicose veins: a varicographic analysis leading to a new practical classification. B J Surg 1995; 82:60–62.

26. Jones L, Braithwaite BD, Selwyn D, Cooke S, Earnshaw JJ. Neovascularisation is the principle cause of varicose vein recurrence: results of a randomised trial of stripping the long saphenous vein. Eur J Vasc Endovascs Surg 1996; 12:442–445.

27. Nyamekye I, Shephard NA, Davies B, Heather BP, Earnshaw JJ. Clinicopathological evidence that neovascularisation is a cause of recurrent varicose veins. Euro J Vasc Endovasc Surg 1998; 15:412–415.

28. van Rij AM, Jones GT, Hill GB, Jiang P. Neovascularisation and recurrent varicose veins: more histologic and ultrasound evidence. J Vasc Surg 2004; 40:296–302.

29. De Maeseneer MG, Giuliani DR, Van Schil PE, De Hert SG. Can interposition of a silicone implant after sapheno-femoral ligation prevent recurrent varicose veins? Euro J Vasc Endovasc Surg 2002; 24:445–449.

30. Bhatti TS, Whitman B, Harradine K, Cooke SG, Heather BP, Earnshaw JJ. Causes of recurrence after polytetrafluoroethylene patch saphenoplasty for recurrent varicose veins. B J Surg 2000; 87:1356–1360.

31. El Wajeh Y, Giannoukas AD, Gulliford CJ, Suvarna SK, Chan P. Saphenofemoral venous channels associated with recurrent varicose veins are not neovascular. Eur J Vasc Endovasc Surg 2004; 28:590–594.

32. Li AKC. A technique for re-exploration of the saphenofemoral junction for recurrent varicose veins. B J Surg 1975; 62:745–746.

33. O'Donnel TF, Burnand KG, Clemenson G, et al. Doppler examination vs clinical and phlebographic detection of incompetent perforating veins. Arch. Surg 1977; 112:31–35.

34. Burnand K, Thomas ML, O'Donnell T, Browse NL. Relationship between postphlebitic changes in the deep veins and results of surgical treatment of venous ulcers. Lancet 1976; 1:936–938.

35. Linton RR. The communicating veins of the lower leg and the operative technique for their ligation. Ann Surg 1938; 107:582–593.
36. Sherman RS. Varicose veins: further findings based on anatomical and surgical dissections. Ann Surg 1949; 130:218–232.
37. Bradbury AW, Ruckley CV. Varicose veins. In: Beard JD GP, ed. Vascular and Endovascular Surgery. London: WB Saunders, 1998:432–459.
38. Wolf B, Brittenden J. Surgical Treatment of Varicose Veins. J R Coll Surg Edin 2001; 46:154–158.
39. Baccaglini U, Spreafico G, Castoro C, Sorrentino P. Sclerotherapy of varicose veins of the lower limbs. Consensus paper. North American Society of Phlebology. Dermatologic Surgery, 1996; 22: 883–889.
40. Rabe E, Pannier-fischer F, Gerlach H, et al. Guidelines for Sclerotherapy of Varicose Veins (ICD 10: I83.0, I83.1, I83.2, and I83.9). Dermatol Surg 2004; 30:687–693.
41. Orbach E. Sclerotherapy of varicose veins: utilisation of intravenous air block. Am J Surg 1944;362–366.
42. Gallagher PH. Varicose veins—Primary treatment of sclerotherapy. J Dermatol Surg Oncol 1992; 18:39–42.
43. Goldman MP. Advances in sclerotherapy treatments of varicose and telangiectatic leg veins. Am J of Cos Surg 1992; 9:235–241.
44. Hauer G. Endoscopic subfascial discussion of perforating veins—preliminary report. German. Vasa 1985; 14:59–61.
45. Pierik EG, van Urk H, Hop WC, Wittens CH. Endoscopic versus open subfascial division of incompetent perforating veins in the treatment of venous leg ulceration: a randomised trial. J Vasc Surg 1997; 26:255–259.
46. Bergan JJ, Murray J, Greason K. Subfascial endoscopic perforator vein surgery: a preliminary report. Ann Vasc Surg 1996; 10:211–219.
47. Gloviczki P, Bergan JJ, Menawat SS, et al. Safety, feasibility and early efficacy of subfascial endoscopic perforator surgery: a preliminary report from the North American registry. J Vasc Surg 1997; 25:94–105.
48. Gloviczki P, Bergan JJ, Rhodes JM, Canton LG, Harmsen S, Ilstrup DM. Mid-term results of endoscopic perforator vein interruption, for chronic venous insufficiency:lessons learned from the North American subfascial endoscopic perforator surgery registry. The North American study group. J Vasc Surg 1999; 29:489–502.
49. TenBrook JA, Iafriati MD, O'Donnell TF, et al. Systematic review of outcomes after surgical management of venous disease incorporating subfascial endoscopic perforator surgery. J Vasc Surg 2004; 39:583–589.
50. Syhrandy JEM, van Gent WB, Pierik EG, Wittens CH. Endoscopic versus open subfascial division of incompetent perforating veins in the treatment of venous leg ulceration: long-term follow-up. J Vasc Surg 2001; 33:1028–1032.
51. Harris E. Radiofrequency ablation of the long saphenous vein without high ligation versus high ligation and stripping for primary varicose veins: pros and cons. Semin Vasc Surg 2002; 15:34–38.
52. Merchant RF, DePalma RG, Kabnick LS. Endovascular obliteration of saphenous reflux: a multicentre study. J Vasc Surg 2002; 35:1190–1196.
53. Rautio TT, Perala JM, Wiik HT, Juvonen TS, Haukipuro KA. Endovenous obliteration with radiofrequency-resistive heating for greater saphenous vein insufficiency: a feasibility study. J Vas Interv Radiol 2002; 13:569–575.
54. Subramonia S, Lees TA, Wyatt MG, Oates C. Radiofrequency ablation in the treatment of varicose veins. In: Wyatt MG WA, ed. Endovascular Intervention. Shrewsbury: tmf Publishing Ltd, 2004:271–276.
55. Lurie F, Creton D, Eklof B, et al. Prospective randomised study of endovenous radiofrequency obliteration (closure procedure) versus ligation and stripping in a selected patient population (EVOLVeS study). J Vasc Surg 2003; 38:207–214.

56. Rautio TT, Ohinmaa A, Perala JM, et al. Endovenous obliteration versus conventional stripping operation in the treatment of primary varicose veins: a randomised controlled trial with comparison of the costs. J Vasc Surg 2002; 35:958–965.

57. Hingorani AP, Ascher E, Markevich N, et al. Deep venous thrombosis after radiofrequency ablation of great saphenous vein: a word of caution. J Vasc Surg 2004; 40:500–504.

58. Pichot O, Kabnick LS, Creton D, et al. Duplex ultrasound scan findings two years after great saphenous vein radiofrequency endovenous ablation. J Vasc Surg 2004; 39:189–195.

59. Navarro L, Min RL, Boné C. Endovenous laser: a new minimally invasive method of treatment for varicose veins—preliminary observations using an 810 nm diode laser. Dermatol Surg 2001; 27:117–122.

60. Min RJ, Zimmet SE, Isaacs MN, Forrestal MD. Endovenous laser treatment of the incompetent greater saphenous vein. J Vasc Interv Radiol 2001; 12:1167–1171.

61. Min RJ, Khilnani N, Zimmet SE. Endovenous laser treatment of saphenous vein reflux: long-term results. J Vasc Interv Radiol 2003; 14:991–996.

62. Scavée V, Theys S, Schoevaerdts JC. Transilluminated powered mini-phlebectomy: early clinical experience. Acta Chir Belg 2001; 101:247–249.

63. Aremu MA, Mahendran B, Butcher W, et al. Prospective randomised controlled trial: conventional versus powered phlebectomy. J Vasc Surg 2004; 39:88–93.

64. Scavée V, Lesceu O, Theys S, Jamart J, Louagie Y, Schoevaerdts JC. Hooh plebectomy versus transilluminated powered phlebectomy for varicose vein surgery: early results. Eur J Endovasc Surg 2003; 25:473–475.

65. Orbach E. Contribution to the therapy of the varicose complex. J Int Coll Surg 1950; 13:765–771.

66. Frullini A, Cavezzi A. Sclerosing foam in the treatment of varicose veins and telangiectases: history and analysis of safety and complications. Dermatol Surg 2002; 28:11–15.

67. Monfreux A. Traitement sclérosant des troncs saphènies et leurs collatérales de gros calibre par la méthode. Phlébologie 1997; 50:351–353.

68. Cabrera Garrido JR, Cabrera Garcia-Olmedo JR, et al. Elargissement des limites de la schlérothérapie:noveaux produits. Sclérosants Phlébologie 1997; 50:181–188.

69. Benigni JP, Sadoun S, Thirion V. Télangiectasies et varices réticulaires. Traitement par la mousse d'Aetoxisclérol a 0.25%. Présentation d'une étude pilote. Phlébologie 1999; 52:283–290.

70. Sadoun S, Benigni JP. The treatment of varicosities and telangiectasias with TDS or Lauromacrgol foam. in XIII World Congress of Phlebology. Sydney 1998.

71. Mingo-Garcia J. Esclerosis venosa con espuma: foam medical system. Revista Español de Medicina y Cirugía Cosmética 1999; 7:29–31.

72. Tessari L, Cavezzi A, Frullini A. Preliminary experience with a new sclerosing foam in the treatment of varicose veins. Dermatol Surg 2001; 27:58–60.

73. Frullini A. New technique in producing sclerosing foam in a disposable syringe Dermatol Surg 2000; 26:705–706.

74. Breu FX, Guggenbichler S. European consensus meeting on foam sclerotherapy. Dermatol Surg 2004; 30:709–717.

75. Jessup G, Lane RJ. Repairing incompetent venous valves: a new technique. Surg Gynaecol Obstet 1994; 8:569–575.

76. Lane RJ. The Correction of Pathological Venous Valves with the Venocuff. Sydney: University of Sydney, 1992:36–62.

77. Lane RJ, McMahon C, Cuzzilla M. The treatment of varicose veins using the venous valve cuff. Phlebology 1994; 9:136–145.

78. Lane RJ, Cuzzilla ML, Coroneos JC. The treatment of varicose veins with external stenting to the saphenofemoral junction. Vasc and Endovasc Surg 2002; 36:179–192.

79. The Royal College of Surgeons of England, Guidelines for Day Case Surgery, Commission on the Provision of Surgical Services. Editor 1992: London.

80. Audit Commission, A short cut to better services. Day surgery in England and Wales. 1990: London.

81. NHS Management Executive. Value for Money Unit, Day Surgery: making it happen. 1991: London.
82. Bevan Report, The Management and Utilisation of Operating Departments. 1989: London.
83. Darzi A, et al. Day Surgery: Operational Guide. London: Department of Health, 2002.
84. Royal College of Nursing, Day Surgery Information: Selection Criteria and Suitability, in Day Surgery Information. 2004: London.

24

Varicose Veins, Pregnancy, and Venous Disorders of the Pelvic Veins

Linda de Cossart
Countess of Chester, NHS Foundation Trust, Chester, U.K.

INTRODUCTION

Myths about varicose veins and pregnancy abound and vascular specialists have done little to educate doctors and the public about this common condition (1). Classification of varicose veins has relied almost exclusively on their clinical presentation and on the opinion of a surgeon to guide treatment. Until the development of duplex scanning, safe and repeated imaging of veins was impossible and the characterization of the underlying abnormality of venous valve reflux which causes them remained a silent contributor to their development.

New imaging technologies are now associating previously unrecognized venous abnormalities with chronic and common conditions such as chronic pelvic pain (CPP) and pelvic congestion syndrome (PCS). As a consequence, new classifications of pelvic venous pathology are being developed and endovascular and surgical procedures pioneered to treat them (2,3). The association of venous dysfunction with chronic non-vascular clinical symptoms is gaining prominence and will challenge vascular specialists to provide new remedies. Women, especially those of child bearing age, form the largest cohort of those affected (4,5). Pregnancy is the common link.

This chapter therefore sets out to provide details of the current understanding about varicose veins with respect to pregnancy, and the developing knowledge of PCS and its association with venous pathology. A scenario is provided at the beginning of each section to set the context.

Each section concludes with challenges to the profession to establish an informed and wise way of managing these conditions and ensure that new interventions are developed, researched and made available to appropriate patients.

VARICOSE VEINS AND PREGNANCY

Typical Scenario

A fit and well 37-year-old woman consults a vascular specialist and says:

> I have had three pregnancies, and my varicose veins have gotten worse with each one. I had phlebitis in the third pregnancy, which was very unpleasant. My GP told me that

I should wait until I have completed my family before having my veins operated on as they will only come back if I get pregnant again. What is your advice?

Factors Contributing to the Development of Varicose Veins

Varicose veins are unique to the human species and most commonly occur in the veins of the lower limbs. Since humans walk in an erect position, blood from the lower limb must return against gravity, back to the heart. The calf muscle pump and the changing pressures in the abdominal compartment are the main agents responsible for forcing the blood back to the heart. The non return valves in the veins of the lower limb facilitate this by closing in a sequential pattern and moving blood upwards. Each time they close they also compartmentalize the column of blood thus preventing venous back pressure being exerted throughout the vascular bed of the leg. They have probably developed this function as an evolutionary process and the body's response to the human posture. There is also emerging knowledge about genetic links and valvular incompetence (6).

Most pathological conditions in the venous system develop in the lower limbs as a consequence of malfunction of the mechanisms which control venous blood flow. They present as a variety of clinical manifestations. Varicose veins develop as a consequence of venous valve malfunction in the superficial veins of the lower limb. This impairs normal venous flow and creates venous back pressure in the veins distal to the incompetent valve, leading to clinically obvious varicose veins. It should be noted, however, that in some cases of reflux in the long saphenous vein there may no visible varicose veins. Pressure increases induced in the capillary bed by this reflux may lead to chronic venous hypertension with its complication of ulceration of the skin, classically in the gaiter area of the leg. The CEAP classification (Clinical manifestations, Etiological factors, Anatomic involvement, Pathophysiological features) is a useful and now widely used method of standardizing the clinical presentation of varicose veins (7).

Prevalence of Varicose Veins

The literature suggests that varicose veins are more prevalent in women and their development is associated with increasing parity, family history and obesity (8–12). However, the Edinburgh Varicose-vein study (mean age 45 yr) reported an age-adjusted frequency for the prevalence of varicose veins as 39.7% in men and 32.2% in women, which challenges the idea of this being a largely female problem (13). The difference in most published data probably reflects how the data is collected and often contains an inherent bias as they are usually on presentations to doctors, rather than being population-based investigations. They have also relied on the clinical manifestation of varicose veins rather than identifying the underlying problem of refluxing valves. If venous valve development is related to an adaptive response to erect posture there is no logic to support a gender difference but genetic associations with varicose veins may turn out to be sex linked. Clinical presentation however is a different matter and is probably genuinely more frequent among women than men especially in the younger age group.

Exploring Advice Given to Women About Varicose Veins

Advice offered to women about varicose veins and pregnancy is drawn from a sparsely populated research base, much of it based on hearsay. Healthcare professionals are responsible for sustaining these ideas, most of which are unproven by investigation.

The particular advice that women should defer any definitive treatment of their varicose veins until their child bearing is over is based on the notion that further pregnancies will create more varicose veins which themselves will require treatment. Out of expediency the advice to treat was combined with that of waiting until child bearing was complete. This takes scant account of the woman's symptoms or risks that may ensue from her varicose veins.

Two recent studies have explored this notion. One investigated the understanding of healthcare practioners about varicose veins and thromboembolic problems in pregnancy; the other the prevalence of venous reflux in pregnant women and its association with some of the commonly held beliefs about varicose veins and pregnancy (2,14).

In the first study, a questionnaire was sent to relevant healthcare professionals in one area in England, and analyzed replies from 849 midwives, 63 obstetricians, 21 vascular surgeons and 77 general practioners. The replies showed that less than half of those surveyed knew the incidence of varicose veins in the general population; only 50% recognized an association between the appearance of varicose veins and multiple pregnancies, and despite the fact that midwives held the strong belief that deep vein thrombosis during gestation was associated with the presence of varicose veins, less than one-third indicted that they would check their mothers for varicose veins. The majority of midwives, obstetricians and general practioners indicated they would prescribe support tights for pregnant women with symptomatic varicose veins despite there being no good evidence for this course of action. The study identified in this community a significant level of ignorance about venous disease and its association with pregnancy. It would be interesting to see if this is isolated to Cheshire (I suspect it is not) by questioning other communities.

The second study, which is the largest reported prospective study of the prevalence of venous reflux in pregnant women, investigated 331 women who, at their first antenatal booking at about twelve weeks gestation, consented to take part (14). The opportunity to scan these women prior to their pregnancy, while desirable, was not feasible. The investigators were experienced in the use of duplex scanning in pregnancy and investigated the women using their standard technique for examining the lower limb venous system, which was to position them on a tilting table at seventy degrees reversed Trendelenberg tilt for the test and to use Valsalva's maneuver and calf squeeze to illicit reflux. Women were examined during their pregnancy and after delivery. Leg symptoms were calculated in all women with and without demonstrable reflux, using the CEAP classification (7).

One in four women had demonstrable superficial venous reflux at between twelve and sixteen weeks gestation. It was assumed that this reflux had been present prior to the pregnancy. This was a higher prevalence of venous reflux than expected but is close to that described by the Edinburgh study (13). The refluxers did not have a higher incidence of a family history of varicose veins when compared with non-refluxers. No reflux developed during pregnancy in any of the veins of the lower limbs which were normal at booking.

Looking at the relationship between body weight and venous reflux the study stratifying 289 women, according to the standard BMI classification, into three groups, non-obese BMI < 25, pre-obese BMI 25.1 to 30 and obese BMI > 30.1. No difference in the incidence of reflux among any of the groups was identified suggesting that obesity is not strongly associated with the presence of varicose veins in pregnant women. A surprize finding, however, was that mothers of normal weight who had reflux had significantly higher CEAP scores than obese women with reflux and they complained more. The explanation for these findings is unclear, but many symptoms of varicose veins are "cosmetic" in nature and relate to the appearance of the veins, leg swelling, and skin pigmentation. Leg swelling may be masked by obesity. Obese women may have areas of skin pigmentation due to obesity and may therefore attribute their symptoms to obesity rather than varicose veins. As might have been predicted, the mothers showing no reflux had negligible CEAP scores. The prevalence of varicose veins in non pregnant women in the same age group would be useful to know, as well as in different ethnic groups, but this suggests that obesity does not predispose to varicose veins.

Multiparous women with reflux were found to have significantly worse venous symptoms than primiparous women (mean CEAP scores for each group 2.14 and 1.5, respectively). Their vein diameters were also greater. By comparison there was no difference in symptoms between multiparous and primiparous women without reflux (CEAP scores 0.37 and 0.29, respectively). This provides a clear link between venous valve reflux and the degree of dilation of the veins and the symptoms experienced by pregnant women.

Venous Changes in Pregnancy

Venous dynamics are altered during pregnancy. This occurs as a response to both the physiological effects induced by pregnancy and the physical effects on venous outflow from the lower limb veins of an enlarging uterus. These physiological changes are essential to allow the mother to develop a circulation which will safely sustain her and the growing fetus throughout gestation. They return to normal following delivery. The mother's circulating blood volume progressively increases by about a third during pregnancy, reaching fifty percent of this increase at thirty-four weeks. This blood volume increase is accommodated by peripheral vasodilatation which is mediated through endothelial-dependent substances such as nitric oxide synthesis upregulated by oestradiol and possibly prostaglandins PGI-2 (15). The presence of oestrogen and progesterone receptors in the vein wall facilitates the changes in tone of the vein wall (16). The role of mast cells and their relationship to vein wall remodeling may also play a part in this process (17).

The dilatation of the vein wall progresses as gestation proceeds appearing to reach a maximum in the superficial and the deep venous systems of the lower limb, at about 34 week (18–20). Most veins return to their pre-pregnancy size after delivery but some varicose veins do not (18). There has for some time been an assumption that along with increased relaxation of the vein wall, the venous valves become temporarily incompetent in order to accommodate these profound, but normal, haemodynamic changes. The persistence after delivery of this newly developed valve incompetence in superficial veins has been thought to lead to the development of varicose veins. Several longitudinal studies have been set up to examine this theory (19,21). They have not been able to demonstrate the phenomenon of a normal venous valve becoming incompetent during pregnancy. This remains the case in over 200 women now investigated for this phenomenon in our vascular laboratory (22). It is largely unrecognized by the healthcare community and even by many vascular specialists. The conclusions to be drawn from these studies are that new venous valve reflux is not created during pregnancy and duplex scanning can identify the problem. The traditional idea that all women with varicose veins should postpone treatment until they have completed their family is therefore inappropriate. Clinical judgement and the opinion of the woman must be taken into account for each case. Obviously not every woman with refluxing valves will either want or even need treatment for their venous reflux.

The physical effects of the growing uterus on the pelvic and abdominal veins are well known to midwives and gynecologists. When a woman in the third trimester of pregnancy lies on her back the enlarged uterus compresses the inferior vena cava and the common iliac veins and even the aorta in what is known as the aorto-caval compression syndrome (23). As a result, venous pressure is increased in the legs and venous flow patterns become less responsive to respiration thus impairing the abdominal and respiratory components of venous return. More significantly, a reduced venous return to the heart created by this effect may cause fainting. The clinical observation of this led to the practice of placing a women on their left side during delivery to avoid this compression. More recent studies have also shown marked velocity changes in lower limb deep veins in the supine position indicating vena cava obstruction (24,25). These obstructive effects however probably have nothing to do with the development of permanent venous problems leading to varicose veins. They are more relevant to the obstetric health of the mother than any vascular problems.

Treatment of Varicose Veins in Women During Pregnancy

In 1964 George Fegan, a pioneer in both injection sclerotherapy and treatment of varicose veins wrote:

> We have been using an injection technique for 14 years for treating varicose veins on 15,000 patients—one-fourth of whom were pregnant at the time (26).

This must be the largest series of pregnant women (3750) who were given inter-ventional treatment during gestation. Today, I believe that vascular specialists do not aim to actively treat varicose veins during pregnancy but aim only to minimize the symptoms of suffering women. An exception to this may be the need to perform a sapheno-femoral or a sapheno-popliteal disconnection for superficial thrombophlebitis which threatens to extend into the deep venous system. This has rarely been reported.

Fegan justified his course of action for treating women when they were pregnant by claiming to deal with their painful problem immediately and further, taking away their need to return to the hospital at a later date for treatment. He further justified his actions by the fact that he had had no thromboembolic complications with this approach. His meticulous bandaging techniques may have contributed to this; however, he provided no evidence to support this statement (27). His treatment was obviously appreciated by his patients and his clinics were full.

Today the most common treatment for symptomatic varicose veins during pregnancy is the prescription of support hosiery. Stansby pointed out that, "the idea that varicose veins may be treated with support hosiery is likely to be costly and to fail" (28). Coughlin presented her findings of a randomized study designed to explore acceptability, compliance and control of the symptoms and venous dilation with the wearing of Class One support tights by pregnant women with venous reflux (14). Eighty-three women with superficial venous reflux and no other identified venous abnormality were randomized. Increasing numbers of women rejected the tights as their pregnancy progressed with the last trimester being the final straw for most. Similar to another study, it showed that Class One support hosiery failed to control completely the superficial and the deep vein dilatation which developed as pregnancy progressed (29). The conclusions by the research team were that careful selection of women was needed before prescribing tights and exploration of other types of garments such as stocking "hold ups" should be considered. Support for the mother by a dedicated team of stocking experts might increase compliance (30).

Pregnancy, Pulmonary Thromboembolism, and Varicose Veins

Pulmonary thromboembolism (PTE) remains the most common *direct* cause of maternal death in the UK (31) with 56 women dying of PE in the five years up to 2002. It was highest in the 25 to 39 years age group. In the latest report of the Confidential Enquiry into Maternal and Child Health (CEMAC), it is reported that in the last 20 years, a demonstrable reduction in other causes, eg., hypertension and anaesthesia have been reported but no such improvement in the rates of death from PTE. Postpartum deaths following Caesarean section have fallen, however, and it is suggested that the adoption of published recommendations on the use of anti-DVT prophylaxis may have contributed to this.

Recommendations for prophylaxis against DVT are published by the Royal College of Obstetricians and Gynecologists (32). These guides indicate three levels of risk *Low, Moderate* and *High* for Cesarean section and these are presented in Table 1. Interestingly, these include in their moderate risk group "gross varicose veins," but they offer no reference to the criteria for such a description or reasons for why they are there. As mentioned below, the risk of superficial thrombophlebitis and its potential development into a DVT needs to be considered further.

Table 1   RCOG UK Risk Factors for Venous Thromboembolism in Pregnancy and the Puerperium

Pre-existing	New onset or transient
Previous VTE	Surgical procedure in pregnancy or
Thrombophilia	puerperium, e.g., evacuation of retained
Congenital	products of conception, postpartum
Antithrombin deficiency	sterilization
Protein C deficiency	Hyperemesis
Protein S deficiency	Dehydration
Factor V Leiden	Ovarian hyperstimulation syndrome
Prothrombin gene variant	Severe infection, e.g., pyelonephritis
Acquired (antiphospholipid syndrome)	Immobility (> 4 days bed rest)
Lupus anticoagulant	Pre-eclampsia
Anticardiolipin antibodies	Excessive blood loss
Age over 35 years	Long-haul travel
Obesity (BMI > 30 kg/m^2) either	Prolonged labour
pre-pregnancy or in early pregnancy	Midcavity instrumental delivery
Parity > 4	Immobility after delivery
Gross varicose veins	
Paraplegia	
Sickle cell disease	
Inflammatory disorders, e.g., inflammatory	
bowel disease	
Some medical disorders, e.g., nephrotic	
syndrome, certain cardiac diseases	
Myeloproliferative disorders, e.g., essential	
thrombocythemia, polycythemia vera	

Source: Modified from Ref. 32.

Factors Contributing to Venous Thrombosis

Venous thromboembolic disease is complex and stimulated by abnormalities of systemic factors and local venous conditions (33,34). It was Virchow who first linked abnormalities of the vein wall, flow and blood constituents as the three things which contribute to venous thrombosis. It is worth considering the vein wall and its contribution to thrombosis with respect to varicose veins because they have an abnormal morphology and do have an association with the body's fibrinolytic system.

The fibrinolytic system is the body's natural defence mechanism against thrombosis and relies on the release of tissue plasminogen activator (TPA), mainly from the vein wall, which then activates circulating plasminogen to plasmin which breaks down fibrin into its soluble fibrin degradation products (FDPs). The presence of FDPs in the blood when a thrombotic process is being lysed is the principle behind the commonly used screening test for DVT, the D Dimer test.

Plasminogen activator was convincingly shown to be present in the vein wall by Todd in 1958 (35). But it was Nilsson who in 1968 postulated the important clinical relationship between thrombosis and the level of plasminogen activator in the vein wall (36). Later with Isacson she suggested that there was a defective release of plasminogen activator in patients with idiopathic thrombosis and went on to hypothesize that deficient supplies of TPA in the vein wall may be a factor in the potential development of thrombosis (37).

The 1960s and 1970s saw extensive research on the vein wall and its relationship to TPA. The demonstration of a fibrinolytic deficiency in patients with venous leg ulcers led to the development of fibrinolytic drugs to treat venous leg ulcers, but they enjoyed a short lifetime of success. The key findings of the time were that lower limb veins had a significantly lower TPA concentration than hand veins; varicose veins had less activity than normal veins, and dilatation of the vein wall depleted it of its TPA reserves (38). This is summarized by de Cossart in her thesis "Plasminogen Activator and Vascular Disease" (39). During pregnancy, a dilated varicose vein, which already has an abnormal wall as well as a reduced TPA level, is subjected to dilatation and significant changes in flow, especially in late pregnancy, when the dilatation is at its peak. These factors all contribute to a thrombogenic environment in the varicose vein, which is therefore a vein waiting to thrombose.

When a varicose vein thromboses, it presents clinically as the painful condition known as superficial thrombophlebitis, and this is a recognized complication of pregnancy. The increasing evidence that superficial thrombophlebitis may extend into the deep veins and even cause pulmonary embolism indicates that it is not the benign condition once thought (40). Superficial thrombophlebitis is commonly recorded as a condition experienced by pregnant women but I have been unable to find any published case which links such events with DVT or PE during pregnancy. I would speculate, however, that some PE deaths in pregnancy may be associated with this condition. The obstetric community needs to be aware of these facts and advise women with varicose veins, especially if they are very dilated to seek advise from a vascular specialist between pregnancies.

Vulval Varicosities

Vulval varicosities are a benign condition, which is usually worse during the last trimester of the pregnancy. They often cause alarm when lumps appear spontaneously on the vulva and defy inspection because of a large abdomen. However, they rarely cause harm and, despite the theoretical risk, do not cause bleeding problems at delivery. Episiotomy, however, is contraindicated. Surprisingly, they rarely thrombose and they usually disappear following delivery. Detailed documentation of their prevalence in different societies is lacking. Before the advent of modern imaging vulval phlebography was pioneered as a useful means of planning a surgical treatment for them. They are associated with PCS, a condition that is very common and multifactorial in etiology.

Challenges to Vascular Specialists Concerning Varicose Veins and Pregnancy

Vascular specialists need to raise awareness in the healthcare community caring for pregnant women about varicose veins and their cause. This is particularly true with respect of the facts that:

- Venous valvular reflux causes varicose veins.
- Research has been unable to demonstrate pregnancy as a cause of valvular reflux.
- Superficial thrombophlebitis may lead to DVT and PE.
- Women are intolerant of support tights.
- There is a need to create a classification of varicose veins with respect to their size as an indicator for treatment to prevent phlebitis.

PELVIC CONGESTION SYNDROME

A Scenario

Recently a 38-years-old woman consulted a vascular surgeon and declared that she had been assured by another doctor that her CPP was most likely be caused by refluxing varicosities in the ovarian veins, which could now be treated successfully by surgery or interventional radiology. She wished to be treated by one of these methods as she had been seeking a cure for many years and had been extensively investigated by the gynecologists who were unable to offer help.

Chronic Pelvic Pain

CPP is common in woman of child bearing age. It falls within the expertise of gynecologists and is reported as being at least ten percent of their outpatient practice. It leads to a significant number of laparoscopies and hysterectomies (41) and is characterized by chronic complaint of lower abdominal/pelvic pain often exacerbated by long periods of standing. Sexual intercourse too is often painful and when dyspareunia is part of the syndrome this tends to reduce the chance of a beneficial outcome from treatment. The exclusion of other pelvic conditions is essential before making the diagnosis and this leads to the high laparoscopic rates in gynecological practice. Absence of a precise cause of this chronic condition limits therapeutic options but high dose progestogen treatment using medroxyprogesterone acetate seems to offer some women symptomatic relief (42). As in many conditions where an objective cause for the symptoms is elusive there is a tendency to disbelieve and even dismiss the woman as a chronic complainer (43). A multidisciplinary approach to the problem which widens deliberation and discussion with these women about their problems has been associated with better management of the condition. Two key papers and a review are recommended for surgeons who would be wise to explore this topic further (4,5,41). PCS is one cause of

CPP and with the emergence of new imaging techniques and potential vascular solutions, is growing in its relevance to vascular specialist (44).

Pelvic Congestion Syndrome

Pelvic Conjestion Syndrome (PCS), also known as pelvic venous incompetence, is a condition resulting from ovarian vein dysfunction either due to reflux caused by abnormal ovarian vein valves or ovarian vein obstruction caused by compression of the left renal vein between the aorta and the superior mesenteric artery, the "nutcracker syndrome" (2). Both of these conditions will result in abnormal venous flow and distal venous hypertension. It will often manifest itself as a plexus of dilated veins around the pelvic structures which can be seen on ultrasound and at laparoscopy. It may also present as varicosities in the lower limbs where no long saphenous or short saphenous valvular reflux can be demonstrated. In the case of renal vein obstruction the venous hypertension may lead to renal failure in this kidney. PCS is one of the recognized causes of chronic pelvic congestion syndrome (41).

The symptoms of PCS are usually thought of as a female problem. The anatomical abnormalities described however are not gender specific. While the condition is twice as common in women, it was in males that the varices were identified as the cause of indentations in the ureter (45,46). Pregnancy undoubtedly imposes its effects on these veins too and probably stimulates further abnormal dilatation of the veins in a similar way to that previously described in the lower limbs (18).

The "Nutcracker Syndrome"

Grant the anatomist first described the obstruction of the ovarian vein by the mesenteric artery. In 1950 this was described more precisely by El Sadr and Mina (47). Later it became known as the "nutcracker syndrome" reflecting the crushing of the renal vein by the artery and likening it to the of action of a nutcracker (48,49). In addition to suffering from symptoms suggestive of PCS, patients with this problem may also suffer renal damage as a complication of renal hypertension. This is characterized by the finding of microscopic hematuria.

The repeated crushing injury to the renal vein also causes physical damage to the vein wall and the development of thickenings and spurs on the outside of the vein wall at the site of the compression (2). Inside the vein, the intimal damage caused by the repeated crushing creates luminal webs surprisingly similar to the changes described by Cockett with respect to the left iliac vein compressed by the right iliac artery in the "iliac vein compression syndrome" (50). Sculteus et al. have elegantly reported an illustrated history of the effects of the "nutcracker" phenomenon and reported a range of interventional therapeutic options (2). Selection of patients for intervention, however, requires a very careful history and examination and good clinical judgement by the vascular specialist about when to intervene and in whom.

Investigation and Treatment of the "Nutcracker Syndrome"

The combined symptoms of PCS with microscopic hematuria and the demonstration of pelvic varices in the female, or a varicocele in the male, are essential to the diagnosis. Thorough investigation of renal function is important because of the likelihood of renal cell damage due to the venous hypertension. Clinical suspicion of the condition should be followed by contrast MRI or CT scan aiming to be able to image distension of the left renal vein as it is compressed between the aorta and the superior mesenteric artery, as well as identifying renal congestion. This clearly defines the anatomical abnormality. Direct venous pressure measurement and the demonstration of a gradient across the obstruction is desirable but obtaining accurate readings is difficult due to variation in measurements when readings are taken in the supine and erect positions. False negative results are also likely in the prone and supine positions. Duplex scanning has a place but the morphology of the patient will affect the imaging (51). Once the problem is defined treatment should be directed by a multidisciplinary group involving vascular, gynaecological and renal specialists. Its aim is to minimize further renal damage by relieving the compression.

The treatment options for this condition include open surgery and transposition of the vein, auto transplantation of the kidney, external stenting of the vein with external supported PTFE and internal stenting (2,51–53). Each of these has pros and cons and selection must be tailored to the individual patient's clinical case. Internal stenting has great attractions due to its less invasive nature but may be complicated by fibromuscular hyperplasia and further obstruction or even occlusion of the left renal vein. The potential for embolisation of endovascular devices are well known in the arterial system and this is likely to be so in the venous system. Deteriorating renal function will be a strong indicator to intervene but vascular specialists must be rigorous in selecting patients for intervention.

Ovarian Vein Reflux

Dilation of the veins in the pelvis and their association with CPP has been demonstrated clinically and at autopsy on many occasions (54–57). Hobbs described ovarian vein reflux and its association with the clinical presentation of vulval and buttock varicosities which develop during gestation and disappear after parturition (59). New imaging technology, which is now both safer and more easily available, is allowing clinicians to investigate patients as never before. These investigations are demonstrating abnormalities in the venous system which are now being associated with chronic conditions not normally considered to be the vascular domain of the vascular specialist. The possibility of being able to treat them is highly seductive but should be approached carefully especially as in a review of CT scans performed for reasons other than investigating ovarian veins, a dilated ovarian venous system was found more often than expected in women without symptoms attributable to CPP (60). Vascular experts will be sent patients who will have a long history of symptoms and who are desperate for a cure.

Intervention for Ovarian Vein Reflux

The traditional treatment for ovarian vein reflux is open surgery to ligate the ovarian vein (59). The procedure may now be carried out minimally invasively and this must be the first choice for surgical intervention in the twenty first century. The question of whether ligation is adequate when compared with excision of the ovarian vein has been raised (3). A claim for the relief of symptoms during pregnancy with phlebotonic agents has been made but is probably of very limited value (61).

Cordts et al. used their standard duplex test with a tilt of twenty degrees reversed Trendelenberg, to illicit reflux in the ovarian and pelvic veins of eleven women with CPP (62). All of the women underwent venography, which is essential in defining the anatomy and patency of the ovarian vein, and was also essential in this study to characterize the ovarian veins that could not be imaged by duplex. CT or MRI was not performed to exclude the "nutcracker syndrome," which may have been a contributing factor to the occluded ovarian veins. Nine cases underwent endovenous embolization of refluxing ovarian veins were carried out. Follow up was short at 13.4 months, but early results are promising, although the authors are honest enough to call for caution in interpreting them. It is a good feasibility study and they call for a randomized study. This will be difficult to do because of the different forms of presentation and the variety of treatments that may be offered. Meticulous recording of important clinical data may contribute more to the understanding of how to manage these conditions especially when combined with pre- and post-assessment questioning of the patients. Agreed datasets should be constructed and there may even be a case for a national registry. Endovenous ovarian vein oblation is possible, however, with minimum morbidity. The greatest challenge to vascular specialists will be to know how to select who to treat. The seductive rush to intervene must be tempered by wise deliberation.

Review of the published literature indicates a multiplicity of possible therapeutic options and the paucity of large studies to create a consistency of approach to treatment (2). The review identified 13 different forms of treatment including: ovarian function suppressing hormones, vasoactive agents, local excision or sclerotherapy of vulval varices, several types of gynecologic surgery, gonadal embolization with coils, glues, balloons, and sclerosants, selective surgical division or catheter embolization of the hypogastric vein tributaries, and extraperitoneal or laparoscopic resection of the gonadal plexus. Long-term follow up, however, is lacking and remains a gap in the knowledge needed to advise and guide treatment in these unfortunate women. The studies to date indicate that patients with mild to moderate symptoms and small vulval varicosities do well with sclerotherapy and gonadal vein resection. The complications of coiling and other endoluminal obliterative therapies are probably underestimated. In this potential huge area of need for treatment there is also a big potential for creating problems rather than resolving them and clinicians need to be systematic in their approach.

The 25 year experience of treating 57 woman with PCS by one unit emphasizes the complexity of the clinical presentations and the many ways of treating them (3). This has led the authors to develop a classification to guide assessment and treatment. It is based on clinical presentation, hemodynamics, and pathophysiology. The four types proposed are:

1. Vulval varices without symptoms of PCS
2. Venous insufficiency of the hypogastric vein and its tributaries (internal pudendal, obturator, round ligament, and gluteal veins)
3. Predominantly gonadal venous insufficiency
4. Obstructed gonadal veins (nutcracker syndrome)

Their range of treatments included injection sclerotherapy and local excision for vulval varices, gonadal vein embolisation for type 2, and gonadal vein resection combined with other modalities for type 3. The management of type 4 has been covered previously (2); physicians intent on treating these conditions should read this paper.

What is obvious from reading the U.S. literature and listening to the experiences of U.S. vascular specialists, is that the U.S. experience is different from that in the United Kingdom. The British literature has few papers on the subject which may either be a reflection of a different clinical need or on the lack of imaging to identify these conditions in the United Kingdom. The clinical presentation in some papers suggests a different population of patients (2,3).

Challenges to Vascular Specialists with Respect to Pelvic Congestion Syndrome

Vascular specialists need to be aware of current understanding with respect to venous abnormalities and their association with PCS. Much of the interventions proposed are untried territories and new knowledge about these conditions is still emerging. There is a need to ensure that interventions are not carried out just because they can be done. The literature does not reveal a standard form of treatment even for the classification offered above. A literature review revealed a lack of uniformity and consensus in the diagnosis and management of patients with pelvic venous disorders. Most series are single cases and there are no randomized studies. The challenges to vascular specialists include:

- Creating a multidisciplinary approach to include vascular surgeons, radiologists, gynecologists, and in the case of renal vein obstruction, urologists
- Approaching interventions in a systematic way and refining the classification above
- Creating a database of known cases and of new ones treated and considering a national registry
- Learning to understand the natural history of the condition in order to learn when to and when not to intervene
- Considering the use of randomized studies once a classification of the venous presentation been has been achieved

Since venous surgery is often considered a cosmetic procedure it is incumbent upon vascular surgeons to lead the way in researching and providing evidence for beneficial interventions. Without such an approach, patients—especially women—will be denied treatments. Used indiscriminately vascular interventions may fall into disrepute. Vascular specialists have a responsibility to their patients and to their profession to get it right.

KEY POINTS

- Advice given to women in the child bearing age group about varicose veins relies on myth rather than fact. There is a need to improve the knowledge and understanding of professional on the known facts.
- Normal lower limb veins dilate during gestation returning to their normal size after delivery but do not develop reflux.
- Refluxing veins of the lower limbs dilate during gestation the maximum changes occurring at about 34 weeks. Many fail to return to their pre-pregnancy size especially after many pregnancies. They are responsible for the appearance of varicose veins following pregnancy.
- PTE remains the most common *direct* cause of maternal death in the UK with 56 women dying of PE in the five years up to 2002.
- Superficial thrombophlebitis in pregnancy may be a cause of PE and even death in pregnant women.
- PCS is a complex problem requiring a careful history, clinical examination and multidisciplinary approach involving vascular surgeons, vascular radiologist and gynecologists to customizing each individual patient's care.
- PCS presents twice as frequently in women compared with men. It has two broad causes, left renal vein obstruction ("nutcracker syndrome") and gonadal vein reflux (valvular dysfunction or absence), and has a wide range of clinical presentations.

- Doppler of vaginal and vulval varices in steep reversed Trendelenberg using Valsalva's maneuvre is useful to illicit reflux, which may indicate the presence of pelvic and ovarian vein reflux.
- CT and/or MRI is necessary in PCS to distinguish the "nutcracker syndrome" from ovarian vein reflux and cinevideo angiography may be useful to vizualise venous connections in the pelvis.
- Pregnancy probably exacerbates the problem of venous reflux in PCS in a similar way to that described in lower limb veins.
- Treatment for PCS, which may include open surgery with transposition of the vein, auto transplantation of the kidney, external stenting of the vein with external supported PTFE, and internal stenting, must be customised for each individual patient.
- Ovarian vein reflux is common in women without symptoms of PCS.
- Symptomatic ovarian vein reflux may be treated with open or minimally invasive surgical intervention or by endovenous techniques. Patient selection is vital.
- Vascular specialists need to develop a system for collecting data on the selection of patients for interventional treatment and of the outcomes achieved.

REFERENCES

1. Gandy R, Coughlin L, Rosser S, de Cossart L. The results of a questionnaire about varicose veins to health professionals involved in the care of pregnant women. Phlebology 2000; 15:89.
2. Scultetus AH, Villavicencio JL, Gillespie DL, Rich NM. The nutcracker syndrome: its role in the pelvic venous disorders. J Vasc Surg 2001; 34:812–819.
3. Scultetus AH, Villavicencio JL, Gillespie DL, Kao TC, Rich NM. The pelvic venous syndromes: analysis of our experience with 57 patients. J Vasc Surg 2002; 36:881–888.
4. Gelbaya TA, El-Halwaggy HE. CME review article 34, focus on primary care: chronic pelvic pain in women. Obstet Gynaecol Surv 2001; 56:757–764.
5. Duffy S. Chronic pelvic pain: defining the scope of the problem. Int J Gynaecol Obstet 2001; 74:S3–S7.
6. Guo Q, Guo C. Genetic analysis of varicose vein of lower extremities. Zhonghua yi xue yi chuan xue za zhi 1998; 15:221–223 (English translation).
7. C.E.A.P. Classification of Venous disorders. www.phlebology.org/syllabus14.htm.
8. Adhikari A, Criqui MH, Wooll V, Denenberg JO, Fronek A, Langer RD. Klauber The epidemiology of chronic venous disease. Phlebology 2000; 15:12–18.
9. Franks PJ, Wright DDI, Moffatt CJ, et al. Prevalence of venous disease. a community study in West London. Eur J Surg 1992; 158:143–147.
10. Callam MJ. Epidemiogy of varicose veins. Br J Surg 1994; 81:167–173.
11. The Management of Chronic Venous Disorders of the leg. An evidence-based report of an international task force. Phlebolgy. 1999; 14:27.
12. Dinelli M, Paraazzini F, Basellini A, Rabaiotti E, Corsi G, Ferrari A. Risk factors for varicose veins before and during pregnancy. Angiology 1993; 44:361–367.
13. Evans CJ, Allan PL, Bradbury AW, Ruckley CV, Fowkes FG. Prevalence of venous reflux in the general population on duplex scanning: the Edinburgh vein study. J Vasc Surg 1998; 28:767–776.
14. Coughlin L, Gandy R, Rosser S, de Cossart L. Factors associated with varicose veins in pregnant women. Phlebology 2001; 16:46.
15. Nelson-Piercy C 2nd ed. Handbook of Obstetric Medicine. London: Pub Martin Dunitz Ltd, 2002.
16. Mashiah A, Berman V, Thole HH, et al. Estrogen and progesterone receptors in normal and varicose saphenous veins. Cardiovasc Surg 1999; 7:327–331.

17. Kakkos SK, Zolota VG, Peristeropoulou P, Apostolopoulou A, Geroukalos G. Increased mast cell infiltration in familial varicose veins: pathogenic implications. Int Angiol 2003; 2:43–49.
18. Sparey C, Haddad N, Sissons G, Rosser S, de Cossart L. The effect of pregnancy on the lower-limb venous system of women with varicose veins. Eur J Vasc Endovasc Surg 1999; 18:294–299.
19. Sparey C, Haddad N, Sissons G, Rosser S, de Cossart L. Serial colour flow duplex scanning of the veins of the lower limb throughout pregnancy. Br J Obstet Gynaecol 1999; 106:557–602.
20. Boivin P, Cornu-Thenard A, Charpak Y. Pregnancy induced changes in lower extremity superficla veins: and ultrasound scan study. J Vasc Surg 2000; 32:570–574.
21. Cordts PR, Gawley TS. Anatomic and physiologic changes in the lower limb extremity venous hemodynamics associated with pregnancy. J Vasc Surg 1999; 24:763–767.
22. de Cossart. Personal communication, 2005.
23. Ker MG, Samuel ES. Studies of the inferior vena cava in late pregnancy. Br Med J 1964; 1:532.
24. Ikard RW, Ueland K, Fo lse R. Lower limb venous dynamics in pregnant women. Surg Gynecol Obstet 1971; 132:483.
25. Macklon N, Greer I, Bowman A. An ultrasound study of gestational and postural changes in the deep venous system of the leg in pregnancy. Br J Obstet Gynaecol 1997; 104:191–197.
26. Fegan WG. The treatment of varicose veins during pregnancy. Pac Med Surg 1964; 72:274–279.
27. Fegan WG. Continuous compression techniques of injecting varicose veins. Lancet 1963; 11:109–112.
28. Stansby G. Women, pregnancy, varicose veins. Lancet 2000; 355:1117–1118.
29. Thaler E, Huch A, Zimmermann R. Compression stockings prophylaxis of emergent varicose veins in pregnancy: a prospective randomised controlled study. Swiss Med Wkly 2001; 131:659–662.
30. Evans, AE. Compliance with compression stockings: a critical anlaysis. MSc dissertation, December 2000. University College Chester.
31. Confidential Enquiry into Maternal and Child Health. Why Mothers Die 2000–2002. CEMACH 2004.
32. Thromboprophylaxis during pregnancy; Report of a Working Party, RCOG 2004. www.rcog.org.uk.
33. Tan KT, Oudkerk M, van Beek EJR. Acute deep venous thrombosis and pulmonary embolism. In: Hallet JW, Mills JL, Earnshaw JJ, Reekers JA, eds. Comprehensive Vascular and Endovascular Surgery, Mosby: London, 2003: 625–663.
34. Guideline Investigations and Management of Heritable Thrombophilia. Br J Haem 2001; 114:512–528.
35. Todd AS. Fibrinolysis autographs. Nature 1958; 4607:495–496.
36. Nilsson IM. Changes in coagulation and fibrinolytic systems predisposing to thrombosis. Acta Chir Scand 1968; 387:15–22.
37. Isacson S, Nilsson IL. Defective fibrinolysis in blood and vein walls in recurrent "Idiopathic" venous thrombosis. Acta Chir Scand 1972; 138:313–319.
38. Wolfe JH, Morland M, Browse NL. The fibrinolytic activity of varicose veins. Br J Surg 1979; 66:185–187.
39. de Cossart, L.M. Plasminogen Activator and Vascular Disease. ChM thesis 1982, University of Liverpool.
40. Jorgensen JO, Hanel KC, Morgan AM, Hunt JM. The incidence of deep venous thrombosis in patients with superficial thrombophlebitis of the lower limbs. J Vasc Surg 1993; 18:70–73.
41. Reiter RC. A profile of women with chronic pelvic pain. Clin Obstet Gynecol 1990; 33:130.
42. Soysal ME, Soysal S, Vicdan K, Ozer S. A randomized controlled trial of goserelin and medroxyprogesteron acetate in treatment of pelvic congestion. Hum Reprod 2001; 16:931–939.
43. Stones RW, Selfe SA, Fransman S, Horn SA. Psychosocial and economic impact of chronic pelvic pain. Best Pract Res Clin Obstet Gynaecol 2000; 14:415–431.
44. Ovarian vein embolisation for pelvic congestion syndrome. AETNA, (2004), clinical policy bulletin 0441. www.aetna.com/cpb/data/CPBA0441.html.
45. Heal MR. Ureteral varicosities—a cause of the corkscrew ureter. Br J Surg 1970; 57:274–276.

46. Zerhouni EA, Siegelmann SS, Walsh PC, White RI. Elevated pressure in the left renal vein in patients with varicocele: preliminary observations. J Urol 1980; 123:512.

47. El Sadr AR, Mina A. Anatomical and surgical aspects of the operative management of varicocoeles. Urol Cutan REV 1950; 54:257–262.

48. de Schepper A. Nutcracker fenomeen van da renalis en veneuz pathologie van de linker nier. J Belge Radiol 1972; 55:507–511.

49. Chait A, Mastasar KW, Fabian CE, Mellins HZ. Vasculkar imopressions on the ureters. Am J Roentgenol Radium Nucl Med 1971; 111:729–749.

50. Cockett FB, Thomas ML. The iliac compression syndrome. Br J Surg 1965; 532:816–821.

51. Park YB, Lim SH, Ahn JH, et al. Nutcracker syndrome: intravascular stenting approach. Nephrol Dial Transplant 2000; 15:99–101.

52. Chuang CK, Chu SH, Lai PC. The nutcracker syndrome managed by autotransplantation. J Urol 1997; 157:1833–1834.

53. Barnes RW, Fleisher HL, III, Rwedman JF, Smith JW, Harshfield DL, Ferris EJ. Mesoaortic compression of the left renal vein (the so-called nutcracker syndrome): repair by a new stenting procedure. J Vasc Surg 1988; 8:415–421.

54. Taylor HC. Vascular congestion and hyperaemia II. The clinical aspect of congestion fibrosis syndrome. Am J Obstet Gynecol 1949; 57:637–653.

55. Taylor HC. Pelvic pain based on a vascular and autonomic nervous system disorder. Am J Obstet Gynecol 1954; 57:1177–1196.

56. Duncan CH, Taylor HC. A psychosomatic study of pelvic congestion. Am J Obstet Gynecol 1952; 64:1.

57. Ahlberg NE, Bartley O, Chidekel N. Right and left gonadal veins: an anatomical and statistical study. Acta Radiol Diagn 1966; 4:593–601.

58. Chidekel N. Female pelvic veins demonstrated by selective renal phlebography with particular reference to pelvic varicosities. Acta Radiol 1968; 7:193–211.

59. Hobbs JT. The pelvic congestion syndrome. Br J Hosp Med 1990; 43:199–206.

60. Rozenblit AM, Ricci ZJ, Tuvia J, Amis ES, Jr. Incompetent and dilated ovarian veins: a common CT finding in asymptomatic parous women. AJR 2001; 176:119–122.

61. Maric C. Varicose vulvaire et grossesse. Rev Fr Gynecol Obstet 1991; 86:184–186.

62. Cordts PR, Eclavea A, Buckley PJ, DeMaioribus CA, Cockerill ML, Yeager TD. Pelvic congestion syndrome: early clinical results after transcatheter ovarian vein embolization. J Vasc Surg 1998; 28:862–868.

25

Superficial Vein Thrombosis: Natural History and Clinical Significance

Athanasios D. Giannoukas
University of Thessaly Medical School and Division of Vascular Surgery, University Hospital of Larissa, Larissa, Greece

Nicos Labropoulos
Vascular Laboratory, Division of Vascular Surgery, New Jersey Medical School, Newark, New Jersey, U.S.A.

Superficial thrombophlebitis (STP) or superficial vein thrombosis most often affects the veins of the lower extremities although it may be found in any superficial vein of the body. Because most physicians consider it as a benign condition, its treatment is usually conservative with elastic stockings (ES), ambulation, antibiotics, and nonsteroidal anti-inflammatory drugs (NSAIDS) (1–4). Patients with STP near to the deep veins have been treated with anticoagulation or ligation.

The main symptoms of STP are pain, erythema, and swelling around a superficial vein. Accessory veins and tributaries with STP become solid and on palpation feel like a cord. However, thrombosis of the main saphenous trunks may be missed on palpation, as they are located in the saphenous canal. STP is often found in patients with varicose veins probably due to blood stasis in these veins, but multiple factors have been implicated with its development (5–10). Its diagnosis can be made based solely on clinical assessment, but the use of duplex ultrasound imaging (DUS) has enabled the accurate detection of its extent and progress (6,11–14).

Additionally, in contrast to the common perception among the physicians that it is a benign condition, this is not always true as there is evidence in the literature suggesting that STP may precipitate or may be associated with deep venous thrombosis (DVT), and it could cause pulmonary embolism (PE). Nevertheless, because there are only a few prospective studies dealing with this condition, the strength of these associations remain unknown.

DEMOGRAPHIC CHARACTERISTICS

The incidence of STP has been reported to be in the range of 3–11% in the general population (15), and in another report the rate clinically recognized STP was 123,000

335

patients per year with a preponderance of the female gender (78%) (16). It is important to mention that both of these studies are old and the diagnosis was clinical, and thus the STP prevalence is probably underestimated because in many patients, the symptoms of STP can be minor and not present for medical attention. Preponderance of females with a ratio of 6 to 4 has been reported in the literature (17–22), attributing this to the higher prevalence of varicose veins in pregnancy (22). Previous thromboembolic episodes, long-haul flight, pregnancy, oral contraceptives, hormone replacement therapy, immobilization, obesity, recent surgery, trauma, and sclerotherapy all have been implicated as potential risk factors. Nevertheless, it is of importance that more than one risk factor has to be present for the development of thrombosis. Of notice is that age is an important factor; the older the patient, the fewer factors are needed (23). In multiple reports the mean age of presentation is around 60 (20,21,24–28).

VARICOSE VEINS, LOCATION, AND STP

The most common location of STP is the saphenous veins and their tributaries in the lower limb. This is followed by the superficial vein system in the upper limb (cephalic and basilic vein), whereas it is uncommon in veins of other parts of the body (20). Patients with varicose veins may develop STP, which in the literature has a wide range varying from 4% to 59% (6,18,22). It appears that the great saphenous vein (GSV) is more often involved (60–80%) than the small saphenous vein (SSV) (10–20%) but none of the lower limbs has a predilection (6). Bilateral involvement is not very common (5–10%) (6,20) but it may be associated with a higher number of complications (8%). GSV thrombosis may also be associated with more complications than thrombosis in other locations (6). In most of the cases STP develops in varicose tributaries rather than in the saphenous trunk (18). As potential pathophysiologic mechanism has been considered the presence of localized defects in the fibrinolysis and platelet aggregation but the current evidence is not definitive and further work is needed (29).

HYPERCOAGULABLE STATES AND STP

While STP confined to varicose tributaries is considered as a complication of varicose vein disease, saphenous trunk thrombosis is often a more significant thromboembolic process (12,24). Many coagulation abnormalities have been reported to be associated with saphenous thrombosis (8,9,24,30). When STP occurs in the absence of varicose veins, autoimmune diseases or malignancy, the risk of STP was found to be six-fold for the Factor V Leiden mutation, 4-fold for the factor II G20210A mutation and 13-fold for antithrombin III, protein C and S deficiencies taken together (7). Anticardiolipin antibodies and increased levels of factor VIII seem to be more prevalent in patients with recurrent STP (30,31). Although there is lack of large studies evaluating the prevalence of hypercoagulable states in different cohorts of patients with STP, it is clear that patients with STP have high prevalence of hypercoagulable states (Table 1) (7,8,24,30–35). Therefore, the development of STP in the absence of varicose veins, or STP extension to the main trunk of the GSV, denotes a possible underline hypercoagulable state, which should be investigated.

Table 1 STP and Hypercoagulable States

Author	Patients	State	Prevalence (%)	Odds ratio (95% CI)	STP
Engesser 1987 (32)	71	Protein S deficiency	72		
Pabinger 1996 (34)	230	Coagulation inhibitor deficiency	↑ in Protein C and S deficiency	–	First episode and recurrent
De Moerloose 1998 (8)	112	Factor V Leiden	14.3	2.51 (1.04–6.24)	First episode
		Factor IIA20210	3.6	3.28 (0.46–36.84)	
Martinelli 1999 (7)	63	Factor VA1691	15.9	6.1 (2.6–14.2)	First episode
		Factor IIG20210A	9.6	4.3 (1.5–12.6)	
		ATIII, Protein C or S deficiency	10.2	12.9 (3.6–46.2)	
de Godoy 2001 (31)	45	Anticardiolipin antibodies	33.3	6.64 (2.48–17.82)	Recurrent
de Godoy 2003 (35)	36	Protein S deficiency	5.2		Recurrent (≥2)
Schonauer 2003 (30)	45	High factor VIII	24% (p=0.004)	4 (2.0–8.6)	Recurrent VTE

Abbreviations: ATIII, antithrombin III deficiency; STP, superficial vein thrombosis.

PREGNANCY AND STP

There are only two studies in this area and both are of retrospective nature. The first investigated 30,040 pregnancies, from which only 14 cases (0.05%) of STP were diagnosed by ultrasonography, mostly presenting within 48 hours of delivery (36). In the other one an incidence of 0.068% (49/72,200 deliveries; 95% CI 0.048–0.088) was found; ten of these cases occurred prior to delivery and the rest (n=39, 0.054%, 95% CI 0.037–0.071) within seven days postpartum (10). A small number of patients with STP (n=24) were tested for thrombophilia, and only one was positive for a Factor V mutation. The limited information on this topic does not allow any meaningful associations.

MALIGNANCY AND STP

The current literature on vascular disorders that preceded the diagnosis of malignancy reveals that the relationship between STP and cancer remains weak (37), and it has been derived from two retrospective studies (13,38). In the first study, the prevalence of malignancy was 13% (14/106), and in 11 patients the malignancy was already diagnosed (13). In the second study, which included 398 limbs, 56 had STP of which only 10 had malignant disease (38). In daily practice when association of STP and cancer is found, usually the latter is diagnosed first. It appears, therefore, that the strength of the association of STP with cancer remains unknown and needs to be further studied.

DVT AND STP

Because most of the studies in this area are retrospective, and some include very small numbers of subjects, the evidence on concomitant STP and DVT and/or PE remains controversial. DVT in association with saphenous thrombosis ranges from 6% to 53%

Table 2 STP and Concomitant VTE

Author	Patients (n)	DVT (%)	PE (%)	Diagnosis	Treatment
Gervais 1956 (39)	64	6	–	Surgery[a]	Surgery
Gjores 1962 (40)	40	32	5	–	Surgery
Zollinger 1962 (21)	335	–	10.1	Clinical	–
Hafner 1964 (41)	133	17	–	Surgery[a]	–
Lofgren 1981 (18)	163	8	–	Clinical	Surgery
Husni 1982 (22)	139	7[b]	–	–	Surgery
Plate 1985 (42)	28	14	–	VNG, VQ	Surgery
Bergqvist 1986 (43)	56	16	–	VNG	–
Skillman 1990 (44)	42	12	–	VNG, SG, DUS	Medical
Lutter 1991 (6)	186	28	4	DUS	–
Pulliam 1991 (14)	20	30	0	DUS	Surgery
Lohr 1992 (46)	43	53	–	DUS	Surgery
Jorgensen 1993 (47)	44	23	–	DUS	–
Ascer 1995 (25)	20[c]	40	0	DUS	Medical
Blumenberg 1997 (48)	213 (220 limbs)	8.6	0.93	DUS	Medical
Bounameaux 1997 (49)	551	5.6 (95% CI 3.8–7.9)	–	VNG, DUS	–
Verlato 1999 (50)	21	–	33.3	DUS, VQ, CXR	
Murgia 1999 (51)	85	25.3	–	DUS	–
Unno 2002 (17)	51	11.8	7.8	DUS	

[a] Free-floating thrombus in the common femoral vein extending from the SFJ was found during surgery.
[b] These thrombi were found in the perforator veins and nothing was mentioned about the deep veins.
[c] These patients were selected to have SFJ thrombosis.
Abbreviations: DUS, duplex ultrasound; STP, superficial vein thrombosis; VNG, venography; SFJ, saphenofemoral junction; VQ, ventilation perfusion lung scan; VTE, venous thromboembolism.

(Table 2) (6,14,17,18,21,22,25,39–51). Thrombus can propagate in a contiguous or non-contiguous fashion. Contiguous extension from the superficial into the deep veins can occur in three ways: from the GSV into the femoral vein, which is the most common (41); from the SSV into the popliteal vein through the saphenopopliteal junction (SPJ) (6,41); through perforating veins to several deep venous structures. In 53 patients with STP and DVT, evidence of direct contiguous propagation was found in 40 cases (75.5%), and the rest was non contiguous calf involvement at the posterior tibial and soleal levels, whereas from 186 DUS scans with evidence of STP, isolated perforating vein involvement was never found (6). It is possible that thrombosis can extend from the deep veins to the superficial ones, but this has not been evaluated in any study.

In another report, 30 (11%) of 263 patients with saphenous thrombophlebitis had documented extension of thrombus into the deep veins: in 21 patients the thrombus extended from the thigh GSV into the common femoral vein (CFV); in three thrombus was extended from the thigh GSV into the femoral vein through thigh perforators; in three there was extension of a below knee saphenous thrombus to the popliteal vein; and in another three patients below-the-knee saphenous thrombi extended via calf perforators to the tibioperoneal veins (26).

The prevalence of DVT in association with STP in the presence of varicose veins was 13% (5/39) and 24.5% (10/41), respectively, in two small studies (44,47).

In another study using ascending venography in 56 patients with clinical evidence of STP, DVT was found in nine patients, but eight of them did not have varicose veins, and thus the prevalence of DVT was 2.6% in patients with varicose veins and 44% in those without (p<0.01) (43). None of these patients with varicose veins developed malignancy on follow-up, whereas two patients without varicosities were subsequently diagnosed with breast cancer and polycythemia vera, respectively.

It appears that the incidence of DVT is higher (17–19%) when STP is confined to above knee segment of the GSV than when STP did not extend above the knee (4–5%) (26,43). Although the site of STP may not point to the presence or absence of DVT (44), propagation of STP to the deep veins by serial DUS has been documented in three studies (14,26,48). Therefore, it appears that most patients with STP should have their deep veins evaluated even if the lowest prevalence of DVT (5.6%) (49) is considered.

PE AND STP

Most of the studies available in the literature include a small number of patients because of the low prevalence of this association. In a report five cases of PE occurred from an embolus originated from the GSV but no evidence of DVT was found (40). Two of them were fatal episodes after prostatectomy and the rest were small and non-fatal. An 18% rate of PE was reported when the thrombotic process was located at the above-the-knee location in the GSV (6). Other investigators found a 1.5% rate of fatal PE in patients with STP (21). PE also has been reported with SSV thrombosis; a 4% rate for SSV involvement and a 7% propagation rate to the popliteal vein (6). A 7.8% rate of PE was found among 51 consecutive patients with STP, chosen from 710 patients referred for treatment of varicose veins, in a risk assessment study, and all cases had involvement of the GSV or SSV (17).

There is only one prospective study in which 21 consecutive patients with STP in the thigh segment of GSV were evaluated by DUS, chest X ray, and perfusion lung scanning, regardless of their symptoms (50). Seven of these patients had high probability of PE (33%; 95% CI, 14.6–57), but only one was symptomatic.

The most important point is that from the existing literature, it remains unclear whether PE associated with STP arises from extension into the deep veins or from a clot that detaches while still in the superficial venous system. This distinction is very important from a treatment point of view as surgical ligation could prevent the latter case, but monitoring with DUS should suffice if the former is more common.

DIAGNOSIS OF STP

Clinical or DUS data can help in the diagnosis of STP. Because thrombosis involves veins located superficially, STP is often easy to diagnose, and its clinical features include the presence of a warm, tender, palpable cord or nodule-like structure following the course of a superficial vein. However, because the correlation between clinical exam and surgical findings is poor, the diagnosis should not be limited to clinical grounds only. The true extent of STP cannot be evaluated by clinical exam as it has been shown from surgical exploration in which the extension of the thrombotic process often reaches 5–10 cm higher than the level clinically diagnosed (40). It is not uncommon in daily practice that DUS often identifies more proximal extension of STP compared to clinical exam. For this reason DUS is recommended not only for confirmation of diagnosis but also for estimation of the extent of thrombosis and for follow-up (11,20,26). In respect to the systematic application of DUS for diagnosis of an associated DVT, there has been criticism based on the low incidence of DVT.

Three broad categories of STP cases can be identified based on DUS and clinical examination, which portends important differences with regard to diagnostic workup and management: a) short segment STP not associated with varicose veins, b) short segment STP associated with varicosities, and c) extensive saphenous thrombophlebitis (12). In the first category, the possibility of the presence of an underlying systematic disease is not uncommon and this should be investigated. No further workup is required in the second category. Treatment should be given to alleviate the symptoms and, if necessary, intervention for the varicosities could be performed. Nevertheless, in this category the patients may still need to be followed-up by clinical exam and DUS in order to confirm the absence of thrombus propagation to the saphenous trunk. Finally, in the third category, the association of STP with DVT and PE is important (Table 2) (6,14,17,18,21,22,25,39–51) and thus prompt management should be applied (12).

Once STP develops, it is important to clarify whether this is confined to varicose saphenous tributaries within the context of pre-existing varicose veins or whether STP involves the saphenous trunk, particularly the thigh segment. Although the former situation may not to require further investigation, as being a localized event complicating varicose vein disease, clinical and DUS follow-up may still be needed to confirm the absence of thrombus propagation to the saphenous trunk. In contrast, the latter situation seems to be more serious, and, as the literature supports, DUS is needed in order to accurately evaluate the extent of thrombus and to exclude the presence of DVT (6,11,13,14,25,26,44–48,55). The clinician should consider the possibility of hypercoagulable states and malignancy in patients without varicose veins who present with STP (43). Thrombophilia screening as a routine can help to identify patients at risk for developing thromboembolic complications (7,8,17,30,52), but some clinicians have adopted in their practice selective screening based on the presence or absence of risk factors (52–54).

Table 3 STP Treatment

Author	Patients (n)	Treatment	Measured outcome	Results	Follow-up (days)
Gjores 1962 (40)	40	Surgery	VTE	8% PE	–
Zollinger 1962 (21)	335[a]	Bed rest + elevation ± Abx Anticoagulation Surgery ± anticoagulation	Ambulation	19% ≤3 days 18% ≤3 days 60% ≤3 days	–
Williams 1964 (56)	92	Surgery	VTE	0	No follow-up
Hafner 1964 (41)	324	Surgery (133) Medical (191)	VTE	PE 2.3% DVT 10.5% –	No follow-up
Husni 1982 (22)	221	Medical (82) Surgery (139)	PE	12%[b] 0	8–28
Lofgren 1981 (18)	163	Surgery	VTE	1.2% PE; 4.3% recurrent STP	365–4380 (median 1825)
Lohr 1992 (46)	41	Surgery	VTE	1 recurrent STP; 1 with PE; 2 with contralateral DVT	Minimum 120
Titon 1994 (57)	117	LMWH, NSAIDs	Signs and symptoms	Greater improvement with LMWH	56
Ascer 1995 (25)	20	Anticoagulation	DUS outcome of thrombosis and PE	N = 13; 92.3% improvement; 7.7% without change	420
Hanson 1998 (24)	17	Medical (NSAIDs, anticoagulation, ES)	DUS thrombus progression	N = 13;46.2% unchanged;46.2% worse; 7.6% improved	?
Belcaro 1999 (19)	444	ES, surgery and anticoagulation in 6 combinations	DVT rate Thrombus extension	No difference Higher with ES; lowest with surgery	180
Beatty 2002 (27)	17	Emergent SFJ division	VTE	5.9% popliteal DVT; no PE	60
Marchiori 2002 (58)	60	UFH low vs. high dose (± NSAIDs)	VTE	20 vs. 3.3% respectively (p=0.05)	180
STENOX 2003 (28)	436	LMWH (2 doses) NSAIDs ES	STP extension and VTE	Best	90

[a] These patients were known to have STP by clinical examination but the number of patients with concomitant DVT was not known. Surgery ± anticoagulation improved patients' signs and symptoms. However, nowadays almost all patients ambulate and this does not seem a good end point for evaluation. Five patients (1.5%) died from PE.

[b] Unknown whether these patients had concomitant DVT.

Abbreviations: ES, elastic stockings; LMWH, low molecular weight heparin; NSAIDS, nonsteroidal antinflammatory drugs; SFJ, saphenofemoral junction; VTE, venous thromboembolism.

MANAGEMENT OF STP

There are several options in the clinician's armamentarium to treat STP including anti-inflammatory agents, anticoagulation, ambulation, ES, and surgery (Table 3) (18,19,21,22,24,25,27,28,34,40,41,46,56–58). Because of the lack of consistency with regards to the measured end points, inadequate follow-up, limited evaluation to rule out venous thromboembolism (VTE), small number of patients studied, and mainly due to the retrospective nature of most of the studies, it appears that the evaluation of medical treatment for STP in the literature yields conflicting results.

Antibiotics have no role in the management of STP, which is supported by the results of bacteriologic studies of thrombi obtained in surgery that revealed a low incidence of microorganisms and a low rate of wound infection (41). In addition, it is important to mention that the role of aspirin and NSAIDS in VTE is not well defined. In general they offer a positive effect in the relief of the local pain and may add anti-inflammatory benefits in STP. Although topical application or oral administration of non-steroidal anti-inflammatory agents, local application of hirudoid and agents with enzymatic action have been used, their efficacy is controversial as they may have only some effect in the alleviation of symptoms and signs (59–63).

Experience with anticoagulation using unfractionated heparin (UFH), low molecular weight heparin (LMWH), coumadin and recently pentasaccharides mostly has been acquired from the treatment of DVT. Since LMWH have proved to be at least as effective and safe as UFH in the treatment of DVT it could be a reasonable alternative (64). Favorable results from LMWH were found only for thrombus extension but were not significant for development of VTE in the only randomized trial that enrolled 436 patients and compared ES, NSAIDS, and two doses of LMWH for 10 days (28).

Surgical management for STP, which includes local thrombectomy, vein ligation, excision or stripping, and sclerotherapy, has shown a PE rate between 0 and 8% (Table 3) (18,19,21,22,24,25,27,28,34,40,41,46,56–58). Although it is possibly an underestimation, given that in most of these studies the diagnosis of PE was made clinically in symptomatic patients only. Also, the rate of recurrent STP varies from 2% to 4.3%, and again it is probably underestimated due to presentation bias. Since there are no randomized control trials against anticoagulation, the selection of patients who have favorable risk/benefit profiles for surgery appears to be a problem in daily practice.

ES is not as effective as anticoagulation (28). ES alone does not prevent thrombus extension and VTE but they may be used as an adjunctive treatment to alleviate pain and swelling. When STP extension remains well away from the SFJ or the SPJ, or STP at lower levels, without evidence of DVT, conservative management using ES, NSAIDS or aspirin is adequate. When concomitant STP and DVT is documented anticoagulation should be started. Surgical removal of the thrombus is an equally good treatment when the thrombus is found in the SPJ or SFJ and extends as free-floating in the CFV or popliteal veins. Anticoagulation is instigated if the thrombus is adherent or non contiguous.

DUS is useful to assess the extent and progression of STP, and it should be performed at about 7–10 days after the original diagnosis. In any case of clinical deterioration or DUS evidence of STP progression, anticoagulation or surgery may be needed.

FINAL REMARKS AND CONCLUSION

STP is generally benign if confined to varicose veins. However, when there is evidence of GSV or SSV involvement, it may be associated with more serious conditions, notably

DVT and PE. Significant association there is also between STP and hypercoagulable states but such a relationship between STP and malignancy or pregnancy remains weak and it should be determined from future studies. It is good practice in all cases to exclude concomitant DVT at presentation and for this reason the diagnosis approach should include assessment with DUS.

Conservative treatment for STP affecting varicose tributaries is sufficient. For more extensive thrombosis affecting the truncal GSV or SSV, anticoagulation or early saphenous ligation is recommended. However, the optimal length and the type of anticoagulation remain unknown.

KEY POINTS

- Superficial thrombophlebitis is not always benign.
- It may be associated with DVT.
- It may be associated with malignancy, pregnancy, and hypercoagulable states.
- It is diagnosed clinically but ultrasound should be performed to define the extent and whether deep veins are involved.
- Follow-up may be needed if the saphenous trunk is involved to assess thrombus propagation.
- Antibiotics have no role in treatment.
- Conservative therapies include anti-inflammatory agents and anticoagulants.
- Surgery is reserved for more extensive involvement.

REFERENCES

1. Ludbrook J, Jamieson GG. Disorders of veins. In: Sabiston DC, Jr., ed. Textbook of Surgery. 12th ed. Philadelphia: WB Saunders, 1981:1808–1827.
2. Hobbs JT. Superficial thrombophlebitis. In: Hobbs JT, ed. The Treatment of Venous Disorders. Philadelphia: JB Lipincott, 1977:414–427.
3. DeWeese MS. Nonoperative treatment of acute superficial thrombophlebitis and deep femoral venous thrombosis. In: Ernst CB, Stanley JC, eds. Current Therapy in Vascular Surgery. 2nd ed. Philadelphia: BC Decker, 1991:952–960.
4. Messmore HL, Bishop M Wehrmacher WH, Acute venous thrombosis. Therapeutic choices for superficial and deep veins. Postgrad Med 1991, 00:73 77
5. Edward EA. Thrombophlebitis of varicose veins. Surg Gynecol Obstet 1938; 66.236 245
6. Lutter KS, Rerr TM, Roedersheimer R, Lohr JM, Sampson MG, Cranley JJ. Superficial thrombophlebitis diagnosed by duplex scanning. Surgery 1991; 100:42–46.
7. Martinelli I, Cattaneo M, Taioli E, De Stefano V, Chiusolo P, Mannucci PM. Genetic risk factors for superficial vein thrombosis. Thromb Haemost 1999; 82:1215–1217.
8. de Moerloose P, Wutschert R, Heinzmann M, Perneger T, Reber G, Bounameaux H. Superficial vein thrombosis of the lower limb: influence of factor V Leiden, factor II G20210A and overweight. Thromb Haemost 1998; 80:239–241.
9. Samlaska CP, James WD. Superficial thrombophlebitis. I. Primary hypercoagulable states. J Am Acad Dermatol 1990; 22:975–989.
10. McColl MD, Ramsay JE, Tait RC, et al. Superficial vein thrombosis: incidence in association with pregnancy and prevalence of thrombophilic defects. Thromb Haemost 1998; 79:741–742.
11. Denzel C, Lang W. Diagnosis and therapy of progressive thrombophlebitis of epifascial leg veins. Zentralbl Chir 2001; 126:374–378.
12. Becker F. Superficial venous thrombosis of the lower limbs. Rev Prat 1996; 46:1225–1228.

13. Barrellier MT. Superficial venous thromboses of the legs. Phlebologie 1993; 46:633–639.

14. Pulliam CW, Barr SL, Ewing AB. Venous duplex scanning in the diagnosis and treatment of progressive superficial thrombophlebitis. Ann Vasc Surg 1991; 5:190–195.

15. Widmer LK, Stahelin HB, Nissen C, da Silva A. Venen-. Arterien-krankheiten, koronare Herzkrankheit bei Berufstatigen: Prospektiv- epidemiologische Untersuchung. Basler studie I–III 1981;1959–1978.

16. Coon WW, Willis PW, III, Keller JB. Venous thromboembolism and other venous disease in the Tecumseh Community Health Study. Circulation 1973; 48:839–846.

17. Unno N, Mitsuoka H, Uchiyama T, et al. Superficial thrombophlebitis of the lower limbs with varicose veins. Surg Today 2002; 32:397–401.

18. Lofgren EP, Lofgren KA. The surgical treatment of superficial thrombophlebitis. Surgery 1981; 90:49–54.

19. Belcaro G, Nicolaides AN, Errichi BM, et al. Superficial thrombophlebitis of the legs: a randomised, controlled, follow-up study. Angiology 1999; 50:523–529.

20. Decousus H, Epinat M, Guillot K, et al. Superficial vein thrombosis: risk factors, diagnosis and treatment. Curr Opin Pulm Med 2003; 9:393–397.

21. Zollinger RW, Williams RD, Briggs DO. Problems in the diagnosis and treatment of thrombophlebitis. Arch Surg 1962; 85:34–40.

22. Husni EA, Williams WA. Superficial thrombophlebitis of lower limbs. Surgery 1982; 91:70–74.

23. Rosendaal FR. Thrombosis in the young: epidemiology and risk factors. A focus on venous thrombosis. Thromb Haemost 1997; 78:1–6.

24. Hanson JN, Ascher E, DePippo P, et al. Saphenous vein trombophlebitis (SVT): A deceptively benign disease. J Vasc Surg 1998; 27:677–680.

25. Ascer E, Lorensen E, Pollina RM, Gennaro M. Preliminary results of a non-operative approach to sapheno-femoral junction thrombophlebitis. J Vasc Surg 1995; 22:616–621.

26. Chengelis DL, Bendick PJ, Glover JL, Brown WO, Ranval TJ. Progression of superficial venous thrombosis to deep veins. J Vasc Surg 1996; 24:745–749.

27. Beatty J, Fitridge R, Benveniste G, Greenstein D. Acute superficial venous thrombophlebitis: does emergency surgery has a role? Int Angiol 2002; 21:93–95.

28. The STENOX study group. A randomized double-blind comparison of low molecular weight heparin, non steroidal anti-inflammatory agent and placebo in the treatment of superficial vein thrombosis. Arch Intern Med 2003; 163:1657–1663.

29. Lee AJ, Lowe GD, Rumley A, Ruckley CV, Fowkes FG. Haemostatic factors and risk of varicose veins and chronic venous insufficiency: Edinburgh Vein Study. Blood Coagul Fibrinolysis 2000; 11:775–781.

30. Schonauer V, Kyrle PA, Weltermann A, et al. Superficial thrombophlebitis and risk for recurrent venous thromboembolism. J Vasc Surg 2003; 37:834–838.

31. de Godoy JM, Batigalia F, Braile M. Superficial thrombophlebitis and anticardiolipin antibodies—report of association. Angiology 2001; 52:127–129.

32. Engesser L, Broekmans AW, Briet E, Brommer EJ, Bertina RM. Hereditary protein S deficiency: clinical manifestations. Ann Intern Med 1987; 106:677–682.

33. Lohr JM, Muck PE, Oliverio EA, Hasselfeld KA, Panke TW. Superficial vein thrombophlebitis: A clinical marker of a hypercoagulable state. Presented at the American Venous Forum.: San Diego, 1992.

34. Pabinger I, Schneider B. Thrombotic risk in hereditary antithrombin III, protein C, or protein S deficiency. A cooperative, retrospective study. Gesellschaft fur Thrombose- und Hamostasefroschung (GTH) Study Group on Natural Inhibitors. Arterioscler Thromb Vasc Biol 1996; 16:742–748.

35. de Godoy JM, Braile DM. Protein S deficiency in repetitive superficial thrombophlebitis. Clin Appl Thromb Henost 2003; 9:61–62.

36. James KV, Lohr JM, Deshmukh RM, Cranley JJ. Venous thrombotic complications of pregnancy. Cardiovasc Surg 1996; 4:777–782.

37. Naschitz JE, Kovaleva J, Shaviv N, Rennert G, Yeshurun D. Vascular disorders preceding diagnosis of cancer: distinguishing the causal relationship based on Bradford-Hill guidelines. Angiology 2003; 54:11–17.
38. Krause U, Kock HJ, Kroger K, Albrecht K, Rudofsky G. Prevention of deep venous thrombosis associated with superficial thrombophlebitis of the leg by early saphenous vein ligation. Vasa 1998; 27:34–38.
39. Gervais M. Les thromboses veineuses superficielles. Lyon Chir 1956; 52:89–96.
40. Gjores JE. Surgical therapy of ascending thrombophlebitis in the saphenous system. Angiology 1962; 13:241–243.
41. Hafner CD, Cranley JJ, Krause RJ, Strasser ES. A method of managing superficial thrombophlebitis. Surgery 1964; 55:201–206.
42. Plate G, Eklof B, Jensen R, Ohlin P. Deep venous thrombosis, pulmonary embolism and acute surgery in thrombophlebitis of the long saphenous vein. Acta Chir Scand 1985; 151:241–244.
43. Bergqvist D, Jaroszewski H. Deep vein thrombosis in patients with superficial thrombophlebitis of the leg. BMJ 1986; 292:658–659.
44. Skillman JJ, Kent KC, Porter DH, Kim D. Simultaneous occurrence of superficial and deep thrombophlebitis in the lower extremity. J Vasc Surg 1990; 11:818–824.
45. Prountjos P, Bastounis E, Hadjinikolaou L, Felekuras E, Balas P. Superficial venous thrombosis of the lower extremities co-existing with deep venous thrombosis. A phlebographic study on 57 cases. Int Angiol 1991; 10:63–65.
46. Lohr JM, McDevitt DT, Lutter KS, Roedersheimer LR, Sampson MG. Operative management of greater saphenous thrombophlebitis involving the saphenofemoral junction. Am J Surg 1992; 164:269–275.
47. Jorgensen JO, Hamel KC, Morgan AM, Hunt JM. The incidence of deep venous thrombosis in patients with superficial thrombophlebitis of the lower limbs. J Vasc Surg 1993; 18:70–73.
48. Blumenberg RM, Barton E, Gelfand ML, Skudder P, Brennan J. Occult deep venous thrombosis complicating superficial thrombophlebitis. J Vasc Surg 1998; 27:338–343.
49. Bounameaux H, Reber-Wasem MA. Superficial thrombophlebitis and deep vein thrombosis. A controversial association. Arch Intern Med 1997; 157:1822–1824.
50. Verlato F, Zuccheta P, Prandoni P, et al. An unexpectedly high rate of pulmonary embolism in patients with superficial thrombophlebitis of the thigh. J Vasc Surg 1999; 30:1113–1115.
51. Murgia AP, Cisno C, Pansini GC, Manfredini R, Liboni A, Zamboni P. Surgical management of ascending saphenous thrombophlebitis. Int Angiol 1999; 18:3430–3437.
52. Guex JJ. Thrombotic complications of varicose veins. A literature review of the role of superficial venous thrombosis. Dermatol Surg 1996; 22:378–382.
53. Gillet JL, Perrin M, Cayman R. Superficial venous thrombosis of the lower limb: prospective analysis in 100 patients. J Mal Vasc 2001; 26:16–22.
54. Tosetto A, Frezzato M, Rodeghiero F. Prevalence and risk factors of non-fatal venous thromboembolism in the active population of the VITA Project. J Thromb Haemost 2003, 1:1724–1729.
55. Welger D, Muller JH. Associated thrombotic processes of the superficial, perforating and intramuscular venous system in patients with acute phlebothrombosis of the lower extremities. Z Gesamte Inn Med 1988; 43:15–18.
56. Williams RD, Zollinger RW. Surgical treatment of superficial thrombophlebitis. Surg Gynecol Obstet 1964; 118:745–747.
57. Titon JP, Auger D, Grange P, et al. Therapeutic management of superficial venous thrombosis with calcium nadroparin. Dosage testing and comparison with a non-steroidal anti-inflammatory agent. Ann Cardiol Angiol 1994; 43:160–166.
58. Marchiori A, Verlato F, et al. High versus low doses of unfractionated heparin for the treatment of superficial thrombophlebitis of the leg. A prospective, controlled, randomized study. Haematologica 2002; 87:523–527.
59. Raake W, Binder M. Treatment of superficial thrombophlebitis. Hamostaseologie 2002; 22:149–153.

60. Ferrari E, Pratesi C, Scaricabarozzi I. A comparison of nimesulide and diclofenac in the treatment of acute superficial thrombophlebitis. Drugs 1993; 46:197–199.
61. Bagliani A, Montalbetti L. Topical treatment of thrombophlebitis with feprazone and benzydamine. Controlled clinical study. Minerva Med 1976; 67:880–884.
62. Bracale G, Selvetella L. Clinical study of the efficacy of and tolerance to seaprose S in inflammatory venous disease. Controlled study versus serratio-peptidase. Minerva Cardioangiol 1996; 44:515–524.
63. Bergqvist D, Brunkwall J, Jensen N, Persson NH. Treatment of superficial thrombophlebitis. A comparative trial between placebo, Hirudoid cream and piroxicam gel. Ann Chir Gynaecol 1990; 79:92–96.
64. Kalodiki E, Nicolaides AN. Superficial thrombophlebitis and low-molecular-weight heparins. Angiology 2002; 53:659–663.

26
Medicolegal Aspects

Bruce Campbell
Royal Devon and Exeter Hospital, Exeter, U.K.

INTRODUCTION

Avoidance and defense of malpractice claims have become increasingly important aspects of medical practice. The boom in medical litigation occurred first in the United States, but other countries like the United Kingdom have followed suit, with a doubling of claims during the 1990s (1).

Some specialists are more vulnerable to medicolegal action than others and this is reflected in premiums for malpractice insurance. Premiums may be related to the number of claims made against a specialty, their potential value (for example huge sums for some obstetric claims), or both. In general surgery (as it was understood in the United Kingdom in the 1990s, including gastrointestinal, vascular and endocrine surgery) the commonest single condition for which claims were made to a major defense organization was varicose veins (2). In addition, medicolegal action relating to venous thromboembolism is common; these claims are frequently against other disciplines, but vascular specialists may become involved in the management of these patients and in providing expert opinions for legal proceedings. Determining the true frequency of medicolegal claims is, however, not straightforward.

DETERMINING THE FREQUENCY OF MEDICOLEGAL CLAIMS

There are several difficulties. First, the words used to describe medicolegal proceedings vary. In the United States "suits" for "malpractice" are the usual terms, while in the United Kingdom "claims" for "negligence" form the basis of any legal action against a doctor or hospital. In this chapter a mid-Atlantic approach will be used, referring to "claims" (because most of the figures cited relate to these) and to "malpractice" (because it is perhaps more easily understood than "negligence").

The second problem in describing numbers of claims is their continual state of flux. Numbers of claims vary from year to year, and each claim develops through a number of stages—from simply being initiated (or notified), to being discontinued because it has no

Table 1 Frequency of Medicolegal Claims After Varicose Vein Surgery

Underlying allegation	Number (%) notified claims
Nerve damage	69 (36)
Incorrect/inadequate/unsatisfactory surgery	38 (20)
Femoral or popliteal vein damage	20 (10)
Infection	11 (6)
Venous thromboembolism	10 (5)
Femoral artery damage	10 (5)
Scarring/blemishing	5 (3)
Tourniquet damage	3 (2)
Miscellaneous	25 (13)
Total	191

Number (% of total) claims notified to the Medical Defense Union (United Kingdom and Republic of Ireland) and the National Health Service Litigation Authority (NHSLA) for England relating to treatment of varicose veins during 1995–2003, classified according to the main underlying allegation.

merit (closed without payment), to being settled (paid) with or without admission of negligence or liability, or (in only a minority) to legal proceedings in court when a judgement is made for or against the hospital or doctor involved. This dynamic situation makes description of claims somewhat difficult and makes it important to be explicit about the types of claims being described.

Another major difficulty is lack of collation of data about medicolegal claims: there is still no single, central database in most countries (3–4). Claims may be handled by a variety of different organizations, even in nationalized health services. In the United Kingdom, National Health Service claims were handled by private defense organizations until 1989, then at regional level until 1995, and since 1995, by a central litigation authority (even since that time, many smaller claims have been handled locally). All this means that there has traditionally been no ready access to national figures. When figures are available, it may be difficult to obtain a reliable or meaningful denominator with which to gauge the risk of litigation.

VARICOSE VEINS

Data from the Medical Defense Union in the United Kingdom (a major indemnity insurer for private surgical practice) showed that varicose veins were the most common reason for litigation against all kinds of general surgeons (2). They remain (in 2004) the most common reason for settled (paid) claims, followed (in descending order) by surgery on the bile ducts, bowel, benign tumours and the breast. A summation of claims notified to the Medical Defense Union and the National Health Service Litigation Authority (NHSLA) for England are shown in Table 1.

There are a number of possible reasons that medicolegal claims for varicose vein treatments have been relatively frequent. Although varicose veins are properly the province of vascular surgeons with special interest and expertise in their management, they have often been dealt with by other disciplines. In the United Kingdom it was normal until the 1990s for varicose veins to be dealt with by any general surgeon and this still applies in many parts of the world. In addition, many "vascular surgeons" have actually been "arterial surgeons" (just as the phrase "peripheral vascular disease" is still used to refer to arterial disease). Many well-known vascular surgeons have, in the past, regarded varicose veins as being insufficiently important or interesting to merit their serious attention. This culture is changing, but it has meant that varicose veins have often been dealt with by surgeons whose expertise may have been insufficient, with resultant problems and legal action.

Many people with varicose veins are troubled largely by their appearance and request treatment in the private sector, where a variety of clinicians may offer treatments which they use infrequently, practicing in isolation. Novel "office based" treatments such as foam sclerotherapy may add to the list of treatments which are used without sufficient expertise, precipitating legal action against clinicians (see below).

The fact that varicose veins are very common and seldom cause medical harm has meant that they are afforded low priority by health services generally. In the United Kingdom they have formed a major component of "waiting lists" and have often been treated by trainees, sometimes without adequate supervision. This is another circumstance with a special risk of adverse events and litigation.

NEW TREATMENTS FOR VARICOSE VEINS

The rapid advance of new treatments for varicose veins may lead to litigation. Each of the new methods (including foam sclerotherapy, radiofrequency, laser, and transilluminated powered phlebectomies) seems relatively safe in experienced hands, but their novelty, their use by relatively inexperienced practitioners, particularly in "office practice," and the need for really good patient counseling all mean that there are special medicolegal risks.

There are uncertainties with any new method—for example the real risk of systemic embolization using sclerosant foam. This may be very rare but if a patient is harmed then litigation may allege that an "experimental" treatment was used, particularly if the patient was not well informed of the known risks and the uncertainties. In the United Kingdom the National Institute for Clinical Excellence (NICE) publishes guidance on the safety and efficacy of new procedures (5). This may help to protect clinicians against allegations of using new procedures inappropriately, so long as they observe NICE advice about informing patients, training, and audit.

The fact that these treatments can be used in an "office" setting increases the risk of litigation: this applies particularly to foam sclerotherapy, which is disseminating very quickly worldwide in the private sector. The published reports of foam sclerotherapy have been from enthusiasts and experts. The apparent simplicity of the technique have led to its rapid adoption not only by vascular specialists, but also by a variety of other doctors with little experience in the treatment of varicose veins. Use of foam sclerotherapy by practitioners working in relative isolation, without great experience in dealing with varicose veins, with predominantly financial motives, and without a mandate for good audit means that substandard practice may well occur. If patients have not been counseled thoroughly about potential risks and benefits, then litigation seems likely.

VENOUS THROMBOEMBOLISM AS A COMPLICATION OF VARICOSE VEIN OPERATIONS

Varicose veins have featured high on some lists of risk factors for DVT, based on evidence of an increased risk of DVT (detected by radioisotope scanning) after major abdominal and pelvic surgery in people with varicose veins (6–7). This has been translated in to a general fear about the specter of DVT as a result of varicose veins, in the minds of both lay people and many doctors. Available evidence suggests that DVT is uncommon after varicose vein surgery (8), but vascular specialists should be mindful of the perceived risk, which probably puts them at increased medicolegal risk if DVT complicates varicose vein surgery (or any other invasive treatment for varicose veins) (9).

Failure to note other risk factors (for example, previous DVT or hormone treatment) and to provide "demonstrable prophylaxis" to patients at risk (including those whose surgery takes more than 30 minutes or who are obese) might well be indefensible if thromboembolism occurs. What constitutes "demonstrable prophylaxis" is a real dilemma: the only practical perioperative measure is low dose heparin, but since most patients are in hospital less than 24 hours, special arrangements need to be made for administration of more than one dose. A record of explicit advice about early mobilization and prescription of anti-embolism stockings in addition would seem sensible and adequate, but controversy between experts is still likely if a high risk patient develops thromboembolism and sues.

VENOUS THROMBOEMBOLISM REQUIRING EXPERT OPINION

Vascular specialists who provide expert opinions in malpractice claims will not infrequently be asked about patients who have suffered DVT or pulmonary embolism following treatment by other doctors. If there has been an obvious failure to provide appropriate prophylaxis then giving a clear opinion is straightforward. It is more difficult when some prophylaxis has been given (see preceding paragraph about varicose veins) to provide a fair and pragmatic opinion about whether this was adequate and what the likelihood would have been of preventing DVT if more had been done. It is important that even the best prophylaxis simply reduces the risk of thromboembolism—it does not guarantee prevention.

SWOLLEN LEGS—POSTPHLEBITIC SYNDROME AND LYMPHATIC DISEASE

These conditions are dealt with together because similar cautions apply from a medicolegal point of view. These patients have chronic and distressing limb swelling (and associated problems) which are difficult to treat and impossible to cure. If the onset of their condition was iatrogenic or associated with any perceived failure of medical management they may have a low threshold for complaint or for medicolegal action against those caring for them. Attempts at treatment by any surgical means may be high risk with limited prospect of improvement. Very careful counseling and recording of such discussions is essential in this.

COMMUNICATING RISKS AND BENEFITS

Medical litigation is often precipitated by poor communication rather than by poor clinical performance (10). A key to avoiding litigation is the rule: "The patient's expectations should be the same as yours." Especially when treatment is being considered for a condition that poses no medical threat—as for most people presenting with varicose veins—a full explanation the good prognosis without treatment, alternative treatments, the likely benefits, and the potential adverse outcomes of treatment are fundamental to avoiding possible litigation (11). The less "severe" the veins, the more thorough this explanation should be. Patients with the smallest "cosmetic" varicosities or with thread veins usually have high expectations and also low thresholds for dissatisfaction if any kind of adverse event occurs.

With regard to likely benefits from treatment, patients need a good explanation of the prognosis if they have no treatment (usually very good). They also need to be told and to understand precisely which of their symptoms are likely to be relieved by treatment. By no means will all discomfort in the legs be cured by treating varicose veins, and patients may be disgruntled to the extent of taking legal action if they are disappointed.

Disclosure of potential risks must be thorough. Clinicians vary greatly in the amount they tell patients by word of mouth (12–13), but there can be no excuse for failing to provide people with really thorough written information about proposed treatment and its risks (13). Provision of this written information needs to be clearly recorded (some doctors ask patients to sign confirming they have received it) and it needs to be archived for reference in case of litigation at a later date (all revisions of written information should be dated and archived for medicolegal use). Unfortunately, documentation of many aspects of doctor–patient consultations in secondary care is often poor (14).

Striking a balance between concise, easily readable information for patients and lengthy screeds of small print is not easy. Provision of really good "patient friendly" information is time consuming, and it is a shame that this is not readily available on a national basis in each country. There certainly do seem to be differences in the general approach to patient information in different countries—large amounts of indigestible information are common in the United States while in parts of Europe a total lack of written information has been common. The provision of thorough information largely parallels and the level of litigation and both are gradually increasing worldwide. There is, however, still a long way to go in supplying patients with good written information to make informed choices and to reduce the chance of litigation if complications occur.

The place and use of consent forms is variable—particularly for "office based" or outpatient treatments. In some medical and legal systems, these are regarded as essential; but a signature on a form will never compensate for proper understanding by the patient or a record of having provided good information, including a warning of whatever damage has prompted a patient to take legal action. Ideally, any consent form should be "dovetailed" with the written information given to the patient (15).

SPOTTING HIGH-RISK CASES

The most unexpected patients may take medicolegal action. However, it is useful to try to spot those patients who are most likely to suffer problems, to complain, or to sue. They merit particularly thorough counseling and recording of discussions. They include:

- Patients with minor cosmetic veins, with odd symptoms, or with bizarre ideas about their veins and the problems associated with them
- Patients who do not seem to want to listen, who seem unable to grasp what they are told, or who press for inappropriate or questionable treatment
- Patients who have complained or taken legal action before
- Patients with a high risk of complications, particularly the obese and those with recurrent varicose veins

- Patients with pale skin—any blemish from treatment is more obvious
- All patients with leg swelling—any intervention runs a risk of making them worse

When talking to patients who seem high risk for litigation, it is always desirable to involve close relatives in discussion, and ideally also another member of the medical or nursing team (record their presence as well as what was said).

WHEN THINGS GO WRONG

When a serious complication occurs, then patients may sue successfully, even if they were warned of the risk beforehand: for example, damage to a major nerve is likely to be construed as malpractice or negligence even if a warning was given. From the moment damage has occurred, first-class management is fundamental to minimize the harm caused; to demonstrate good care to the patient; and to reduce both the likelihood and magnitude of any medicolegal claim. This damage limitation should include:

- Immediate repair, by the most appropriate person (for example, repair of the common peroneal nerve by a plastic surgeon or repair of the femoral vein by a senior vascular surgeon)
- All adjunctive measures to reduce harm or disability (for example, neurological advice, splinting, early physiotherapy for nerve injury; or prophylactic anti-coagulants, compression hosiery, mobilization or foot pump after venous injury)
- Advising the patient fully and sympathetically about exactly what has happened and what is being done to correct the situation. It is entirely appropriate to apologize
- Reporting the problem without delay to clinical incident or legal liaison teams (when treatment took place in a hospital or clinic). In private practice indemnity insurers should be informed at an early stage, and it seems wise to involve all colleagues who might be able to offer help to the patient and support to the responsible clinician
- Being sure that the patient is followed up assiduously by the responsible clinician and all others who can offer help

These measures not only lay the foundations for the best possible medicolegal defense, they will hopefully avoid litigation altogether if the patients feel that they have been dealt with in a thoroughly professional and caring way.

THE UNCERTAINTIES OF MEDICOLEGAL DECISIONS

Unfortunately, there are no dependable rules for the judgements made in medicolegal cases. Some—for example a recent English court decision against the liability of manufacturers for venous thromboembolism from third generation oral contraceptives (16)—may seem illogical based on objective appraisal of the evidence. Courts may be swayed by persuasive and biased presentation of evidence by experts, and different judges may reach apparently different conclusions. These vagaries of the law are particularly disturbing to clinicians who are used to scientific objectivity. They also mean that it is difficult to provide unequivocal guidance or confident answers to many questions about specific medicolegal matters. The best that a chapter like this can achieve is to highlight particular areas of risk and to give advice on how best to avoid and to defend medicolegal claims. The fundamentals remain good communication; good record keeping; meticulous technique; and thoughtful management when adverse outcomes do occur.

KEY POINTS

- Varicose veins are the most common reason for litigation against general and vascular surgeons. Nerve damage is the most frequent complaint.
- Counseling patients thoroughly about the risks and potential benefits of treatment (including written information) and good documentation reduce the chance of successful litigation.
- Problems following treatment for small varicose veins and cosmetic concerns may well be followed by medicolegal action. Remember: "The patient's expectations should be the same as yours."
- Spotting patients at high risk allows special care in counseling and record keeping. When problems do occur, damage limitation by good remedial treatment and thorough explanation may avoid or minimize medicolegal consequences.
- New treatments for varicose veins may pose special risks—for example, foam sclerotherapy if done by inexperienced practitioners in an "office based" practice.

REFERENCES

1. Fenn P, Diacon S, Gray A, Hodges R, Rickman N. Current cost of medical negligence in NHS hospitals: analysis of claims database. BMJ 2000; 320:1567–1571.
2. Goodwin H. Litigation and surgical practice in the UK. Br J Surg 2000; 87:977–979.
3. Rotker J, Trosch F, Deng MC, Roeder N, Scheld HH. Medical liability disputes involving thoracic and cardiovascular surgeons. Thorac Cardiovasc Surg 2001; 49:60–63.
4. Campbell WB, France F, Goodwin HM. On behalf of the Research and Audit Committee of the Vascular Surgical Society of Great Britain and Ireland Medico-legal claims in vascular surgery. Ann R Coll Surg Engl 2002; 84:181–184.
5. National Institute for Health and Clinical excellent intervention procedures; avilable at www.nice.org.uk/ip.
6. Thromboembolic Risk Factors (THRIFT) Consensus Group. Risk of and prophylaxis for venous thromboembolism in hospital patients. BMJ 1992; 305:567–574.
7. European Consensus Statement. Prevention of Venous Thromboembolism. London: Med-Orion, 1992.
8. van Rij AM, Chai J, Hill GB, Christie RA. Incidence of deep vein thrombosis after varicose vein surgery. Br J Surg 2004; 91:1582–1585.
9. Campbell WB, Ridler BMF. Varicose veins and deep vein thrombosis. Br J Surg 1995; 82:1494–1497.
10. Fischer JE. The effect of litigation on surgical practice in the USA. Br J Surg 2000; 87:833–834.
11. Reference Guide to Consent for Examination or Treatment. London: Department of Health, 2001.
12. Meredith P, Emberton M. The NHS patient information lottery: it is whom you see rather than what you need. Ann R Coll Surg 2000; 82:217–222.

13. McManus PL, Wheatley KE. Consent and complications: risk disclosure varies widely between individual surgeons. Ann R Coll Surg Engl 2003; 85:79–82.
14. Fernando KJ, Siriwardena AK. Standards of documentation of the surgeon–patient consultation in current surgical practice 2001; 88:309–312.
15. Campbell B. Informed consent. Ann R Coll Surg Engl 2004; 86:457–458.
16. Skegg DCG. Oral contraceptives, venous thromboembolism and the courts. BMJ 2002; 325:504–505.

27

Pathophysiology of Leg Ulceration

Peter J. Pappas, Brajesh K. Lal, and Walter N. Durán
New Jersey Medical School, Newark, New Jersey, U.S.A.

Frank T. Padberg, Jr.
New Jersey Health Care System–Veterans Affairs Medical Center, East Orange, New Jersey, U.S.A.

Robert W. Zickler
UMDNJ–New Jersey Medical School, Newark, New Jersey and New Jersey Health Care System–Veterans Affairs Medical Center, East Orange, New Jersey, U.S.A.

INTRODUCTION

Ten to 35% of adults in the United States have some form of chronic venous insufficiency (CVI) with venous ulcers affecting 4% of people over the age of 65 (1,2). Treatment of patients with CVI and venous ulcers cost the U.S. government over one billion dollars a year. In addition, 4.6 million work days per year are lost secondary to chronic venous disease (3,4). The recurrent nature of the disease, the high cost to the healthcare system and the ineffectiveness of current treatment modalities, underscore the need for CVI related research. The past decade has refined our understanding of leukocyte mediated injury and elucidated the role of inflammatory cytokines in lower extremity dermal pathology. In addition, our understanding of pathologic cellular function and the molecular regulation of these processes is increasing. This chapter will discuss the potential causes of varicose vein and venous ulcer formation and the scientific evidence supporting these theories.

THE VENOUS MACROCIRCULATION

Unlike arteries, veins are thin walled, low pressure conduits whose function is to return blood from the periphery to the heart. Muscular contractions in the upper and lower extremities propel blood forward and a series of intra-luminal valves prevent retrograde flow or reflux. Venous reflux is observed when valvular destruction or dysfunction occurs. Valvular reflux causes an increase in ambulatory venous pressure and a cascade of pathologic events that manifest themselves clinically as varicose veins, lower extremity edema, pain, itching, skin discoloration, and in its severest form, venous ulceration. These clinical signs and symptoms collectively refer to the disorder known as chronic venous insufficiency (CVI) (5). Classification of CVI according to the signs and severity of the disease is discussed elsewhere in this book.

Primary valvular incompetence can involve all veins participating in the macro-circulation: the superficial, deep and the perforating venous systems, alone or in combination. In patients with post-thrombotic syndrome, destruction of the valves results in secondary valvular incompetence. Chronic obstruction of deep veins due to previous deep vein thrombosis is another important etiology of persistent ambulatory venous hypertension. The role of the perforating veins is still under much debate.

VARICOSE VEINS

Etiology

Age, gender, pregnancy, weight, height, race, diet, bowel habits, occupation, posture, previous deep venous thrombosis (DVT) and genetics have all been proposed as pre-disposing factors associated with varicose vein formation (6). Except for previous deep vein thrombosis and genetics, there is poor evidence that indicates a causative relationship between these predisposing factors and the formation of varicose veins.

The Role of Genetics

There are few reported epidemiologic investigations that suggest a relationship between varicose vein formation and a genetic predisposition (7,8). It was previously thought that axial destruction of venous valves led to transmission of ambulatory venous hypertension causing reflux and varix formation (6). However, a publication by Labropoulos et al. indicated that the most frequent location for initial varicose vein formation was in the below knee great saphenous vein (GSV) and its tributaries, followed by the above knee GSV, and the saphenofemoral junction (9). This study clearly indicates that vein wall degeneration with subsequent varix formation can occur in any segment of the superficial and deep systems at any time and suggests a genetic component to the disease. In 1969, Gunderson and Hauge reported on the epidemiology of varicose veins observed in their vein clinic in Malmo, Sweden over a two month period (7). Of 250 patients, 154 female and 24 male patients provided complete survey information on their parents and siblings. Although biased by the predominance of women and dependence on survey data, this report suggested that patients with varicose veins had a higher likelihood of developing varicosities if their fathers had varicose veins. Furthermore, the risk of developing varicose veins increases if both parents had varicosities. Cornu-Thenard et al. prospec-tively examined 67 patients and their parents. Patients non-affected spouses and parents were used as controls for a total of 402 subjects (8). These investigators reported that the risk of developing varicose veins was 90% when both parents were affected, 25% for males and 62% for females if one parent is affected and 20% when neither parent is affected. These data suggest an autosomal dominant with variable penetrance mode of genetic transmission. The decreased incidence in males with an affected parent and the spontaneous development in patients without affected parents, suggests that males are more resistant to varix formation and that other multi-factorial etiologies in patients with pre-dispositions to the disease must exist. To further elucidate the genetic component of the disease, molecular analyses with gene chip technologies is required. The chromosome responsible for the disease and its protein by-products are currently unknown.

The Role of DVT

An injury to the venous endothelium or local pro-coagulant environmental factors, leads to thrombus formation in the venous system. It is currently well accepted that a venous thrombus initiates a cascade of inflammatory events that contributes to or causes vein wall fibrosis (10). Thrombus formation at venous confluences and valve pockets leads to activation of neutrophils and platelets. Activation of these cells leads to formation of inflammatory cytokines, pro-coagulants and chemokines leading to thrombin activation and further clot formation. Production of inflammatory mediators creates a cytokine/chemokine gradient leading to leukocyte invasion of the vein wall at the thrombus wall interface and from the surrounding adventitia. Up-regulation of adhesion molecules perpetuates this process, eventually leading to vein wall fibrosis, valvular destruction and alteration of vein wall architecture (10,11). Although the mechanisms associated with vein wall damage secondary to venous thrombosis are beginning to be unraveled, the majority of varicose veins occur in patients with no prior history of deep venous thrombosis. The etiology of primary varicose veins continues to be a mystery.

Vein Wall Anatomy and Histopathology

Whatever the initiating event, several unique anatomic and biochemical abnormalities have been observed in patients with varicose veins. Normal and varicose great saphenous veins (GSVs) are characterized by three distinct muscle layers within their walls. The media contains an inner longitudinal and an outer circular layer, while the adventitia contains a loosely organized outer longitudinal layer (12–14). In normal GSVs, these muscle layers are composed of smooth muscle cells (SMCs) which appear spindle shaped (contractile phenotype) when examined with electron microscopy (Fig. 1) (15). These cells lie in close proximity to each other, are in parallel arrays and surrounded by bundles of regularly arranged collagen fibers.

In varicose veins, the orderly appearance of the muscle layers of the media is replaced by an intense and disorganized deposition of collagen (15–17). Collagen deposits separate the normally closely opposed SMCs and are particularly striking in the media. SMCs appear elliptical, rather than spindle shaped and demonstrate numerous collagen containing vacuoles imparting a secretory phenotype (Fig. 2) (15). What causes SMCs to dedifferentiate from a

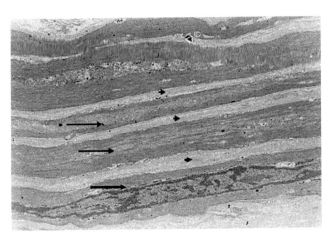

Figure 1 Electron micrograph of normal greater saphenous vein (magnification 11,830×). Note organized structure of alternating smooth muscle cells (*long arrows*) with spindle shaped contractile phenotype, interspersed by longitudinally arranged collagen bundles (*short arrows*).

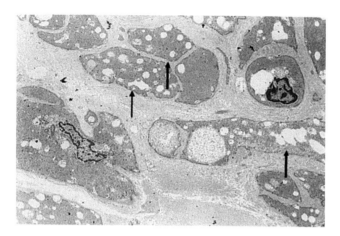

Figure 2 Electron micrograph of varicosed greater saphenous vein (magnification 4240✕). Smooth muscle cells exhibit prominent vacuoles (*arrows*) and an elliptical appearance consistent with a secretory phenotype. Smooth muscle cells are separated by diffusely deposited collagen bundles, which impart a disorganized architectural appearance to the vein wall.

contractile to a secretory phenotype is currently unknown. It has been suggested that SMC dedifferentiation may be related to alterations in apoptosis mediators such as bax and PARP (Poly ADP-ribose polymerase) and/or increased phosphorylation of differentiation mediators such as the retinoblastoma protein (13,18,19). The molecular regulation of vein wall degeneration is currently ill-defined and requires further research.

Vein wall remodeling has been consistently observed in histologic varicose vein specimens (12,14–17,20). Gandhi et al. quantitatively demonstrated an increase in collagen content and a decrease in elastin content compared to normal GSVs (20). The net increase in the collagen/elastin ratio suggested an imbalance in connective tissue matrix regulation. As a result, several investigators have observed alterations in matrix metalloproteinase and fibrinolytic activity in varicose veins. TIMP-1 and MMP-1 protein levels are increased at the saphenofemoral junction compared to normal controls whereas MMP-2 levels are decreased (21). No overall differences in MMP-9 protein or activity levels have been identified. However, the number of cells expressing MMP-9 by immunohistochemistry has been reported to be elevated in varicose veins compared to normal veins (22,23). There are conflicting reports regarding the role of plasmin activators and their inhibitors. Shireman et al. reported that uPA (urokinase plasminogen activator) levels are increased three to five times compared to normal controls in the media of vein specimens cultured in an organ bath system (24). No differences were noted in tPA (Tissue Plasminogen Activator) or PAI-1 (Plamin Activator Inhibitor-1) levels. However, other investigations have reported a decrease in uPA and tPA activity by enzyme zymography in varicose veins (22,25). These data suggest that the plasminogen activators may play a role in matrix metalloproteinase activation leading to vein wall fibrosis and varix formation.

Abnormal Vein Wall Function in Varicose Veins

Varicose veins clearly demonstrate abnormal contractile properties. The contractile responses of varicose and normal GSV rings to noradrenaline, potassium chloride, endothelin, calcium ionophore A23187, angiotensin II and nitric oxide have been evaluated by several investigators (26,27). These studies have demonstrated decreased contractility of varicose veins when stimulated by noradrenaline, endothelin and potassium chloride. Similarly, endothelium dependent and independent relaxations after A23187 or nitric oxide administration were diminished compared to normal GSVs, respectively. The mechanisms responsible for decreased varicose vein contractility appear to be receptor mediated (27,28). Utilizing Sarafotoxin S6c (selective pharmacologic inhibitor of endothelin B) and competitive inhibition receptor assays with ^{131}I-endothelin-1, a decrease in endothelin B receptors have been observed in varicose veins compared to normal GSVs (28). Feedback inhibition of receptor production secondary to increased endothelin-1 is postulated to mediate the decreased receptor content in varicose vein walls. Other possible mechanisms for decreased contractility appear related to cAMP levels and the ratio of prostacyclin to thromobxane-A2 (29). Cyclic-AMP is increased in varicose vein specimens compared to normal GSVs. In addition, the ratio of prostacyclin to throboxane-A2 is increased although no difference in absolute protein levels between normal veins and varicosities were observed. Whether venodilation of varicosities is caused by diminished endothelin receptor levels and responsiveness to cAMP or a secondary effect of varix formation is not known. However, it is clear that with the development of vein wall fibrosis, varicose veins demonstrate decreased contractile properties that probably exacerbate the development of ambulatory venous hypertension.

HISTORICAL THEORIES OF CVI

In the twentieth century numerous theories have been postulated regarding the etiology and pathophysiology of CVI and the cause of venous ulceration. The venous stasis, arteriovenous fistula and diffusion block theories have been disproven over time and are discussed here for historical interest only. The etiology for dermal skin pathology is primarily a chronic inflammatory process and the events regulating these events are discussed below.

Venous Stasis Theory

In 1917, John Homans published a manuscript entitled The Etiology and Treatment of Varicose Ulcer of the Leg in *Surgery, Gynecology and Obstetrics* (30). This work was a clinical treatise on the diagnosis and management of patients with CVI. Homans coined the term post-phlebitic syndrome and speculated that venous ulceration was secondary to venous stasis (30). This hypothesis resulted in a generation of investigators trying to seek a causal relationship between hypoxia, stagnant blood flow and the development of CVI.

The first investigator to address the question of hypoxia and CVI scientifically was Alfred Blalock (31). He obtained venous samples from the femoral, greater saphenous and varicose veins in 10 patients with CVI isolated to one limb and compared their oxygen content to samples taken from corresponding veins in the opposite limb. Seven of the patients had active ulcers at the time. All samples were collected in the recumbent and standing positions. He reported that in patients with unilateral CVI the oxygen content was higher in the femoral vein of the affected limb. He speculated that this observation may be reflective of increased venous flow rather than stagnation.

Arteriovenous Fistula Theory

The concept of increased venous flow in the dermal venous plexus was expanded upon by Pratt who reported that increased venous flow in patients with CVI could be clinically observed (32). He attributed the development of venous ulceration to the presence of arteriovenous connections and coined the term "arterial varices." He reported that in a series of 272 patients with varicose veins who underwent vein ligation, 24% had arteriovenous connections. Of the 61 patients who developed recurrences, 50% occurred in patients with arteriovenous communications identified clinically by the presence of arterial pulsations in venous conduits. Pratt hypothesized that increased venous flow shunted nutrient and oxygen rich blood away from the dermal plexus leading to areas of ischemia and hypoxia and resulting in venous ulceration. Pratt's clinical observations however, have never been confirmed with objective scientific evidence. Experiments with radioactively labeled microspheres have never demonstrated shunting and have therefore cast serious doubts on the validity of this theory.

Diffusion Block Theory

Hypoxia and alterations in nutrient blood flow were again proposed as the underlying etiology of CVI in 1982 by Burnand et al. (33). These authors performed histologically analyzed skin biopsies from 109 limbs of patients with CVI and 30 limbs from patients without CVI and measured venous pressure at rest and after heel raises. The authors reported that venous hypertension was associated with increased numbers of capillaries in the dermis of patients with CVI. Similarly, in a canine hind limb model, the same authors were able to induce enlargement in the number of capillaries with experimentally induced hypertension (34). This important investigation was one of the first studies to demonstrate a direct effect of venous hypertension on the venous microcirculation. In a later study, Browse and Burnand noted that the enlarged capillaries observed on histologic examination exhibited pericapillary fibrin deposition and coined the term "fibrin cuff" (35). They speculated that venous hypertension led to widening of endothelial gap junctions with subsequent extravasation of fibrinogen leading to the development of fibrin cuffs. These authors theorized that the cuffs acted as a barrier to oxygen diffusion and nutrient blood flow, resulting in epidermal cell death. Although pericapillary cuffs do exist, it has never been demonstrated that they act as a barrier to nutrient flow or oxygen diffusion.

Leukocyte Activation

Dissatisfaction with the fibrin cuff theory and subsequent observations of decreased circulating leukocytes in blood samples obtained from the greater saphenous veins in patients with CVI led Coleridge Smith and colleagues to propose the leukocyte trapping theory (36). This theory proposes that circulating neutrophils are trapped in the venous microcirculation secondary to venous hypertension. The subsequent sluggish capillary blood flow leads to hypoxia and neutrophil activation. Neutrophil activation leads to degranulation of toxic metabolites with subsequent endothelial cell damage. The ensuing heterogenous capillary perfusion causes alterations in skin blood flow and eventual skin damage. The problem with the leukocyte trapping theory is that neutrophils have never been directly observed to obstruct capillary flow therefore casting doubt on its validity. However, there is significant evidence that leukocyte activation plays a major role in the pathophysiology of CVI.

Role of Leukocyte Activation and Function

In 1988, Thomas et al. reported that 24% fewer white cells left the venous circulation after a period of recumbency and that packed red blood cell volume increased in patients with CVI compared to normal patients (37). They also noted that the relative number of white cells, were significantly decreased compared to control and primary varicose vein patients (28% vs. 5%, $p < 0.01$). The authors concluded that the decrease in white cell number was due to leukocyte trapping in the venous microcirculation secondary to venous hypertension. They further speculated that trapped leukocytes may become activated resulting in release of toxic metabolites causing damage to the microcirculation and overlying skin. These important observations were the first to implicate abnormal leukocyte activity in the pathophysiology of CVI.

The importance of leukocytes in the development of dermal skin alterations was emphasized by Scott et al. (38). These authors obtained punch biopsies from patients with primary varicose veins, lipodermatosclerosis, and patients with lipodermatosclerosis and healed ulcers and reported the median number of white blood cells (WBCs) per high power field ($40\times$ magnification) in each group. No patients with active ulcers were included and no attempt to identify the type of leukocytes was made. The authors reported that in patients with primary varicose veins, lipodermatosclerosis and healed ulceration there was a median of 6, 45 and 217 WBCs per mm^2 respectively. This study demonstrated a correlation between clinical disease severity and the number of leukocytes in the dermis of patients with CVI.

The types of leukocytes involved in dermal venous stasis skin changes are controversial. T-lymphocytes, macrophages and mast cells have been observed on immunohistochemical and electronmicroscopic examinations (39,40). The variation in types of leukocytes observed may reflect the types of patients investigated. Wilkerson et al. biopsied patients with erythematous and eczematous skin changes whereas Pappas et al. predominantly evaluated older patients with dermal fibrosis. Patients with eczematous skin changes may have an autoimmune component to their CVI whereas patients with dermal fibrosis may experience pathologic alterations consistent with chronic inflammation and altered tissue remodeling (Fig. 3).

Extracellular Matrix Alterations

Once leukocytes have migrated into the extracellular space they localize around capillaries and post-capillary venules. The perivascular space is surrounded by extracellular matrix alterations (ECM) proteins and forms a perivascular "cuff." Adjacent to these perivascular cuffs and throughout the dermal interstitium is an intense and disorganized collagen deposition (33,40). Perivascular cuffs and the accompanying collagen deposition are the sine qua non of the dermal microcirculation in CVI patients (Fig. 4). The perivascular cuff was originally thought to be the result of fibrinogen extravasation and erroneously referred to as a "fibrin cuff." It is now known that the cuff is a ring of ECM proteins consisting of collagens type I and III, fibronectin, vitronectin, laminin, tenascin and fibrin (41). The role of the cuff and its cell of origin is not completely understood. The investigation by Pappas et al. suggested that the endothelial cells of the dermal microcirculation were responsible for cuff formation (40). The cuff was once thought to be a barrier to oxygen and nutrient diffusion however, recent evidence suggests that cuff formation is an attempt to maintain vascular architecture in response to increased mechanical load (42). Although perivascular cuffs may function to preserve microcirculatory architecture, several pathologic processes may be related to cuff formation. Immunohistochemical analyses have demonstrated transforming growth factor-β_1 (TGF-β_1) and α_2-macroglobulin in the interstices of perivascular cuffs (43). It has been suggested that these "trapped" molecules are abnormally distributed in the dermis leading to altered tissue remodeling and fibrosis. Cuffs may also serve as a lattice for capillary angiogenesis explaining the capillary tortuosity and increased capillary density observed in the dermis of CVI patients.

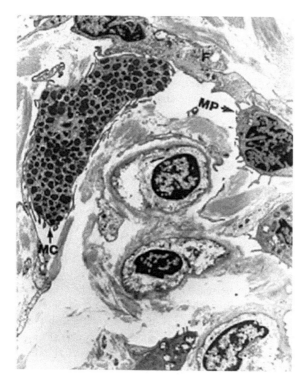

Figure 3 Electron micrograph (magnification 4300×) of mast cells (MC), macrophages (MP), and Fibroblast (F) surrounding a central capillary from dermal biopsy of a patient with CEAP class 4 chronic venous insufficiency.

Pathophysiology of Stasis Dermatitis and Dermal Fibrosis

The mechanisms modulating leukocyte activation, fibroblast function and dermal extra-cellular matrix alterations have been the focus of investigation in the 1990s. CVI is a disease of chronic inflammation due to a persistent and sustained injury secondary to

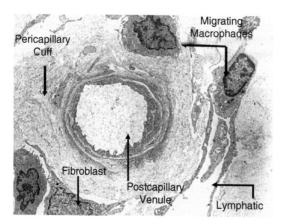

Figure 4 Electron micrograph (magnification 4300×) of a well-developed perivascular cuff in close proximity to a fibroblast in a patient with CEAP class 6 chronic venous insufficiency. The long arrow points to macrophages that appear to be entering a lymphatic lumen.

venous hypertension. It is hypothesized that the primary injury is extravasation of macromolecules (i.e., fibrinogen and α_2-macroglobulin) and red blood cells (RBCs) into the dermal interstitium (33,34,43–45). RBC degradation products and interstitial protein extravasation are potent chemoattractants and presumably represent the initial underlying chronic inflammatory signal responsible for leukocyte recruitment. It has been assumed that these cytochemical events are responsible for the increased expression of ICAM-1 (intercellular adhesion molecule-1) on endothelial cells of microcirculatory exchange vessels observed in CVI dermal biopsies (39,46). ICAM-1 is the activation dependent adhesion molecule utilized by macrophages, lymphocytes and mast cells for diapedesis. As stated above, all these cells have been observed by immunohistochemistry and electron microscopy in the interstitium of dermal biopsies (39,40).

Cytokine Regulation and Tissue Fibrosis

Several authors have attempted to identify cytokines and growth factors involved in the pathophysiology of CVI. As stated above, CVI is a chronic inflammatory disease characterized by leukocyte recruitment, tissue remodeling and dermal fibrosis. These physiologic processes are prototypical of disease states regulated by TGF-β_1. TGF-β_1 is present in pathologic quantities in the dermis of patients with CVI and increases with disease severity (47). TGF-β_1 is secreted by interstitial leukocytes and bound to dermal fibroblasts and extracellular matrix proteins (Figs. 3 and 5). Whether or not perivascular cuffs bind TGF-β_1 is controversial (47).

The distribution and location of several other growth factors in the skin of CVI patients has also been investigated. Peschen et al. reported on the role of platelet derived growth factor receptor alpha and beta (PDGFR-α and β) and vascular endothelial growth factor (VEGF) (48). These authors reported that PDGFR-α and β and VEGF expression was strongly increased in the stroma of CVI patients with eczema and active ulcers compared to patients with reticular veins and pigmentation changes only (48). To a lesser degree, patients with lipodermatosclerosis demonstrated immunoreactivity to PDGFR-α and β and VEGF as well. PDGFR-α and β expression was considerably elevated in the capillaries and surrounding fibroblasts and inflammatory cells of venous eczema patients.

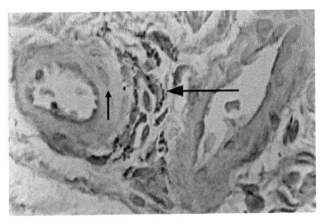

Figure 5 Immunohistochemistry (magnification 575×) of dermal skin biopsy demonstrating transforming growth factor-β1 positive granules (*long arrow*) in leukocytes surrounding a peri-vascular cuff and leukocytes migrating through a peri-vascular cuff (*short arrow*).

In addition, immunoreactivity was increased in dermal fibroblasts, smooth muscle cells and vascular cells of lipodermatosclerosis patients compared to patients with reticular veins only. The greatest expression of PDGFR-α and β was observed in mesenchymal cells and vascular endothelial cells of patients with active venous ulcers. VEGF immunoreactivity correlated with disease severity. VEGF positive capillary endothelial cells and pericapillary cells increased in patients with venous eczema, lipodermato-sclerosis and active venous ulceration respectively. In a subsequent investigation, these authors reported that with progression of CVI dermal pathology, the endothelial cell adhesion molecules intercelluar and vascular adhesion molecules (ICAM-1, VCAM-1) and their corresponding leukocyte ligands LFA-1 and VLA-4 increased (46). Based on these observations, the authors speculated that leukocyte recruitment, capillary proliferation and interstitial edema in CVI patients may be regulated through PDGF and VEGF by upregulation of adhesion molecules leading to leukocyte recruitment, diapadesis and release of chemical mediators (46).

In summary, the above investigations indicate that progression of CVI dermal pathology is mediated by a cascade of inflammatory events. Venous hypertension causes extravasation of macromolecules like fibrinogen and red blood cells which act as potent inflammatory mediators. These mediators cause an upregulation of adhesion molecules and the expression of growth factors like PDGF and VEGF which result in leukocyte recruitment. Monocytes and mast cells travel to the site of injury which activate or release TGF-β_1 and probably other undiscovered chemicals as well. What effect growth factor binding has on fibroblast and endothelial cell function has been the focus of numerous investigations in the 1990s.

Dermal Fibroblast Function

Several studies have reported aberrant phenotypic behavior of fibroblasts isolated from venous ulcer edges when compared to fibroblasts obtained from ipsilateral thigh biopsies of normal skin in the same patients. Hasan et al. reported that collagen production was increased by 60% in a dose dependent manner in control fibroblasts whereas venous ulcer fibroblasts were unresponsive. This unresponsiveness was associated with a fourfold decrease in TGF-β_1 type II receptors (49). In a follow-up report, Kim et al. indicated that the decrease in TGF-β_1 type II receptors was associated with a decrease in phosphorylation of the TGF-β_1 receptor substrates SMAD 2 and 3 as well as p42/44 mitogen activated protein kinases (50). A similar investigation reported a decrease in collagen production from venous ulcer fibroblasts and similar amounts of fibronectin production when compared to normal controls (51).

Fibroblast responsiveness to growth factors was further delineated by Stanley et al. (52). These investigators reported that venous ulcer fibroblast growth rates were markedly suppressed when stimulated with bFGF, EGF and IL-1β. In a follow-up investigation these authors noted that the previously observed growth inhibition could be reversed with bFGF (53). Lal et al. reported that the proliferative responses of CVI fibroblasts to TGF-β_1, correlated with disease severity (54). Fibroblasts from patients with CEAP class 2–3 disease retain their agonist induced proliferative capacity. Class 4 and 5 fibroblasts demonstrated diminished agonist induced proliferation whereas class 6 (venous ulcer fibroblasts) did not proliferate after TGF-β_1 stimulation confirming the observations made by previous investigators. Phenotypically, venous ulcer fibroblasts appear morphologically similar to fibroblasts undergoing cellular senescence. Therefore, the blunted growth response of CVI venous ulcer fibroblasts appears related to the development of cellular senescence (52,55).

Other characteristics of senescent cells are an overexpression of matrix proteins such as fibronectin (cFN) and enhanced activity of β-galactosidase (SA-β-Gal). In an evaluation of seven patients with venous stasis ulcers, it was noted that a higher percentage of SA-β-Gal positive cells in venous ulcers compared to normal controls (6.3% vs. 0.21%, p 0.0.6) (53). It was also reported that venous ulcer fibroblasts produced one to four times more cFN by western blot analysis compared to controls (55). These data support the hypothesis that venous ulcer fibroblasts phenotypically behave like senescent cells. However, senescence is probably the end manifestation of a wide spectrum of events that leads to proliferative resistance and cellular dysfunction. Diminished telomere length and telomerase activity are the sine qua non of truly senescent cells. To date, there are no reported studies indicating an abnormality in CVI fibroblast telomere length or telomerase activity. Absent these investigations, the true role of senescence in CVI remains ill-defined.

Role of Matrix Metalloproteinases and Their Inhibitors in CVI

The signaling event responsible for the development of a venous ulcer and the mechanisms responsible for prolonged wound healing are poorly understood. Wound healing is an orderly process that involves inflammation, re-epithelialization, matrix deposition and tissue remodeling. Tissue remodeling and matrix deposition are processes controlled by matrix metalloproteinases (MMPs) and tissue inhibitors of matrix metalloproteinases (TIMPs). In general, MMPs and TIMPs are not constitutively expressed. They are induced temporarily in response to exogenous signals such as various proteases, cytokines or growth factors, cell–matrix interactions and altered cell–cell contacts. TGF-β_1 is a potent inducer of TIMP-1 and collagen production and inhibitor of MMP-1 through regulation of gene expression and protein synthesis. Several studies have demonstrated that prolonged and continuous TGF-β_1 production causes tissue fibrosis by stimulating ECM production and inhibiting degradation by affecting MMP and TIMP production. Alterations in MMP and TIMP production may similarly modulate the tissue fibrosis of the lower extremity in CVI patients. Several investigators have reported that the gelatinases MMP-2 and 9 as well as TIMP-1 are increased in the exudates of patients with venous ulcers compared to acute wounds (56–58). However, analyses of biopsy specimens have demonstrated variable results. Herouy et al. reported that MMP-1,2 and TIMP-1 are increased in patients with lipodermatosclerosis compared to normal skin (59). In a subsequent investigation, biopsies from venous ulcer patients were found to have increased levels of the active form of MMP-2 compared to normal skin (60). In addition, increased immunoreactivity to EMMPRIN (Extracelluar inducer of MMP), MT1-MMP (Membrane Type 1) and MT2-MMP in the dermis and perivascular regions of venous ulcers (61). Saito et al. were unable to identify differences in overall MMP-1, 2, 9 and TIMP-1 protein levels or activity in CVI patients with CEAP class 2 through 6 disease compared to normal controls or CVI groups (62). However, within a clinical class, MMP-2 levels were elevated compared to MMP-1, 9 and TIMP-1 in patients with class 4 and class 5 disease. These data indicate that active tissue remodeling is occurring in patients with CVI. Which matrix metalloproteinases are involved and how they are activated and regulated is currently unclear. It appears that MMP-2 may be activated by urokinase plasminogen activator (uPA). Herouy et al. observed increased uPA and uPAR mRNA and protein levels in patients with venous ulcers compared to normal skin (63). The elevated levels of active TGF-β_1 in the dermis of CVI patients suggests a regulatory role for TGF-β_1 in MMP and TIMP synthesis and activity. However, there is currently no direct evidence indicating such a relationship.

CONCLUSION

The mechanisms regulating varicose vein development and the subsequent dermal skin sequelae caused by chronic ambulatory venous hypertension have only recently been investigated. It is clear that varicose vein formation has a genetic component that is linked to environmental stimuli. Susceptible patients develop vein wall fibrosis and loss of valvular competence that lead to venous hypertension. The transmission of high venous pressures to the dermal microcirculation causes extravasation of macromolecules and red blood cells that serve as the underlying stimulus for inflammatory injury. Activation of the microcirculation results in cytokine and growth factor release leading to leukocyte migration into the interstitium. At the site of injury, a host of inflammatory events is set into action. TGF-β_1 appears to be a primary regulator of CVI induced injury. TGF-β_1 secretion from leukocytes with subsequent binding to dermal fibroblasts is associated with intense dermal fibrosis and tissue remodeling. In addition, decreased TGF-β_1 type II receptors on venous ulcer fibroblasts, are associated with diminished fibroblast proliferation. Fibroblast proliferation diminishes with disease progression ultimately leading to senescence and poor ulcer healing. In addition, increases in MMP-2 synthesis, appear to increase tissue remodeling and further impede ulcer healing. As our understanding of the underlying cellular and molecular mechanisms that regulate CVI and ulcer formation increase, improved therapeutic interventions for treatment and prevention will ultimately follow.

KEY POINTS

- It seems probable that varicose vein formation has a genetic component that is linked to environmental stimuli.
- The relevant gene(s) have not yet been identified.
- DVT results in valvular destruction and sustained venous hypertension.
- In chronic venous insufficiency (CVI) there is actually increased venous flow rather than stagnation.
- Pericapillary fibrin cuffs exist but have never been demonstrated to act as a barrier to nutrient flow or oxygen diffusion.
- The signaling events responsible for the development of a venous ulcer and the mechanisms responsible for prolonged wound healing are still poorly understood.
- The transmission of high venous pressures to the dermal microcirculation causes extravasation of macromolecules and red blood cells that serve as the underlying stimulus for inflammatory injury.
- At the site of injury, a host of inflammatory events is set into action.
- Activation of the microcirculation results in cytokine and growth factor release leading to leukocyte migration into the interstitium causing local injury.
- TGF-β_1 appears to be a primary regulator of CVI induced injury.
- Fibroblast proliferation diminishes with disease progression ultimately leading to senescence and poor ulcer healing.
- Increase in MMP-2 synthesis appear to increase tissue remodeling and further impede ulcer healing.
- A deeper understanding of the mechanism involved in CVI may lead to new treatment strategies in the future.

REFERENCES

1. White GH. Chronic venous insufficiency. In: Veith F, Hobson RW, II, Williams RA, Wilson SE, eds. Vascular Surgery. New York: McGraw-Hill Inc, 1993:865–888.
2. Callam MJ. Epidemiology of varicose veins. Br J Surg 1994; 81:167–173.
3. Hume M. Presidential address: a venous renaissance? J Vasc Surg 1992; 6:947–951.
4. Lawrence PF, Gazak CE. Epidemiology of chronic venous insufficiency. In: Gloviczki P, Bergan JJ, eds. Atlas of Endoscopic Perforator Vein Surgery. London: Springer-Verlag, 1998:31–44.
5. Porter JM. International Consensus Committee on Chronic Venous Disease. Reporting Standards in venous disease: an update. J Vasc Surg 1995; 21:635–645.
6. Varicose veins: pathology. In: Browse NL, Burnand KG, Irvine AT, Wilson NM, eds. Diseases of the Veins. London and New York: Oxford University Press, 1999:145–162.
7. Gunderson J, Hauge M. Hereditary factors in venous insufficiency. Angiology 1969; 20:346–355.
8. Cornu-Thenard A, Boivin P, Baud MM, De Vincenzi I, Carpentier PH. Importance of the familial factor in varicose disease: clinical study of 134 families. J Derm Surg Onc 1994; 20:318–326.
9. Labropoulos N, Giannoukas AD, Delis K, et al. Where does the venous reflux start. J Vasc Surg 1997; 26:736–742.
10. Wakefield TM, Strietert RM, Prince MR, Downing LJ, Greenfield LJ. Pathogenesis of venous thrombosis: a new insight. Cardiovasc Surg 1997; 5:6–15.
11. Takase S, Bergan JJ, Schmid-Schonbein G. Expression of adhesion molecules and cytokines on saphenous veins in chronic venous insufficiency. Ann Vasc Surg 2000; 14:427–435.
12. Rose A. Some new thoughts on the etiology of varicose veins. J Cardiovasc Surg 1986; 27:534–543.
13. Pappas PJ, Gwertzman GA, DeFouw DO, et al. Retinoblastoma protein: a molecular regulator of chronic venous insufficiency. J Surg Res 1998; 76:149–153.
14. Travers JP, Brookes CE, Evans J, et al. Assessment of was structure and composition of varicose veins with reference to collagen, elastin and smooth muscle content. Eur J Vasc Endovasc Surg 1996; 11:230–237.
15. Jurukova Z, Milenkov C. Ultrastructural evidence for collagen degradation in the walls of varicose veins. Exp and Molec Path 1982; 37:37–47.
16. Venturi M, Bonavina L, Annoni F, et al. Biochemical assay of collagen and elastin in the normal and varicose vein wall. J Surg Res 1996; 60:245–248.
17. Maurel E, Azema C, Deloly J, Bouissou H. Collagen of the normal and the varicose human saphenous vein: a biochemical study. Clinica Chimica Acta 1990; 193:27–38.
18. Ascher E, Jacob T, Hingorani A, Gunduz Y, Mazzariol F, Kallakuri S. Programmed cell death (Apoptosis) and its role in the pathogenesis of lower extremity varicose veins. Ann Vasc Surg 2000; 14:24–30.
19. Ascher E, Jacob T, Hingorani A, Tsemekhin B, Gunduz Y. Expression of molecular mediators of apoptosis and their role in the pathogenesis of lower-extremity varicose veins. J Vasc Surg 2001; 33:1080–1086.
20. Gandhi RH, Irizarry E, Nachman GB, Halpern JJ, Mulcare RJ, Tilson MD. Analysis of the connective tissue matrix and proteolytic activity of primary varicose veins. J Vasc Surg 1993; 18:814–820.
21. Parra JR, Cambria RA, Hower CD, et al. Tissue inhibitor of metalloproteinase-1 is increased in the saphenofemoral junction of patients with varices in the leg. J Vasc Surg 1998; 28:669–675.
22. Kosugi I, Urayama H, Kasashima F, Ohtake H, Watanabe Y. Matrix metalloproteinase-9 and urokinase-type plasminogen activator in varicose veins. Ann Vasc Surg 2003; 17:234–238.
23. Woodside KJ, Hu M, Burke A, et al. Morphologic characteristics of varicose veins: Possible role of metalloproteinases. J Vasc Surg 2003; 38:162–169.
24. Shireman PK, McCarthy WJ, Pearce WH, et al. Plasminogen activator levels are influenced by location and varicosity in greater saphenous vein. J Vasc Surg 1996; 24:719–724.

25. Badier-Commander C, Verbeuren T, Lebard C, Michel J, Jacob M. Increased TIMP/MMP ratio in varicose veins: a possible explanation for extracellular matrix accumulation. J Path 2000; 192:105–112.

26. Lowell RC, Gloviczki P, Miller VM. In vitro evaluation of endothelial and smooth muscle function of primary varicose veins. J Vasc Surg 1992; 16:679–686.

27. Rizzi A, Quaglio D, Vasquez G, et al. Effects of vasoactive agents in healthy and diseased human saphenous veins. J Vasc Surg 1998; 28:855–861.

28. Barber DA, Wang X, Gloviczki P, Miller VM. Characterization of endothelin receptors in human varicose veins. J Vasc Surg 1997; 26:61–69.

29. Nemcova S, Gloviczki P, Rud KS, Miller VM. Cyclic nucleotides and production of prostanoids in human varicose veins. J Vasc Surg 1999; 30:876–884.

30. Homans J. The etiology and treatment of varicose ulcer of the leg. SG&O 1917; 24:300–311.

31. Blalock A. Oxygen content of blood in patiens with varicose veins. Arch Surg 1929; 19:898–905.

32. Pratt GH. Arterial varices; a syndrome. Am J Surg 1949; 77:456–460.

33. Burnand KG, Whimster I, Naidoo A, Browse NL. Pericapillary fibrin deposition in the ulcer bearing skin of the lower limb: the cause of lipodermatosclerosis and venous ulceration. Br Med J 1982; 285:1071–1072.

34. Burnand KG, Clemenson G, Gaunt J, Browse NL. The effect of sustained venus hypertension in the skin and capillaries of the canine hind limb. Br J Surg 1981; 69:41–44.

35. Browse NL, Burnand KG. The cause of venous ulceration. The Lancet 1982; 2:243–245.

36. Smith PDC, Thomas P, Scurr JH, Dormandy JA. Causes of venous ulceration: a new hypothesis. Br Med J 1988; 296:1726–1727.

37. Thomas P, Nash GB, Dormandy JA. White cell accumulation in dependent legs of patients with venous hypertension: a possible mechanism for trophic changes in the skin. Br Med J 1988; 296:1693–1695.

38. Scott HJ, Smith PDC, Scurr JH. Histological study of white blood cells and their association with lipodermatosclerosis and venous ulceration. Br J Surg 1991; 78:210–211.

39. Wilkinson LS, Bunker C, Edward JCW, Scurr JH, Smith PDC. Leukocytes: their role in the etiopathogenesis of skin damage in venous disease. J Vasc Surg 1993; 17:669–675.

40. Pappas PJ, DeFouw DO, Venezio LM, et al. Morphometric assessment of the dermal microcirculation in patients with chronic venous insufficiency. J Vasc Surg 1997; 26:784–795.

41. Herrick S, Sloan P, McGurk M, Freak L, McCollum CN, Ferguson WJ. Sequential changes in histologic pattern and extracellular matrix deposition during the healing of chronic venous ulcers. Am J Pathol 1992; 141:1085–1095.

42. Bishop JE. Regulation of cardiovascular collagen deposition by mechanical forces. Molec Med Today 1998; 4:69–75.

43. Higley HR, Kassander GA, Gerhardt CO, Falanga V. Extravasation of macromolecules and possible trapping of transforming growth factor-β1 in venous ulceration. Br J Surg 1995; 132:79–85.

44. Leu HJ. Morphology of chronic venous insufficiency-light and electron microscopic examinations. Vasa 1991; 20:330–342.

45. Wenner A, Leu HJ, Spycher M, Brunner U. Ultrastructural changes of capillaries in chronic venous insufficiency. Expl Cell Biol 1980; 48:1–14.

46. Peschen M, Lahaye T, Gennig B, Weyl A, Simon JC, Wolfgang V. Expression of the adhesion molecules ICAM-1, VCAM-1, LFA-1 and VLA-4 in the skin is modulated in progressing stages of chronic venous insufficiency. Acta Derm Venereol 1999; 79:27–32.

47. Pappas PJ, You R, Rameshwar P, et al. Dermal tissue fibrosis in patients with chronic venous insufficiency is associated with increased transforming growth factor-β_1 gene expression and protein production. J Vasc Surg 1999; 30:1129–1145.

48. Peschen M, Grenz H, Brand-Saberi B, et al. Increased expression of platelet-derived growth factor receptor alpha and beta and vascular endothelial growth factor in the skin of patients with chronic venous insufficiency. Arch Dermatol Res 1998; 290:291–297.

49. Hasan A, Murata H, Falabella A, et al. Dermal fibroblasts from venous ulcers are unresponsive to the action of transforming growth factor-β1. J Dermatol Sci 1997; 16:59–66.

50. Kim B, Kim HT, Park SH, et al. Fibroblasts from chronic wounds show altered TGF-β signaling and decreased TGF-β type II receptor expression. J Cell Physil 2003; 195:331–336.

51. Herrick SE, Ireland GW, Simon D, McCollum CN, Ferguson MW. Venous ulcer fibroblasts compared with normal fibroblasts show differences in collagen but not in fibronectin production under both normal and hypoxic conditions. J Invest Dermatol 1996; 106:187–193.

52. Stanley AC, Park H, Phillips TJ, Russakovsky V, Menzoian JO. Reduced growth of dermal fibroblasts from chronic venous ulcers can be stimulated with growth factors. J Vasc Surg 1997; 26:994–1001.

53. Mendez MV, Stanley A, Park H, Shon K, Phillips TJ, Menzoian JO. Fibroblasts cultured from venous ulcers display cellular characteristics of senescence. J Vasc Surg 1998; 28:876–883.

54. Lal BK, Saito S, Pappas PJ, et al. Altered proliferative responses of dermal fibroblasts to TGF-β1 may contribute to chronic venous stasis ulcers. J Vasc Surg 2003; in press.

55. Mendez MV, Stanley A, Phillips TJ, Murphy M, Menzoian JO, Park H. Fibroblasts cultured from distal lower extremities in patients with venous reflux display cellular characteristics of senescence. J Vasc Surg 1998; 28:1040–1050.

56. Weckroth M, Vaheri A, Lauharanta J, Sorsa T, Konttinen YT. Matrix metalloproteinases, gelatinase and collagenase, in chronic leg ulcers. J Invest Dermatol 1996; 106:1119–1124.

57. Wysocki AB, Staiano-Coico L, Grinell F. Wound fluid from chronic leg ulcers contains elevated levels of metalloproteinases MMP-2 and MMP-9. J Invest Dermatol 1993; 101:64–68.

58. Bullen EC, Longaker MT, Updike DL, et al. Tissue inhibitor of metalloproteinases-1 is decreased and activated gelatinases are increased in chronic wounds. J Invest Dermatol 1995; 104:236–240.

59. Herouy Y, May AE, Pornschlegel G, et al. Lipodermatosclerosis is characterized by elevated expression and activation of matrix metalloproteinases: Implications for venous ulcer formation. J Invest Dermatol 1998; 111:822–827.

60. Herouy Y, Trefzer D, Zimpfer U, Schopf E, Vanscheidt W, Norgauer J. Matrix metalloproteinases and venous leg ulceration. Eur J Dermatol 2000; 9:173–180.

61. Norgauer J, Hildenbrand T, Idzko M, et al. Elevated expression of extracellular matrix metalloproteinase inducer (CD 147) and membrane-type matrix metalloproteinases in venous leg ulcers. Br J Dermatol 2002; 147:1180–1186.

62. Saito S, Trovato MJ, You R, et al. Role of matrix metalloproteinases 1, 2, and 9 and tissue inhibitor of matrix metalloproteinase-1 in chronic venous insufficiency. J Vasc Surg 2001; 34:930–938.

63. Herouy Y, Trefzer D, Hellstern MO, et al. Plasminogen activation in venous leg ulcers. Br J Dermatol 2000; 143:930–936.

28

Compression Therapy and Nursing Care for Venous Leg Ulcers

Jill Robson
Freeman Hospital, Newcastle upon Tyne, U.K.

Hany Hafez
St. Richard's Hospital, Chichester, U.K.

BACKGROUND

Patients with leg ulcers should expect to have a full assessment carried out by a competent healthcare professional (1). In most cases the ulcer will be found to be due to venous insufficiency, and should respond to treatment with sustained graduated compression, which remains the preferred method of treatment worldwide (2). There are different ways of applying this amount of compression, and healthcare professionals who carry out these treatments should demonstrate their competence to do so. The choice of compression method should be based on the patient's condition, the patient's preference and the availability of suitable, evidence-based equipment. As with any intervention, patient consent must be sought.

Most leg ulcers are due to venous incompetence. The incidence of venous ulceration is in the region of 0.3% and is responsible for 90% of all leg ulcers. Venous ulceration can result from superficial venous insufficiency, deep venous insufficiency, or both. "Stasis" ulceration can also occur secondary to excessive obesity, immobility with prolonged leg dependency, and poor calf muscle pump function. These ulcers often benefit from treatment aimed at improving venous return. Compression therapy is currently the most effective way of doing this (3). There are, however, other causes for leg ulceration which, although less common, can have serious consequences if treated inappropriately. These causes include arterial insufficiency, diabetes, skin malignancy, vasculitis, and autoimmune disease such as rheumatoid arthritis. Every patient presenting with a leg ulcer should therefore be carefully assessed to determine the etiology prior to proceeding with compression therapy.

The Venous System in the Leg and Principles of Compression

Leg venous flow to the heart is mainly maintained by the combined action of the muscle pump and venous valvular directional regulation. When the calf muscles contract, pressure is exerted on the deep veins which are responsible for 75% of the venous return from the leg. During relaxation, blood is prevented from gravitating in the veins by the action of competent valves. Failure of one or both components of this system, such as damaged valves or poor muscle function or inability to move the ankle joint, can lead to *venous hypertension*. Over a period of time venous hypertension can lead to skin devitalisation and ulceration. The principle behind compression therapy for venous ulceration is to counteract the venous hypertension effects on the skin. This is achieved by the direct physical pressure of the dressing and by augmenting the calf muscle pump action (4). The ideal levels of compression to reverse venous hypertension are 35–40 mmHg at the ankle, graduating down to 17–20 mmHg under the knee.

Several methods of applying such pressure have been tried, these include:

1. Multilayer elastic compression bandage
2. Inelastic short stretch bandage
3. Two layer Vari-stretch® bandage (Proguide®)
4. Elastic compression hosiery

As the degree of compression is inversely proportional to the circumference of the limb, i.e., more compression is exerted on a thinner part of the leg than on a wider part (Laplace's law), the effectiveness of any graduated compression method will rely on the shape of the leg being conical. The leg should therefore be thinner at the ankle than it is below the knee. If the leg is not naturally this shape, then the padding layer should be used to reshape it before the compression is applied (Fig. 1).

It is important that *none* of these methods of compression are used *if there is any evidence of arterial insufficiency, as indicated by an ankle brachial pressure index of less than .85*. Reduced compression may, however, be appropriate for some patients with mixed disease. All patients must be fully assessed and etiology determined before a plan of care can be made (5).

ASSESSMENT

All patients require full assessment, preferably using a written pro forma. Particular attention should be paid to the following issues (6).

Predisposing History for Venous Disease

Carefully question the patient and use medical records if available.

- Patients may already have history of venous disease and surgery. The type of previous surgery should be sought. Similarly, patients may have had deep venous thrombosis (DVT) in the past; details of this should also be sought.

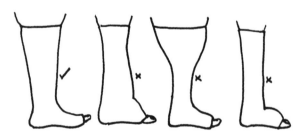

Figure 1   Correct and incorrect appearance of leg before application of compression.

- An undiagnosed DVT in the past should be investigated. Relevant history includes history of major leg orthopedic trauma or surgery, known DVT risks such as concurrent malignancy, thrombophilia, and morbid obesity.
- Any occupation that involves long periods of standing can aggravate or lead to varicose veins and so an occupational history should be taken.

Predisposing History for Arterial Disease

- Smoking is the most significant risk factor for arterial disease and should always be asked about.
- Arterial disease often affects other vessels such as coronary arteries, carotid or renal arteries. Symptoms related to these vessels such as angina, myocardial infarction, stroke or hypertension should be sought. Some patients may have already been diagnosed with peripheral arterial disease.
- Diabetes can be associated with medium and small vessel disease.
- Rheumatoid arthritis and other autoimmune diseases can lead to vasculitic changes.

Presenting Clinical Signs and Symptoms of Venous Disease

- *Varicose veins*, if present, are easily visible under the skin.
- *Inverted champagne bottle shape* is the characteristic shape of the leg, due to long term venous insufficiency. This is due to gradual loss of muscle bulk and lipodermatosclerosis.
- *Lipodermatosclerosis* is the term given to the hard "woody," scaly, appearance of the skin due to gradual hardening of the dermis and fibrosis of the subcutaneous fat, a side effect of long-term venous hypertension.
- *Venous eczema* also known as varicose eczema, is similar in appearance to eczema. It is the term given to red, very itchy patches that weep clear fluid. This is due to small splits in the skin, as it is unable to stretch and accommodate edema.
- *Ankle flare* also known as telangiectasia, is often seen as a result of venous insufficiency. As the veins and venules become more and more congested, they become distended and visible as a crop of purple vessels under the skin on the foot or ankle.
- *Edema* in venous disease is usually accompanied by one or more other symptoms. It is not "pitting," and care must be taken to ensure that it is not a result of congestive cardiac failure.
- *Atrophie blanche* is another symptom of venous disease. It refers to the ivory white patches of scarred looking skin, often stippled with the red dots of distended capillary loops, due to a loss of the capillaries' ability to transfer oxygen to the tissues. This condition can be very painful and is often mistaken as an arterial symptom.
- The *skin pigmentation* associated with venous insufficiency is due to microhemorrhages leading to a build up of hemosiderin deposition. This causes the skin to become brown or black in the area most affected. The gaiter area of the leg is usually most affected (Fig. 2).

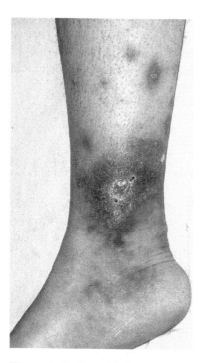

Figure 2 Patient with chronic venous insufficiency showing skin pigmentation, venous ulceration, and patchy lipodermatosclerosis in the gaiter area.

Presenting Signs and Symptoms of Arterial Disease

- *Intermittent claudication* is the term given to a severe cramp-like pain usually in the calf but sometimes in the thigh or buttock. The pain comes on during walking or other exercise, and stops after a few minutes of rest. This is due to poor perfusion of muscles and is an indicator of arterial disease.
- *Ischemic rest pain* also known as just "rest pain," is usually in the foot or lower part of the leg. It comes on whenever the limb is elevated. This is due to critical foot arterial supply, which relies on gravity to draw the arterial blood into the foot. The limb may also *lose color on elevation*. Patients with this condition often have to sleep in a chair or hang their leg out of the bed. This is not to be confused with night cramps, a benign condition suffered by many elderly people with or without peripheral arterial disease.
- The *location of the ulcer* is important. Any ulcer on the toes or foot, below the level of the malleolus, must be suspected of being arterial or diabetic in origin. Occasionally, however, patients may present with pressure ulcers on the foot, which have the appearance of arterial ulcers, so this should be eliminated as a cause.
- *Delayed capillary refilling*, when combined with other features of arterial disease, can be a useful sign. The perfusion of the skin is often poor in arterial disease. To test capillary refill time, gently apply pressure to the toenail bed until it blanches, then release the pressure and count the number of seconds until the color returns. As a rule, refill time over 3 seconds may indicate poor perfusion.

- *Atrophic shiny skin*, when combined with other signs and symptoms of arterial disease, can add to the overall picture of long-term arterial insufficiency. This sign can also occur with long-term steroid therapy.
- The *appearance of the ulcer* is important, as arterial ulcers are usually deeper, have a "punched out" edge, and often have evidence of *tissue necrosis* such as eschar or slough.

Mixed Arterial and Venous Disease

As previously mentioned, most patients with ulcers have venous insufficiency, and will benefit from compression therapy. Careful history taking and physical examination can determine those whose ulcers are due to arterial disease who must not have compression therapy. There are, however, some patients who present with all the features of venous disease, but who have underlying arterial disease not immediately apparent. It is therefore imperative that further investigation is carried out to determine this, before potentially dangerous bandaging is started.

Ankle to Brachial Pressure Index (ABPI)

This procedure is used widely to assess arterial blood flow in the arteries in the leg, and must be done for all patients presenting with a leg ulcer, and have absent palpable ankle pulses before any compression is used (7). Ankle to brachial pressure index (ABPI) is a comparison of the ankle systolic arterial blood pressure with the brachial systolic arterial blood pressure. The procedure should be explained to the patient and verbal consent obtained. Make sure the patient is lying flat for at least 10 minutes before starting.
Prepare the equipment:

- Doppler machine
- Sphygmomanometer and suitably sized cuff
- Ultrasound gel or other water-based gel
- Tissues
- Light waterproof dressing to cover the ulcer

Secure the cuff around the arm as if taking a blood pressure reading in the normal manner. Apply gel over the brachial pulse. Hold the Doppler probe over the brachial pulse, at an angle of 60° to the skin, tucked into the gel. Move the probe carefully until a good signal is obtained. Inflate the cuff until the signal disappears, then gradually inflate until the signal returns. Note the pressure reading on the sphygmomanometer. Repeat on the other arm. Make a note of the higher of the two readings. This is the *brachial systolic pressure*.

Place a light dressing over the ulcer, look for foot pulses in the shown positions (Fig. 3). Apply gel to the search area. Secure the cuff around the leg just above the ankle. Hold the Doppler probe in the gel over the dorsalis pedis area at an angle of 60°, and look for a signal. Once a signal is found, keep the probe in position and inflate the cuff until the signal disappears. Deflate gradually until the signal returns. Note the pressure reading on the sphygmomanometer. Repeat the procedure for the posterior tibial signal. Make a note of the higher of the two readings. This is the *ankle systolic pressure*. Use the tissues to remove gel from patient's skin. To work out the ABPI, divide the ankle systolic pressure by the brachial systolic pressure. If the ankle pressure is the same as the

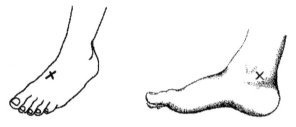

Figure 3   Sites of dorsalis pedis and posterior tibial arteries.

brachial, the ABPI will be 1.0. If the ankle pressure is lower than the brachial, then the ABPI will be less than 1.0. To allow for a small margin of error, any reading of between 0.85 and 1.2, where all the assessment criteria point to there being no arterial disease, is considered normal and compression can be used (8).

In patients with *diabetes*, *renal disease* or severe *arteriosclerosis*, the ankle pressure reading may be significantly higher than the brachial systolic pressure. These conditions can lead to calcification of the arterial walls, making them impossible to occlude with the sphygmomanometer cuff. It is therefore important that all readings are interpreted with care.

An ABPI of between 0.6 and 0.85 indicates a moderate degree of arterial insufficiency. It is not considered safe to apply full compression, but in some circumstances light compression can be applied. It is advisable to seek advice from a specialist practitioner before doing so.

An ABPI of less than 0.6 usually indicates more severe arterial disease; *no compression* should be applied to these patients under any circumstances. They will require referral to the vascular service for further investigations.

Recognizing Rare Causes for Leg Ulceration

There are several unusual causes for ulcers that will be difficult for less experienced practitioners to recognize. Some are listed here:

- *Neuropathic diabetic foot ulcers* will need to be referred to the diabetic podiatry service. Initial treatment will be centered on relief of pressure, and prevention and treatment of infection. Compression is not advised.
- *Pyoderma gangrenosum* can occur anywhere on the body, but particularly on the leg. It is due to a vasculitic response to a systemic autoimmune disease such as Crohn's disease or ulcerative colitis. The ulcer often has a necrotic appearance and may have a purple border around it. Treatment is usually offered though the dermatology unit.
- *Rheumatoid ulcers* often have a punched out appearance with tissue necrosis. Treatment of the underlying rheumatoid disease along with local wound care is advised. *Malignancy* can occur on the skin of the leg or develop within an existing ulcer. If malignancy is suspected then the patient should be referred urgently to the dermatology department.
- *Factitious* ulcers are those caused by the patient self-harming. This is a complex problem requiring sensitive management. Psychological support may be required.

- *Tropical ulcers* are due to infection with any one of a number of tropical organisms, causing tissue necrosis. The infection should be treated and help should be sought from microbiology or the department of tropical diseases.

If any of these unusual causes is suspected, the patient should be referred to the appropriate specialist and simple local wound care continued.

Assessing the Ulcer and Surrounding Skin

The size of the ulcer should be documented either with a ruler or tape measure, making a tracing, or taking a photograph. Remember that the patient's consent is required before photographs may be taken, and this must be documented.

As with other chronic wounds, good wound bed preparation is important. The wound should be assessed to determine the presence of necrotic material or slough, the bacterial burden on the wound surface and the level and type of exudate. Patients with leg ulceration often develop skin sensitivities to various preparations used to treat their ulcers or their dry scaly skin. If skin sensitivity or allergy is suspected, then the preparation should be discontinued and referral to dermatology considered so that the source of the sensitivity can be determined. A pain assessment form should also be completed for all patients. As with all patients suffering from chronic illness, it is important that they are adequately nourished. Obesity can also be a contributing factor to the leg ulceration and should be treated. Dietetic referral may be appropriate in these circumstances.

TREATMENT

The leg should be washed in warm tap water and the ulcer and surrounding skin treated before dressings are applied. The type of primary dressing should be chosen according to the nature of the wound bed. As a general rule it is best to choose the simplest dressing, such as non-adherent knitted viscose. There may be circumstances where the wound bed requires modification.

1. An anti-microbial dressing may help to reduce the bacterial burden
2. An odor control dressing may be used if odor is a problem

Hydrogels and other dressings with high water content are not usually appropriate under a compression bandage as they can cause maceration of the surrounding skin.

Where there is a large amount of exudate, it is important to get the compression profile correct, so padded dressings are to be avoided. These can alter the shape of the limb and make the problem worse (Fig. 1). A simple absorbent pad can be applied *on top of* the bandage if "strike through" occurs.

COMPRESSION

The first graduated compression stockings were introduced by Conrad Jobst more than 40 years ago and now bandaging systems and hosiery of various types are available. The common forms of compression used today are:

1. Multi-layer elastic compression bandages; e.g., Profore®, K four®, Ultra four®, System 4®, Hospifour®
2. Short stretch inelastic bandages; e.g., Comprilan®, Rosidal K®, Actiban®, Silkolan®, Varex®

3. Multi-layer Varistretch® elastic compression bandage; e.g., Proguide®
4. Elastic compression hosiery

Application Methods

The methods used should be in conjunction with the manufacturers instructions for use and alongside supervized practical instruction. All patients should receive careful explanation of the procedure. If written information is given, this must be documented.

Multi-Layer Elastic Compression Bandages (9)

Measure the patient's ankle circumference. Most kits are only suitable for ankles that are 18–25 centimeters in circumference. Narrower ankles will need more padding, and wider ankles will need bandages with more power to provide enough compression.

The patient and nurse should be comfortably positioned so that the patient's foot is at right angles to the leg throughout, and the nurse can reach around the leg without having to lift it or bend his/her back. The padding layer should be applied in a spiral. The first turn starting at the base of the toes, the next turn cupping the heel, returning over the top of the instep, down under the foot and then continuing up the leg to just below the knee. If the leg is thin, then more padding may be required to protect any bony prominences. Extra padding will also be required if the leg needs reshaping. The leg should then be twice as wide under the knee as it is at the ankle (Fig. 1).

The next layer is a crepe bandage used to smooth out the padding layer. It is applied in a similar fashion to the first layer. Cut off any excess and secure with tape under the knee. The third layer is a light compression bandage. This is applied around the foot in the same way as the first two layers, using only enough stretch to take up the slack and make it fit snugly over the crepe layer. Overstretching at this point will be very uncomfortable for the patient and can lead to tissue damage. Once the ankle is covered, then the bandage should be stretched by 50% and applied in a figure-of-eight technique with 50% overlap. Once the knee is reached, cut off the excess and secure with tape.

The final layer is a cohesive compression bandage. It is applied over the foot as before, just taking up the slack; then at the ankle stretching by 50% and continuing in a spiral with 50% overlap. Cut off the excess. Make sure the patient can move the ankle joint (Fig. 4).

Short Stretch Inelastic Bandages

These bandages cannot accommodate any change in the limb circumference. They work as the pressure beneath the bandage increases as the calf muscle is activated. The bandage reinforces the action of the calf muscle pump. Because they rely on this calf muscle action and have low resting pressures, they are unsuitable for immobile patients or those who have fixed ankles due to arthritis. A recent randomized trial has suggested that they are less effective in ulcer healing than four-layer bandaging (10).

The method of application depends upon the size and shape of the limb. The width of bandage is also dependent upon the circumference of the limb. An easy way to gauge this is to choose a bandage with a similar width to the diameter of the widest part of the leg. Padding should be used over any bony prominences and to fill any concave areas such as behind the malleoli.

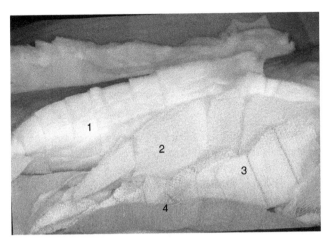

Figure 4 Standard four-layer compression: 1) cotton wool padding, 2) crepe, 3) light compression bandage, and 4) cohesive bandage.

Starting at the toes the bandage should be applied at full stretch with one anchoring turn around the foot. The next turn should go around the heel, mostly above the heel. The next goes over the instep and back around the heel, mostly below it. The bandage can then be wound around the leg at full stretch to just below the knee. It must not be cut, as it would fray. Instead it can be brought back down the leg and secured with tape. If a second bandage is required to treat a large limb, it should be applied in the opposite direction to the first. Pieces of tape around the toes and heel can prevent the bandage rolling or slipping. As these bandages have no elastic they may not stay in place on some patients.

If this happens then use the "knee lock" method. The bandage is applied on the foot as before. It is then taken at a steep angle up to the knee where an anchoring turn is made around the knee. The bandage is then wound down the leg to be secured at the ankle with tape.

Multi-Layer Varistretch® Bandages

These elastic bandages employ new technology, which reduces the margin for error in applying the correct amount of compression. There are three sizes of kit so it is important to measure the ankle and choose the correct one. The first layer is padding, which is applied toe to knee. This is to protect bony prominences and absorb exudate. Extra padding may be used to reshape the limb as with the other multi-layer bandages.

The other layer has a guide printed on it to enable the nurse to tell if the bandage has been extended by the correct amount. The bandage should be applied around the foot as in the other methods, without any extension. At the ankle the bandage should be stretched until the oval guide printed on it becomes circular. Continue using this degree of stretch in a spiral method at 50% overlap until the knee is reached. Cut off the excess and secure with tape.

Although there is a printed guide, there is no need to worry too much about using an exact amount of stretch, as the bandage itself has been developed to deliver 35–40 mmHg compression at the ankle, even if it has not been stretched quite enough or a little too much.

All compression bandaging techniques will reduce edema in the limb if correctly applied. It is important, therefore, to reassess the limb circumference in the initial stages of treatment to ensure the patient has the correct bandage system. Once the edema is controlled, the bandages should stay in place for up to one week.

Elastic Compression Hosiery

Compression hosiery can be used to prevent recurrence of venous leg ulcers once they have healed. In some circumstances, such as patient preference and when there is only a small ulcer, they can be used to provide a treatment for venous ulcer disease.

Treating ulcers and controlling venous edema requires a similar amount of compression to an elastic compression bandage; i.e., up to 35 mmHg at the ankle. A continental class 2 stocking will provide this, or a U.K. class 3 stocking (the classifications are different). If the patient cannot tolerate this, then a lower compression class can be used but will not be as effective. Below-knee stockings are adequate in most cases.

Correct measurement is important. This should be done with the patient barefoot and standing on a flat surface. Measurements should be taken in three places: at the ankle just above the level of the malleolus, around the widest part of the calf, and the length from the top of the stocking under the knee to the ground. The correctly sized stocking can then be fitted. Some patients find stockings very difficult to apply, particularly if they have arthritis or cannot reach their feet. Application aids are available. Stockings should be replaced every 3–6 months; and continued compression may prevent recurrence (11). It is advisable to ensure that the patient has not developed any arterial disease in the interim before supplying new stockings.

Choice of Compression Method

In light of the multitude of compression therapies available, several trials have been conducted to study the efficacy of each method. Table 1 summarizes some of these trials.

Most authors therefore believe that four-layer compression therapy achieves the best results. There are however other factors that might cause delayed or failed healing with compression. These factors include an ulcer size greater than 10 cm and a duration of more than 12 months (16,17).

Table 1 Trials of Types of Compression

Study	Type (No. of patients)	Compression used				Conclusion
		Four-layer	Short-stretch	Two-layer	Other	
Nelson et al. (10)	Randomized (387)	X	X			Healing is quicker with four-layer compression
Franks et al. (12)	Randomized (156)	X	X			Healing speed similar between both
Ukat et al. (13)	Randomized (89)	X	X			Healing is quicker with four-layer compression
O'Brien et al. (14)	Randomized (200)	X			X	Four-layer is most effective treatment
Moffat et al. (15)	Randomized (112)	X		X		Four-layer is better tolerated, and less expensive

KEY POINTS

- Most venous ulcers can be effectively treated using compression therapy.
- Patients with leg ulcers should have a full assessment by an experienced practitioner.
- Arterial insufficiency should be excluded by clinical assessment and measurement of the ankle: brachial pressure index (ABPI).
- The dressing should be simple, non-adherent and not padded or bulky.
- Compression bandages should be carefully applied to ensure graduated compression from ankle upward.
- Compression hosiery can be used to prevent recurrence of venous leg ulcers once they have healed.

REFERENCES

1. Royal College of Nursing Clinical Practice Guidelines. The Management of Patients with Venous Leg Ulcers. RCN Institute, 1998.
2. Moneta GL, Nicoloff AD, Porter JM. Compression treatment of chronic venous ulceration: a review. Phlebology 2000; 15:162–168.
3. Cullum N, Nelson EA, Fletcher AW, Sheldon TA. Compression for venous leg ulcers Cochrane Database Syst Rev 2001; (2):CD000265. Update of: Cochrane Database Syst Rev 2000; (3):CD000265.
4. Partsch H. Compression therapy in venous leg ulcers. How does it work. J Phlebol 2002; 2:129–136.
5. Marston W, Vowden KR. Compression therapy: a guide to safe practice. In: Understanding Compression Therapy (EWMA position document). MEP, 2003.
6. Morrison M, Moffatt C. A Colour Guide to the Assessment and Management of Leg Ulcers. 2nd ed. London: Mosby, 1994.
7. Stubbings NJ, Bailey P, Poole M. Protocol for the accurate assessment of ABPI in patients with leg ulcers. J Wound Care 1997; 6:417–418.
8. Scottish Intercollegiate Guideline Network. The Care of Patients with Chronic Leg Ulcers. SIGN secretariat, 1998.
9. Ruckley CV, Dale JJ, Gibson B, Brown D, Lee AJ, Prescott RJ. Multi-layer compression: comparison of four different four-layer bandage systems applied to the leg. Phlebology 2003; 18:123–129.
10. Nelson EA, Iglesias CP, et al. Randomized clinical trial of four-layer and short-stretch compression bandages for venous leg ulcers (VenUS I). Br J Surg 2004; 91:1292–1299.
11. Nelson EA, Bell-Syer SE, Cullum NA. Compression for preventing recurrence of venous ulcers. Cochrane Database Syst Rev 2000; (4):CD002303.
12. Franks PJ, Moody M, et al. Randomized trial of cohesive short-stretch versus four-layer bandaging in the management of venous ulceration. Wound Repair Regen 2004; 12:157–162.
13. Ukat A, Konig M, et al. Short-stretch versus multilayer compression for venous leg ulcers: a comparison of healing rates. J Wound Care 2003; 12:139–143.
14. O'Brien JF, Grace PA, et al. Randomized clinical trial and economic analysis of four-layer compression bandaging for venous ulcers. Br J Surg 2003; 90:794–798.
15. Moffatt CJ, McCullagh L, et al. Randomized trial of four-layer and two-layer bandage systems in the management of chronic venous ulceration. Wound Repair Regen 2003; 11:166–171.
16. Meaume S, Couilliet D, et al. Prognostic factors for venous ulcer healing in a non-selected population of ambulatory patients. J Wound Care 2005; 14:31–34.
17. Margolis DJ, Allen-Taylor L, et al. The accuracy of venous leg ulcer prognostic models in a wound care system. Wound Repair Regen 2004; 12:163–168.

29

Surgical Therapies for Chronic Venous Disease: Superficial Venous Surgery

Frank C. T. Smith
Bristol Royal Infirmary, Bristol, U.K.

INTRODUCTION

The term chronic venous insufficiency embraces a variety of disorders of the lower limb veins, ranging from simple varicose veins to skin changes and venous ulceration. The broad condition is characterized by long-term failure of venous return due to reflux in the superficial, perforating or deep veins, or to combinations of these, failure of the calf muscle pump, or due to venous outflow obstruction. These conditions lead to ambulatory or dependent venous hypertension and sequelae of pain, discomfort, swelling, varicose eczema, lipodermatosclerosis or ulceration.

The condition is widespread and has enormous economic impact. Between 2–9% of the adult population are affected (1). The prevalence of active ulceration in the United Kingdom is approximately 1.9 per 1000 in adults over the age of 45 years, with an annual incidence of 3.5 per 1000 in the same age group, a figure that increases with age (2). Open venous ulcers occur in approximately 0.3% of the population and a history of open or healed ulceration, exists in around 1% (3). In the United Kingdom, the cost of chronic venous insufficiency to the National Health Service is estimated to be between £230–600 million per annum (4). In the United States 4.6 million workdays are lost each year due to chronic venous disease. Up to 5% of affected patients may suffer job losses (5).

Appropriate surgical treatment for chronic venous disease should be directed at the underlying causes of venous hypertension. This is dependent on accurate diagnosis of predisposing factors. This chapter deals specifically with superficial venous surgery.

THE ROLE OF SUPERFICIAL INCOMPETENCE IN CHRONIC VENOUS INSUFFICIENCY

The CEAP classification of venous disease outlines three aetiologies for chronic venous insufficiency: congenital, primary and secondary (6,7).

Although the stigmata of chronic venous insufficiency have traditionally been associated with a post-phlebitic picture, it is now evident that these may also occur due to isolated primary deep or superficial reflux, with or without perforator incompetence, or as a result of multisystem incompetence involving at least two of these three systems. Primary valvular incompetence accounts for approximately 70% of cases of advanced chronic venous insufficiency and can be diagnosed in the absence of history of previous deep venous thrombosis (DVT), and where duplex ultrasound or venography fails to demonstrate signs suggestive of previous DVT (5).

Secondary incompetence usually affects the deep or perforating veins and most frequently arises as a result of deep venous thrombosis. Incompetence rather than venous obstruction is the more common cause of chronic venous insufficiency in the latter group. Symptoms of persisting deep venous obstruction include leg swelling and venous claudication.

Various studies have identified the extent of involvement of isolated and mixed incompetence in patients with chronic venous insufficiency although published evidence has been conflicting.

In a duplex study of patients with venous ulceration, Hanrahan et al. demonstrated isolated superficial venous incompetence in only 17% of 91 limbs (8). Lees and Lambert, also using duplex, found isolated superficial reflux in 57% of limbs. In patients with more than one site of reflux, 77% had involvement of the superficial system, with the deep system implicated in 39% of cases (9). Darke and Penfold employed ascending and descending venography, detecting superficial reflux in 39% and deep reflux in 57% of 213 legs (10). In an overview of 12 studies involving 1084 limbs with chronic venous disease, examined with a variety of techniques, Kalra and Gloviczki noted that isolated superficial incompetence occurred in 10%, the superficial system was affected as part of multisystem disease in a further 73% of cases and that isolated deep venous incompetence occurred in only 11% of cases (5). The role of superficial venous incompetence in chronic venous insufficiency, particularly in the absence of previous DVT, has therefore clearly been established.

Key techniques used for pre-operative assessment of the extent and nature of reflux include duplex Doppler imaging, venography, plethysmography and ambulatory venous pressure measurements. These have been discussed in detail elsewhere in this book.

SURGERY FOR SUPERFICIAL VENOUS REFLUX

Aims of Surgical Treatment

The aims of superficial venous surgery are to alleviate the component of chronic venous insufficiency which is due to superficial reflux and to promote ulcer healing, or to prevent further skin changes or symptoms such as swelling and pain, by reducing venous ambulatory hypertension. The ESCHAR study suggested that while surgery confers no benefit over multilayer elastic compression, in terms of healing of venous ulcers, it does lead to reduction of ulcer recurrence in patients with isolated superficial venous reflux (11). Haemodynamic benefits from superficial surgery, in patients with coexisting segmental deep venous reflux, have been clearly demonstrated in other studies (12,13). These results are reflected by improvement in quality of life, as assessed by both disease-specific and generic questionnaires (14–16).

In each case, surgery will be tailored to the individual patient on the basis of findings from clinical examination and the results of non-invasive or invasive investigations. In the case of superficial incompetence this may be achieved by attenuation of reflux in the long or short saphenous systems, and by removal of incompetent varicose veins, (phlebectomies).

Various interventional techniques have been employed to ablate superficial venous reflux. These include surgery, radio-frequency ablation, laser ablation of the saphenous vein and ultrasound-guided foam sclerotherapy. Subfascial endoscopic perforator surgery (SEPS) has been used to deal with incompetent perforators. This chapter deals with superficial surgery alone and the other therapeutic modalities are addressed elsewhere in this book.

Medico-Legal Aspects of Venous Surgery

Venous surgery is the most common source of medico-legal claims arising from vascular surgery. In 424 vascular claims notified to the National Health Service Litigation Authority and Medical Defence Union from 1990–1999, 244 arose from varicose vein surgery (nerve damage 76; incorrect or unsatisfactory surgery 35; damage to femoral vein 16, or artery 13) (17). Prior to undertaking superficial venous surgery, the operating surgeon must therefore explain the proposed procedure to the patient in detail, outlining specific risks. These include haematoma formation, wound infection, recurrence and the possibility that not all varicosities affecting the patient will be excised or ameliorated. Flare veins may occasionally be exacerbated. Risks of injury to the saphenous nerve during stripping of the long saphenous vein with resultant anesthesia, paraesthesia or neuralgia should be explained. Where short sapheno-popliteal surgery is proposed, the risks of associated sural or peroneal nerve injury should also be outlined. Discussion of these risks should be documented. Best practice dictates that the patient should be provided with a comprehensive information leaflet, but this alone will not provide a defence against litigation.

Factors increasing thrombotic tendency, particularly the oral contraceptive pill and hormone replacement therapy, should be considered with the patient. These medications should either be stopped for an adequate period before elective surgery, or, if patient and surgeon elect to continue with treatment, the deliberation and rationale for this course of management and potential treatment with other anti-thrombotic measures should also be carefully documented.

Day-Case or In-Patient Surgery?

The majority of patients undergoing long or short saphenous vein surgery can be treated as day cases. Patient fitness is usually assessed by the clinician in the out-patient department. Routine pre-operative evaluation can be undertaken by a nurse specialist. If day-case surgery is carried out, then adequate time must be taken to explain the consequences of surgery to the patient and to ensure that questions are answered. It is important to ensure that adequate post-operative analgesia is prescribed and that the patient is fully conversant with treatment protocols detailing dressing removal, use of compression hosiery, bathing, exercise, driving and resumption of employment.

Factors militating against successful day-case surgery include long procedures entailing prolonged anesthesia, obesity and co-morbidity. Age, fitness, and the availability of a care-giver in the early post-operative period should also be considered. Some day-case units will not undertake bilateral procedures or revision surgery and in these cases, admission to a short-stay unit (<24 hr) may be a viable option. The patient's wishes should also be considered.

Factors contributing to a successful outcome of day-case surgery include adequate local anesthetic infiltration of wounds, judicious use of non steroidal anti-inflammatory drugs and avoidance of opiates, which may help to reduce post-operative nausea (18). Early telephone follow-up by a specialist nurse or medical practitioner, together with printed contact details of who to contact in case of post-operative problems, may help to allay any residual patient fears.

Skin Marking

The operating surgeons should carry out preoperative marking of varicosities to their own satisfaction. Where revision surgery is being undertaken, when perforators play a significant part in the pattern of incompetence, as an aid to marking the variable level of the sapheno-popliteal junction, or where any doubt exists as to the source of incompetence, pre-operative duplex scanning and mapping provides an invaluable aid to surgery. Each surgeon adopts their own approach to marking of varicosities, but a common theme will be to avoid placing markings where cuts or stab incisions might predispose to skin tattooing. It is worth noting that alcohol-based skin preparations may prove a frustrating solvent for many proprietary skin markers, resulting in the outline of carefully mapped varicosities disappearing before the surgeon's eyes! On completion of marking, the patient should always be asked whether any varicosities of concern to them have been missed.

Anesthesia

The majority of superficial venous surgery performed in the United Kingdom is undertaken under general anesthesia. This is not necessarily the case in other parts of the world, for instance in areas of Europe, where regional and local anesthesia are sometimes prevalent alternatives. The latter techniques may have particular merit when dealing with high-risk, elderly or pregnant patients. A femoral nerve block can be used when stripping the long saphenous vein, but prolonged effects may prevent early postoperative discharge from the hospital. Many surgeons opt to infiltrate the path of the long saphenous vein with a solution of dilute local anesthesia and adrenaline, which promotes vasoconstriction, reducing bleeding and haematoma formation. Flush ligation and division of the sapheno-femoral junction, with localised distal ligation/division of the long saphenous vein can be performed under local anesthetic infiltration and may be a valuable adjunct to ulcer healing, particularly in elderly or frail patients. When employing extensive infiltration with local anesthetics, it is important that compliance with maximal dosage is adhered to, in order to avoid potential problems with overdose toxicity.

Positioning

The patient is placed supine for long saphenous surgery, but ideally, is turned prone for short saphenous surgery and popliteal explorations. The anaesthetist may entreat the surgeon to undertake the latter surgery with the patient in a lateral position, the affected leg lying uppermost, or from underneath with the knee flexed, but this allows the veins to retreat from the skin surface into the depths of the popliteal fossa and provides sub-optimal access. When the patient is placed prone for surgery under general anesthesia, adequate chest support and use of a cuffed endotracheal tube, to protect the airway, will be necessary. The patient should be warned about the possibility of a postoperative "sore throat" before surgery. A head-down position reduces venous pressure and bleeding.

Sapheno-Femoral Ligation and Stripping of the Long Saphenous Vein

Flush ligation of the long saphenous vein at the sapheno-femoral junction, with division of the vein and stripping to the level of the knee, reduces risk of recurrence (19,20) and remains the preferred surgical procedure for treatment of sapheno-femoral incompetence.

A 2 cm oblique incision is placed in, or just above, the groin skin crease, medial to the femoral pulse. In obese patients, access should not be hampered by a diminutive incision. The skin may be lifted with a small self-retaining retractor allowing the adventitial tissue and fat to be swept away distally from the saphenous opening in the fascia lata, exposing the long saphenous vein and tributaries. All tributaries are dissected to facilitate division and ligation distant to the saphenous vein. (So named long saphenous vein tributaries in the femoral triangle include the superficial epigastric, the superficial external pudendal, the superficial circumflex iliac veins and the lateral and medial femoral branches). If these vessels are not divided at some distance from the long saphenous vein, then persistent branches may form a residual network of veins, a common source of recurrence. When approaching the sapheno-femoral junction care should be taken to prevent bleeding from the external pudendal artery which usually passes from lateral to medial in the angle between the long saphenous vein and femoral vein.

The most important part of the groin dissection is clear visualization of the sapheno-femoral junction with demonstration of the descending portion of the femoral vein. Inadvertent ligation or stripping of the femoral vein (or even the artery) is well recognized as a cause for successful litigation, and demonstration of the junction will help the surgeon avoid this potentially disastrous pitfall.

Ligation of the sapheno-femoral junction should be undertaken flush with the femoral vein, avoiding creation of a stenosis. Techniques of ligation are a matter of surgeon preference, as are suture materials, but ligation in continuity reduces the risk of bleeding from the femoral vein defect if a securing vascular clip slips and some authors have argued that employment of a non-absorbable polypropylene transfixion suture reduces risk of recurrence due to neovascularisation.

Traction on the divided proximal end of the long saphenous vein and retraction on the lower border of the skin incision should enable access to and ligation of, the postero-medial and anterior thigh veins, further potential sources of recurrence.

Stripping of the long saphenous vein reduces risk of recurrence compared to high ligation alone. Historically, stripping of the full length of vein to the ankle was associated with a significant incidence of saphenous nerve injury (10%) and disabling saphenous nerve neuralgia in approximately 1% of cases. Current recommendations suggest stripping of the long saphenous vein to just below the level of the knee. This ablates the major effect of truncal incompetence, allows disruption of the thigh perforators and confers some protection to the saphenous nerve which joins the long saphenous vein at a variable distance below the knee. Proponents advocate stripping from groin to knee but there is no good prospective evidence to support the hypothesis that this results in fewer nerve injuries. However, risk of inadvertent passage of the stripper into the deep veins is less likely using this technique. The technique of PIN-stripping, with inversion of the vein, allows retrieval of the long saphenous vein through a small distal incision at the knee and may result in less local damage to the vein tract than passage of a stripper with a terminal "olive."

The presence of dense scar tissue may hamper exploration of the groin during revision varicose vein surgery. A persistent sapheno–femoral junction can be approached from laterally, having dissected down to the femoral artery and then having identified the femoral vein medially. A clean plane of dissection on the surface of the femoral vein can usually be developed above and below the sapheno-femoral junction, allowing eventual circumferential control of the junction, which can be divided and transfixed with a non-absorbable suture. If the long saphenous vein is still present, identification of the proximal end in scar tissue in the groin may be facilitated by passing a stripper up the vein, proximally.

On completion of surgery, local anesthetic infiltration of groin and stripper retrieval wounds with a preparation such as 0.5% Marcain reduces postoperative discomfort.

Use of Tourniquets

Some surgeons advocate use of a tourniquet to reduce postoperative haematoma caused by stripping of the long saphenous vein (21,22). An autoclavable Boazul/Loefqvist-type pneumatic tourniquet, inflated to 40–50 mmHg above systolic arterial pressure, can be employed both to exsanguinate the leg during application and then, when secured at upper thigh level, to prevent bleeding. Proponents suggest that this encourages the operating surgeon to carry out more effective phlebectomies, but a Cochrane Database review found only three prospective randomized trials, with small sample sizes, concluding that although blood loss was reduced, there was no evident reduction in complications or morbidity (23).

Short Sapheno-Popliteal Surgery

The sapheno-popliteal junction has a variable anatomical location (24–26). The short saphenous vein terminates within 5 cm of the knee skin crease in approximately 60% of subjects but at a higher level in the thigh, in the vein of Giacomini (12%) or in the femoro-popliteal or other vein, in up to 40% of patients. Pre-operative marking of the sapheno-popliteal junction with duplex Doppler ultrasound will allow the operating surgeon to employ a smaller, appropriately placed incision.

With the patient lying prone, unless otherwise marked, a 2–3 cm transverse skin incision is made in the skin creases of the popliteal fossa. The Short Saphenous Vein is usually found beneath the popliteal fascia whose fibers run in a transverse plane. Some surgeons advocate dividing this fascia longitudinally, allowing proximal and distal access to the sapheno-popliteal junction. However, with confidence in the location of the sapheno-popliteal junction inspired by ultrasound mapping, splitting the fascial fibers transversely is the less disruptive surgical technique and facilitates subsequent repair. Great care should be taken to avoid damage to the common peroneal nerve, (with the potential consequence of foot-drop), which may be closely related to the short saphenous vein as it courses through the popliteal fossa. The vein of Giacomini should be ligated and divided.

Classical surgical teaching advocates dissection of the short saphenous vein to its anastomosis with the popliteal vein at the sapheno-popliteal junction. However recent comprehensive discussion at the Venous Forum of the Royal Society of Medicine in the United Kingdom, a study undertaken by the Joint Vascular Research Group (JVRG), to be published shortly, and a survey of members of the Vascular Surgical Society of Great Britain and Ireland all indicate widespread variation in surgical practices with respect to this part of the procedure (27).

The sapheno-popliteal junction can be difficult to access in a proportion of patients, increasing risk of neurovascular damage if dissection is pursued. In these cases discretion may be the better part of surgical valour and ligation of the short saphenous vein short of the sapheno-popliteal junction may be advisable. Wherever possible a gastrocnemius vein, entering the short saphenous vein a short distance before its anastomosis with the popliteal vein, should be ligated to eliminate a potential source of recurrence.

Discussion persists on whether to tie and divide the short saphenous vein alone, excise a short segment, or strip to mid-calf or ankle, with greater potential risk of sural nerve injury. However there is little in the way of prospective evidence to inform debate. The prospect of a randomized trial of stripping versus no stripping, with sufficient power to provide a definitive solution, may well be hampered by the potential impact of foam sclerotherapy as a potential therapeutic alternative. Where stripping is undertaken, the surgeon should attempt to ensure that the sural nerve is separated from the short saphenous vein before the stripper is retrieved. Retrograde stripping may reduce risk of nerve injury.

Phlebectomies

Phlebectomies to remove troublesome varicosities are undertaken via fine stab incisions in the skin creases, which are made with a pointed size 11 blade or an ophthalmic scalpel. An "Oesch"-type or similar vein hook is used to pull a loop of the varicosity through the incision. This is separated from adherent tissue, the afferent and efferent ends controlled with fine haemostatic clips and the vein divided at the mid-point of the loop. Both ends of the vein are then avulsed by gentle traction.

Care should be taken with avulsions to reduce risks of nerve injury. Areas particularly prone to this risk include the path of the short saphenous vein in the posterior calf where the sural nerve can be damaged, the region of the neck of the fibula laterally, where the peroneal nerve is at risk, the long saphenous trunk and related saphenous nerve in the calf and the nerves accompanying the anterior and posterior tibial arteries at the ankle.

Ligation of cut ends of the vein with a fine absorbable tie is an alternative when haemostasis is a particular concern. A short period of pressure over the phlebectomy site usually quells bleeding and the incision is closed with an adhesive paper suture strip.

While placement of Steri-Strips® over phlebectomy sites may appear to be the most innocuous part of the surgical procedure, application of these adhesive dressings by an over-zealous assistant may result in "pinching" of skin if they are applied under tension. This has resulted in friction burns, which can have a long-lasting, cosmetically debilitating effect and has been a source for litigation. Any intolerance or allergy to adhesive dressings should have been noted pre-operatively.

Post-operative bandaging after leg-elevation is carried out using either crepe, or elastic bandages. The foot is included to prevent swelling. Pressure should be adequate to staunch venous bleeding but not overly tight so as to compromise arterial circulation.

Pedal Varicosities

Traditionally many surgeons have shied away from surgical treatment of pedal varicosities because of a perceived risk of associated cutaneous nerve injury. Venous hypertension associated with such varicosities can cause significant skin changes including haemosiderin pigmentation, varicose eczema and occasionally, a corona phlebectatica. The patient may well complain of pain or swelling in the foot, particularly after prolonged dependency or in association with venodilation, for instance after bathing. Pedal varicosities can be dealt with via discrete stab incisions in the lines of the skin creases, gentle extrusion of the varicosity with a vein hook and then by division, segmental excision and ligation of the divided ends of the veins with fine absorbable ties. This reduces the volume of pedal haematoma postoperatively.

Perforator Surgery

Incompetent calf perforating veins may be abolished by superficial venous surgery in the absence of specific perforator surgery (28). Specific perforator surgery should be reserved for the few (2–3%) of patients with isolated perforator incompetence. Open surgery for incompetent perforators was popularized by Linton, who described subfascial dissection and ligation of perforating veins in the calf (29). Subsequently a number of modifications to this procedure were introduced by surgeons, including Cockett, who described an extrafascial approach, and Dodd (30,31). Popularity of open procedures, which entailed long incisions with associated morbidity and high ulcer recurrence rates, has waned with the advent of subfascial endoscopic perforator surgery (SEPS), which is described elsewhere in this book.

Postoperative Care

Prior to discharge, bandages should be taken down and wounds inspected. Where dressings or Steri-Strips® have lifted, these should be replaced and the leg cleaned. Management protocols vary from surgeon to surgeon, but usually the patient will be asked to wear a full-length elastic compression stocking continuously for one week and to mobilise as soon as possible. Patients with ulcers may well require dressing changes in the interim. Oral analgesia is prescribed and the patient should be given clear contact details of who to contact in case of a query. In contrast to uncomplicated varicose vein surgery, where it is rarely necessary to subject the patient to further formal outpatient follow-up, patients with stigmata of chronic venous disease, or ulceration, will usually be reviewed within four to six weeks after surgery.

KEY POINTS

- Chronic venous disease remains a major socio-economic problem in modern healthcare.
- Surgical intervention should be directed at correcting underlying causes of ambulatory venous hypertension.
- Superficial, or mixed superficial and deep incompetence, play a significant part in the etiology of chronic venous disease.
- Appropriate superficial venous surgery in chronic venous disease is associated with hemodynamic benefits, improved quality of life and reduced ulcer recurrence rates.
- Risks of litigation specifically associated with superficial venous surgery can be reduced by good communication, fully informed consent, scrupulous pre-operative assessment and awareness of potential for nerve injuries.
- A future role for superficial venous surgery, in the context of alternative potentially effective minimally-invasive therapies, remains to be seen.

REFERENCES

1. Evans CJ, Fowkes FG, Ruckley CV, Lee AJ. Prevalence of varicose veins and chronic venous insufficiency in men and women in the general population: Edinburgh vein study. J Epidemiol Commun Health 1999; 53:149–153.
2. Lees TA, Lambert D. Prevalence of lower limb ulceration in an urban health district. Br J Surg 1992; 79:1032–1034.
3. Fowkes FG, Lee AJ, Evans CJ, Allan PL, Bradbury AW, Ruckley CV. Lifestyle risk factors for lower limb venous reflux in the general population: Edinburgh Vein Study. Int J Epidemiol 2001; 30:846–852.
4. Bosanquet N. Costs of venous ulcers: from maintenance therapy to investment programmes. Phlebology 1992; 7:44–46.
5. Kalra M, Gloviczki P. Surgical treatment of chronic venous insufficiency. In: Hallett JW, Mills JL, Earnshaw JJ, Reekers JA, Mosby, eds. Comprehensive Vascular and Endovascular Surgery, 2004:601–624.
6. Porter JM, Moneta GL. Reporting standards in venous disease: an update. International consensus committee on chronic venous disease. J Vasc Surg 1995; 21:635–645.
7. Beebe HG, Bergan JJ, Bergqvist D, et al. Classification and grading of chronic venous disease in the lower limbs. A consensus statement. Eur J Vasc Endovasc Surg 1996; 12:487–491.
8. Hanrahan LM, Araki CT, Rodriguez AA, Kechejian GJ, LaMorte WW, Menzoian JO. Distribution of valvular incompetence in patients with venous stasis ulceration. J Vasc Surg 1991; 13:805–811.
9. Lees TA, Lambert D. Patterns of venous reflux in limbs with skin changes associated with chronic venous insufficiency. Br J Surg 1993; 80:725–728.
10. Darke SG, Penfold C. Venous ulceration and saphenous ligation. Eur J Vasc Surg 1992; 6:4–9.
11. Barwell JR, Davies CE, Deacon J, et al. Comparison of surgery and compression with compression alone in chronic venous ulceration (ESCHAR study): randomised controlled trial. Lancet 2004; 363:1854–1859.
12. Adam DJ, Bello M, Hartshorne T, London NJ. Role of superficial venous surgery in patients with combined superficial and segmental deep venous reflux. Eur J Vasc Endovasc Surg 2003; 25:469–472.
13. MacKenzie RK, Allan PL, Ruckley CV, Bradbury AW. The effect of long saphenous vein stripping on deep venous reflux. Eur J Vasc Endovasc Surg 2004; 28:104–107.
14. MacKenzie RK, Paisley A, Allan PL, Lee AJ, Ruckley CV, Bradbury AW. The effect of long saphenous vein stripping on quality of life. J Vasc Surg 2002; 35:1197–1203.
15. Mackenzie RK, Lee AJ, Paisley A, et al. Patient, operative, and surgeon factors that influence the effect of superficial venous surgery on disease-specific quality of life. J Vasc Surg 2002; 36:896–902.
16. Sam RC, MacKenzie RK, Paisley AM, Ruckley CV, Bradbury AW. The effect of superficial venous surgery on generic health-related quality of life. Eur J Vasc Endovasc Surg 2004; 28:253–256.
17. Campbell WB, France F, Goodwin HM. Research and audit committee of the vascular surgical society of Great Britain and Ireland. Medicolegal claims in vascular surgery. Ann R Coll Surg Engl 2002; 84:181–184.
18. Onuma OC, Beam PE, Khan U, Malluchi P, Adiseshiah M. The influence of effective analgesia and general anesthesia on patient's acceptance of day-case varicose vein surgery. Phlebology 1993; 8:29–31.
19. Sarin S, Scurr JH, Coleridge Smith PD. Stripping of the long saphenous vein in the treatment of primary varicose veins. Br J Surg 1994; 81:1455–1458.
20. Dwerryhouse S, Davies B, Harradine K, Earnshaw JJ. Stripping the long saphenous vein reduces the rate of reoperation for recurrent varicose veins: five-year results of a randomized trial. J Vasc Surg 1999; 29:589–592.
21. Robinson J, Macierewicz J, Beard JD. Using the Boazul cuff to reduce blood loss in varicose vein surgery. Eur J Vasc Endovasc Surg 2000; 20:390–393.

22. Sykes TC, Brookes P, Hickey NC. A prospective randomised trial of tourniquet in varicose vein surgery. Ann R Coll Surg Engl 2000; 82:280–282.
23. Rigby KA, Palfreyman SJ, Beverley C, Michaels JA. Surgery for varicose veins: use of tourniquet. Cochrane Database Syst Rev 2002;CD001486.
24. Moosman DA, Hartwell SW. The surgical significance of the subfascial course of the lesser saphenous vein. Surg Gynecol Obstet 1964; 118:761–766.
25. Nabatoff RA. The short saphenous vein. Surg Gynecol Obstet 1979; 149:49–53.
26. Engel AF, Davies G, Keeman JN, von Dorp TA. Colour flow imaging of the normal short saphenous vein. Eur J Vasc Surg 1994; 8:179–181.
27. Winterborn RJ, Campbell WB, Heather BP, Earnshaw JJ. The management of short saphenous varicose veins: a survey of the members of the vascular surgical society of Great Britain and Ireland. Eur J Vasc Endovasc Surg 2004; 28:400–403.
28. Gohel MS, Barwell JR, Wakely C, et al. The influence of superficial venous surgery and compression on incompetent calf perforators in chronic venous leg ulceration. Eur J Vasc Endovasc Surg 2005; 29:78–82.
29. Linton RR. The post-thrombotic ulceration of the lower extremity: its etiology and surgical treatment. Ann Surg 1953; 138:415–433.
30. Cockett FB. The pathology and treatment of venous ulcers of the leg. Br J Surg 1955; 43:260–278.
31. Dodd H. The diagnosis and ligation of incompetent ankle perforating veins. Ann R Coll Surg Engl 1964; 34:186–196.

30

Surgical Therapies in Chronic Venous Insufficiency: Deep Venous Surgery/ Valve Transplantation/SEPS

Michael C. Dalsing
Indiana University School of Medicine, Indianapolis, Indiana, U.S.A.

INTRODUCTION

Chronic venous disease is common in Western countries. Over 30 million U.S. citizens are affected with some manifestation of venous disease while skin changes suggestive of the disease are noted in about 6 million and venous ulcers are observed in up to 2% of those with chronic venous insufficiency (about one half million patients) (1–3). Recent population studies confirm these observations (4). The annual cost of treating venous ulcers is estimated to be greater than one billion dollars in the United States (5).

Although many theories abound to explain the sequelae of chronic venous disease, venous hypertension and the resulting stasis of venous blood are key to the pathophysiology. The goal when treating significant chronic venous insufficiency is to diminish venous hypertension on the target organ such that the sequelae of the disease is prevented or minimized. External compression is the mainstay of conservative management even in patients with venous ulceration but the recurrence rate is 70%–100% in non-compliant patients and 30–40% in those who faithfully comply and in only a few years (6,7). In depth evaluation is not required if therapy is restricted to conservative measures but if intervention is contemplated then confirmatory diagnostic studies must differentiate those patients without venous disease from those with superficial, perforator, deep disease or any combination thereof. Valvular insufficiency accounts for 85% of symptomatic chronic venous disease cases with the majority primarily superficial and 30% primarily deep venous insufficiency (8,9). Isolated superficial and/or perforator venous insufficiency has been observed to cause advanced manifestations of venous disease, but in approximately two-thirds of these advanced cases, the deep system is insufficient alone, or more commonly, in association with superficial/perforator disease (10–13). In patients with superficial/perforator and deep venous insufficiency, removal of pathologic superficial and/or perforator veins can result in prolonged venous ulcer healing (14). The hemodynamic importance of perforator vein insufficiency is currently controversial but, in a clinical sense, the "ankle blow-out syndrome" has been recognized for years in patients with advanced clinical disease (15,16). Certainly, in patients with clinically advanced disease ($C_{5,6}$), postoperative incompetent perforator veins are a risk factor for recurrence (17). About one-third of patients with primary deep venous insufficiency and 70% of those with the post-thrombotic syndrome will experience ulcer recurrence after removal of essentially all other significant insufficiency demonstrating the importance of the deep venous component (9,14). Venous obstruction accounts for a minority of venous ulcers observed in our practices (2–20%) (8,10,11), can be managed by various interventional means and is not further considered in this chapter.

ETIOLOGY/PATHOPHYSIOLOGY OF VALVULAR DAMAGE

In the past, perforating veins were named for their discoverer (e.g., Crockett's, Boyd's perforators) but more descriptive terms describing location are now preferred (18). The anatomy of the perforating veins becomes extremely important when considering surgery aimed at preventing reflux in the lower leg. For example, not recognizing the presence of paratibial perforators can result in an unsuccessful operation aimed at preventing calf perforator reflux (19). The etiology of perforator vein insufficiency mimics other major venous tributaries in having similar primary and secondary causes.

Deep venous insufficiency is rarely due to a congenital absence of the valves (20). Syndromes associated with venous abnormalities can have associated venous aplasia or dysplasia. These syndromes are uncommon, and seldom require deep venous valvular reconstruction. Primary deep venous insufficiency occurs as a result of a structural elongation of the valve cusps or stretching of the vein wall without apparent histologic damage (21,22). Floppy, redundant valves permit valve leaflet prolapse and poor coaptation (21). Alternatively, an enlarged venous diameter can prevent a normal valve cusps from coapting properly (23,24). On standing or with other causes of increased intravenous pressure, blood refluxes through the architecturally preserved valve cusps. An in situ repair is possible since all necessary valve architecture is available and competency can be realized. Approximately 40% to 70% of deep vein valvular dysfunction occurs as a consequence of DVT (deep venous thrombosis), whereas the remainder appear to be of a primary etiology (8,21,25). As a result of the destructive process of thrombosis, inflammation and scarring can cause shortening and fibrosis of the valve leaflets, recannulation can result in small channels replacing the normal vein and valve, or valve adhesions can cause luminal narrowing (21). This is the post-thrombotic syndrome. These valves are often so damaged that an in situ repair is not feasible. This leaves only the options of venous valve transplantation, transposition, or the use of "valve substitutes" to address the pathologic reflux.

This classical differentiation between "primary" and "secondary" pathology is fleeting when subjected to direct observation of veins and valves at surgery. In fact, as noted decades ago, the two conditions can be present in the same patient (26). In some cases during surgery, the vein wall has been noted to be thickened/fibrotic at the valve station or there is thickening of the valve cusps and/or intima. Pathologic study of eleven such veins demonstrated post-thrombotic changes in six, but non-thrombotic phlebosclerosis was found in the remainder (21). Preservation of a normal valve architecture can be explained if "primary" reflux with resultant high pressure on the wall is the cause since stretching without destruction could be the process of cusp incompetence. Another theory is that rapid resolution of acute thrombi may leave the valves undamaged, or alternatively, the valve itself may not have been directly involved in the thrombotic process (27–29). The fibrotic process involves the vein wall only and the cusps become floppy because of a diminished diameter consistent with a thickened, non-compliant vein wall (21). The valve remains architecturally intact and can be repaired surgical, a situation once thought impossible in the post-thrombotic patient (21).

DIAGNOSIS

Patients with chronic deep and/or perforator vein reflux present with signs and symptoms typical of the sequelae of long standing venous hypertension. The patient may experience dependent edema, leg fatigue and a feeling of "fullness" especially after long periods of standing. There may be progression to skin changes such as eczema, cellulitis, hyperpigmentation, lipodermatosclerosis, and stasis ulcers. During the physical examination all of these signs may be observed alone or in combination. The history should concentrate on venous disease especially prior DVT, clotting abnormalities or prior venous interventions. Some estimate of how the disease process is affecting the patient's life should be gathered. Significant arterial disease can generally be ruled in or out as a contributing problem as can other causes of similar skin changes such as diabetic ulcers, simple eczema or skin cancers. The CEAP (clinical (C), etiologic (E), anatomic (A), and pathophysiologic (P))classification system should be used to describe patients as they currently present in the spectrum of the disease process (30). An extension of the clinical classification can aid in quantifying the disease process to allow evaluation of treatment response (31,32). Similarly, the patients' clinical outcome scores can be evaluated according to a grading scheme (31). An improved method of determining the change in disease severity following intervention has been developed but awaits overall utility in the clinical arena (32). Quality of life surveys can quantify the impact of the venous disease on the patient's life and effect of therapy on the patient's overall well-being (33). Using these tools and the diagnostic studies discussed below, the physician can precisely define the disease process and can formulate a reasonable treatment plan.

Further diagnostic studies provide the surgeon with information to complete the CEAP classification to its fullest extent. The venous duplex ultrasound study can clarify the etiology (E of CEAP; congenital, primary, or secondary), better define the anatomic location (A of CEAP;), and help to determine the pathophysiology (P of CEAP; reflux, obstruction, or both) of the venous disease. Venous duplex imaging can provide rather impressive imaging of individual valve cusps in many patients and can determine the presence or absence of reflux past a given valve following provocative studies: A prolonged reflux time of >0.5 seconds is considered abnormal and indicative of pathologic reflux if a rapidly deflating distal cuff is used as the provocative tent, while >1.0 seconds is considered abnormal when manual compression is used (34,35). A recent study suggests that these values may be appropriate for the deep calf veins but that 1.0 seconds should be the cut-off of the larger femoropopliteal veins even when using the rapidly deflating distal cuff method (36). The examination is performed in the upright position in these reports. Suffice it to say, many other provocative maneuvers to generate venous reflux exists (Valsalva, standardized Valsalva, etc) in addition to performing the test in different positions (15% Tredelenberg, sitting, etc.) (37). Each may be acceptable if standardized for your laboratory. Incompetent perforating veins are generally larger in diameter than normal perforators, thereby allowing a larger volume of blood flow during reflux, and are considered to demonstrate reflux with a reflux time greater than 0.5 seconds (38). There is some thought that this cut-off should be decreased to 0.35 seconds (39). Of course, isolated deep venous valvular insufficiency may have little clinical impact on a given patient and therefore clinicians have attempted to quantify the pathology by adding segmental disease, determining mean duration of reflux, determining peak reverse flow velocity, etc. (34,40). Although, average scores and means do correlate with disease severity, individual results have little predictive value and have not been widely adopted. The issue of common standards for the performance and interpretation of venous duplex studies still plagues efforts to defining venous disease (37), but many find duplex imaging the most versatile and reproducible imaging device currently available in clinical use (37,41). Imaging the entire lower extremity venous system, provides a detailed roadmap of all veins and a means of determining if obstruction or valvular reflux is present.

Plethysmography can assess overall lower extremity venous hemodynamics. Air plethysmography (APG) can measure several venous hemodynamic parameters and is the most common device currently utilized in the clinical setting. A venous filling index of 2 mL/s or less is indicative of a competent venous system and higher values suggest venous insufficiency (42,43). The use of tourniquets to separate superficial from deep or perforator disease has not been reliable (44), but it can be useful in specific cases. The residual volume fraction is relatively equivalent to the ambulatory venous pressure (5,44). Several other plethysmographic methods (impedance, photo, etc.) and even light reflex rheography have evaluated similar venous parameters. These plethysmographic methods can differentiate severe chronic venous insufficiency (class 3 or greater) from disease absence but is unreliable in less severe disease (37). Because these studies do not provide an anatomic image of the venous system or evaluate individual venous valve function, most physicians combine one of these estimates of global hemodynamics with ultrasonography to complete the non-invasive venous evaluation of patients with advanced disease.

Although intravenous pressure measurements and venography were once the gold standard for evaluating venous disease, duplex scanning and plethysmographic techniques are the anatomic and functional tests of choice in current medical practice (42).

Patients with significant deep venous valvular reflux contemplating surgery generally have a venographic study for proper operative planning. Ascending venography is useful in demonstrating the anatomy of the deep venous system and helps eliminate obstruction as a major contributing or confounding factor (21,45). It provides a road map to allow selection of the most disease-free portion of lower extremity venous system for valve transplantation if that becomes necessary. Simultaneous intravenous AVP measurements can be obtained to provide an estimate of the magnitude of reflux (5). The magnitude of the AVP correlates with the presence of venous ulceration such that each 10 Torr increase above 30 Torr corresponding to a 10 to 15 percent increase in the incidence of venous ulceration (46). If the VRT is less than 20 seconds, overall valvular reflux throughout the lower leg is evident.

Descending venography is used to determine valve leaflet integrity, anatomic location, and demonstrate the extent of reflux (47). Assessment of profunda femoris venous system competence in addition to the femoral system is mandatory. Either system may be a source of a competent valve for the transposition procedure, or may indicate potential success with an isolated proximal femoral vein repair in the case of profunda venous valve competence (48–50). It can fail in its attempt to determine the presence or absence of a normal valve (21). Raju, et al. reports that the descending venogram misrepresented the presence of a valve in 11% of cases (no valve was present at operation), and missed an intact valve in 25% of cases (a valve thought absent was present) (21). When combined with non-invasive venous imaging, descending venography is the best method available to determine preoperatively if an in situ reconstruction will be possible.

INDICATIONS AND GOALS FOR SURGICAL INTERVENTION

In general, patients presenting for intervention of incompetent perforator and/or deep venous insufficiency have attempted conservative measures to control the disease process and have generally undergone superficial surgery if incompetence was also located there. Likewise, proximal venous obstruction has usually been addressed. One study in patients with combined superficial reflux and "segmental deep venous reflux" showed that superficial venous surgery alone corrected deep venous reflux in about 50% of limbs involved and allowed ulcer healing in 77% of limbs after one year of follow-up (51). This study cannot be generalized to include patients with severe and extensive deep venous reflux but it is interesting that treatment of superficial disease can impact the deep venous system in such a positive manner. Failure of these measures, especially with recurrent symptoms of advanced disease, requires consideration for further surgical intervention.

The precise candidate for the correction of perforator insufficiency is often difficult to define since many reports in the literature have combined perforator surgery with superficial saphenous ablation making comment on the effect of isolated perforator incompetence hard to substantiate. Certainly, in those rather rare cases of isolated perforator incompetence, treatment may be the only option available to correct venous hypertension causing the sequelae such as venous ulceration. It is becoming increasing evident that perforator vein incompetence is very common in patients with venous ulcers being noted in about 60% of patients (12,13,52). It is clearly difficult to differentiate the hemodynamic effect of perforator vein incompetence when deep disease is also present, as it generally is in patients with advanced disease. Isolated perforator disease is really quite unusual (12). It does appear, however, that incompetent perforators can result in significant supramalleolar venous pressure with calf contraction (16). Furthermore, increasing number and size of perforating veins does correlate with worsening chronic venous insufficiency and, more importantly, the presence of incompetent perforating veins is a risk factor for recurrent venous ulcers after attempted surgical correction of hemodynamic derangements (17,38,53). Keeping in mind that the goal of therapy is alleviation of venous hypertension on the target organ (the ankle skin), the data is mounting that correction of perforator vein incompetence may be beneficial especially in the patient with venous ulceration. The goal of treatment in perforator surgery is to remove the influence of incompetent perforator veins on the lower leg and this implies removal of all incompetent perforating veins.

Patients considered for deep venous valvular surgery generally are end-stage patients with C3 C6 disease with only deep venous disease remaining untreated. However, as the results of surgery demonstrate improving long-term success, some surgeons consider intervention in patients with disabling life-style symptoms like severe edema. When the decision has been made to treat deep venous valvular incompetence, the goal is to prevent axial reflux into the lower leg. If one ignores the rule of correcting all axial reflux in patients with deep venous insufficiency, for example by ignoring reflux in the profunda femoris vein, femoral vein valvular reconstruction alone will be clinically unsuccessful and lower limb venous hemodynamics will not be improved (54). However, with profunda femoris venous valvular competence, repair of femoral vein incompetence alone can improve chronic lower limb venous hemodynamics (54,55). Tremendous enlargement of the profunda femoris vein following femoral vein DVT has been clearly demonstrated by venography and other methods, repair of both the femoral and profunda vein valvular reflux is required for a successful outcome if both demonstrate incompetence (56). The popliteal vein is the gateway through which all thigh venous reflux must pass and, therefore, another way of correcting axial reflux may be to position any valve reconstruction in the popliteal vein location (48,57,58). One group of investigators feels that multiple valve repairs in the same axial system (e.g., two in the femoral vein) may decrease the risk of long-term failure (59), but most surgeons use solitary valve repair with similar success. One investigator has even performed multiple tibial vein valve repairs to correct axial reflux (59).

TREATMENT OPTIONS AND RESULTS

Perforator Vein Ligation

Perforator vein ligation can be performed via an open or minimally invasive endoscopic technique. A Linton type procedure utilizes an incision along the medial or posterior lower leg and the creation of subfascial flaps to allow exposure of the perforators (60–62). The perforating veins are directly ligated and divided. The best scenario allows for healing of any ulceration prior to operation to minimize the risk of infection in the flap area, but if a skin ulcer is recalcitrant, it will likely require simultaneous debridement. If a large amount of soft tissue and/or fascia is involved, a skin graft can aid in healing. DePalma used multiple incisions orientated along skin lines and the development of bipedicle flaps between each to allow ligation of perforating veins (63). Possibly a historical preamble to endoscopic perforator surgery was Edwards use of a phlebotome placed subfascially via a proximal, medial knee incision utilizing blind advancement to the medial malleolus to disrupt encountered perforator veins (64). Infection concerns or lack of visualization resulted in a technical switch with advancements in technology.

An endoscopic technique (SEPS or Subfascial Endoscopic Perforator Surgery) can be employed (65,66). Following slight knee flexion, two small (10–15 mm) incisions are made on the medial aspect of the lower leg near the knee proximal to areas of induration and inflammation. Subfascial dissection is performed using sharp and blunt balloon dissection. Some surgeons place a tourniquet on the upper leg to be inflated prior to subfascial insufflation of carbon dioxide (CO_2), which is used to improve visualization and to prevent CO_2 emboli. Other surgeons feel this step unnecessary because the venous system is better visualized with blood within the perforator veins and because the risk of embolism is minimal. Under video enhanced imaging, the perforating veins are ligated with clips and divided. Some physicians have utilized mediastinoscopes and long clip applier to obviate the need for second incision (67,68). The closeness of the light source and clipping mechanism within the same port can sometimes make it difficult to dissect with three-dimensional clarity. Most surgeons preoperatively mark the perforating veins with duplex scanning to assure that all offending veins are identified at the time of surgery. Recognizing the impact of paratibial perforator veins, which require a fascial incision to visualize, has prevented the need for subsequent operations to address missed perforators (19). Recent adventures into subfascial endoscopic perforating vein surgery for laterally located veins with associated venous ulceration have been reported with some but less impressive clinical success (69,70). Venous ulceration in this locale accounts for less than 10% of cases but can be a problem when encountered and awareness of potential treatments is useful.

Safety and early efficacy of SEPS has been demonstrated (65,66). A mid-term evaluation of patients undergoing SEPS demonstrated the patients to have decreased symptoms and a near 90% ulcer healing rate at two years (71). Information on current SEPS literature reports that wound complications are less common after the SEPS (0–10%) than the open method (12–53%) with comparable outcomes (72). These findings were confirmed by the only prospective, randomized study comparing SEPS with the

Linton procedure (68). 53% of patients undergoing the Linton procedure had wound complications while none in the SEPS group experienced this complication. At four years of follow-up, 22% of the patients in the Linton group had recurrent venous ulceration while 12% were so affected in the SEPS cohort (73). Whether SEPS is required in addition to saphenous surgery for advanced chronic venous disease when both systems demonstrate insufficiency remains debatable but a trend to more aggressive use to control all potential venous hypertension is being seen in the literature (72).

Deep Venous Reconstructions

General Comments

During the performance of deep venous reconstruction, several observations influence what the surgeon can do for a given patient. If manipulation of an in situ valve results in vasoconstriction and secondary competence (the "strip test" becomes normal), then an external valvuloplasty or a prosthetic sleeve technique may be a good repair for the patient (74). If a valve requires an in situ repair, careful adventitial dissection of the valve attachment lines facilitates appropriate venotomy, preventing damage to the delicate valve leaflets, and helps to verify the feasible of an in situ repair (75). A lack of clear valve attachment lines can signify valve destruction as a component of the post-thrombotic syndrome prompting other than an in situ repair (75).

Prophylactic antibiotics should be given prior to skin incision, generally a first-generation cephalosporin, and continued postoperatively for two to three days. Intra-operative heparin is administered (2,000 to 10,000 units) based on the need to open the vein and duration of clamping. Heparin is generally not reversed at the end of the procedure. Pneumatic compression devices may be helpful postoperatively to decrease swelling and may increase flow over the valve repair during inactivity. Low molecular weight heparin or low-dose intravenous heparin should be started immediately postoperatively and may influence the use of closed drainage to avoid hematoma formation. Warfarin is generally begun on postoperative day one to help decrease the hospital length of stay. A target INR of 2.0 to 2.5 is applied for the first six weeks with a decreased to 1.7 to 2.0 for four months at which point it is stopped with adjustments for any increased risk of thrombosis. One suggested long-term regiment of anticoagulation is "minidose" warfarin using daily doses of 1 mg to 2.5 mg to prevent thrombosis (75,76). Many surgeons encourage the use of compressive support following surgery but many patients fail to comply and yet have a good clinical result (21,26).

Internal Valvuloplasty

An internal valvuloplasty, open direct valve repair, has been a mainstay for the repair of primary venous valvular reflux for over 40 years. This technique requires a venotomy and suturing of the floppy valve leaflets under direct visualization with 7-0 or 6-0 polypropylene suture to tighten the valve cusps. Kistner reported success with a longitudinal venotomy extending through the valve commissure in 1968 (77). Raju uses a supracommissural approach involving a transverse venotomy beginning atleast 2.5 cm above the valve (78). Sottiurai devised a hybrid "T"-shaped venotomy using a supravalvular transverse venotomy with distal extension into a valve sinus (79). Tripathi and his associates now champion a "trapdoor" approach involving two transverse incisions (80). One incision is above and one below the valve connected by a single vertical incision through the commissure (80). The suturing of the valve leaflets remains essentially the same no matter what opening in the vein is made and plication of about 20% of the valve leaflet length seems to restore valve competency in most cases (81).

External Valvuloplasty

The technique of external valvuloplasty offers the advantage of valve repair without venotomy (82). It is performed by placing sutures completely through the valve attachment lines such that when the sutures are tied the commissural angle is narrowed and the valve becomes competent. Although some reports suggest that it may be less durable than the more precise open valvuloplasty, patient selection likely plays a key role in success realized (48). A modification uses a limited anterior plication which involves only anterior vein wall dissection and reefing of the cusps using a running mattress suture. The suture is begun at a point 3–4 mm above the angle of the valve cusp insertion lines and progresses to the angle of valve cusp insertion (83). About 3 mm of the vein wall is incorporated into the stitch to narrow the cusps. The aim is to decrease the vein wall dissection and therefore to hopefully reduce the progressive dilatation of the vein sometimes noted after valvuloplasty. It has been described in conjunction with saphenous vein stripping and limited to the femoral vein valve station. Results after ten-year follow-up demonstrated improved venous refilling time and decreased ambulatory venous pressures in patients with moderate deep venous valvular incompetence (83). Thus, it shows promise as a mode of therapy for highly selected patients. Another modification of the external technique features the use of an angioscope which therefore adds a component of intralumenal visualization (84). A side branch of the GSV allows introduction of an angioscope, which is advanced into the femoral vein above the incompetent valve allowing external sutures to be placed under direct vision (84). Following a learning curve which involved use of the angioscope, Raju and colleagues demonstrated good clinical and competency data with the "transcommissural" technique without the use angioscopy in a study with 30 months of follow-up (85).

External Banding

External banding has been employed when dissection vasospasm renders a valve spontaneously competent. The technique uses an external sleeve made of synthetic material [polytetraflouroethylene (PTFE) or polyester (Dacron)] wrapped circumferentially around the vein at the valve and tightened to diminish the vein diameter until the valve becomes competent. The sleeve is anchored to the adventitia by sutures to prevent slippage. It has achieved good results when used in very select patients (48).

Venous Valve Transplantation

Venous valve transplantation is sometimes the only option when an in situ valve is absent or destroyed. This procedure was first reported clinically by Taheri early in the 1980's (86). A 2–3 cm segment of upper extremity vein containing a valve is first removed. Approximately 40% of axillary vein valves are incompetent at the time of explant and therefore require bench repair prior to implant (75,81). Should a bench repair be necessary, the transcommissural external valvuloplasty technique appears to have better results than the standard external valvuloplasty (75), and some success has been achieved with internal valvuloplasty (87). The incompetent femoral vein is exposed in routine fashion from below the takeoff of the profunda femoris vein and for at least several centimeters distally to allow removal of appropriate femoral vein such that the axillary vein segment can be sutured into place without tension or laxity. The popliteal location may be more appropriate if the femoral location does not completely control axial reflux, for example, if the profunda femoral vein system is also incompetent. The proximal anastomosis may be accomplished first to allow distention and lengthening of the vein and to confirm competence of the valve prior to and as an aid to completing the distal anastomosis. Trabeculated post-thrombotic veins were once thought unacceptable for valve transplantation but investigators have described excision of intraluminal synechiae to create an acceptable lumen for transplantation (88). An interrupted sutures technique is recommended by most surgeons to avoid suture line stenosis (81). Valve competence is determined by intraoperative strip testing. An external sleeve can then be placed around the segment to prevent later dilation of the segment.

Valve Transposition

Valve transposition is another option in management of patients with the post-thrombotic syndrome. If a venous valve is competent in one of the axial thigh venous systems, then a transposition procedure can be used to place the incompetent venous system below the competent valve. Most commonly, the femoral system is incompetent and the profunda femoris valve remains competent. The incompetent femoral vein can be transected and reimplanted distal to the competent valve in the profunda femoris vein. Alternatively, the incompetent femoral system can be reimplanted below a competent greater saphenous vein valve. When the profunda femoris venous system is dysfunctional, it may be placed distal to a competent valve in either the femoral vein or the greater saphenous vein. A technique has been described for transposition of the ipsilateral valve-competent greater saphenous vein to the femoral vein with subsequent ligation of the femoral vein proximally yet distal to the takeoff of the profunda femoris vein to escape problems with diameter mismatch (89). At ten years, 55% of the patients were reported to be ulcer-free (89).

Results of Standard Methods of Deep Venous Reconstructions

Valve repair procedures have a low morbidity and essentially zero mortality in most series (9). Hematoma and seroma formation is seen in up to 15% of cases, with some expected variation in the rate of hematoma formation dependent on the intensity of anticoagulation (26,81,90,91). Deep venous thrombosis occurs in less than 10% of cases in most series (26,75,81,90,91). Although one series had an incidence of thrombosis (often not occlusive nor extensive) in the extremity of repair of approximately 20% as detected by ascending venogram two days postoperatively. These events did not appear to have an impact on clinical results (92). Wound infections have been seen in 2–4% of cases (26,75,81).

In general, reported results have been separated by the method of deep venous reconstruction. Kistner and colleagues have followed their patients requiring internal valvuloplasty for decades and have reported their results in life-table format with excellent results (93,94). Valve competency is approximately 70% at five years in most series (21,26,48,54,78,80,92–97). A patent and competent valve translates into clinical improvement and a healed ulcer in general, while recurrent reflux is associated with clinical failure. A similar commentary can be made about all types of venous valvular reconstruction.

Valve transposition has reported clinical improvement of 50–60% of patients so treated with three to five years of follow-up (9,26,89,96). The valve competency rate varies from 30–80% and is clearly reflected in the clinical improvement noted (9,26,89,96).

Valve transplantation operations are performed in patients with the most difficult anatomy and most damaged deep venous system. Clinical improvement is seen in about 50% of patients even at eight years of follow-up, and remains a viable and acceptable option in cases where other techniques are not possible (8,9,81).

There does not appear to be a difference between reported competency rates or clinical results when considering the location of valve transplantation (femoral verses popliteal) but, in general, the competency rates reported for all other repairs are inferior to internal valvuloplasty (57,58,77,96,98–102). Some of the difference in results can be attributed to the more severe disease (damage inflicted by DVT) noted in patients requiring transplantation or a transposition operation when compared to those requiring valvuloplasty (generally a primary etiology) (26). Although Raju and associates find little difference between the post-thrombotic and primary patient results in their series (48), this may simply reflect a delay in the appearance of ulceration following valve failure. These same investigators are one of a few with sufficiently high volume in a variety of venous valve repairs to report a difference in valve competence based on method of repair. It would appear that there is decreasing durability as one progresses from internal valvuloplasty, to external valvuloplasty, and finally, to a need for transplantation (48).

Valve Substitutes

For those end-stage patients with chronic deep venous insufficiency and no autogenous valve available, the only option is a valve substitute. Ingenious and creative methods have been invented to address these patients. Dr. Raju and associates have reported a small series of patients receiving de novo valve reconstruction procedures with rather good clinical results (75). These procedures involve the use of donor vein wall from which semilunar cusps are made after trimming adventitia and part of the media. The valve "cusps" are sutured into the recipient vein with the nonendothelial surface directed intralumenally to hopefully decrease the risk of thrombosis. Another attempt to use autogenous vein as a valve substitute has been reported by Plagnol et al. (103). This approach invaginates a stump of the greater saphenous vein into the femoral vein to form a bicuspid valve. The invaginated component of the greater saphenous vein is tacked to the opposite femoral vein wall with prolene suture to maintain its structure. They report 19 of 20 reconstructions to be patent and competent at a mean of ten months (103). One valve demonstrated reflux. The invagination of an adventitial surface into the venous lumen is of some concern, a fear not upheld in this one report. Pushing the limits even further, an Italian vascular surgeon has reported a series of bicuspid or monocusp venous valves made from dissecting the intimal/medial wall from the thickened post-phlebitic vein to form cusps. The initial seven cases were reported in 2002 with acceptable preliminary results (104). A more robust report was given at the recent American Venous Forum meeting in 2005 (105). Eighteen venous valves were constructed in 16 patients with recurrent or non-healing venous ulcers due to post-thrombotic chronic deep venous insufficiency. The patients were anticoagulated for six months. Early thrombosis below the valve occurred in two patients and there was one late occlusion after beginning oral contraceptives. Therefore, 83.3% of treated segments at a mean 22 months of follow-up remained patent primarily with significantly improved duplex and air plethysmographic results. This technique certainly seems promising if others can duplicate these results.

Psathakis and Psathakis reported on a substitute "valve" operation using a Silastic tendon designed to produce an external compression of the popliteal vein and thereby prevent reflux with relaxation of the calf muscles (106). Perrin has attempted this procedure in nine patients but poor clinical and hemodynamic results were obtained. He stopped using this procedure after one year (92). The technique has not gained wide acceptance.

Many experimental attempts using allografts and synthetics have been unsuccessful (107,108). A cadaveric cryopreserved pulmonary monocusp patch has been described with reasonable clinical results in a very small group of patients (109). None of these valve substitutes have been proven clinically useful to date.

Most recently, a bioprosthetic (small intestinal submucosa architecture), bicuspid square stent-based venous valve was developed and placed percutaneously in the external jugular vein of sheep (110). The valve appears to be somewhat resistant to thrombosis and does become repopulated with recipient endothelial cells following implantation (110,111). This technique shows promise as a minimally invasive synthetic valve and continues in research and development (personal communication).

SUMMARY

The surgical treatment of CVI is a maturing field with various options available to the patient based on specific preoperative evaluation. The majority of patients treated have $C_{5,6}$ clinical disease, but with improving results some surgeons have extended the indications to symptoms disabling to the patients in their daily lives. Noninvasive studies, most notably duplex imaging, can provide detailed information about perforator and deep venous valvular insufficiency. Perforator venous insufficiency is recommended in patients with advanced disease, with or without associated superficial or deep disease, either as primary treatment or to prevent recurrence due to missed perforator disease. In many cases, descending venography provides an invasive but easy visualization of options available for the treatment of deep venous insufficiency. Primary deep vein valve incompetence is most commonly treated by internal valvuloplasty due to its adaptability and long track record, followed by external banding or external valvuloplasty in select patients. Transcommissural valvuloplasty may achieve superior results to a standard external valvuloplasty. For management of the post-thrombotic syndrome, valve transplantation is the most versatile option with transposition remaining useful in a select patient cohort. Some autogenous valve substitutes have reached very limited clinical use, most probably in cases where all other options were simply not possible. The search for off-the-shelf valve substitutes continues with little success to date. Proper follow-up with appropriate measurement tools to analyze success must be the goal of future study to determine the best treatment for any given cohort of patients.

KEY POINTS

- Chronic venous disease affects 30 millions U.S. citizens with 2% experiencing the disability of venous ulceration.
- Although the majority are affected primarily by superficial venous insufficiency, approximately 30% have primarily deep venous insufficiency with associated perforator disease in both, especially if the symptom is venous ulceration (60%).
- Patients with disabling symptoms unresponsive to compression or less invasive treatments (i.e., superficial saphenous ablation) are candidates for perforator or deep venous insufficiency surgery.

- The etiology of primary venous valvular insufficiency is dilation of valve cusps or the vein wall with preservation of valve architecture, while secondary valvular insufficiency is generally the result of the scarring and fibrosis of deep venous thrombosis. Differentiating the impact of each is blurred in individual patients.
- An accurate picture of the patient's condition is critical to develop a proper treatment plan and evaluate it. The CEAP classification, severity scores, and quality of life surveys aid in this task and in wide spread acceptance of any treatment.
- Currently, the two most useful non invasive diagnostic studies to clarify the location and impact of venous insufficiency are the Duplex venous imaging study and air plethysmographic (APG) evaluation.
- Descending venography is still utilized by many surgeons prior to deep venous reconstruction to determine reflux degree and clarify valve anatomy.
- Perforator vein insufficiency surgery is warranted when demonstrated objectively (generally by duplex imaging) and the patient has advanced disease especially venous ulceration.
- Deep venous reconstruction is warranted when other less invasive methods have failed and disabling symptoms remain (often recalcitrant or recurrent venous ulceration).
- SEPS (Subfascial Endoscopic Perforator Surgery) is currently the recommended method of treating perforator disease due to less wound complications than Linton type procedures with equivalent clinical results.
- Internal Valvuloplasty is the best studied and most versatile technique for treating primary deep venous valvular insufficiency with a 70% valve competence rate, which translates into a similar rate of clinical success. Various techniques of external valvuloplasty and external banding are useful for select patients and when chosen well are also effective.
- Venous valve transplantation is the most versatile method of treating secondary deep venous insufficiency while the transposition operation has limited application. Clinical success is about 50% at five to eight years.
- In the treatment of deep venous insufficiency, the location and number of valve reconstructions must aim to eliminate all major axial reflux into the calf.
- Preliminary reports using autogenous valve substitutes in difficult cases show quite acceptable early results.
- Nonautogenous valve substitutes have fared poorly to date in the clinical arena.

REFERENCES

1. Brand FN, Dannenberg AL, Abbott RD, Kannel WB. The epidemiology of varicose veins: the Framingham Study. Am J Prev Med 1988; 4:96–101.
2. Coon WW, Willis PW, Keller JB. Venous thromboembolism and other venous disease in the tecumseh community health study. Circulation 1973; 48:839–846.
3. Baker SR, Stacey MC, Jopp-McKay AG, et al. Epidemiology of chronic venous ulcers. Br J Surg 1988; 78:864–867.
4. Heit JA, Rooke TW, Silverstein MD, et al. Trends in the incidence of venous stasis syndrome and venous ulcer: a 25-year population-based study. J Vasc Surg 2001; 33:1022–1027.
5. Nicolaides AN. Investigation of chronic venous insufficiency: a consensus statement. Circulation 2000; 102:e126–e163.

6. Mayberry JC, Moneta GL, Taylor LM, Jr., Porter JM. Fifteen-year results of ambulatory compression therapy for chronic venous ulcers. Surgery 1991; 109:575–581.

7. Erickson CA, Lanza DJ, Karp DL, et al. Healing of venous ulcers in an ambulatory care program: the roles of chronic venous insufficiency and patient compliance. J Vasc Surg 1995; 22:629–636.

8. O'Donnell TF. Chronic venous insufficiency: an overview of epidemiology, classification, and anatomic considerations. Sem Vas Surg 1988; 1:60–65.

9. Eklof BG, Kistner RL, Masuda EM. Venous bypass and valve reconstruction: long-term efficacy. Vasc Med 1998; 3:157–164.

10. Darke SG, Penfold C. Venous ulceration and saphenous ligation. Eur J Vasc Surg 1992; 6:4–9.

11. Barwell JR, Taylor M, Deacon J, et al. Surgical correction of isolated superficial venous reflux reduces long-term recurrence rate in chronic venous leg ulcers. Eur J Vasc Endovasc Surg 2000; 20:363–368.

12. Labropoulos N, Leon M, Geroulakos G, et al. Venous hemodynamic abnormalities in patients with leg ulceration. Am J Surg 1995; 169:572–574.

13. Hanrahan LM, Araki CT, Rodriguez AA, et al. Distribution of valvular incompetence in patients with venous stasis ulceration. J Vasc Surg 1991; 13:805–811.

14. Kalra M, Gloviczki P. Surgical treatment of venous ulcers: role of subfascial endoscopic perforator vein ligation. Surg Clin North Am 2003; 83:671–705.

15. Crockett FB, Jones BD. The ankle blow-out syndrome: a new approach to the varicose ulcer problem. Lancet 1953; 1:17–23.

16. Negus D, Friedgood A. The effective management of venous ulceration. Br J Surg 1983; 70:623–627.

17. TenBrook JA, Jr., Iafrati MD, O'Donnell TF, et al. Systematic review of outcomes after surgical management of venous disease incorporating subfascial endoscopic perforator surgery. J Vasc Surg 2004; 39:583–589.

18. Caggiati A, Bergan JJ, Gloviczki P, et al. Nomenclature of the veins of the lower limbs: an international interdisciplinary consensus statement. J Vasc Surg 2002; 36:416–422.

19. Mozes G, Gloviczki P, Menawat SS, Fisher DR, Carmichael SW, Kadar A. Surgical anatomy for endoscopic subfascial division of perforating veins. J Vasc Surg 1996; 24:800–808.

20. Plate G, Brudin L, Eklof B, et al. Physiologic and therapeutic aspects in congenital vein valve aplasia of the lower limb. Ann Surg 1983; 198:229–233.

21. Raju S, Fredericks RK, Hudson CA, et al. Venous valve station changes in "primary" and postthrombotic reflux: an analysis of 149 cases. Ann Vasc Surg 2000; 14:193–199.

22. Budd TW, Meenaghan MA, Wirth J, Taheri SA. Histopathology of veins and venous valves of patients with venous insufficiency syndrome: ultrastructure. J Med 1990; 21:181–199.

23. Sandri JL, Barros FS, Pontes S, et al. Diameter-reflux relationship in perforating veins of patients with varicose veins. J Vasc Surg 1999; 30:867–873.

24. Clarke H, Smith SR, Vasdekis SN, et al. Role of venous elasticity in the development of varicose veins. Br J Surg 1989; 76:577–580.

25. Kistner RL, Eklof B, Masuda EM. Deep venous valve reconstruction. Cardiovasc Surg 1995; 3:129–140.

26. Masuda EM, Kistner RL. Long-term results of venous valve reconstruction: a four to twenty-one year follow-up. J Vasc Surg 1994; 19:391–403.

27. Killewich LA, Bedford GR, Beach KW, Strandness DE, Jr. Spontaneous lysis of deep venous thrombi: rate and outcome. J Vasc Surg 1989; 9:89–97.

28. Masuda EM, Kessler DM, Kistner RL, et al. The natural history of calf vein thrombosis: lysis of thrombi and development of reflux. J Vasc Surg 1998; 28:67–73.

29. McLafferty RB, Moneta GL, Passman MA, et al. Late clinical and hemodynamic sequelae of isolated calf vein thrombosis. J Vasc Surg 1998; 27:50–56.

30. Prepared by the Executive Committee, chaired by Andrew N. Nicolaides, of the ad hoc committee, American Venous Forum, 6th Annual Meeting. February 22–25, 1994, Maui,

Hawaii: Classification and grading of chronic venous disease in the lower limbs: a consensus statement. In: Gloviczki P, and Yao JST, eds. Handbook of Venous Disorders. London: Chapman & Hall;1991:653–656.

31. Porter JM, Moneta GL. An international consensus committee on chronic venous disease. Reporting standards in venous disease: an update. J Vasc Surg 1995; 21:634–645.

32. Rutherford RB, Padberg FT, Jr., Comerota AJ, et al. Venous severity scoring: an adjunct to venous outcome assessment. J Vasc Surg 2000; 31:1307–1312.

33. Lamping DL, Schroter S, Kurz X, et al. Evaluation of outcomes in chronic venous disorders of the leg: development of a scientifically rigorous, patient-reported measure of symptoms and quality of life. J Vasc Surg 2003; 37:410–419.

34. Mattos MA. Direct noninvasive tests (duplex scan) for the evaluation of chronic venous obstruction and valvular incompetence. In: Gloviczki P, Yao JST, eds. Handbook of Venous Disorders. London: Arnold, 2001:120–131.

35. vanBemmelen PS, Bedford G, Beach K, et al. Quantitative segmental evaluation of venous valvular reflux with duplex ultrasound scanning. J Vasc Surg 1989; 10:425–431.

36. Labropoulos N, Tiongson J, Pryor L, et al. Definition of venous reflux in lower-extremity veins. J Vasc Surg 2003; 38:793–798.

37. Lynch TG, Dalsing MC, Ouriel K, et al. Developments in diagnosis and classification of venous disorders: non-invasive diagnosis. Cardiovasc Surg 1999; 7:160–182.

38. Labropoulos N, Mansour MA, Kang SS, et al. New insights into perforator vein incompetence. Eur J Vasc Endovasc Surg 1999; 18:228–234.

39. Labropoulos N, Tiongson J, Pryor L, et al. Definition of venous reflux in lower-extremity veins. J Vasc Surg 2003; 38:793–798.

40. Danielsson G, Eklof B, Grandinetti A, et al. Deep axial reflux, an important contributor to skin changes or ulcer in chronic venous disease. J Vasc Surg 2003; 38:1336–1341.

41. Mantoni M, Larsen L, Lund JO, et al. Evaluation of chronic venous disease in the lower limb: comparison of five diagnostic methods. Br J Surg 2002; 75:578–583.

42. Bays RA, Healy DA, Atnip RG, et al. Validation of air plethysmography, photoplethysmography, and duplex ultrasonography in the evaluation of severe venous stasis. J Vasc Surg 1994; 20:721–727.

43. Nicolaides AN, Christopoulos D. Quantification of venous reflux and outflow obstruction with air-plethysmography. In: Bernstein EF, ed. Vascular Diagnosis. U.S.A: St. Louis: Mosby, 1993:915–921.

44. Criado E, Farber MA, Marston WA, et al. The role of air plethysmography in the diagnosis of chronic venous insufficiency. J Vasc Surg 1998; 27:660–670.

45. Raju S. New approaches to the diagnosis and treatment of venous obstruction. J Vasc Surg 1986; 4:42–54.

46. Nicolaides AN, Hussein MK, Szendro G, et al. The relation of venous ulceration with ambulatory venous pressure measurements. J Vasc Surg 1993; 17:414–419.

47. Kistner RL, Ferris EB, Randhawa G, Kamida C. A method of performing descending venography. J Vasc Surg 1986; 4:464–468.

48. Raju S, Fredericks RK, Neglen PN, et al. Durability of venous valve reconstruction techniques for "primary" and postthrombotic reflux. J Vasc Surg 1996; 23:357–367.

49. Cheatle TR, Perrin M. Venous valve repair: early results in fifty-two cases. J Vasc Surg 1994; 19:404–413.

50. Kistner RL, Sparkuhl MD. Surgery in acute and chronic venous disease. Surgery 1979; 85:31–43.

51. Adam DJ, Bello M, Hartshorne T, London NJ. Role of superficial venous surgery in patients with combined superficial and segmental deep venous reflux. Eur J Endovasc Surg 2003; 25:469–472.

52. Myers KA, Ziegenbein RW, Zeng GH, Matthews PG. Duplex ultrasonography scanning for chronic venous disease: patterns of venous reflux. J Vasc Surg 1995; 21:605–612.

53. Stuart WP, Adam DJ, Allan PL, et al. The relationship between the number, competence, and diameter of medial calf perforating veins and the clinical status in healthy subjects and patients with lower-limb venous disease. J Vasc Surg 2000; 32:138–143.

54. Eriksson I, Almgren B. Influence of the profunda femoris vein on venous hemodynamics of the limb. Experience from thirty-one deep vein valve reconstructions. J Vasc Surg 1986; 4:390–395.

55. Queral LA, Whitehouse WM, Jr., Flinn WR, et al. Surgical correction of chronic deep venous insufficiency by valvular transposition. Surgery 1980; 87:688–695.

56. Raju S, Fountain T, Neglen P, Devidas M. Axial transformation of the profunda femoris vein. J Vasc Surg 1998; 27:651–659.

57. O'Donnell TF, Mackey WC, Shepard AD, et al. Clinical, hemodynamic, and anatomic follow-up of direct venous reconstruction. Arch Surg 1987; 122:474–482.

58. Bry JD, Muto PA, O'Donnell TF, Isaacson LA. The clinical and hemodynamic results after axillary-to-popliteal vein valve transplantation. J Vasc Surg 1995; 21:110–119.

59. Raju S. Multiple-valve reconstruction for venous insufficiency: Indications, optimal technique, and results. In: Veith FJ, ed. Current Critical Problems in Vascular Surgery. 4th ed. St. Louis, U.S.A: Quality Medical Publishing, 1992:122–125.

60. DePalma RG. Management of incompetent perforators: conventional techniques. In: Gloviczki P, Yao JST, eds. Handbook of Venous Disorders. 2nd ed. London: Arnold, 2001:384–390.

61. Linton RR. The post-thrombotic ulceration of the lower extremity: its etiology and surgical treatment. Ann Surg 1953; 138:415–432.

62. Dodd H. The diagnosis and ligation of incompetent ankle perforating veins. Ann R Coll Surg Engl 1964; 34:186–196.

63. DePalma RG. Surgical therapy for venous stasis: results of a modified linton operation. Am J Surg 1979; 137:810–813.

64. Edwards JM. Shearing operation for incompetent perforating veins. Br J Surg 1976; 63:885–886.

65. Gloviczki P, Bergan JJ, Menawat SS, et al. Safety, feasibility, and early efficacy of subfascial endoscopic perforator surgery: a preliminary report from the north American registry. J Vasc Surg 1997; 25:94–105.

66. Conrad P. Endoscopic exploration of the subfascial space of the lower leg with perforator interruption using laparoscopic equipment: a preliminary report. Phlebology 1994;154–157.

67. Bergan JJ, Murray J, Greason K. Subfascial endoscopic perforator vein surgery: a preliminary report. Ann Vasc Surg 1996; 10:211–219.

68. Pierik EG, van Urk H, Hop WC, Wittens CH. Endoscopic versus open subfascial division of incompetent perforating veins in the treatment of venous leg ulceration: a randomized trial. J Vasc Surg 1997; 26:1049–1054.

69. de Rijcke PA, Schenk T, van Gent WB, Kleinrensink GJ, Wittens CH. Surgical anatomy for subfascial endoscopic perforating vein surgery of laterally located perforating veins. J Vasc Surg 2003; 38:1349–1352.

70. de Rijcke PA, Hop WC, Wittens CH. Subfascial endoscopic perforating vein surgery as treatment for lateral perforating vein incompetence and venous ulceration. J Vasc Surg 2003; 38:799–803.

71. Gloviczki P, Bergan JJ, Rhodes JM, et al. Mid-term results of endoscopic perforator vein interruption for chronic venous insufficiency: lessons learned from the north American subfascial endoscopic perforator surgery registry. The north American study group. J Vasc Surg 1999; 29:489–502.

72. Kalra M, Gloviczki P. Subfascial endoscopic perforator vein surgery: who benefits? Semin in Vasc Sur 2002; 15:39–49.

73. Sybrandy JE, van Gent WB, Pierck EG, Wittens CH. Endoscopic versus open subfascial division of incompetent perforating veins in the treatment of venous leg ulceration: long-term follow-up. J Vasc Surg 2001; 33:1028–1032.

74. Camilli S, Guarnera G. External banding valvuloplasty of the superficial femoral vein in the treatment of primary deep valvular incompetence. Int Angiology 1994; 13:218–222.

75. Raju S, Hardy JD. Technical options in venous valve reconstruction. Am J Surg 1997; 173:301–307.

76. Poller L, McKernan A, Thomson JM, et al. Fixed minidose warfarin: a new approach to prophylaxis against venous thrombosis after major surgery. Br Med J 1987; 295:1309.

77. Kistner RL. Surgical repair of a venous valve. Straub Clin Proc 1968; 24:41–43.

78. Raju S. Venous insufficiency of the lower limb and stasis ulceration: changing concepts and management. Ann Surg 1983; 197:688–697.

79. Sottiurai VS. Technique in direct venous valvuloplasty. J Vasc Surg 1988; 8:646–648.

80. Tripathi R, Ktenidis KD. Trapdoor internal valvuloplasty: a new technique for primary deep vein valvular incompetence. Eur J Vasc Endovasc Surg 2001; 22:86–89.

81. Raju S, Fredericks R. Valve reconstruction procedures for nonobstructive venous insufficiency: rationale, techniques, and results in 107 procedures with two-to eight-year follow-up. J Vasc Surg 1988; 7:301–310.

82. Kistner RL. Surgical technique of external venous valve repair. The Straub Found Proc 1990; 55:15.

83. Belcaro G, Nicolaides AN, Ricci A, et al. External femoral vein valvuloplasty with limited anterior plication (LAP): a 10-year randomized, follow-up study. Angiology 1999; 50:531–536.

84. Gloviczki P, Merrell SW, Bower TC. Femoral vein valve repair under direct vision without venotomy: a modified technique with use of angioscopy. J Vasc Surg 1991; 14:645–648.

85. Raju S, Berry MA, Neglen P. Transcommissural valvuloplasty: technique and results. J Vasc Surg 2000; 32:969–976.

86. Taheri SA, Lazar L, Elias SM, Marchand P. Vein valve transplant. Surgery 1982; 91:28–33.

87. Sottiurai VS. Supravalvular incision for valve repair in primary valvular insufficiency. In: Bergan JJ, Kistner RL, eds. Atlas of Venous Surgery. Philadelphia: W.B. Saunders, 1992:137–138.

88. Raju S, Neglen P, Doolittle J, Meydrech EF. Axillary vein transfer in trabeculated postthrombotic veins. J Vasc Surg 1999; 29:1050–1064.

89. Cardon JM, Cardon A, Joyeux A, et al. Use of ipsilateral greater saphenous vein as a valved transplant in management of post-thrombotic deep venous insufficiency: long-term results. Ann Vasc Surg 1999; 13:284–289.

90. Welch H, McLaughlin RL, O'Donnell TF. Femoral vein valvuloplasty: intraoperative angioscopic evaluation and hemodynamic improvement. J Vasc Surg 1992; 16:694–700.

91. Jamieson WG, Chinnick B. Clinical results of deep venous valvular repair for chronic venous insufficiency. Can J Surg 1997; 40:294–299.

92. Perrin M. Reconstructive surgery for deep venous reflux: a report on 144 cases. Cardiovasc Surg 2000; 8:246–255.

93. Kistner RL. Surgical repair of the incompetent femoral vein valve. Arch Surg 1975; 110:1336–1342.

94. Ferris EB, Kistner RL. Femoral vein reconstruction in the management of chronic venous insufficiency: a 14-year experience. Arch Surg 1982; 117:1571–1579.

95. Lurie F, Makarova NP, Hmelniker SM. Results of deep-vein reconstruction. Vasc Surg 1997; 31:275–276.

96. Perrin MR. Results of deep-vein reconstruction. Vasc Surg 1997; 31:273–275.

97. Perrin M, Hiltbrand B, Bayon JM. Results of valvuloplasty in patients presenting deep venous insufficiency and recurring ulceration. Ann Vasc Surg 1999; 13:524–532.

98. Taheri SA, Lazar L, Elias SM, Marchand P. Vein valve transplant. Surgery 1982; 91:28–33.

99. Taheri SA, Elias SM, Yacobucci GN, et al. Indications and results of vein valve transplant. J Cardiovasc Surg 1986; 27:163–168.

100. Nash T. Long term results of vein valve transplants placed in the popliteal vein for intractable post-phlebitic venous ulcers and pre-ulcer skin changes. J Cardiovasc Surg 1988; 29:712–716.

101. Rai DB, Lerner R. Chronic venous insufficiency disease. Its etiology. A new technique for vein valve transplantation. Int Surg 1991; 76:174–178.

102. Sottiurai VS. Results of deep-vein reconstruction. Vasc Surg 1997; 31:276–278.

103. Plagnol P, Ciostek P, Grimaud JP, Prokopowicz SC. Autogenous valve reconstruction technique for post-thrombotic reflux. Ann Vasc Surg 1999; 13:339–342.

104. Maleti O. Venous valvular reconstruction in post-thrombotic syndrome. A new technique. J des Mal Vasculaires 2002; 27:218–221.
105. Lugle, M, Maleti, O. Neovalve Construction in Postthrombotic Syndrome. Presented at American Venous Forum 17th Annual Meeting, San Diego, California, February 9–13, 2005.
106. Psathakis ND, Psathakis DN. Surgical treatment of deep venous insufficiency of the lower limb. Surg Gynecol Obstet 1988; 166:131–141.
107. Dalsing MD, Ricotta JJ, Wakefield T, et al. Animal models for the study of lower extremity chronic venous disease: lessons learned and future needs. Ann Vasc Surg 1998; 12:487–494.
108. Neglen P, Raju S. Venous reflux repair with cryopreserved vein valves. J Vasc Surg 2003; 37:552–557.
109. Garcia-Rinaldi R, Soltero E, Gaviria J, et al. Implantation of cryopreserved allograft pulmonary monocusp patch: to treat nonthrombotic femoral vein incompetence. Tex Heart Inst J 2002; 29:92–99.
110. Pavcnik D, Uchida BT, Timmermans HA, et al. Percutaneous bioprosthetic venous valve: a long-term study in sheep. J Vasc Surg 2002; 35:598–602.
111. Brountzos E, Pavcnik D, Timmersmans HA, et al. Remodeling of suspended small intestinal submucosa venous valve: an experimental study in sheep to assess the host cells' origin. J Vasc Interv Radiol 2003; 14:349–356.

31

Management of Deep Venous Obstruction of the Lower Extremity: Endovascular Intervention and Surgery

Peter Neglén and Seshadri Raju
River Oaks Hospital and University of Mississippi Medical Center, Jackson, Mississippi, U.S.A.

INTRODUCTION

The treatment of chronic outflow obstructions has previously been largely neglected because of diagnostic difficulties and lack of appropriate surgical interventions. The open venous bypass surgery has been unattractive for several reasons and restricted to a minority of patients with severe disabling symptoms. Endovascular treatment of venous outflow obstruction with percutaneous stenting has drastically changed the treatment and view on venous outflow obstruction. The introduction of venous stenting has refocused the interest on the role of venous outflow obstruction in patients with chronic venous disorders, and has renewed interest in the nature and pathophysiology of venous obstruction in itself and in tests for detection of hemodynamically significant lesions. Iliac venous stenting has already largely replaced surgery as the "method of choice" for treatment of venous blockage. However, venous stenting is still under development, and there are several issues regarding diagnosis, methods of assessment and selection of patients, which needs to be resolved.

VENOUS OUTFLOW OBSTRUCTION

Venous obstruction may have many causes, such as a remaining stenosis after thrombolysis of acute iliofemoral venous thrombosis, complete occlusion or stenosis in chronic postthrombotic disease, nonthrombotic iliac vein compression syndrome, retroperitoneal fibrosis, and malignant venous obstruction. The majority of lower extremity outflow obstructions are observed following acute deep vein thrombosis (DVT) with subsequent absent or poor venous recanalization. Remaining obstruction is the principal cause of symptoms in approximately one-third of postthrombotic limbs. Obstruction is observed combined with reflux in 55% of symptomatic patients with CVI (1,2). This combination is most harmful. It leads to the highest levels of venous hypertension and the most severe symptoms as compared to either alone (3,4). It appears that proximal obstruction of the venous outflow, especially the iliac vein, is more symptomatic as compared to lower segmental blockage (5,6). The collateral formation is relatively poor around an iliofemoral obstruction contrary to blockage of the femoral-popliteal vein. Following proximal DVT, only 20–30% of iliac veins completely recanalize spontaneously, while the remaining veins recanalize partly and develops varying degrees of collaterals (7,8). Although postthrombotic obstruction is most frequent, an iliac vein obstruction may be "primary" or nonthrombotic in nature (May-Thurner syndrome (9) or iliac vein compression syndrome (10)). The compression is caused by arteries compressing the pelvic veins frequently resulting in secondary intraluminal lesions, and it is probably more common than previously thought (11). These limbs may have had a subclinical isolated iliac vein thrombosis, which was initiated at the vessel crossing and then propagated distally into the external iliac vein. On the other hand, limbs with obvious postthrombotic disease may have had an underlying iliac vein compression resulting in a clinical iliofemoral vein thrombosis (12). Whatever the chain of events, it will remind us that those patients with signs and symptoms of chronic venous insufficiency and absent history and findings of previous DVT may still have iliac vein obstruction, even in the presence of primary venous reflux (13).

DIAGNOSIS AND SELECTION OF PATIENTS

Unfortunately, there are no reliable tests to measure a hemodynamically significant stenosis. In fact, it is not known what degree of narrowing constitutes a "critical stenosis" in the venous system. This lack of "gold standard" is the major obstacle to assess the importance of chronic outflow obstruction, select limbs for treatment, and evaluate the outcome.

Non-invasive duplex Doppler and plethysmography have been helpful in the diagnosis of acute complete obstruction. However, in chronic venous obstruction, ultrasound investigation and outflow fractions obtained by air and strain gauge plethysmography have been shown to be inaccurate to measure hemodynamically important obstruction. Significant blockage may be present with normal findings (14–16).

Invasive pressures, i.e., hand/foot pressure differential and reactive hyperemia pressure increase, and indirect resistance calculations appear better than non-invasive studies (17–19), but these tests are also relatively insensitive and do not define the level of obstruction (16). Venous pressures may also be measured during venographic evaluation or at surgery as a pressure differential over the obstruction or a pressure increase on exercise or induced hyperemia. The difficulty does not arise when these pressure gradients are high, but when the pressure differentials are near normal. Although a positive hemodynamic test may indicate hemodynamic significance, a normal test does not exclude it.

It is presently impossible to detect potentially hemodynamically important borderline obstructions. Therefore, the diagnosis of outflow obstruction has to be made by morphological investigations. Although a positive non-invasive or invasive test may support to proceed with venography, a negative test should not exclude it. The key for the physician is to be aware of the importance and possibility of venous blockage combined with increased suspicion in patients with history and clinical signs and symptoms suggestive of outflow obstruction. Certainly patients with severe CVI and leg ulcer must undergo morphological studies. Transfemoral ascending (antegrade) venography is the standard method to image the venous outflow tract, showing the site of obstruction and the presence of collaterals. Collaterals appear to be poor substitutes for the original obstructed vein. Collateral development on venogram should perhaps instead be considered an indicator of a significant obstruction (17,18,20). To increase diagnostic accuracy, it is important to take images in multiple-planes including lateral views. Important lesions at the iliocaval junction may otherwise be missed. Intravascular ultrasound (IVUS) is superior to standard single-plane and multi-plane venography for estimating the morphological degree and extent of iliac vein stenosis and visualize details of intraluminal lesions (20–22). Patients with significant signs and symptoms of CVI need to have a transfemoral venography, or preferably an IVUS, performed in addition to routine non-invasive reflux investigations. Arbitrarily, we consider to stent limbs with ilio-caval vein stenosis with more than 50% reduction of the luminal cross-cut area as measured by IVUS, especially if pre- or intra-operative pressures gradients indicate hemodynamic significance. Pressure changes are not decisive to allow stenting, but markedly increased venous pressure levels have been considered compulsory to perform open surgery.

OPEN SURGICAL RECONSTRUCTION

Open surgical bypasses can be performed to alleviate severe venous outflow obstruction. The operations most frequently used are femoro-femoral crossover or unilateral ilio-caval bypass for proximal iliofemoral vein occlusion, and, rarely, sapheno-popliteal bypass for distal femoro-popliteal obstruction. For short left iliac venous stenosis at the vessel crossing (iliac vein compression syndrome) right iliac artery transposition and iliac vein patch angioplasty have been used in selected patients (23).

The results following open reconstructions are usually presented in series with small numbers of treated limbs and with poor reporting standards; rarely are cumulative patency and success rates given. The outcome of open surgery has not been so convincing as to make a major impact on the routine treatment outflow obstruction and has only been limited to a selective group of patients with the most severe clinical condition. The general problem with bypass grafting is relatively poor long-term patency. The reasons for this are several. The grafts tend to clot because the area of insertion has low velocity flow, external compression of the low pressure bypass may occur, non-saphenous graft material is inherently thrombogenetic, and the distal inflow is often poor due to extensive distal disease. The best clinical results has been achieved with large-diameter polyterafluoro-ethylene (PTFE) graft (10 mm) with external support (ringed), adjunct use of an arteriovenous fistulae and meticulous perioperative anticoagulation (24,25). The arteriovenous fistula is left in place and anticoagulation continued as long as no side effects occur and the bypass stays patent. Life-long anticoagulation is usually necessary to keep the bypass open. If the graft suddenly occludes with a functioning fistula, symptoms of pain and swelling are accentuated and the fistula has to be disconnected.

THE CROSS-OVER BYPASS

The cross-over bypass can be constructed either by using the contralateral saphenous vein or a prosthetic graft (Fig. 1). The donor vein is exposed and then rotated at the sapheno-femoral junction to cross to the other side [classic Palma technique (26)] or used as a free femoro-femoral graft. This free saphenous graft appears to do better than rotation of the vein avoiding kinking at the sapheno-femoral junction (27). The autogenous cross-femoral venous bypass appears to be less thrombogenetic with better patency than prosthetic grafts (28). The cross-over reconstruction has been reported to be durable with good symptom relief, so called "clinical" and venographic patency ranging from 44% to 100%

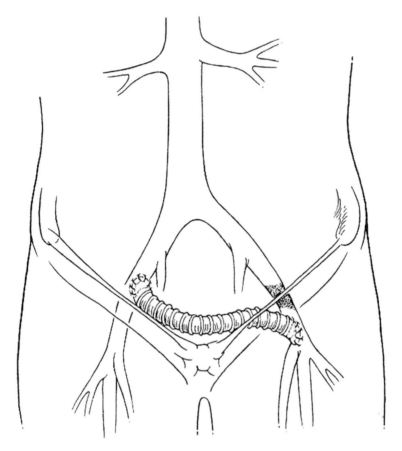

Figure 1 Femoro-iliac cross-over bypass with ringed PTFE-graft, usually constructed with temporary arteriovenous fistula. *Source*: From *Atlas of Venous Surgery*, (eds) Bergan JJ, Kistner RL, W.B. Saunders.

with a follow-up of five years (27–37). Most series have small number of patients with inconsistent clinical and venographic follow-up (Tables 1 and 2).

Halliday et al. performed the only cumulative analysis existing, showing a 75% cumulative venographic patency rate at five years (30). This excellent result has not been reproduced elsewhere. Clinical improvement is unfortunately not necessarily related to graft patency. Superior results are achieved if the inflow channel is normal. Despite remaining patent the saphenous grafts may give poor symptom relief owing to its small

Table 1 Results of Saphenous Vein Femoro-Femoral Bypass

Author	Number of limbs	Follow-up (months)	Clinical success (%)	Patency (%)
Husni (32)	78	7–144	74	73
Hutschenreiter et al. (34)	20	6–28	69	44
O'Donnell et al. (31)	6	24	100	100
Halliday et al. (30)	47	60	89	75
AbuRahma et al. (29)	24	66	88	75

Table 2 Results of Prosthetic Femoro-Femoral Bypass

Author	Number of limbs	Follow-up (months)	Clinical success (%)	Patency (%)
Eklof et al. (25)	7	2–31	86	17
Yamamoto et al. (35)	5	1–18	60	60
Comerota et al. (36)	3	40–60	67	67
Gruss and Hiemer (37)	32		85	85

cross-cut area and relatively large resistance to flow. It has been shown that at least a 4.0 mm diameter vein is necessary to adequately relieve the iliac vein outflow obstruction (24). This is the reason for recommended size of a 10 mm PTFE graft for femoral cross-over bypass as an alternative to the absence or an inadequate size of the saphenous vein.

THE IN-LINE BYPASS

Anatomic in-line bypass reconstruction can be used in the femoro-ilio-caval axial outflow axis with segmental obstruction in the presence of a sufficient venous in- and outflow of

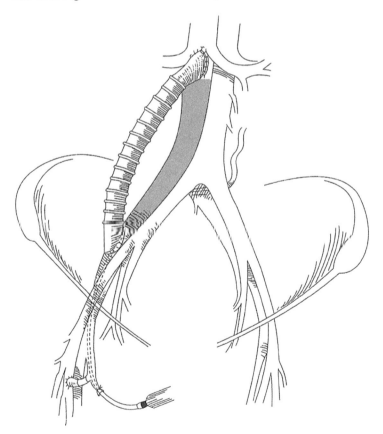

Figure 2 In-line ilio-caval bypass with ringed PTFE-graft and arterivenous fistula. *Source*: Ref. 39.

Table 3 Results of Femoro-Caval/Ilio-Caval Prosthetic Bypass Grafting

	Number of limbs	Follow-up (months)	Clinical success (%)	Patency (%)
Husfeldt (44)	4	4–30	100	100
Dale et al. (43)	3	1–30	100	100
Ijima et al. (40)	5	22–36	60	60
Eklof et al. (25)	7	2–31	86	29
Plate et al. (38)	3	1–11	67	33
Okadome et al. (41)	4	17–48	100	100
Gloviczki et al. (39)	12	1–60	67	58
Alimi et al. (42)	8	10–45	88	88
Jost et al. (28)	13	1–150	49	54

the graft (Fig. 2). As with cross-over bypasses, the in-line reconstructions, especially when starting in the groin, are constructed with a concomitant arteriovenous fistula, and life-long anticoagulation is usually necessary for patency. Patency rates during follow-up from 1–150 months vary from 29–100% (Table 3) (38–44).

The only cumulative study by Jost et al. shows a secondary patency rate of 54% at two years for prosthetic in-line bypass (28). This should be compared to 83% for saphenous vein femoro-femoral cross-over bypass in the same study. Early patency for caval reconstruction with excision of the cava and interposition graft for malignant disease is better than in-line bypasses for postthrombotic obstruction (45).

SAPHENO-POPLITEAL BYPASS

Sapheno-popliteal vein bypass is a rarely performed surgery for outflow obstruction. It is possible to perform only in extremely selected limbs with chronic segmental occlusion confined to the femoro-popliteal vein segment. The saphenous vein cannot be involved in the phlebitic process, which is very unusual. Limbs for treatment must have a patent, non-varicose great saphenous vein with competent valves and a patent tibial inflow tract (essentially normal calf views on venography). In addition, the results are not impressive. The few reported series of patients (29,32,46,47), show a clinical success and patency rates of 31–58% and 56–67%, respectively, at follow-up of one to five years.

FEMORO-ILIO-CAVAL STENTING

The surgical treatment of limbs with suspected venous outflow obstruction has been limited to a minority of patients with chronic venous insufficiency owing to the invasiveness and magnitude of the described operations, continuous anticoagulation with inherent risk of complications, and uncertain long-term results. Strict criteria for selection, including severe disabling symptoms and markedly increased venous pressure levels, have been used, and, for technical reasons, the saphenous vein in order to be utilized must be unaffected by any disease. Inadequate size, phlebitic obstruction or valve incompetence are factors often precluding the use of the autogenous vein. The introduction of percutaneous iliac venous balloon dilation and stenting has dramatically changed the premises for treatment.

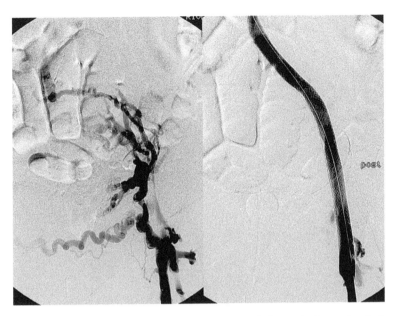

Figure 3 Recanalization of a postthrombotic iliofemoral obstruction before and after stent placement. While the initial venogram suggests otherwise, it is more often than not possible to transverse this type of occlusion.

The endovascular technique makes it possible to correct pelvic and caval vein obstruction more safely and less invasively, and, therefore, can be offered to a larger group of patients. Venous stenting has been used to successfully treat iliac vein obstruction of various etiologies (Figs. 3–5). The complication rate related to the endovascular intervention is minimal and comprises mostly cannulation site hematoma, but a minimal number of acquired arteriovenous fistula when the cannulation site is distal on the thigh

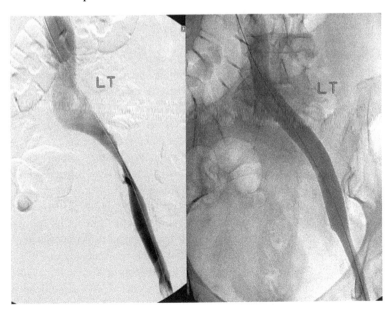

Figure 4 Images of stenting of a complex nonthrombotic obstruction due to iliac compression syndrome (common iliac vein compressed in the frontal and external iliac vein in the sagital plane).

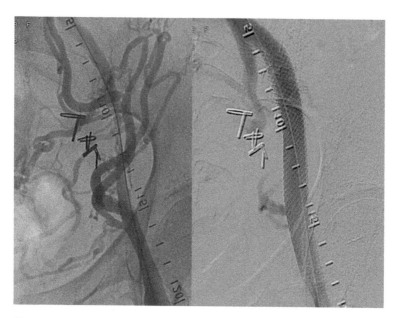

Figure 5 Patient with recurrent ovarial carcinoma resulting in external iliac vein obstruction. The patency of the stent is mostly related to the behavior of the malignancy.

has been observed and a few cases of retroperitoneal hematoma requiring blood transfusions have been described (14,48). The utilization of ultrasound guided cannulation and closure of the cannulation site with collagen plugs have largely abolished these problems. The mortality has been nil.

Studies of venous stenting in peer review publications often have similar short comings as reports for open surgery. Most studies are case reports and few are sizable, the follow-up is short-term and patency not reported in cumulative fashion, stented sites in the upper and lower extremities are mixed, and the majority of the reports series have not differentiated between etiologies or in management of acute and chronic conditions. In a group of patients, Nazarian et al. reported a one-year primary assisted patency rate of 66% of 29 iliac obstructions of mixed etiologies (49). The lower patency rate may be explained by the selection of patients (13/29 had complete occlusion and 16/19 were caused by malignancy). Interestingly, few occlusions occurred after six months, and the patency rate remained the same at one- and four-year follow-up. The same group has also reported an overall primary and secondary one-year primary and secondary patency rate of 50% and 81%, respectively, in a mixed population including 56 patients with iliac obstruction caused by malignancy, trauma, pregnancy, and postoperative stenosis (50).

Binkert et al. reported a 100% patency at an average follow-up time of three years in eight patients with chronic and acute pelvic vein obstruction (in four limbs following surgical thrombectomy) with resolution or substantial improvement of symptoms in most patients (51). Similarly, O'Sullivan et al. have reported a one-year patency of 79% in a retrospective analysis of 39 patients (52). Only half of the patients was stented for chronic symptoms (12/20 had adjuvant lysis); the remaining half presented with acute deep vein thrombosis and was treated after successful thrombolysis. Excluding initial technical failures, the stented patients had a one-year patency of 94% and 92% in respective group. The clinical results were excellent in the stented limbs.

Juhan et al. stented 15 limbs (six following open thrombectomy) and showed a venographic primary and secondary venographic patency of 87% and 93%, respectively, at mean follow-up of 24 mo (range 5–52). More than 80% of patients had satisfactory result and mean clinical and severity score decrease substantially to less than one (53). Lamont et al. inserted 15 flexible stents in 15 limbs (9 following acute DVT removal) and achieved cumulative secondary patency rate of 87% at 41 mo as measured by Duplex ultrasound (54). Similarly to Juhan et al. 80% (12/15) were asymptomatic. Symptoms were only mild in the three symptomatic limbs (Fig. 4).

ILIOCAVAL STENTING FOLLOWING THROMBOLYSIS/ THROMBECTOMY FOR ACUTE DVT

An unveiled proximal chronic obstruction of the iliac vein following thrombectomy or lysis is known to decrease future patency if not treated. Juhan et al. reported in patients undergoing surgical thrombectomy a low rethrombosis rate of 7% in limbs without stenosis versus 56% in limbs with severe stenosis (55). Mickley et al. found a rethrombosis rate of 13% if the underlying stenosis was stented as compared to 73% when not treated (56). In a retrospective study of thrombectomized limbs (1985–1995) Wohlgemuth et al. showed that there was no difference in patency rate between venous balloon angioplasty alone and stenting (approximately 66%) in 34 limbs (57). The evaluation was not prospective and only 7/34 limbs had stenting. However, the rethrombosis rate increased form 14% to 57% when remaining thrombosis or lesions were found on angioscopy post-thrombectomy. None of these papers relate the clinical result to any remaining partial obstruction.

In the report introducing thrombolysis as a valuable treatment option for acute iliofemoral venous thrombosis, Semba et al. performed balloon angioplasty and stent placement in more than 50% of limbs with an early patency rate of 85% (58). A gigantic multi-center registry collected data on 473 limbs with iliofemoral thrombosis treated by a wide variety of endovascular techniques (59). Limbs with ilio-caval stent placement had a greater one-year patency as compared to limbs undergoing only balloon angioplasty (74% and 53%, respectively).

It appears that the patency rates after stent placement following immediate removal of acute thrombosis and in treatment of chronic postthrombotic disease are similar. Presently the general consensus is to treat any underlying remaining stenosis after clot removal (thrombolysis, mechanical clot removal or open thrombectomy) by percutaneous stenting. Balloon angioplasty alone appears to be insufficient.

STENTING OF CHRONIC NONMALIGNANT OBSTRUCTION

Blättler and Blättler reported in 1999 treatment of chronic venous and neurogenic claudication due to pelvic venous blockage and achieved 100% patency in 11 successfully stented limbs with a mean follow-up of 15 months (range 1–43 months). The clinical success rate was 81% (9/11) (60). A group of 18 patients were reported by Hurst et al. (14). Twelve limbs were treated for chronic obstruction. The primary patency rates at 12 and 18 months were 79% and 79%, respectively. Most patients (72%) had resolution or substantial improvement of leg swelling and pain. However, five remaining patients continued to have pain despite resolved swelling and widely patent stents on venogram.

Several reports have been published by our group describing results after stenting of pelvic and caval veins in patients with chronic non malignant occlusions without any pre-treatment of acute deep vein thrombosis (48,61–64). Cumulative patency rates based on venographic findings as defined by reporting standards of SVS/ISCVS (65), frequency of in-stent recurrent stenosis, clinical results assessing pain, swelling and ulcer healing, and limited quality-of-life data are available. The obstructive lesion in these reports was considered postthrombotic when the patient had a known history of DVT or when postthrombotic changes was found on venography or ultrasound at any level of the lower extremity. The remaining limbs were considered non-thrombotic ("primary"). No obstructions due to malignancy were included.

Transfemoral venogram was performed after treatment in 324/455 limbs which underwent iliac vein stenting between 1997 and 2001 (61,62,66). Cumulative primary, assisted-primary and secondary patency rates at four years were 72%, 92% and 93%, respectively. The stented limbs with non-thrombotic disease appeared to fare significantly better than did those with thrombotic disease (primary, assisted-primary and secondary cumulative patency rates of 89%, 100% and 100%, and 65%, 85% and 88% at 36 months, respectively) (Table 4).

Although some degree of in-stent recurrent stenosis (ISR) is common (only 23% were completely free of any stenosis at 42 months), severe in-stent recurrent stenosis, i.e., > 50% diameter decrease on single plane anterior-posterior venogram, is infrequent (only 15% present in 42 months) (66). Several factors, which may potentially influence the development of ISR, were analyzed. Gender and sidedness of limb involvement did not affect outcome. Cumulative higher rates of severe IRS occurred with treatment of thrombotic than in nonthrombotic limbs (23% and 4%, respectively) at 36 months, and in the presence of thrombophilia (18% and 12%, respectively). The data concerning the length of stented area and extension of stent system to below the inguinal ligament appears intimately connected. Length of stented area 13–35 cm and extension of stent to below the inguinal ligament had a cumulative rate of severe ISR of 25% at 36 months and 40% at 24 months, respectively.

The strong impact of the thrombotic disease on development of in-stent restenosis appears to be reflected in the analysis of other potential contributing factors. There was an overrepresentation of limbs with thrombotic disease in patients with thrombophilia, long

Table 4 Cumulative Patency Rates and Frequency of In-Stent Restenosis After Iliofemoral Venous Stenting

	Follow-up time (months)	Cumulative patency rate (%)		
		Primary	Primary-assisted	Secondary
All limbs (n=324)	36	75	92	93
Thrombotic limbs (n=175)	36	65	85	88
Nonthrombotic limbs (n=147)	36	89	100	100

	Follow-up time (months)	Cumulative in-stent restenosis rate (%)		
		0	>20	>50
All limbs (n=316)	42	23	61	15
Thrombotic limbs (n=156)	36	–	63	23
Nonthrombotic limbs (n=145)	36	–	41	4

stents, and stents terminating below the inguinal ligament, which all had higher rates of in-stent restenosis. The result may reflect treatment of a more severe and extensive disease seen in limbs with thrombotic disease.

Although groups of limbs with multiple follow-up venograms do not unequivocally show an increase of stenosis over time, there is no doubt that there may be significant progress in individual cases. Whether the late occlusions occur due to acute recurrent thrombosis or due to gradual development of true intimal hyperplasia requires further study. The three major risk factors for development of ISR and late occlusion appear similar. At 24 months post-stenting, limbs with the three risk factors outlined above showed a 61% rate of severe in-stent restenosis, while none developed in their absence. No conclusion regarding a cause–effect relationship can be drawn from this paper.

As alluded to above, the reports describing patency rates indicate clinical improvement in most patients (>80%) (51,52). Hurst et al. showed resolution or substantial improvement in 72% of limbs (14). In addition to assessment of ulcer healing, Raju and Neglén have evaluated pain, swelling and quality-of-life. The degree of swelling was assessed by physical examination (Grade 0: none, Grade 1: pitting, not obvious, Grade 2: ankle edema Grade 3: obvious swelling involving the limb), the level of pain was measured by the visual analogue scale method (67), and quality-of-life by a questionnaire, validated for assessment of chronic venous insufficiency (68). The incidence of ulcer healing after iliac vein balloon dilation and stent placement in 41 limbs with active ulcer was 68% and the cumulative ulcer recurrence-free rate at two years was 62% (61). During the observation period no additional surgery was performed to treat reflux. Median swelling and pain severity scores decreased significantly (grade 2 to 1 and 4 to 0, respectively). The frequency of limbs with any swelling decreased significantly from 88% to 53% and limbs with any pain fell from 93% to 29%. The improvement of pain and swelling was significant in both ulcerated and non-ulcerated limbs, indicating that the ulcer was not the only cause of pain and swelling. Using a quality-of-life questionnaire assessing subjective pain, sleep disturbance, morale and social activities, routine and strenuous physical activities, the patients indicated significant improvement in all major categories after venous stenting. The clinical outcome is favorable in the intermediate term. The results clearly indicate a significant symptom relief after balloon angioplasty and stent placement to treat iliac venous outflow obstruction.

ENDOVASCULAR TECHNIQUE

Balloon angioplasty with stenting of the venous system is minimally invasive and straightforward to perform, but attention to details is important to achieve satisfactory results. The detailed technique is described elsewhere (48,52,63,64). Venous stenting is fundamentally a different procedure from stenting in the arterial system, e.g., the "kissing" balloon technique and the confluence of the common iliac veins or insertion of bilateral stents is not necessary. The cannulation of the femoral vein under ultrasound guidance has largely eliminated access complications. There is no problem of hemostasis, even in the middle of the thigh, as would be encountered after arterial puncture.

It has previously been shown that simple balloon dilation leads to early restenosis and an immediate recoil of the iliac vein has been observed intraoperatively in the majority of limbs (69–71). Therefore, stenting is advised of most dilated obstructions, especially when immediate significant recoil occur or the external compression is excessive. The intravascular ultrasound (IVUS) is invaluable, both as a diagnostic tool and as an intra-operative aid to direct placement of the stent.

Table 5 Technical Recommendations

1. Venous balloon angioplasty and stenting is conceptually different from that employed in the arterial system.
2. The "kissing" balloon technique and insertion of bilateral stents necessary at the aortic bifurcation is superfluous at the confluence of the common iliac veins.
3. Balloon angioplasty is most often insufficient in the venous system and stenting routine.
4. Ultrasound to guide cannulation of the femoral vein prevents complications.
5. IVUS is invaluable, both as a diagnostic tool and as an intra-operative aid, to direct stent placement.
6. Braided stents adjacent to the confluence of the common iliac veins must be placed well into the IVC to avoid early restenosis (retrograde migration).
7. Insertion of a large diameter stent (14–16 mm wide) is recommended. Unlike the artery, the vein accepts extensive dilation without clinical rupture.
8. Post insertion stent dilation is vital to prevent migration.
9. The most common cause of early restenosis is inadequate stenting of the lesion. The obstructive vein segment is usually more extensive than shown on venography. Cover the entire diseased venous segment as outlined by IVUS.
10. Avoid short skip areas (<5 cm) between two stents since these are prone to develop secondary stenosis.

If a braided stent, e.g., Wallstent®, is used, it should be placed well into the IVC in stenosis closed to the confluence of the common iliac veins. Owing to its inherent properties it is otherwise frequently displaced ("squeezed") distally and a proximal restenosis may develop (48). This IVC placement raises concern for risk of occlusion of the contralateral limb. The stent does, however, not appear to significantly impair the flow from the contralateral limb resulting in thrombosis. Only a few cases of contralateral limb DVT has been observed and appear to be caused by recurrent attacks of thrombosis.

Insertion of a self expanding flexible large stent (14–16 mm diameter) is recommended. The vein seems to accept extensive dilation without clinical rupture contrary to the artery. No clinical rupture of the vein has so far been reported, even when a total occlusion is recanalized and dilated up to 16 mm width. Re-dilatation after stent insertion is mandatory to achieve a good wall apposition as evaluated by IVUS.

The inflow and outflow of the stent can not be impeded to ensure long-term patency. Therefore, it is vital to cover the entire obstruction as outlined by the IVUS. Short skip areas in between two stents should be avoided. There should be no hesitation to extend the stent below the inguinal ligament if the lesion reaches the common femoral vein. The occlusion rate does not appear to be related to the length of stent or metal load per se, but to incomplete treatment or other factors (Table 5).

The perioperative thrombosis prophylaxis is fairly standardized in all patients. The patient received 2500 units subcutaneously of dalteparin preoperatively. During the procedure, 5.000 units of unfractionated heparin and 30 mg ketorolac were administered intravenously. All patients were admitted for less than 23 hours. Postoperatively, a foot compression device was applied, dalteparin 2500 units administered subcutaneously in the recovery room; and a ketorolac injection and dalteparin 5000 units repeated in the morning before discharge. Low dose aspirin (81 mg p.o.) daily was started immediately postoperatively and continued. Most patients did not have additional anticoagulation. Only patients already on warfarin preoperatively owing to prior recurrent deep vein thrombosis and/or thrombophilia or those with significant thrombophilia discovered preoperatively were anticoagulated postoperatively. These were a minority, often on life-long anticoagulation. Warfarin was routinely discontinued prior to surgery, and 5000 units of dalteparin were injected during the days warfarin had been discontinued.

SUMMARY

Interest in venous outflow obstruction is increasing with the emergence of practical treatment alternatives. The lack of accurate objective non-invasive or invasive test for evaluation of hemodynamically significant obstruction makes the selection of patients difficult. Presently patients have to be selected on clinical signs and symptoms with a high index of suspicion, and final diagnosis and treatment has to be based on morphological investigations. Transfemoral venography (multi-plane if possible), or preferably IVUS, should probably be utilized more generously in the work-up of patients with significant signs and symptoms of chronic venous disorder, especially in patients with leg ulcer or previous thrombosis.

Venous balloon angioplasty and stenting appears to be a safe, relatively simple, and efficient method to treat ilio-caval vein obstruction, at least in the mid-term. An immediate or late failure of the procedure does not preclude later open surgery to correct the obstruction. Associated reflux may be controlled subsequently when necessary. Open bypass surgery will probably be reserved for those patients in whom stenting initially could not be performed for technical reasons, late failures which can not be adequately disobliterated, and long total occlusions, which appear to have a poorer result.

Although venous stenting appears to be a promising treatment some caveats are necessary. The technology is relatively recent; thus, the follow-up period is limited. The long-term effects of stents in the venous system are not fully known. Several more years of monitoring is required to assess the efficacy and safety of this therapeutic modality in venous disease. In addition, further research on understanding the nature of venous obstruction and development of reliable methods to test hemodynamic consequences are needed.

KEY POINTS

- The lack of accurate objective non-invasive or invasive test for evaluation of hemodynamically significant obstruction makes the selection of patients difficult.
- Transfemoral multi-plane venography or, preferably, intravascular ultrasound should be utilized more generously in the work-up of patients with significant signs and symptoms of chronic venous disorder.
- Venous balloon angioplasty and stenting appears to be a safe, relatively simple, and efficient method to treat iliocaval vein obstruction.
- An immediate or late failure of the endovenous procedure does not preclude later open surgery to correct the obstruction.
- Open bypass surgery is mostly reserved for patients in whom stenting initially could not be performed for technical reasons, late failures which can not be adequately disobliterated, and long total occlusions, which appear to have a poorer result.

REFERENCES

1. Johnson BF, Manzo RA, Bergelin RO, Strandness DE, Jr. The site of residual abnormalities in the leg veins in long-term follow-up after deep vein thrombosis and their relationship to the development of the post-thrombotic syndrome. Int Angiol 1996; 15:14–19.
2. Johnson BF, Manzo RA, Bergelin RO, Strandness DE, Jr. Relationship between changes in the deep venous system and the development of the postthrombotic syndrome after an acute episode of lower limb deep vein thrombosis: a one- to six-year follow-up. J Vasc Surg 1995; 21:307–312; discussion 313.
3. Nicolaides AN, Hussein MK, Szendro G, Christopoulos D, Vasdekis S, Clarke H. The relation of venous ulceration with ambulatory venous pressure measurements. J Vasc Surg 1993; 17:414–419.
4. Nicolaides AN, Sumner DS. Investigations of patients with deep vein thrombosis and chronic venous insufficiency. Los Angeles, CA: Med-Orion Publishing Co, 1991.
5. May R. Anatomy. Surgery of the veins of the leg and pelvis. Stuttgart, Germany: Georg Thieme Verlag, 1979:1–36.
6. Mavor GE, Galloway JM. Collaterals of the deep venous circulation of the lower limb. Surg Gynecol Obstet 1967; 125:561–571.
7. Plate G, Akesson H, Einarsson E, Ohlin P, Eklof B. Long-term results of venous thrombectomy combined with a temporary arteriovenous fistula. Eur J Vasc Surg 1990; 4:483–489.
8. Mavor GE, Galloway JM. Iliofemoral venous thrombosis. Pathological considerations and surgical management. Br J Surg 1969; 56:45–59.
9. May R, Thurner J. The cause of the predominantly sinistral occurrence of thrombosis of the pelvic veins. Angiology 1957; 8:419–427.
10. Cockett FB, Thomas ML. The iliac compression syndrome. Br J Surg 1965; 52:816–821.
11. Raju S, Neglen P. Laser, "Closure," stents and other new technology in the treatment of venous disease. J Miss State Med Assoc 2004; 45:290–297.
12. Cockett FB, Thomas ML, Negus D. Iliac vein compression—Its relation to iliofemoral thrombosis and the post-thrombotic syndrome. Br Med J 1967; 2:14–19.
13. Neglen P, Thrasher TL, Raju S. Venous outflow obstruction: An underestimated contributor to chronic venous disease. J Vasc Surg 2003; 38:879–885.
14. Hurst DR, Forauer AR, Bloom JR, Greenfield LJ, Wakefield TW, Williams DM. Diagnosis and endovascular treatment of iliocaval compression syndrome. J Vasc Surg 2001; 34:106–113.
15. Labropoulos N, Volteas N, Leon M, et al. The role of venous outflow obstruction in patients with chronic venous dysfunction. Arch Surg 1997; 132:46–51.
16. Neglen P, Raju S. Detection of outflow obstruction in chronic venous insufficiency. J Vasc Surg 1993; 17:583–589.
17. Raju S. A pressure-based technique for the detection of acute and chronic venous obstruction, Phlebology 1988; 3:207–216.
18. Raju S, Fredericks R. Venous obstruction: an analysis of one hundred thirty-seven cases with hemodynamic venographic, and clinical correlations. J Vasc Surg 1991; 14:305–313.
19. Nicolaides AN. In: Outflow obstruction. Los Angeles, CA: Med-Orion Publishing Co, 1991:56–62.
20. Neglen P, Raju S. Intravascular ultrasound scan evaluation of the obstructed vein. J Vasc Surg 2002; 35:694–700.
21. Forauer AR, Gemmete JJ, Dasika NL, Cho KJ, Williams DM. Intravascular ultrasound in the diagnosis and treatment of iliac vein compression (May-Thurner) syndrome. J Vasc Interv Radiol 2002; 13:523–527.
22. Satokawa H, Hoshino S, Iwaya F, Igari T, Midorikawa H, Ogawa T. Intravascular Imaging Methods for Venous Disorders. Int J Angiol 2000; 9:117–121.
23. Taheri SA, Williams J, Powell S, et al. Iliocaval compression syndrome. Am J Surg 1987; 154:169–172.
24. Lalka SG, Lash JM, Unthank JL, et al. Inadequacy of saphenous vein grafts for cross-femoral venous bypass. J Vasc Surg 1991; 13:622–630.
25. Eklof B, Albrechtson U, Einarsson E, Plate G. The temporary arteriovenous fistula in venous reconstructive surgery. Int Angiol 1985; 4:455–462.

26. Palma EC, Esperon R. Vein transplants and grafts in the surgical treatment of the postphlebitic syndrome. J Cardiovasc Surg (Torino) 1960; 1:94–107.
27. Danza R, Navarro T, Baldizan J. Reconstructive surgery in chronic venous obstruction of the lower limbs. J Cardiovasc Surg (Torino) 1991; 32:98–103.
28. Jost CJ, Gloviczki P, Cherry KJ, Jr., et al. Surgical reconstruction of iliofemoral veins and the inferior vena cava for nonmalignant occlusive disease. J Vasc Surg 2001; 33:320–327 discussion 327–8.
29. AbuRahma AF, Robinson PA, Boland JP. Clinical, hemodynamic, and anatomic predictors of long-term outcome of lower extremity venovenous bypasses. J Vasc Surg 1991; 14:635–644.
30. Halliday P, Harris J, May J. Femoro-femoral crossover grafts (Palma operation): A long-term follow-up study. Surgery of the veins. Orlando, FL: Grune & Stratton 1985:241–254.
31. O'Donnell TF, Jr., Mackey WC, Shepard AD, Callow AD. Clinical, hemodynamic, and anatomic follow-up of direct venous reconstruction. Arch Surg 1987; 122:474–482.
32. Husni EA. In: Clinical experience with femoropopliteal venpus reconstruction. Chicago, IL: Yearbook Medical Publishers, 1978:485–491.
33. Gruss JD. In: Venous bypass for chronic venous insufficiency. Philadelphia, PA: WB Saunders, 1991:316–330.
34. Hutschenreiter S, Vollmar J, Loeprecht H, Abendschein A, Rodl W. Rekonstruktive Eingriffe am Venensystem: Spatergebnisse unter Kritischer Bewertung funktioneller und gefassmorphologischer Kriterien. Chirurg 1979; 50:555–563.
35. Yamamoto N. Reconstruction with insertion of expanded polytetrafluoroethylene (PTFE) graft for iliac venous obstruction. J Cardiovasc Surg 1986; 27:697–702.
36. Comerota AJ, Aldridge SC, Cohen G, Ball DS, Pliskin M, White JV. A strategy of aggressive regional therapy for acute iliofemoral venous thrombosis with contemporary venous thrombectomy or catheter-directed thrombolysis. J Vasc Surg 1994; 20:244–254.
37. Gruss JD, Hiemer W. Bypass procedures for venous obstruction: Palma and May-Husni bypasses, Raju perforator bypass, prosthetic bypasses, and primary and adjunctive arteriovenous fistulae. In: Surgical management of venous disease. Baltimore, MD: Williams & Wilkins, 1997:289–305.
38. Plate G, Einarsson E, Eklof B, Jensen R, Ohlin P. Iliac vein obstruction associated with acute iliofemoral venous thrombosis. Results of early reconstruction using polytetrafluoroethylene grafts. Acta Chir Scand 1985; 151:607–611.
39. Gloviczki P, Pairolero PC, Toomey BJ, et al. Reconstruction of large veins for nonmalignant venous occlusive disease. J Vasc Surg 1992; 16:750–761.
40. Ijima H, Kodama M, Hori M. Temporary arteriovenous fistula for venous reconstruction using synthetic graft: a clinical and experimental investigation. J Cardiovasc Surg (Torino) 1985; 26:131–136.
41. Okadome K, Muto Y, Eguchi H, Kusaba A, Sugimachi K. Venous reconstruction for iliofemoral venous occlusion facilitated by temporary arteriovenous shunt. Long-term results in nine patients. Arch Surg 1989; 124:957–960.
42. Alimi YS, DiMauro P, Fabre D, Juhan C. Iliac vein reconstructions to treat acute and chronic venous occlusive disease. J Vasc Surg 1997; 25:673–681.
43. Dale WA, Harris J, Terry RB. Polytetrafluoroethylene reconstruction of the inferior vena cava. Surgery 1984; 95:625–630.
44. Husfeldt KJ. Venous replacement with Gore-tex prosthesis: experimental and first clinical results. In: Pelvic and abdominal veins: Progress in diagnostics and therapy. Amsterdam: Excerpta Medica, 1981:249–258.
45. Bower TC, Nagorney DM, Cherry KJ, Jr., et al. Replacement of the inferior vena cava for malignancy: an update. J Vasc Surg 2000; 31:270–281.
46. Husni EA. In situ saphenopopliteal bypass graft for incompetence of the femoral and popliteal veins. Surg Gynecol Obstet 1970; 130:279–284.
47. Frileux C, Pillot-Bienayme P, Gillot C. Bypass of segmental obliterations of ilio-femoral venous axis by transposition of saphenous vein. J Cardiovasc Surg (Torino) 1972; 13:409–414.

48. Neglen P, Raju S. Balloon dilation and stenting of chronic iliac vein obstruction: technical aspects and early clinical outcome. J Endovasc Ther 2000; 7:79–91.

49. Nazarian GK, Austin WR, Wegryn SA, et al. Venous recanalization by metallic stents after failure of balloon angioplasty or surgery: four-year experience. Cardiovasc Intervent Radiol 1996; 19:227–233.

50. Nazarian GK, Bjarnason H, Dietz CA, Jr., Bernadas CA, Hunter DW. Iliofemoral venous stenoses: effectiveness of treatment with metallic endovascular stents. Radiology 1996; 200:193–199.

51. Binkert CA, Schoch E, Stuckmann G, et al. Treatment of pelvic venous spur (May-Thurner syndrome) with self-expanding metallic endoprostheses. Cardiovasc Intervent Radiol 1998; 21:22–26.

52. O'Sullivan GJ, Semba CP, Bittner CA, et al. Endovascular management of iliac vein compression (May-Thurner) syndrome. J Vasc Interv Radiol 2000; 11:823–836.

53. Juhan C, Hartung O, Alimi Y, Barthelemy P, Valerio N, Portier F. Treatment of nonmalignant obstructive iliocaval lesions by stent placement: mid-term results. Ann Vasc Surg 2001; 15:227–232.

54. Lamont JP, Pearl GJ, Patetsios P, et al. Prospective evaluation of endoluminal venous stents in the treatment of the May-Thurner syndrome. Ann Vasc Surg 2002; 16:61–64.

55. Juhan CM, Alimi YS, Barthelemy PJ, Fabre DF, Riviere CS. Late results of iliofemoral venous thrombectomy. J Vasc Surg 1997; 25:417–422.

56. Mickley V, Schwagierek R, Rilinger N, Gorich J, Sunder-Plassmann L. Left iliac venous thrombosis caused by venous spur: treatment with thrombectomy and stent implantation. J Vasc Surg 1998; 28:492–497.

57. Wohlgemuth WA, Weber H, Loeprecht H, Tietze W, Bohndorf K. PTA and stenting of benign venous stenoses in the pelvis: long-term results. Cardiovasc Intervent Radiol 2000; 23:9–16.

58. Semba CP, Dake MD. Iliofemoral deep venous thrombosis: aggressive therapy with catheter-directed thrombolysis. Radiology 1994; 191:487–494.

59. Mewissen MW, Seabrook GR, Meissner MH, Cynamon J, Labropoulos N, Haughton SH. Catheter-directed thrombolysis for lower extremity deep venous thrombosis: report of a national multicenter registry. Radiology 1999; 211:39–49.

60. Blattler W, Blattler IK. Relief of obstructive pelvic venous symptoms with endoluminal stenting. J Vasc Surg 1999; 29:484–488.

61. Raju S, Owen S, Jr., Neglen P. The clinical impact of iliac venous stents in the management of chronic venous insufficiency. J Vasc Surg 2002; 35:8–15.

62. Neglen P. Endovascular treatment of chronic iliofermoral venous obstruction - A review. Phlebolymphology 2003; 43:204–211.

63. Neglen P, Berry MA, Raju S. Endovascular surgery in the treatment of chronic primary and post-thrombotic iliac vein obstruction. Eur J Vasc Endovasc Surg 2000; 20:560–571.

64. Raju S, McAllister S, Neglen P. Recanalization of totally occluded iliac and adjacent venous segments. J Vasc Surg 2002; 36:903–911.

65. Porter JM, Moneta GL. Reporting standards in venous disease: an update. International Consensus Committee on Chronic Venous Disease. J Vasc Surg 1995; 21:635–645.

66. Neglen P, Raju S. In-stent recurrent stenosis in stents placed in the lower extremity venous outflow tract. J Vasc Surg 2004; 39:181–187.

67. Scott J, Huskisson EC. Graphic representation of pain. Pain 1976; 2:175–184.

68. Launois R, Reboul-Marty J, Henry B. Construction and validation of a quality of life questionnaire in chronic lower limb venous insufficiency (CIVIQ). Qual Life Res 1996; 5:539–554.

69. Marzo KP, Schwartz R, Glanz S. Early restenosis following percutaneous transluminal balloon angioplasty for the treatment of the superior vena caval syndrome due to pacemaker-induced stenosis. Cathet Cardiovasc Diagn 1995; 36:128–131.

70. Neglen P, al-Hassan HK, Endrys J, Nazzal MM, Christenson JT, Eklof B. Iliofemoral venous thrombectomy followed by percutaneous closure of the temporary arteriovenous fistula. Surgery 1991; 110:493–499.

71. Wisselink W, Money SR, Becker MO. Comparison of operative reconstruction and percutaneous balloon dilatation for central venous obstruction. Am J Surg 1993; 166:200–204; discussion 204–5.

32

Upper-Extremity Venous Thrombosis

Klaus Overbeck and Shankat N. Khan
Northern Vascular Centre, Freeman Hospital, Newcastle upon Tyne, U.K.

Gerard Stansby
University of Newcastle upon Tyne, Newcastle upon Tyne, U.K.

Nicos Labropoulos
Vascular Laboratory, Division of Vascular Surgery, New Jersey Medical School, Newark, New Jersey, U.S.A.

INTRODUCTION

Of all cases of deep venous thrombosis (DVT), the veins of the upper limb are involved in 1–4% (1–6) with "Primary thrombosis" or Paget-Schroetter Syndrome (PSS), accounting for approximately 20% of these in recent series. When Paget and Schroetter independently described their syndrome the underlying causes were mostly obscure but by now an underlying pathology can often be found. These include an association with inherited or acquired disorders of coagulation and abnormality or variations in the anatomy of the thoracic outlet (7). Approximately 40% of upper limb DVT is secondary to indwelling catheters. This form of thrombosis is referred to as secondary thrombosis.

ETIOLOGY

Primary Upper-Extremity Venous Thrombosis

The anatomical arrangement of the thoracic outlet is complex. Three main spaces have been described (8).

- The prescalene space (clavicle anteriorly and the anterior scalene muscle posteriorly)
- The costoclavicular space (the triangular space bounded anteriorly by the inner half of the clavicle and subclavius muscle and posteromedially by the first rib)
- The retropectoralis minor space (defined anteriorly by the posterior border of the pectoralis minor and posteriorly by the subscapularis muscle)

All of these are narrowed during elevation and hyperabduction of the arm resulting in compression of the axillary/subclavian vein (8,9). It has been postulated that such movement can cause repeated mechanical injury to the vein, augmented by adjoining bone, ligament and muscle structures (10–12).

In addition to compression by "normal" anatomical structures, anatomic anomalies or variants may also play a role in the aetiology of PSS. Such anatomical abnormalities have been found in up to 92% of certain series (13,14) and include intrinsic webs or bands, cervical ribs, abnormal costocoracoid ligaments, anterior or accessory phrenic nerves and a persistent axillopectineal ligament (10,13–21).

Secondary Venous Thrombosis

Central venous catheterization (CVC) can cause thrombosis due to several factors. Underlying malignancy and thrombophilia are associated with catheter induced thrombosis (22,23). Puncture of a vein is by nature traumatic and often repeated punctures may be required. The insertion of the catheter causes abrasion of endothelium as it slides along the wall sometimes with considerable force. These injuries are short lived, and due to the ability of the endothelium to resurface the damaged vein, are not a major factor in the development of a upper extremity venous thrombosis (24). Rather, the duration of the catheterization is the major factor associated with a DVT. Martin et al. found no thrombosis of the axillary vein if the catheter had been in situ less than six days in 60 cases but three after up to two weeks and five after more than two weeks duration (24). De Cicco et al. found in cancer patients phlebographic incidence of a DVT in 64% and 98% at eight and 30 days after CVC line insertion (25).

The length of the catheter may also influence the incidence of upper extremity venous thrombosis. Everitt et al. found in a randomized controlled trial using fine bore feeding catheters of different length inserted into the arm no difference in the incidence of a thrombosis (26). There is evidence that long peripherally induced central venous catheters (PICC) are more thrombogenic when compared with catheters inserted into a central vein directly (27). Allen et al. found a overall thrombosis rate of 38% for PICC. The incidence of thrombosis by site was cephalic 57%, basilic 14%, and brachial 10% (28). The size of PICC may be important: Grove et al. found no thrombosis with less than 3 F catheters (29). Large dialysis access lines are more prone to cause thrombosis. The clearest association between upper extremity venous thrombosis and thrombosis risk is related to the anatomical site. Larger veins with higher flow are less likely to thrombose. Kearns et al. found a increased thrombosis risk with tips in the axillo-subclavian-innominate vein compared with the superior vena cava (60% vs. 21%, $p < .05$) (27).

The precise position of the tip of the catheter is also important. Koolen found a 66.7% incidence of catheter tip malposition in patients who developed a upper extremity venous thrombosis following insertion of a Hickman line (30). The correct placement in the distal SVC reduced the thrombosis rate very significantly (31). The material the catheters are made of is important with polyvinyle chloride or polyethylene catheters being most thrombogenic. Polyvinyl chloride catheters were intermediate and hydromer coated polyurethane catheters being the least thrombogenic, followed closely by silicone catheters (32–34). Silicon catheters are also the least stiff devices (35). There is a benefit in using heparin bondage catheters in children (36). The implantation of permanent electrodes or pacing wires into a central vein also not surprisingly leads to venous thrombosis in a significant number of cases. Venous thrombosis has been demonstrated inside the innominate or subclavian veins in up to 40% of such cases with a 20% occlusion rate at two years after implantation. These thromboses are invariably asymptomatic (37,38).

CLINICAL PRESENTATION

Primary Upper-Extremity Venous Thrombosis

The diagnosis should be suspected in the setting of an acute onset of symptomatic upper extremity swelling, often with an antecedent episode of repetitive or sustained ipsilateral abduction and external rotation in an otherwise healthy individual (39,40). The condition is sometimes called "effort thrombosis." Other frequent symptoms and signs include heaviness, redness, increased limb temperature, and the presence of subcutaneous venous collaterals at the shoulder girdle. Pain is usually aching in nature and may be referred to the arm or axilla. Generally the patients are young, healthy and active and more often male than female with a ratio approaching 2:1 and an average age of 31 (41). Symptoms often are sufficiently dramatic that most patients present promptly for treatment (12,42,43). A history of antecedent strenuous or repetitive activities is present in more than 75% of the patients (2,15,44–46) and approximately 75% of the cases occur in the dominant extremity (10,12,17,44,47–50).

Resumption of normal activity after a period of recuperation (following an episode of thrombosis) frequently leads to symptoms of upper extremity venous hypertension exacerbated by using the arms in the overhead position. If not detected at an early stage symptomatic patients may sustain chronic disability from venous obstruction, with arm swelling, pain, and early exercise fatigue (12,42,43,45,51). This may lead to significant loss of occupational productivity and quality of life (52).

Paget-Schroetter Syndrome (PSS) can present as pulmonary embolism although fatal pulmonary embolism is rare (53–55). Presentations like phlegmasia cerulea dolens and frank venous gangrene are also rare (56–58).

Secondary Upper-Extremity Venous Thrombosis

Secondary thrombosis due to catheterization presents differently to PSS. First of all the patients tend to be older and more unwell, since CVC is used to monitor the critically ill and for nutritionally challenged patients. A second subgroup is oncological patients—adults and children—receiving chemotherapy via tunnelled lines with or without implanted ports. The third group consists of patients requiring central venous access for dialysis either temporarily while waiting for a surgical access to be performed or mature. Percutaneous dialysis access using catheters may also be required permanently when the surgical options are exhausted. Thrombosis related to implanted pacemakers or implantable cardiac defibrillators (ICD) rarely becomes symptomatic. An incidence of 1–5% of patients experiencing a symptomatic thrombosis has been quoted (59,60). Symptomatic SVC or innominate vein thrombosis is rare 1–3% (38,61,62). Most patients therefore present at the time of revision of the pacemaker with venographic evidence of a upper extremity venous thrombosis. The presence of a pulmonary embolism in a patient with a pacemaker or ICD should cause concern about the presence of an upper extremity venous thrombosis (59).

There is an association between permanent pacemaker implantation thrombosis and infection of the implants (63). The thrombosis may well be asymptomatic or there may be arm swelling, cyanosis and pain. Presentation as a PE is rare.

If the SVC is involved the patient may present with facial oedema vertigo, blurred vision or dyspnoea. These patients may present with a tachycardia, cyanosis of the involved extremity and as well as neck vein distension, with distended collateral veins over the chest and upper arm.

ASSESSMENT

A full blood count, thrombophilia screen, x-rays of the thoracic outlet and a chest X ray should be obtained routinely. In addition the thrombosis should be proven by specific imaging.

Ultrasound

For specific confirmation of upper limb venous thrombosis, duplex ultrasonography has a sensitivity of 94% to 100% and a specificity of 96% as compared to venography and has established itself the first choice of imaging technique in suspected cases (64–66). Thrombosis can be diagnosed by ultrasound using compression by the transducer at all veins but the subclavian and brachiocephalic. For these veins imaging is performed by color. Thrombosed vein segments are partially compressible or non compressible, and have filling defects on color mode. New thrombi are more echolucent (dark) compared to old thrombi that are more echogenic (bright). In old thrombosis large vein collaterals are seen bypassing the obstructed segment. Imaging of the distal subclavian vein is performed by placing the transducer over the clavicle. In this way the vein immediately before and right after the clavicle is seen. Stenosis at that level fixed or at different positions of the upper extremity can be diagnosed by the increased velocity after the stenosis. Complete occlusion interrupts the flow. Thrombus around the catheter is easily seen as the catheter is more echogenic than the blood and the thrombus. The vein lumen is also compressible around the catheter. Failure to compress the vein around the catheter is diagnostic for thrombosis. Intravascular ultrasound has been used to identify the aetiology of residual stenosis following thrombolysis (67).

Digital Subtraction Venography

Digital subtraction venography is a mainstay investigation in upper extremity thrombosis (68,69). Positional or provocative venography, by showing the costoclavicular compression of the subclavian/axillary vein on abduction and external rotation of the upper extremity, helps in identifying those patients who are at risk of recurrent thrombosis (70,71). Lee et al. (72) have emphasized looking for evidence of compression of the collateral vessels, as well as the main vein with provocative maneuvers. This helps to determine not only the haemodynamic significance but also the chronicity of the occlusion. Although venography is used as the "gold standard," false positive results are possible from inadequate positioning of the patient or by the inflow of nonopacified blood. Many surgeons use venography only if an intervention is planned or likely or if duplex ultrasound has provided inadequate information.

Magnetic Resonance Venography

Magnetic resonance angiography (MRA) is highly sensitive in detecting not only thrombosis but also venous stenosis in the central veins of the upper extremities (73–75). Short occlusions of the proximal portion of the left subclavian vein may be missed by duplex scanning but are occasionally seen with magnetic resonance imaging (MRI). MRI and duplex are inferior to venography in detecting non occlusive mural thrombi (66). MRI is highly reliable in ruling out the presence of a thrombotic process in the subclavian vein but it may on occasion fail to detect the presence of isolated subclavian thrombi. For this reason, in cases with suspected subclavian vein thrombosis MRI may not be used as the only modality. MRI has been shown to be suitable to analyze both vascular and musculoskeletal structures of the thoracic outlet. It may show significant narrowing of the costoclavicular space after positional manoeuvring in symptomatic patients (76). We suspect that with technical improvements in the future MRA may become the investigative modality of choice in many units.

MANAGEMENT

Management of Primary Thrombosis

As there have been no controlled therapeutic trials in Paget-Schroetter Syndrome the standard approach to management remains controversial (39,52,77–79). Rutherford and Hurlbert (50) in 1996 administered a questionnaire to a panel of experts from the United States with a special interest in subclavian vein thrombosis. The majority agreed upon (80) early clot removal for active, healthy patients with a need/desire to use the involved limb in work or sport. Catheter-directed thrombolysis was suggested as initial therapy with further therapy being based on follow-up positional venography. A brief period of anticoagulation followed by surgery was recommended once venous compression had been documented. If post-lysis venography showed either no extrinsic compression or a short residual occlusion surgery was not recommended but intervention for residual intrinsic lesions with over 50% narrowing. For residual symptomatic occlusion, 66% favored jugular vein turndown; only 10% would perform first rib removal. According to a similar questionnaire sent by Khan et al. in 2001 (81) to the members of Vascular Surgical Society of Great Britain and Ireland, only 17% still managed PSS conservatively. Thrombolysis was the most common intervention (86.7%) usually followed by elective thoracic outlet decompression delayed by 6–12 weeks. First rib resection was the most commonly performed operation (58%), usually by the transaxillary approach (55%).

Conservative Management with Anticoagulation

Anticoagulation is believed to protect the collateral vessels and interrupt the period of active clot propagation resulting leading to a better functional result than would be expected from the natural history. Conventional management of lower limb DVT involves anticoagulation for three to six months. This practice has been carried over to the initial conservative treatment of upper-extremity venous thromboses without direct evidence as there are no studies assessing benefit and duration of anticoagulation in PSS. Therapeutic unfractionated or low molecular weight heparin followed by at least three months of oral anticoagulants is the commonly used regime (39,77–79,82). There is good evidence from several larger long-term follow up studies that conservative treatment alone leads to persistent sequelae and disability in 33% to 85% of cases. This includes arm swelling, pain, disability, and even in rare cases venous gangrene (2,10,12,15,45,51,83).

Thrombolysis

Systemic or local thrombolysis with urokinase, tissue-plasminogen activator and streptokinase are used for the treatment of PSS (47,84,85). Thrombolysis is used mainly in the acute setting and around 90% success rates have been reported when employed within the first week of onset of thrombosis (6,84,86). It is significantly less successful two to four weeks after the diagnosis when the beginning organization of the thrombus hinders the recanalization of the vein (87). It has little, if any, role to play in chronic thrombosis. Physiological recanalization is associated with marked valvular damage and valvular insufficiency, and in contrast thrombolysis tends to preserve this valvular function (88). The use of thrombolytic therapy ultimately has improved the overall efficacy of oral anticoagulation therapy and may partially explain the improved results of more current oral anticoagulation series over historical studies.

Usually a bolus dose of the lytic agent is given which is followed by an infusion. The length of infusion time depends upon the degree of lysis observed on serial venography. The actual dose and the infusion regimens tend to vary from center to center. From a catheter directed urokinase infusion into the thrombus at a dose of 100,000 to 250,000 units for 24 to 72 hours to a bolus dose ranging from 100,000 to 1000,000 followed by a continuous infusion ranging from 50,000 to 240,000 units (89) have been used. Streptokinase has been given from at 10,000 to 100,000 unit per hour (90) for up to 96 hours (80). Continuous infusions of thrombolytics, especially streptokinase, may be associated with fever, headaches, allergic reactions including anaphylaxis, and hemorrhage (1). Hemorrhage is the most feared complication, although in the upper limb, it has been claimed major, bleeding events including intracerebral hemorrhage are no more frequent than with conventional heparin therapy (91). Allergic reactions are mostly associated with streptokinase. Urokinase is preferred because of its effectiveness and its avoidance of systemic effects and allergic reactions (17). Pulse-spray recombinant tissue-type plasminogen activator is a safe and effective alternative (92). *p*-Anisoylated streptokinase–plasminogen complex has also been successfully employed as a lytic agent in SAVT (93,94). Machleder found urokinase as the most effective pharmacologic agent for clot lysis (p=0.003) in his series of 50 patients (44).

Systemic thrombolysis has been replaced by catheter directed thrombolysis. It allows the evaluation of the progress of thrombolysis, exposure of the clot to higher concentration of the thrombolytic agent, less time to dissolve the clot, decreased incidence of systemic complications and the benefit of subsequent venography following completion of thrombolysis. Restoration of initial patency is the most significant factor in establishing final venous patency determined venographically (44). Successful thrombolysis is helpful in recognizing areas of stenosis and extrinsic compression at the thoracic outlet that may predispose to thrombosis (48,95). In a recent study Schmacht et al. demonstrated residual stenosis in six and occlusion in one axillosubclavian venous segments following catheter-directed thrombolysis in a series of seven patients (96).

Variable long-term outcomes have been associated with thrombolysis alone. In cases of residual symptoms and stenosis it carries poor long term results (10,21,97–102). In a series reported by Lokanathan et al. 22 out of the 25 patients had complete recanalization of the vein following catheter directed pulse spray method of thrombolysis (89). Twelve of the 13 patients who had intrinsic venous narrowing underwent percutaneous transluminal angioplasty to 12 mm. Three of these reoccluded 17 months after the initial diagnosis. Two patients developed PSS on the contralateral side. However, used alone rethrombosis of the subclavian or axillary vein following recanalization has been reported between 6–18% (4,16,49,84,103).

Although some authors have reported long-term symptom relieve it seems reasonable to suggest that thrombolysis alone may be inadequate when residual internal, external or positional obstruction has been demonstrated (13,16,44,83,97).

Balloon Angioplasty and Stenting

Residual stenosis after completion venography following successful thrombolysis commonly represents extrinsic compression from fixed, musculoskeletal structures of the thoracic outlet. Balloon angioplasty alone has therefore little to offer in patients with preoperative dynamic compression of the subclavian or axillary vein in the costoclavicular space (44,72,104,105). Angioplasty has, however, been found useful in cases of residual stenosis following surgical thoracic outlet decompression (106).

Kreienberg et al. recommend percutaneous transluminal angioplasty and subclavian vein stenting in short segment venous strictures following thrombolysis after their experience with 23 patients (107). However Azakie et al. and Lokanathan et al. have played down the role of venoplasty in the relief of venous compression or in the prevention of venous thrombosis (70,89). It may even increase the risk of subsequent rethrombosis (44,108). Machleder reports immediate rethrombosis in seven of the 12 venoplasties performed before thoracic decompression (44). Lee et al. tried balloon angioplasty of stenotic costoclavicular level venographic lesions in 12 of 22 cases and stenting in one (72). None of the 12 angioplasties resulted in any significant venographic improvement, and in the case of the stent it fractured at the site of previous stenosis.

Rethrombosis or restenoses is likely to occur without thoracic decompression (47,84,95,105). Venous stenoses are composed of large amount of elastin and collagen and are likely to be resistant to balloon dilatation. These are unlikely to fracture and remodel as the atherosclerotic lesions do (108). In the presence of external compression of the vein, stenting is not effective and invariably fails since the stent is simply crushed in the thoracic outlet (70,72,103,109–111). There may be a place for the use of stents after the surgical thoracic outlet decompression as the subclavian vein may still be subjected to intermittent compression (112).

Surgery

Long-term functional outcome is dependent on the early re-establishment of venous patency and the prevention of recurrent thrombosis and its sequelae. Recurrent thrombosis has been documented in one-third of the cases when the underlying abnormality has not been corrected surgically (44,70). The recurrence of symptoms suggests the aetiology lies in the narrow thoracic outlet and the functional anatomy of the region (44,113,114). This has therefore led to surgical correction of the abnormal anatomy as treatment. The early surgical procedures of venolysis, perivenous and periarterial sympathectomies, cervical sympathectomy and venous segment excision proved unsuccessful until the importance of thoracic outlet decompression was realized (13,17,41,71,104).

The advent of thrombolytic therapy has obviated the need of early thrombectomy. Thrombectomy initially showed some good short-term results but as rethrombosis was common unless accompanied by thoracic decompression. It has largely been abandoned (11,14,15,17). However thrombectomy may be favored if failure of thrombolysis has failed or is contraindicated (115).

In case of residual occlusion or stenosis following thrombolysis, the symptomatic patient may require more extensive surgery than the simple thoracic decompression like a bypass, crossover or internal jugular turndown (116–123). Molina advocated first rib resection and operative thrombectomy with vein patch angioplasty (49). In his series of 19 patients all had immediate success with four patients later requiring balloon angioplasty. Limited success rates (37%) have been reported when the venous lesion is more than two cm in length (16). These may require a bypass. Saphenous vein and synthetic material like polytetrafluoroethylene have been used for bypass with variable results (103,118,122,123). With a view to avoid occlusion of these bypass grafts many authors have placed an arteriovenous fistula distal to the bypass for a limited time (103,118,122–124). This type of surgery is only recommended for patients with severe disabling symptoms and whose part of the major veins proximal to elbow are patent. The risks of surgery are small but include brachial plexus injury, Horner's syndrome, long thoracic and phrenic nerve injuries, pneumothorax, chronic postoperative pain syndromes, chylothorax, as well as the possibility of arterial, venous and lymphatic injuries.

Timing of the Surgery. The timing of first rib resection following initial successful thrombolysis is controversial. Some authorities advocate thoracic outlet decompression shortly after the vein has been recanalised and a few days of heparin therapy have been administered. The rationale for this is to decompress the vein before it reoccludes. In addition early surgical decompression of the thoracic allows the patient to go home earlier and resume their work or desired activities avoiding a second admission. The second option, is to maintain warfarin therapy for six weeks to six months and then perform a first rib resection for persistent and significant symptoms or when there is continuing evidence of compression (44,125,126). The rational for delayed surgical intervention has been the assumption that acute phlebitic process resolves under the protection of oral anticoagulation over three months. At the end of that time it can be determined more effectively which patients require additional therapy. This interval allows for healing of the endothelium and avoidance of thrombosis at the time of surgery. Further, it gives the time to evaluate the need for surgery based on residual symptoms following the return of full arm movement (17).

Angle et al. advocate an abbreviated course where thrombolytic therapy is followed by early surgical decompression during the same admission, followed by a period of anticoagulation (127). In a clinical trial they compared early versus late surgery and found that thrombolysis followed by early surgery does not result in increased perioperative morbidity or mortality. Urschel and Razzuk recommend expeditious thrombolytic therapy and early surgery (first rib resection) reporting excellent results with thrombolysis plus prompt first rib resection in 199 extremities within a month and only fair results if treatment was delayed more than a month. However, they associate poor functional outcome with an occluded venous repair and extensive venous thrombosis on initial presentation and justified the use of multimodal intervention in patients with PSS presenting with recurrent thrombosis and significant residual disease after thrombolysis (128). In another series based on 3000 patients with 800 recurrent cases for thoracic outlet syndrome, Urschel has again recommended prompt thrombolysis followed by transaxillary first rib resection with no long term anticoagulation as standard management (129). Molina has advocated early decompression to prevent chronic fibrous narrowing of the vein and to limit the formation of collateral vessels as they may adversely affect the patency of a operative angioplasty or subsequent stent (16,49). Others have waited a month before the rib resection without adversely affecting the long-term outcomes (4,47,84,103). Adelman from New York University Medical Centre reported 18 cases (out of a series of 38 with upper extremity venous thrombosis) of PSS (84). Urokinase was used for thrombolysis in 17 of the 18 patients (94.4%) with complete lysis in 14 (82.4%). Clot lysis revealed axillary vein compression secondary to a thoracic outlet syndrome in 11 patients, and these underwent staged transaxillary thoracic outlet decompression by first rib resection. All 17 patients had a mean follow-up of 21 months, and none receiving lytic therapy reoccluded.

Machleder also recommended three months of anticoagulation following thrombolysis before transaxillary first rib resection and decompression (44). He recruited fifty consecutive patients into a sequential treatment program for spontaneous axillary-subclavian vein thrombosis. Forty-three had initial thrombolytic or anticoagulant treatment followed by longer-term warfarin therapy. Thirty-six (72%) underwent surgical correction of the underlying structural abnormality, and nine patients had postoperative balloon angioplasty. After surgical correction there were no episodes of recurrent thrombosis in a mean follow-up period of 3.1 years.

Surgical Approaches.   There is no standard approach. It is a matter of personal preference and experience of the surgical team.

Supraclavicular approach.   The advocates of this approach highlight its provision of excellent exposure, allowing the accurate identification of the specific compressive elements and decompression, with complete removal of the first rib along with the scalene and subclavius muscles, and at the same time complete circumferential venolysis (72,104,118). However, the supraclavicular incision places the major collaterals from the subclavian to the jugular vein at risk. These can be more easily avoided with a transaxillary or infraclavicular approach. At times it is necessary to remove the very proximal rib and cartilage at the sternochondral junction in order to completely free up the proximal vein and prevent recurrent symptoms. This cannot be safely reached via the supraclavicular incision alone.

Infraclavicular approach.   The infraclavicular approach allows adequate exposure of the subclavian vein and the costoclavicular space. It gives space to undertake any venous reconstruction procedures like endovenectomy and vein patching for stenotic lesions that come into limelight following lysis and first rib resection. Molina et al. described extension of the infraclavicular incision to involve a limited transverse sternotomy to allow the adequate exposure of the subclavian and brachiocephalic vein junction. This allows one to deal with any stenosis of the vein in that region (130).

Paraclavicular approach.   This term has been coined for a combination of supra and infraclavicular approaches. This allows the satisfactory completion of the surgical decompression and any additional procedures if so desired. In low-lying subclavian veins additional procedures may be necessary to gain adequate exposure.

Axillary approach.   This is currently the more favored approach. Its advantages over the supraclavicular route are relatively good exposure of the anterior end of the first rib and limitation of any damage on the collaterals. If only the portion of rib under the vein is removed, postoperative fibrosis and the residual rib remnant, especially anteriorly, can compromise the vein lumen and cause rethrombosis. To avoid this, first rib resection to the costosternal junction is advocated and this is easier through the axillary approach (70). It allows adequate subclavian vein exposure for venolysis but provides limited exposure for more extensive procedures. It produces an excellent cosmetic result. Disadvantages are that views can be poor and as a result bleeding may be difficult to deal with.

Miscellaneous approaches.   Green et al. have described a medial claviculectomy approach (131). They recommend that an early subclavian venous repair performed through a medial claviculectomy is a durable operation with excellent long-term functional results. Ohtsuka et al. have developed a thoracoscopic first rib resection technique by using a harmonic scalpel, rongeurs and an endoscopic drill (132).

Management of Upper Extremity Venous Thrombosis Due to Catheterization

The treatment of upper extremity venous thrombosis begins with therapeutic dose infusion of unfractionated heparin or LMWH for five to seven days and is continued with anticoagulation with Warfarin. If possible a catheter should be removed.

A more aggressive approach would include local or systemic thrombolysis and/or thrombectomy. This approach may be contemplated with young or very symptomatic patients. The catheter or access line does not necessarily have to be removed, in particular the electrodes of pacemakers or ICDs, unless there is evidence of infection, catheter damage, or malposition. Even in cases of thrombosis of the SVC stents can be safely placed over the electrodes left in situ. The catheter can be removed at the end of the lysis, which has been recommended if there is a high venous pressure due to, e.g., a SVC stenosis to avoid bleeding (133).

Systemic thrombolysis has been largely abandoned because of its high complication rate. Local or catheter directed lysis is the technique of choice. A small sheet is introduced into a superficial arm vein and a multiside hole catheter advanced to or even into the thrombus. A sub therapeutic heparin infusion is continued to reduce thrombus formation along the catheter. An average of two to three days of treatment may be required.

A further adjunct is the use of a thrombectomy. Venous thrombectomy is now rarely performed as an open procedure but can have good results (134). The more common practice is the percutaneous thrombectomy with one of the many available thrombectomy devices. There are two types; wall contact and nonwall contact devices, which both are used in venous thrombectomy. Once flow is restored the residual stenosis can be treated by angioplasty. Although venous strictures tend to offer far higher resistance to balloon dilatation than arterial stenoses, the results of angioplasty, even of the central vein, are acceptable and offer at least temporary relief. Re-intervention is commonly required. Oderich et al. reported a primary patency rate of 85%, 27%, and 9% at 3, 12, and 24 months, respectively; the secondary patency rate was reported as 91%, 71%, and 39% at 3, 12, and 24 months, respectively (135).

NATURAL HISTORY

There are only a few reports with a relatively small number of patients studying the natural history of upper extremity DVT. In a recent systematic review, the reported prevalence of postthrombotic signs and symptoms was 15% with a range of 7% to 46% (136). The risk of developing signs and symptoms and recurrent thrombosis is lower compared to the lower extremity DVT (137). Reflux has not been demonstrated after thrombosis in the upper extremity veins. The signs and symptoms are related to the residual obstruction rather than the extent of thrombosis (137). There is little work on the impact of upper extremity DVT on the quality of life. There are specific questionnaires that have been validated for this purpose. Prevention or reduction of the postthrombotic events needs to be evaluated.

CONCLUSIONS

For PSS use of the terms "primary" or "idiopathic" do not seem appropriate as there is growing evidence of functional or positional anatomical defects, which lead to subtle intimal injury and a tendency to recurrence or poor outcome. Despite this, and with no randomized data, it is difficult to give clear guidelines as to management and we suspect large numbers of patients are still treated conservatively based on protocols established for lower limb DVT. However, the majority of the recent literature recommends active treatment with thrombolysis followed by thoracic outlet decompression. Thrombolytic therapy appears to be a safe and efficacious method of establishing immediate patency of the axillary/subclavian vein. The timing of surgery remains controversial and is likely to remain an unresolved issue until level one evidence is available.

Secondary upper extremity thrombosis has replaced thoracic outlet syndrome as the most common cause of thrombosis. Catheterization is performed for drug infusion, monitoring of the critically ill patient, and long-term nutrition. In patients with underlying malignancy the risk of thrombosis is increased. Unlike in patients with thoracic outlet obstruction anticoagulation followed by angioplasty, which can be performed repeatedly, is effective. The incidence of thrombosis due to indwelling catheters causing thrombosis is related to site, duration, tip position, diameter and material. There is evidence that the ideal central venous catheter is placed via the right internal jugular vein into the SVC at the level of the atrium and made of silicon or polyurethane.

KEY POINTS

- Catheterization, malignancy, thrombophilia and throacic outlet obstruction are the most common causes of upper extremity venous thrombosis.
- Upper extremity venous thrombosis caused by extrinsic obstruction (PSS) of the thoracic outlet requires active invention.
- Thrombolysis and surgical decompression is the treatment of choice.
- The treatment should be performed by a team of vascular surgeons and interventional radiologist.
- Secondary thrombosis due to catheterization is the most common cause of thrombosis of the upper extremity veins.
- Intervention usually requires removal of the catheter and therapy is required if the patient is symptomatic.
- Treatment consists of anticoagulation, thrombolysis and angioplasty/stenting of a residual stenosis.
- Secondary upper extremity venous thrombosis due to catheterization responds well to endovascular therapy alone.

REFERENCES

1. Hill SL, Berry RE. Subclavian vein thrombosis: a continuing challenge. Surgery 1990; 108:1–9.
2. Coon WW, Willis PW, III. Thrombosis of axillary and subclavian veins. Arch Surg 1967; 94:657–663.
3. Horattas MC, Wright DJ, Fenton AH, et al. Changing concepts of deep venous thrombosis of the upper extremity report of a series and review of the literature. Surgery 1988; 104:561–567.
4. Hood DB, Kuehne J, Yellin AE, Weaver FA. Vascular complications of thoracic outlet syndrome. Am Surg 1997; 63:913–917.
5. Lindblad B, Tengborn L, Bergqvist D. Deep vein thrombosis of the axillary-subclavian veins: epidemiologic data, effects of different types of treatment and late sequelae. Eur J Vasc Surg 1988; 2:161–165.
6. Prescott SM, Tikoff G. Deep venous thrombosis of the upper extremity: a reappraisal. Circulation 1979; 59:350–355.
7. Leebeek FW, Stadhouders NA, van Stein D, Gomez-Garcia EB, Kappers-Klunne MC. Hypercoagulability states in upper-extremity deep venous thrombosis. Am J Hematol 2001; 67:15–19.
8. Demondion X, Boutry N, Drizenko A, Paul C, Francke JP, Cotten A. Thoracic outlet: anatomic correlation with MR imaging. AJR Am J Roentgenol 2000; 175:417–422.
9. Remy-Jardin M, Remy J, Masson P, et al. Helical CT angiography of thoracic outlet syndrome: functional anatomy. AJR Am J Roentgenol 2000; 174:1667–1674.

10. AbuRahma AF, Sadler D, Stuart P, Khan MZ, Boland JP. Conventional versus thrombolytic therapy in spontaneous (effort) axillary-subclavian vein thrombosis. Am J Surg 1991; 161:459–465.
11. Aziz S, Straehley CJ, Whelan TJ, Jr. Effort-related axillosubclavian vein thrombosis. A new theory of pathogenesis and a plea for direct surgical intervention. Am J Surg 1986; 152:57–61.
12. Swinton NW, Jr, Edgett JW, Jr., Hall RJ. Primary subclavian-axillary vein thrombosis. Circulation 1968; 38:737–745.
13. Thompson RW, Schneider PA, Nelken NA, Skioldebrand CG, Stoney RJ. Circumferential venolysis and paraclavicular thoracic outlet decompression for "effort thrombosis" of the subclavian vein. J Vasc Surg 1992; 16:723–732.
14. DeWeese JA, Adams JT, Gaiser DL. Subclavian venous thrombectomy. Circulation 1970; 41:II158–II164.
15. Adams JT, DeWeese JA. "Effort" thrombosis of the axillary and subclavian veins. J Trauma 1971; 11:923–930.
16. Molina JE. Surgery for effort thrombosis of the subclavian vein. J Thorac Cardiovasc Surg 1992; 103:341–346.
17. Kunkel JM, Machleder HI. Treatment of Paget-Schroetter syndrome. A staged, multidisciplinary approach. Arch Surg 1989; 124:1153–1157, discussion 1157–1158.
18. Daskalakis E, Bouhoutsos J. Subclavian and axillary vein compression of musculoskeletal origin. Br J Surg 1980; 67:573–576.
19. Sundqvist SB, Hedner U, Kullenberg HK, Bergentz SE. Deep venous thrombosis of the arm: a study of coagulation and fibrinolysis. Br Med J (Clin Res Ed) 1981; 283:265–267.
20. Stevenson IM, Parry EW. Radiological study of the aetiological factors in venous obstruction of the upper limb. J Cardiovasc Surg (Torino) 1975; 16:580–585.
21. Steed DL, Teodori MF, Peitzman AB, McAuley CE, Kapoor WN, Webster MW. Streptokinase in the treatment of subclavian vein thrombosis. J Vasc Surg 1986; 4:28–32.
22. Van Rooden CJ, Rosendaal FR, Meinders AE, Van Oostayen JA, Van Der Meer FJ, Huisman MV. The contribution of factor V Leiden and prothrombin G20210A mutation to the risk of central venous catheter-related thrombosis. Haematologica 2004; 89:201–206.
23. Kuter DJ. Thrombotic complications of central venous catheters in cancer patients. Oncologist 2004; 9:207–216.
24. Martin C, Viviand X, Saux P, Gouin F. Upper-extremity deep vein thrombosis after central venous catheterization via the axillary vein. Crit Care Med 1999; 27:2626–2629.
25. De Cicco M, Matovic M, Balestreri L, et al. Central venous thrombosis: an early and frequent complication in cancer patients bearing long-term silastic catheter. A prospective study. Thromb Res 1997; 86:101–113.
26. Everitt NJ, McMahon MJ. Influence of fine-bore catheter length on infusion thrombophlebitis in peripheral intravenous nutrition: a randomised controlled trial Ann R Coll Surg Engl 1997; 79:221–224.
27. Kearns PI, Coleman S, Wehner JH. Complications of long arm-catheters: a randomized trial of central vs peripheral tip location. JPEN J Parenter Enteral Nutr 1996; 20:20–24.
28. Allen AW, Megargell JL, Brown DB, et al. Venous thrombosis associated with the placement of peripherally inserted central catheters. J Vasc Interv Radiol 2000; 11:1309–1314.
29. Grove JR, Pevec WC. Venous thrombosis related to peripherally inserted central catheters. J Vasc Interv Radiol 2000; 11:837–840.
30. Koolen DA, van Laarhoven HW, Wobbes T, Punt CJ. Single-centre experience with tunnelled central venous catheters in 150 cancer patients. Neth J Med 2002; 60:397–401.
31. Cadman A, Lawrance JA, Fitzsimmons L, Spencer-Shaw A, Swindell R. To clot or not to clot? That is the question in central venous catheters Clin Radiol 2004; 59:349–355.
32. Borow M, Crowley JG. Prevention of thrombosis of central venous catheters. J Cardiovasc Surg (Torino) 1986; 27:571–574.
33. Monreal M, Raventos A, Lerma R, et al. Pulmonary embolism in patients with upper extremity DVT associated to venous central lines—a prospective study. Thromb Haemost 1994; 72:548–550.

34. Bozzetti F, Terno G, Bonfanti G, et al. Prevention and treatment of central venous catheter sepsis by exchange via a guidewire. A prospective controlled trial. Ann Surg 1983; 198:48–52.

35. Cervera M, Dolz M, Herraez JV, Belda R. Evaluation of the elastic behaviour of central venous PVC, polyurethane and silicone catheters. Phys Med Biol 1989; 34:177–183.

36. Pierce CM, Wade A, Mok Q. Heparin-bonded central venous lines reduce thrombotic and infective complications in critically ill children. Intensive Care Med 2000; 26:967–972.

37. Stoney WS, Addlestone RB, Alford WC, Jr., Burrus GR, Frist RA, Thomas CS, Jr. The incidence of venous thrombosis following long-term transvenous pacing. Ann Thorac Surg 1976; 22:166–170.

38. Spittell PC, Hayes DL. Venous complications after insertion of a transvenous pacemaker. Mayo Clin Proc 1992; 67:258–265.

39. Prandoni P, Polistena P, Bernardi E, et al. Upper-extremity deep vein thrombosis. Risk factors, diagnosis, and complications. Arch Intern Med 1997; 157:57–62.

40. Ninet J, Demolombe-Rague S, Bureau du Colombier P, Coppere B. Les thromboses veineuses profondes des membres supérieurs. Sang Thrombose Vaisseaux 1994; 6:103–114.

41. Hurlbert SN, Rutherford RB. Primary subclavian-axillary vein thrombosis. Ann Vasc Surg 1995; 9:217–223.

42. Adams J, McEvoy RK, DeWeese J. Primary deep vein thrombosis of upper extremity. Arch Surg 1968; 91:29–42.

43. Kleinsasser L. "Effort" thrombosis of the axillary and subclavian veins. Arch Surg 1949; 59:258–274.

44. Machleder HI. Evaluation of a new treatment strategy for Paget-Schroetter syndrome: spontaneous thrombosis of the axillary-subclavian vein. J Vasc Surg 1993; 17:305–315; discussion 316–317.

45. Tilney ML, Griffiths HJ, Edwards EA. Natural history of major venous thrombosis of the upper extremity. Arch Surg 1970; 101:792–796.

46. Campbell CB, Chandler JG, Tegtmeyer CJ, Bernstein EF. Axillary, subclavian, and brachiocephalic vein obstruction. Surgery 1977; 82:816–826.

47. Sheeran SR, Hallisey MJ, Murphy TP, Faberman RS, Sherman S. Local thrombolytic therapy as part of a multidisciplinary approach to acute axillosubclavian vein thrombosis (Paget-Schroetter syndrome). J Vasc Interv Radiol 1997; 8:253–260.

48. Machleder HI. Effort thrombosis of the axillosubclavian vein: a disabling vascular disorder. Compr Ther 1991; 17:18–24.

49. Molina JE. Need for emergency treatment in subclavian vein effort thrombosis. J Am Coll Surg 1995; 181:414–420.

50. Rutherford RB, Hurlbert SN. Primary subclavian-axillary vein thrombosis: consensus and commentary. Cardiovasc Surg 1996; 4:420–423.

51. Donayre CE, White GH, Mehringer SM, Wilson SE. Pathogenesis determines late morbidity of axillosubclavian vein thrombosis. Am J Surg 1986; 152:179–184.

52. Becker DM, Philbrick JT, Walker FBT. Axillary and subclavian venous thrombosis. Prognosis and treatment. Arch Intern Med 1991; 151:1934–1943.

53. Monreal M, Lafoz E, Ruiz J, Valls R, Alastrue A. Upper-extremity deep venous thrombosis and pulmonary embolism. A prospective study. Chest 1991; 99:280–283.

54. Black MD, French GJ, Rasuli P, Bouchard AC. Upper extremity deep venous thrombosis. Underdiagnosed and potentially lethal. Chest 1993; 103:1887–1890.

55. Harley DP, White RA, Nelson RJ, Mehringer CM. Pulmonary embolism secondary to venous thrombosis of the arm. Am J Surg 1984; 147:221–224.

56. Smith BM, Shield GW, Riddell DH, Snell JD. Venous gangrene of the upper extremity. Ann Surg 1985; 201:511–519.

57. Chandrasekar R, Nott DM, Enabi L, Bakran A, Harris PL. Upper limb venous gangrene, a lethal condition. Eur J Vasc Surg 1993; 7:475–477.

58. Kammen BF, Soulen MC. Phlegmasia cerulea dolens of the upper extremity. J Vasc Interv Radiol 1995; 6:283–286.

59. Phibbs B, Marriott HJ. Complications of permanent transvenous pacing. N Engl J Med 1985; 312:1428–1432.

60. Thompson MF, Arnold RM, Bogart DB, Earnest JB, Bailey RE. Symptomatic upper extremity venous thrombosis associated with permanent transvenous pacemaker electrodes. Chest 1983; 83:274–275.

61. Barakat K, Robinson NM, Spurrell RA. Transvenous pacing lead-induced thrombosis: a series of cases with a review of the literature. Cardiology 2000; 93:142–148.

62. Van Vleet JF, Schollmeyer MP, Engle WR, Tacker WA, Jr., Bourland JD. Cardiovascular alterations induced by chronic transvenous implantation of an automatic defibrillator electrode catheter in dogs. J Electrocardiol 1981; 14:67–72.

63. Pavia S, Wilkoff B. The management of surgical complications of pacemaker and implantable cardioverter-defibrillators. Curr Opin Cardiol 2001; 16:66–71.

64. Koksoy C, Kuzu A, Kutlay J, Erden I, Ozcan H, Ergin K. The diagnostic value of colour Doppler ultrasound in central venous catheter related thrombosis. Clin Radiol 1995; 50:687–689.

65. Baxter GM, Kincaid W, Jeffrey RF, Millar GM, Porteous C, Morley P. Comparison of colour Doppler ultrasound with venography in the diagnosis of axillary and subclavian vein thrombosis. Br J Radiol 1991; 64:777–781.

66. Haire WD, Lynch TG, Lund GB, Lieberman RP, Edney JA. Limitations of magnetic resonance imaging and ultrasound-directed (duplex) scanning in the diagnosis of subclavian vein thrombosis. J Vasc Surg 1991; 13:391–397.

67. Chengelis DL, Glover JL, Bendick P, Ellwood R, Kirsch M, Fornatoro D. The use of intravascular ultrasound in the management of thoracic outlet syndrome. Am Surg 1994; 60:592–596.

68. Kinnison ML, Kaufman SL, Chang R, Kadir S, Mitchell SE, White RI, Jr. Upper-extremity venography using digital subtraction angiography. Cardiovasc Intervent Radiol 1986; 9:106–108.

69. Baarslag HJ, van Beek EJ, Tijssen JG, van Delden OM, Bakker AJ, Reekers JA. Deep vein thrombosis of the upper extremity: intra- and interobserver study of digital subtraction venography. Eur Radiol 2003; 13:251–255.

70. Azakie A, McElhinney DB, Thompson RW, Raven RB, Messina LM, Stoney RJ. Surgical management of subclavian-vein effort thrombosis as a result of thoracic outlet compression. J Vasc Surg 1998; 28:777–786.

71. Rutherford RB. Primary subclavian-axillary vein thrombosis: the relative roles of thrombolysis, percutaneous angioplasty, stents, and surgery. Semin Vasc Surg 1998; 11:91–95.

72. Lee WA, Hill BB, Harris EJ, Jr., Semba CP, Olcott CI. Surgical intervention is not required for all patients with subclavian vein thrombosis. J Vasc Surg 2000; 32:57–67.

73. Kroencke TJ, Taupitz M, Arnold R, Fritsche L, Hamm B. Three-dimensional gadolinium-enhanced magnetic resonance venography in suspected thrombo-occlusive disease of the central chest veins. Chest 2001; 120:1570–1576.

74. Fielding JR, Nagel JS, Pomeroy O. Upper extremity DVT. Correlation of MR and nuclear medicine flow imaging. Clin Imaging 1997; 21:260–263.

75. Thornton MJ, Ryan R, Varghese JC, Farrell MA, Lucey B, Lee MJ. A three-dimensional gadolinium-enhanced MR venography technique for imaging central veins. AJR Am J Roentgenol 1999; 173:999–1003.

76. Demondion X, Bacqueville E, Paul C, Duquesnoy B, Hachulla E, Cotten A. Thoracic outlet: assessment with MR imaging in asymptomatic and symptomatic populations. Radiology 2003; 227:461–468.

77. Hingorani A, Ascher E, Lorenson E, et al. Upper extremity deep venous thrombosis and its impact on morbidity and mortality rates in a hospital-based population. J Vasc Surg 1997; 26:853–860.

78. Elliott G. Upper-extremity deep vein thrombosis. Lancet 1997; 349:1188–1189.

79. Hicken GJ, Ameli FM. Management of subclavian-axillary vein thrombosis: a review. Can J Surg 1998; 41:13–25.

80. Albrechtsson U, Anderson J, Einarsson E, Eklof B, Norgren L. Streptokinase treatment of deep venous thrombosis and the postthrombotic syndrome. Follow-up evaluation of venous function. Arch Surg 1981; 116:33–37.

81. Khan SN, Stansby G. Current management of Paget-Schroetter syndrome in the UK. Ann R Coll Surg Engl 2004; 86:29–34.

82. Savage KJ, Wells PS, Schulz V, et al. Outpatient use of low molecular weight heparin (Dalteparin) for the treatment of deep vein thrombosis of the upper extremity. Thromb Haemost 1999; 82:1008–1010.

83. Urschel HC, Jr., Razzuk MA. Improved management of the Paget-Schroetter syndrome secondary to thoracic outlet compression. Ann Thorac Surg 1991; 52:1217–1221.

84. Adelman MA, Stone DH, Riles TS, Lamparello PJ, Giangola G, Rosen RJ. A multidisciplinary approach to the treatment of Paget-Schroetter syndrome. Ann Vasc Surg 1997; 11:149–154.

85. Haire WD, Atkinson JB, Stephens LC, Kotulak GD. Urokinase versus recombinant tissue plasminogen activator in thrombosed central venous catheters: a double-blinded, randomized trial. Thromb Haemost 1994; 72:543–547.

86. Kolodinsky SD, Brandschwei FH. Axillary vein thrombosis in a female backpacker: Paget-Schroetter syndrome. Can Assoc Radiol J 1989; 40:230–231.

87. Francis CW, Marder VJ. Fibrinolytic therapy for venous thrombosis. Prog Cardiovasc Dis 1991; 34:193–204.

88. Comerota AJ, White JV, Grosh JD. Intraoperative intra-arterial thrombolytic therapy for salvage of limbs in patients with distal arterial thrombosis. Surg Gynecol Obstet 1989; 169:283–289.

89. Lokanathan R, Salvian AJ, Chen JC, Morris C, Taylor DC, Hsiang YN. Outcome after thrombolysis and selective thoracic outlet decompression for primary axillary vein thrombosis. J Vasc Surg 2001; 33:783–788.

90. van Leeuwen PJ, Huisman AB, Hohmann FR. Selective low-dose thrombolysis in patients with an axillary-subclavian vein thrombosis. Eur J Vasc Surg 1990; 4:503–506.

91. Rogers LQ, Lutcher CL. Streptokinase therapy for deep vein thrombosis: a comprehensive review of the English literature. Am J Med 1990; 88:389–395.

92. Chang R, Horne MK, 3rd, Mayo DJ, Doppman JL. Pulse-spray treatment of subclavian and jugular venous thrombi with recombinant tissue plasminogen activator. J Vasc Interv Radiol 1996; 7:845–851.

93. Ruckley CV, Boulton FE, Redhead D. The treatment of venous thrombosis of the upper and lower limbs with "APSAC" (p-anisoylated streptokinase-plasminogen complex). Eur J Vasc Surg 1987; 1:107–112.

94. Pires LA, Jay G. Upper-extremity deep-vein thrombosis: thrombolytic therapy with anistreplase. Ann Emerg Med 1993; 22:748–750.

95. Becker GJ, Holden RW, Rabe FE, et al. Local thrombolytic therapy for subclavian and axillary vein thrombosis. Treatment of the thoracic inlet syndrome. Radiology 1983; 149:419–423.

96. Schmacht DC, Back MR, Novotney ML, Johnson BL, Bandyk DF. Primary axillary-subclavian venous thrombosis: is aggressive surgical intervention justified? Vasc Surg 2001; 35:353–359.

97. Wilson JJ, Zahn CA, Newman H. Fibrinolytic therapy for idiopathic subclavian-axillary vein thrombosis. Am J Surg 1990; 159:208–210; discussion 210–211.

98. Taylor LM, Jr, McAllister WR, Dennis DL, Porter JM. Thrombolytic therapy followed by first rib resection for spontaneous ("effort") subclavian vein thrombosis. Am J Surg 1985; 149:644–647.

99. Smith-Behn J, Althar R, Katz W. Primary thrombosis of the axillary/subclavian vein. South Med J 1986; 79:1176–1178.

100. Landercasper J, Gall W, Fischer M, et al. Thrombolytic therapy of axillary-subclavian venous thrombosis. Arch Surg 1987; 122:1072–1075.

101. Strange-Vognsen HH, Hauch O, Andersen J, Struckmann J. Resection of the first rib, following deep arm vein thrombolysis in patients with thoracic outlet syndrome. J Cardiovasc Surg (Torino) 1989; 30:430–433.

102. Zimmermann R, Morl H, Harenberg J, Gerhardt P, Kuhn HM, Wahl P. Urokinase therapy of subclavian-axillary vein thrombosis. Klin Wochenschr 1981; 59:851–856.

103. Meier GH, Pollak JS, Rosenblatt M, Dickey KW, Gusberg RJ. Initial experience with venous stents in exertional axillary-subclavian vein thrombosis. J Vasc Surg 1996; 35:974–981; discussion 981–983.

104. Lee MC, Grassi CJ, Belkin M, Mannick JA, Whittemore AD, Donaldson MC. Early operative intervention after thrombolytic therapy for primary subclavian vein thrombosis: an effective treatment approach. J Vasc Surg 1998; 27:1101–1107; discussion 1107–1108.

105. Beygui RE, Olcott CT, Dalman RL. Subclavian vein thrombosis: outcome analysis based on etiology and modality of treatment. Ann Vasc Surg 1997; 11:247–255.

106. Perler BA, Mitchell SE. Percutaneous transluminal angioplasty and transaxillary first rib resection. A multidisciplinary approach to the thoracic outlet syndrome. Am Surg 1986; 52:485–488.

107. Kreienberg PB, Chang BB, Darling RC, 3rd, et al. Long-term results in patients treated with thrombolysis, thoracic inlet decompression, and subclavian vein stenting for Paget-Schroetter syndrome. J Vasc Surg 2001; 33:S100–S105.

108. Glanz S, Gordon DH, Lipkowitz GS, Butt KM, Hong J, Sclafani SJ. Axillary and subclavian vein stenosis: percutaneous angioplasty. Radiology 1988; 168:371–373.

109. Urschel HC, Jr., Patel AN. Paget-Schroetter syndrome therapy: failure of intravenous stents. Ann Thorac Surg 2003; 75:1693–1696; discussion 1696.

110. AbuRahma AF, Robinson PA. Effort subclavian vein thrombosis: evolution of management. J Endovasc Ther 2000; 7:302–308.

111. Molinari AC, Castagnola E, Mazzola C, Piacentino M, Fratino G. Thromboembolic complications related to indwelling central venous catheters in children with oncological/haematological diseases: a retrospective study of 362 catheters. Support Care Cancer 2001; 9:539–544.

112. Hall LD, Murray JD, Boswell GE. Venous stent placement as an adjunct to the staged, multimodal treatment of Paget-Schroetter syndrome. J Vasc Interv Radiol 1995; 6:565–569; discussion 569–570.

113. Hughes E. Venous obstruction in the upper extremity. Br J Surg 1949; 36:155–163.

114. Machleder H. Upper Extremity Venous Occlusion. Current Therapy in Vascular Surgery. 3rd ed. Hamitton, Ontario: BC Decker. 1995. 958–963.

115. Hulbert S, Rutherford RB. Subclavian-axillary vein thrombosis. Vasc Surg 2000; 5:1208–1221.

116. Feugier P, Aleksic I, Salari R, Durand X, Chevalier JM. Long-term results of venous revascularization for Paget-Schroetter syndrome in athletes. Ann Vasc Surg 2001; 15:212–218.

117. Hashmonai M, Schramek A, Farbstein J. Cephalic vein cross-over bypass for subclavian vein thrombosis: a case report. Surgery 1976; 80:563–564.

118. Sanders RJ, Cooper MA. Surgical management of subclavian vein obstruction, including six cases of subclavian vein bypass. Surgery 1995; 118:856–863.

119. Malatinsky J, Faybik M, Samel M, Majek M. Surgical, infectious and thromboembolic complications of central venous catheterization. Resuscitation 1983; 10:271–281.

120. Inahara T. Surgical treatment of "effort" thrombosis of the axillary and subclavian veins. Am Surg 1968; 34:479–483.

121. Rabinowitz R, Goldfarb D. Surgical treatment of axillosubclavian venous thrombosis: a case report. Surgery 1971; 70:703–706.

122. Hansen B, Feins RS, Detmer DE. Simple extra-anatomic jugular vein bypass for subclavian vein thrombosis. J Vasc Surg 1985; 2:921–923.

123. Currier CB, Jr., Widder S, Ali A, Kuusisto E, Sidawy A. Surgical management of subclavian and axillary vein thrombosis in patients with a functioning arteriovenous fistula. Surgery 1986; 100:25–28.

124. Malcynski J, O'Donnell TF, Jr., Mackey WC, Millan VA. Long-term results of treatment for axillary subclavian vein thrombosis. Can J Surg 1993; 36:365–371.

125. Rauwerda JA, Bakker FC, van den Broek TA, Dwars BJ. Spontaneous subclavian vein thrombosis: a successful combined approach of local thrombolytic therapy followed by first-rib resection. Surgery 1988; 103:477–480.

126. Pittam MR, Darke SG. The place of first rib resection in the management of axillary-subclavian vein thrombosis. Eur J Vasc Surg 1987; 1:5–10.

127. Angle N, Gelabert HA, Farooq MM, et al. Safety and efficacy of early surgical decompression of the thoracic outlet for Paget-Schroetter syndrome. Ann Vasc Surg 2001; 15:37–42.

128. Urschel HC, Jr., Razzuk MA. Paget-Schroetter syndrome: what is the best management? Ann Thorac Surg 2000; 69:1663–1668; discussion 1668–1669.

129. Urschel HC, Jr. The transaxillary approach for treatment of thoracic outlet syndromes. Semin Thorac Cardiovasc Surg 1996; 8:214–220.

130. Molina JE. Approach to the confluence of the subclavian and internal jugular veins without claviculectomy. Semin Vasc Surg 2000; 13:10–19.

131. Green RM, Waldman D, Ouriel K, Riggs P, Deweese JA. Claviculectomy for subclavian venous repair: long-term functional results. J Vasc Surg 2000; 32:315–321.

132. Ohtsuka T, Wolf RK, Dunsker SB. Port-access first-rib resection. Surg Endosc 1999; 13:940–942.

133. Sharafuddin MJ, Sun S, Hoballah JJ. Endovascular management of venous thrombotic diseases of the upper torso and extremities. J Vasc Interv Radiol 2002; 13:975–990.

134. Lacroix H, Van Belle K, Nevelsteen A, Suy R. The venous thrombectomy: obsolete or forgotten? Acta Chir Belg 1998; 98:14–17.

135. Oderich GS, Treiman GS, Schneider P, Bhirangi K. Stent placement for treatment of central and peripheral venous obstruction: a long-term multi-institutional experience. J Vasc Surg 2000; 32:760–769.

136. Elman EE, Kahn SR. The post-thrombotic syndrome after upper extremity deep venous thrombosis in adults: a systematic review. Thromb Res Epub ahead of print. July 2005.

137. Prandoni P, Bernardi E, Marchiori A, et al. The long term clinical course of acute deep vein thrombosis of the arm: prospective cohort study. BMJ 2004; 329:484–485.

33
Mesenteric and Portal Vein Thrombosis

Klaus Overbeck
Northern Vascular Centre, Freeman Hospital, Newcastle upon Tyne, U.K.

Derek Manas
Hepatic Surgery Unit, Freeman Hospital, Newcastle upon Tyne, U.K.

Gerard Stansby
University of Newcastle upon Tyne, Newcastle upon Tyne, U.K.

INTRODUCTION

Mesenteric venous thrombosis (MVT), although rare, can be associated with a high rate of morbidity and mortality. Portal vein thrombosis (PVT) has better prognosis but, it is like MVT, difficult to diagnose and can be found in combination with MVT.

MVT was first described as early as 1876 by Fagge (1) at Guy's Hospital in a patient with a previous deep venous thrombosis and subsequently by Elliot (2) in 1895 who reported the first successful resection for MVT. PVT was first describes 8 years earlier by Balford and Steward (3) in a case of an enlarged spleen and ascitis.

Because of their rarity many aspects of their diagnosis and management still remain controversial or unclear. In this chapter we aim to summarise current knowledge and recent advances relating to MVT and PVT.

MESENTERIC VENOUS THROMBOSIS

Etiology and Classification

Anatomy

Venous blood from the left colon and rectum drains into the inferior mesenteric vein (IMV), which in turn joins the splenic vein. The superior mesenteric vein (SMV) drains blood via the ileal and jejunal veins from the small intestine as well as from the caecum, the ascending and the transverse colon. The SMV then joins with the splenic vein behind the neck of the pancreas to form the portal vein.

The SMV or IMV alone may be thrombosed (isolated MVT) or it may be associated with PVT (4,5). Patients with isolated MVT are more likely to have an underlying thrombophilia and are more likely to require surgery (4).

Thrombosis of the mesenteric veins are usually segmental and as the vasa recta and venous arcades act as collaterals, infarction is more common if these vessels are also involved (6). Rhee et al. (7) found in a series of cases of MVT that the ileum and jejunum were infarcted in 81.1% and 83.3% of cases respectively. In contrast colonic infarction was found in only 13% of cases. This may be due to the colon possessing additional drainage via the middle and inferior rectal veins into the iliac veins.

Incidence of Mesenteric Venous Thrombosis

In his literature review of 273 cases of MVT (1911–1984), Abdu (8) found that the condition was most common in the sixth and seventh decades of life. By contrast a more recent series of 170 cases (1993–2000) by Endean found the average age to be 43 years (range 20–63) (9) although MVT can affect even young children (10,11). Of the 170 patients described by Endean (9) found with thrombotic acute intestinal ischemia, MVT accounted for 26% (15/58). In addition Clavien (12) reported a 13.2% incidence in 89 cases (13/98). Other reports identify MVT as the cause of intestinal ischemia in 5–25% of cases (7,13). Although the true overall incidence of MVT is not clear, one autopsy study found 0.5–1.5% of the mesenteric veins thrombosed (14).

Etiology and Classification of Mesenteric Venous Thrombosis

MVT are conventionally described as "primary" or "secondary." However, the proportion of true primary MVT cases in more recent series is in decline due to the increasing recognition of specific inherited or acquired thrombotic and hypercoagulopathic disorders. In current series "primary" MTV accounts only for 10–21% of all cases (15,7,16). Because of this it is probably more sensible to classify MVT into "spontaneous" and "secondary." "Spontaneous" then includes cases where thrombosis is secondary to a coagulation disorder or where no specific cause is found.

Coagulation abnormalities covering the whole spectrum of inherited and acquired forms of thrombophilia have been described as causes of MVT. They include hereditary disorders like antithrombin III deficiency (17–19), Protein C deficiency (20–22), Protein S deficiency (23,24), Factor V Leiden (25–27) and 20210A mutation in the prothrombin gene (28,29). Acquired prothrombitic forms of thrombophilia are also described, including Anticardiolipin antibodies (30,31), Antiphospholipid syndrome (APS) (32), Hyperhomocysteinemia (33,29) and Plasminogen activator deficiency. Oral contraceptives are responsible for up to 18% of MVT cases in some series (8,34–36). Nephrotic syndrome (37–40), myeloproliferative disorders (41), polycythemia vera (42), Essential thrombocythemia (43), Paroxysmal nocturnal hemoglobinuria (44,45) and pregnancy (46) have all also been found to be associated with MVT.

Secondary MVT describes the other group of conditions known to cause MVT. Malignancy (4) leads to paraneoplastic syndrome (47) and external compression of the portal vein or SMV. Inflammatory disorders like pancreatitis (48–50) and Crohn's disease (51) are also well known to lead to MVT. Postoperative splenectomy MVT is well described (52,53), Appendicitis is associated with MVT in cases of portal pyemia (54,55) and laparoscopic surgery has been reported to trigger MVT (56,57). In a retrospective review Fichera (58) found that 4.8% 4/83 of patients after a total colectomy for inflammatory bowel disease had developed a symptomatic MVT. Sclerotherapy related propagation of thrombus leading to MVT is well described (59,60). Portal hypertension and cirrhosis are also part of the long list of causes (Table 1) (66).

Table 1   Causes of Mesenteric Venous Thrombosis

"Spontaneous" MVT
Hereditary Thrombophilia
Antithrombin III deficiency (17–19)
Protein C deficiency (20–22,61), Protein S deficiency (23–27,62) and 20210A mutation in the
prothrombin gene (28,29)
Acquired Thrombophilia
Anticardiolipin antibodies (30,31,63)
Antiphospholipid syndrome (32)
Hyperhomocysteinemia (29,33) and
Plasminogen activator deficiency
Oral contraceptives (8,34–36)
Nephrotic syndrome (37–40,61)
Myeloproliferative disorders (41)
Polycythemia vera (42)
Essential thrombocythemia (64)
Paroxysmal nocturnal hemoglobinuria (44,45)
Pregnancy (46)
Secondary MVT
Malignancy (4)
Paraneoplastic syndrome (65)
Inflammatory disorders
Pancreatitis (48–50)
Crohn's disease (51)
Post-Splenectomy (52,53)
Appendicitis (54,55)
Laparoscopic surgery (56,57)
Colectomy for inflammatory bowel disease (58)
Sclerotherapy (59,60)
Portal hypertension and cirrhosis (66)

Abbreviation: MVT, mesenteric venous thrombosis.

Kumar et al. (4) have suggested a further possible classification. They noted that "the location of the thrombus may be determined on the basis of the underlying cause." With intra-abdominal causes the thrombosis tends to start in the large vessels at the site of compression and then progresses peripherally to involve the smaller venous arcades and arcuate channels. In prothrombotic states the thrombosis begins in the smaller vessels and progresses to involve the larger veins. Subsequently the same authors have published a retrospective review of 69 cases of acute MVT in which two groups were identified (4). In the *isolated* group only the small vessels and SMV were involved and in the second group or *combined group* the SMV and the portal or splenic vein were thrombosed. In the subgroup analysis in the *isolated* group signs of peritonitis were more likely to be seen (p = 0.009) and surgical intervention was required in 70% versus 26% of cases (p = 0.0002). Thrombophilia was five times more common in the *isolated* group.

Clinical Features of Mesenteric Venous Thrombosis

The clinical picture can vary greatly. MVT can present acute with sudden onset of symptoms, subacute with symptoms lasting for days or weeks and chronic where the patient presents with complications of MVT such as oesophageal variceal bleeding (67). The most common clinical presentation is with abdominal pain (83–91%) often out of proportion with the physical findings. MVT causes anorexia in 49%, nausea or vomiting in 36–70%, diarrhoea in 15–42% and melena in 22%. Up to 21% developed upper GI bleeding in acute MVT and in 50% the fecal occult blood test is positive (68,7). The initial pain is usually central and colicky in nature. The presentation depends on whether primarily the large or the small veins are involved and to what degree the bowel wall is ischemia. If the ischemia is limited to the mucosa abdominal pain and diarrhoea are common and the patient rarely develops transmural infarction. If the ischemia has caused transmural infarction and necrosis MVT will present as peritonitis. This is then followed by signs of a progressing systemic sepsis. A systemic pressure of <90 mmHg is a sign of a poor prognosis (68). At presentation 33–43% patients have clinical signs of peritonitis and most patients have symptoms lasting longer than 48 hours (7,4) with an average of 5–7 days (4).

Differential Diagnosis of Mesenteric Venous Thrombosis

Arterial mesenteric ischemia is the main differential diagnosis of MVT. However, a more insidious onset and longer duration of symptoms may suggest MVT. Occlusive and non occlusive arterial mesenteric ischemia accounts for 75–95% of cases of mesenteric ischemia (7) but a strangulated internal hernia or bowel ischemia due to adhesions can also present with similar symptoms. 15–44% of patients give a history of a previous DVT or PE or known coagulopathy which should alert the clinician toward suspecting MVT in a patient with somewhat unspecific abdominal signs and symptoms (69,70) whilst underlying atrial fibrillation or known PVD or atherosclerosis points more at an arterial mesenteric event. Archibald described a case of a 32-year-old male who presented with abdominal pain and rectal bleeding due to ischemic colitis caused by a SMV thrombosis (71). Roman highlighted a case of pseudo-obstruction with a grossly dilated colon caused by MVT (72).

Investigations

Blood Tests

The WBC can be raised. Rhee found 50.9% of patients of acute MVT had a leucocytosis and similarly 44.4% with chronic MVT exhibited a leucocytosis (7). Lactate levels are a sensitive but nonspecific marker of bowel ischemia. The rise in lactate levels is temporary and returns to normal within hours after the onset of ischemia (73–78). Rhee (7) found in his review of MVT a raised lactate in 28.3% of patients with acute cases, but in chronic MVT in only 5.3%.

Plain X-Ray

Plain X-ray studies are usually unhelpful. Possible findings are ground glass appearance with ascitis and thickening of the bowel wall, air in the bowel wall and portal vein and free gas may be seen if perforation has occurred (79,80).

Duplex Ultrasound

Duplex ultrasound is useful for the assessment of the portal and mesenteric vein flow but is often limited by bowel gas, has a low sensitivity to detect slow flow and is highly operator dependant. Despite these limitations it has a good sensitivity for PVT 84% (81). In a recent review the diagnosis of port-MVT was made with duplex sonography in 57% of 23 cases (43).

Computer Tomography and Magnetic Resonance Angiography

Spiral abdominal computer tomography (CT) and magnetic resonance (MR) angiography are becoming the investigation of choice for the diagnosis of MVT. Recent fast acquisition, high resolution breath holding imaging can compete with venous phase DSA angiography except for the distal mesenteric branches. Sensitivity reaches 100% in several series (70). These techniques also are readily available, non-invasive, and also provide morphological and functional information (82). Kreft found no statistical difference in comparing MR angiography with intra-arterial DSA of the portal venous system in 36 patients with portal hypertension. The overall sensitivity, specificity, and accuracy for the detection of thrombosis were 100%, 98%, and 99% for MR angiography and 91%, 100%, and 96% for DSA (83).

Management of Mesenteric Venous Thrombosis

If the diagnosis is made preoperatively the patient should be started on intravenous heparin. Laparotomy is required only if the patient displays signs of peritonitis and or there is radiological evidence of perforation. Laparoscopy may be useful to identify patients who need resection (84). At laparotomy resection should be performed only of clearly non viable bowel since bowel may potentially recover once venous drainage is restored (85). The use of fluorescein may be useful to identify bowel that is still viable (86). A second look laparotomy should be performed at 24–48 hours. Surgical thrombectomy may be attempted but has a high recurrence rate. Transjugular intrahepatic portosystemic shunt (TIPS) and thrombolysis combined with or without laparotomy/scopy appears to be a attractive technique (87–92). Long-term anti-coagulation is usually required.

Outcome of Mesenteric Venous Thrombosis

The mortality of venous mesenteric thrombosis is significantly lower than for arterial mesenteric ischemia. Wang (93) reported a 7/16 (43%) mortality in patients with MVT, Morasch (70) reported a 7/31 (22.1%) 30 day mortality and Rhee (7) a 27% 30 day mortality. Survival at 3 years was 36% for acute MVT and 83% for chronic MVT (7).

Conclusions

The mortality of MVT is significant, but lower than the mortality of arterial mesenteric ischemia. History and clinical examination are unreliable and often inconclusive. A high index of suspicion is required to make the diagnosis early. A conservative approach with anticoagulation, as long there is no evidence of infarction is indicated and may reduce the mortality of a MVT compared with a primary surgical approach. Reports of thrombolysis and thrombectomy have been promising but the rarity of the condition has so far prevented the evaluation of these techniques in larger series or a randomised trial.

PORTAL VEIN THROMBOSIS

Etiology and Incidence of Portal Vein Thrombosis

Thrombosis of the portal vein can occur either outside of the liver (extrahepatic) or within the liver (intrahepatic). The etiology of PVT is heterogeneous and its occurrence can be influenced by both local and systemic etiological factors.

Local factors comprise disorders leading to decreased portal flow. This is commonly seen in adult patients with cirrhosis—(25%). The annual incidence in patients with cirrhosis is less than 1%, although this risk increases with more advanced liver disease. In the presence of the mutation 20210 of the prothrombin gene the incidence increases fivefold (62).

Other commonly associated conditions include hepatobiliary malignancies such as HCC (62) and cholangio-carcinoma (94) usually as a result of direct tumour invasion. Bland thrombosis of the extrahepatic PV may also result from occlusion by enlargement of hilar lymph nodes, inflammation of the portal vein due to ascending pylephlebitis secondary to infection in the appendix or colon, ascending cholangitis, intra-abdominal sepsis, and ulcerative colitis. Portal and splenic vein thrombosis is a common complication secondary to complicated pancreatitis (95–102).

Systemic risk factors for PVT consist mainly of acquired and inherited abnormalities leading to hypercoagulability. This may be general prothrombotic states like hyperhomocysteinemia, myeloproliferative syndromes—especially polycythemia rubra vera, APS, antithrombin deficiency, protein C or S deficiencies, or factor II, factor V gene mutations. Collagen vascular diseases, such as lupus have been implicated as well as pregnancy and women on the OC Pill. The disorder usually results from the association of causal factors, which should all be investigated. In addition profound dehydration may worsen a hypercoagulable state.

Table 2   Causes of Portal Vein Thrombosis

1. Inherited prothrombotic states
Antithrombin III deficiency (103)
Factor V Leiden mutation (104)
Prothrombin gene mutation (104)
Protein C deficiency (104)
Protein S deficiency (105)
Antithrombin deficiency (106,107)
Factor II (PTHR A ^{20210} mutation) (108)
2. Acquired prothrombotic states
Liver cirrhosis (109)
Hepatocellular carcinoma (62)
Antiphospholipid syndrome (110)
Cholangiocarcinoma (94)
Pancreatic carcinoma (111) and gastric carcinoma (112)
Splenectomy (113)
Intra abdominal sepsis (101,113)
Myeloproliferative disorders
Oral contraceptives (114)
Pregnancy (115)
Trauma (116)
Acute pancreatitis (95)
Appendicitis (54)
Inflammatory bowel disease (117)
Diverticulitis (102)
Ascending cholangitis (118)
Cholecystitis (119)
Following liver transplantation (120)
3. Idiopathic

Less commonly it is seen following liver transplantation (1–3% in adult whole grafts and up to 6% in split/pediatric grafts), or secondary to abdominal surgery such as splenectomy and shunt surgery (Table 2) (113,121–124).

Finally, it may simply be idiopathic. Up to 30% of patients with PVT do not have a clear etiology, although approximately 70% of patients will have an identifiable hypercoagulable condition. Importantly, PV involvement may be complete or partial and may involve any portion of the portal venous system.

Pathophysiology of Portal Vein Thrombosis

The portal vein forms from the junction of the SMV and the splenic vein and divides into two main intrahepatic branches followed by a further segmental division to each lobe. The portal vein provides approximately two thirds of the total hepatic blood flow and about 50% of its oxygen delivery under normal circumstances.

Acute PVT may not produce acute manifestations. Immediately there is vasodilatation of the hepatic arterial supply (125). Thrombosis due to intrahepatic causes originates distally and extends into the extrahepatic portal vein as found in cirrhosis and hepatic malignancies. In most of the other causes the thrombus forms proximally and propagates distally. Portal venous obstruction due to cirrhosis can be complicated by thrombosis due to the low flow state. Tumor invasion of the portal vein is found in hepatocellular carcinomas leading to thrombosis.

Recent thrombosis of the portal vein is characterized by a thrombus, which may not give rise to any symptoms or may be associated with a systemic inflammatory syndrome or with intestinal ischemia syndrome. Old thrombosis of the portal vein is usually only recognizable by its anatomic consequences—the cavernoma. The cavernoma is made up of multiple collateral veins linking the venous bed upstream from the obstacle to the venous bed downstream. The cavernoma still represent an obstruction to portal blood flow, causing portal hypertension (Fig. 1).

The main complication of chronic PVT is gastrointestinal bleeding and is due to the rupture of the varices or portal hypertensive gastropathy. The intrahepatic venous pressure is normal, but hepatic blood flow is usually reduced in comparison to both normal subjects and patients with cirrhosis.

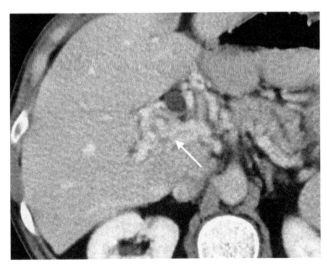

Figure 1 Cavernous transformation of the portal vein. *Source*: Freeman hospital archive.

Symptoms

Up to 40% of patients will be asymptomatic and may be overshadowed by those of the underlying cause. Symptoms often develop from complications of portal hypertension such as variceal bleeding. The location of the gastroesophageal varices often correlates with the segment of the portal vasculature that is occluded.

Splenic vein thrombosis for example, often results in gastric varices in the fundus. PVT is renowned for causing ectopic varices outside of the gastroesophageal region. Splenomegaly often develops as a result of long standing presinusoidal portal hypertension. Occasionally, abdominal pain and/or intestinal infarction may result from concomitant mesenteric vein involvement. Other symptoms include nausea, vomiting, anorexia, weight loss, diarrhoea (126). Liver function testes are usually normal.

Ascites is not a prominent feature of presinusoidal hypertension because of the greater compliance of the gastric and intestinal interstitium compared with the liver, which permits more fluid to be accommodated in the interstitium before it spills in to the peritoneal cavity. The large capacity of intestinal lymphatics accommodates the increases in intestinal lymph production due to filtration of fluid in the intestinal capillaries. The ultra structure of the layers of the intestine allows preferential passage of fluid filtered into the submucosal capillary network and then to the mucosal surface and then the lumen rather than to the serosal surface and the peritoneal cavity.

Imaging and Investigations in Portal Vein Thrombosis

Since the advent of modern cross sectional imaging invasive diagnostic methods like portal venography and selective mesenteric arteriography have been replaced.

Color Duplex ultrasound will reveal flow direction and echogenic structure within the portal vein, enlargement of the thrombosed portion of the portal vein. Cavernous transformation of the portal vein produces characteristic patterns on color duplex (127). However, a recently formed thrombus in the portal vein can show an anechoic or hypoechoic structure. CT is an excellent method for demonstrating thrombosis of the

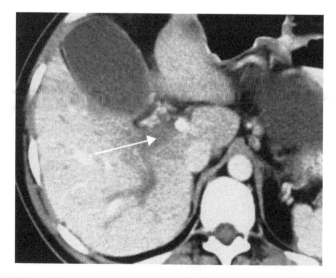

Figure 2   Computer tomography image of an acute portal vein thrombosis. *Source*: Freeman hospital archive.

portal vein. On the precontrast scan the portal vein is enlarged and an increased attenuation of the portal vein contents may indicate recent thrombus (Fig. 2).

Postcontrast CT images reveal rim enhancement of the wall of the portal vein but lack of enhancement of its contents if the occlusion is due to thrombus. If, however, a tumour thrombus is present inhomogeneous or streaky enhancement within the portal vein may be observed. With chronic PVT numerous small enhancing structures, representing venous collaterals, surround the portal vein.

Moreover, CT may show perfusion changes as either decreased parenchyma enhancement during the portal venous phase or transiently increased segmental or lobar enhancement seen during the late arterial and early portal venous phases. This localized increased enhancement is explained by compensatory hepatic arterial flow or arterioportal shunting towards the segment or the lobe supplied by the portal vein branch, which is thrombosed.

MRI is at least as good as CT in showing PVT by demonstrating absence of flow. Transient segmental or lobar enhancement, similar to that seen on contrast-enhanced CT can be visualized with gadolinium-enhanced T1-weighted images (128–130).

Treatment

Since most cases are identified incidentally and the natural history is unclear, treatment usually focuses on the underlying condition. Treatment is more important in recent PVT. In the absence of severe liver disease or major contraindication to anticoagulation, antithrombotic therapy should be initiated on presentation and continued for approximately six months. After initial intravenous heparin infusion anticoagulant therapy is commenced, which generally allows recanalization of the thrombosed veins in recently constituted thrombosis (106,131).

Permanent anticoagulant treatment is recommended when a permanent prothrombotic state exists, even in patients with a history of gastrointestinal bleeding. Prognosis is good.

In rare cases of acute portal vein thrombus with total occlusion, thrombolysis with TIPS placement has been shown to be feasible and efficacious (132–134).

It is still a matter of debate if anticoagulation is of benefit in patients with chronic PVT (104,135). The patient with PVT is at risk of bleeding as well as thrombosis. Condat (136) found in 136 adults with non-malignant, non-cirrhotic PVT the incidence of bleeding at 1.25% per year and the risk of thrombosis 0.55% per year. 85 of his patients received anticoagulation therapy without increasing the bleeding incidence. In patients with intraabdominal sepsis spontaneous resolution of the PVT has been observed. Transjugular or transhepatic thrombolysis and thrombectomy have been used successfully (137–142). That said, the data come from small case series some of which involve liver transplant patients.

Bleeding can be treated in most cases by beta-adrenergic blockade, endoscopic ligation, or endoscopic sclerosis of varices.

If PVT is complicated by recurrent variceal bleeding and hypersplenism reconstituting the portal vein by stent insertion across the occluded segment of the portal vein with or without a transjugular portosystemic shunt (TPIS) may be beneficial (143,144). Shunt surgery especially splenorenal (Warren) shunts may still be a successful treatment in exceptional cases where endoscopic management and TIPS have failed to control variceal bleeding (145,146).

Outcome of Portal Vein Thrombosis

The overall outcome of extrahepatic PVT is good with an overall mortality of 13% or less. Janssen (147) found in a review of 172 cases of extrahepatic PVT that in absence of cancer, cirrhosis, and mesenteric vein thrombosis the 1 year survival can be as high as 95%. PVT due to pylephlebitis has a high mortality without prompt antibiotic therapy. Bacteraemia (often polymicrobial) is present in up to 88% of the patients. The most common blood isolate were bacteroides species (148).

Variceal bleeding is associated with a significant better prognosis if the portal hypertension is due to PVT rather than liver cirrhosis. Poor outcome of PVT is related rather to the underlying disease than the PVT itself (136,149).

KEY POINTS

- PVT is often a asymptomatic condition.
- PVT in itself is a benign condition, but can be associated with a high mortality due to the underlying conditions.
- Cross sectional imaging techniques are available, sensitive, and diagnostic in most cases.
- Bleeding due to PVT has a more benign character than that caused by portal hypertension due to liver cirrhosis.
- Treatment is primarily anticoagulation and sufficient in most of the cases.
- Addressing the underlying condition is essential.

REFERENCES

1. Fagge C. Mesenteric venous thrombosis. Trans Path Soc London 1876;27.
2. Elliot J. The operative relieve of gangrene of intestine due to occlusion of the mesenteric vessels. Ann Surg 1895; 21:9–23.
3. Balford G, Stuard TG. Case of enlarged spleen complicated with ascitis, both depending upon varicose dilatation and thrombosis of the portal vein. Edinburg Med J 1869; 14:589–598.
4. Kumar S, Kamath PS. Acute superior mesenteric venous thrombosis: one disease or two? Am J Gastroenterol 2003; 98:1299–1304.
5. Mahmoud AE, Elias E, Beauchamp N, Wilde JT. Prevalence of the factor V Leiden mutation in hepatic and portal vein thrombosis. Gut 1997; 40:798–800.
6. Johnson C, Baggenstoss A. Mesenteric vascular occlusion I: study of 99 cases of occlusion of the veins. Proc Staff Meet Mayo Cllnic 1949, 24:628–636.
7. Rhee RY, Gloviczki P, Mendonca CT, et al. Mesenteric venous thrombosis: still a lethal disease in the 1990s. J Vasc Surg 1994; 20:688–697.
8. Abdu RA, Zakhour BJ, Dallis DJ. Mesenteric venous thrombosis—1911 to 1984. Surgery 1987; 101:383–388.
9. Endean ED, Barnes SL, Kwolek CJ, Minion DJ, Schwarcz TH, Mentzer RM, Jr. Surgical management of thrombotic acute intestinal ischemia. Ann Surg 2001; 233:801–808.
10. Azarow K, Connolly B, Babyn P, Shemie SD, Ein S, Pearl R. Multidisciplinary evaluation of the distended abdomen in critically ill infants and children: the role of bedside sonography. Pediatr Surg Int 1998; 13:355–359.
11. Ludwig DJ, Hauptmann E, Rosoff L, Jr., Neuzil D. Mesenteric and portal vein thrombosis in a young patient with protein S deficiency treated with urokinase via the superior mesenteric artery. J Vasc Surg 1999; 30:551–554.
12. Clavien PA, Durig M, Harder F. Venous mesenteric infarction: a particular entity. Br J Surg 1988; 75:252–255.

13. Andersson R, Parsson H, Isaksson B, Norgren L. Acute intestinal ischemia. A 14-year retrospective investigation. Acta Chir Scand 1984; 150:217–221.

14. Grendell JH, Ockner RK. Mesenteric venous thrombosis. Gastroenterology 1982; 82:358–372.

15. Ortega Diaz de Ceballos A, Jaber Ismail AR, Estrada Saiz RV. Primary mesenteric venous thrombosis. An Med Interna 1990; 7:361–363.

16. Balthazar EJ, Gollapudi P. Septic thrombophlebitis of the mesenteric and portal veins: CT imaging. J Comput Assist Tomogr 2000; 24:755–760.

17. el Kouri D, Potel G, Hamidou M, Sadr FB, Fressinaud E, Armstrong O. Mesenteric venous thrombosis and antithrombin III deficiency: diagnosis before an acute digestive hemorrhage. J Mal Vasc 1997; 22:361–363.

18. Grewal HP, Barrie WW. Congenital antithrombin III deficiency causing mesenteric venous infarction: a lesson to remember—a case history. Angiology 1992; 43:618–620.

19. Pokorney BH, Eyster ME, Jeffries GH. Antithrombin III deficiency appearing as mesenteric vein thrombosis. Am J Gastroenterol 1981; 76:534–537.

20. Green D, Ganger DR, Blei AT. Protein C deficiency in splanchnic venous thrombosis. Am J Med 1987; 82:1171–1174.

21. Yates P, Cumber PM, Sanderson S, Harrison BJ. Mesenteric venous thrombosis due to protein C deficiency. Clin Lab Haematol 1991; 13:137–139.

22. Momoi A, Komura Y, Kumon I, et al. Mesenteric venous thrombosis in hereditary protein C deficiency with the mutation at Arg169 (CGG-TGG). Intern Med 2003; 42:110–116.

23. Blanc P, Rouanet C, Donadio D, Paleirac G, Michel H. Hereditary protein S deficiency responsible for digestive vascular thrombosis. Presse Med 1990; 19:416–419.

24. Inagaki H, Sakakibara O, Miyaike H, Eimoto T, Yura J. Mesenteric venous thrombosis in familial free protein S deficiency. Am J Gastroenterol 1993; 88:134–138.

25. Bergenfeldt M, Svensson PJ, Borgstrom A. Mesenteric vein thrombosis due to factor V Leiden gene mutation. Br J Surg 1999; 86:1059–1062.

26. Pinar A, Saenz R, Rebollo J, et al. Portal and mesenteric vein thrombosis in a patient heterozygous for a mutation (Arg506—>Gln) in the factor V gen (factor V Leiden). J Clin Gastroenterol 1998; 27:361–363.

27. Al-Juburi A, Scott MA, Shah HR, Raufman JP. Heterozygosity for factor V Leiden and G20210A prothrombin genotypes in a patient with mesenteric vein thrombosis. Dig Dis Sci 2002; 47:601–606.

28. Marie I, Levesque H, Le Cam-Duchez V, Borg JY, Ducrotte P, Philippe C. Mesenteric venous thrombosis revealing both factor II G20212A mutation and hyperhomocysteinemia related to pernicious anemia. Gastroenterology 2000; 118:237–238.

29. Silingardi M, Ghirarduzzi A, Galimberti D, Iorio A, Iori I. Mesenteric-portal vein thrombosis in a patient with hyperhomocysteinemia and heterozygous for 20210A prothrombin allele. Thromb Haemost 2000; 84:358–359.

30. Blanc P, Barki J, Fabre JM, et al. Superior mesenteric vein thrombosis associated with anticardiolipin antibody without autoimmune disease. Am J Hematol 1995; 48:137.

31. Higa M, Kojima M, Ohnuma S, et al. Portal and mesenteric vein and inferior vena cava thrombosis associated with antiphospholipid syndrome. Intern Med 2001; 40:1245–1249.

32. Kaushik S, Federle MP, Schur PH, Krishnan M, Silverman SG, Ros PR. Abdominal thrombotic and ischemic manifestations of the antiphospholipid antibody syndrome: CT findings in 42 patients. Radiology 2001; 218:768–771.

33. Varela Ruiz F, Fernandez-Sosbilla JM, Espinosa R. Mesenteric thrombosis, hyperhomocysteinemia and oral contraceptive agents intake. An Med Interna 2003; 20:221.

34. Abet D, Pietri J. Portal and superior mesenteric venous thrombosis secondary to oral contraceptive treatment. Two cases (author's transl). J Mal Vasc 1982; 7:59–63.

35. Civetta JM, Kolodny M. Mesenteric venous thrombosis associated with oral contraceptives. Gastroenterology 1970; 58:713–716.

36. Hassan HA. Oral contraceptive-induced mesenteric venous thrombosis with resultant intestinal ischemia. J Clin Gastroenterol 1999; 29:90–95.

37. De Luca M, Dugo M, Arduini R, Liessi G. Acute venous thrombosis of spleno-mesenteric portal axis: an unusual localization of thromboembolism in the nephrotic syndrome. Am J Nephrol 1991; 11:260–263.

38. McGregor DO, Bailey RR. Mesenteric arterial thrombosis complicating the nephrotic syndrome. N Z Med J 1997; 110:62–63.

39. Lin JL. Massive hemorrhagic necrosis of small intestine due to mesenteric vein thrombosis: an unusual complication of nephrotic syndrome. Nephron 1992; 61:230–231.

40. Draganic BD, Clark DA. Venous infarction of the jejunum secondary to the nephrotic syndrome. Aust N Z J Surg 1997; 67:902–903.

41. De Stefano V, Teofili L, Leone G, Michiels JJ. Spontaneous erythroid colony formation as the clue to an underlying myeloproliferative disorder in patients with Budd-Chiari syndrome or portal vein thrombosis. Semin Thromb Hemost 1997; 23:411–418.

42. Edmondson HT. Mesenteric vein thrombosis secondary to polycythemia vera. J Med Assoc Ga 1972; 61:159–161.

43. Rieu V, Ruivard M, Abergel A, et al. Mesenteric venous thrombosis. A retrospective study of 23 cases. Ann Med Interne (Paris) 2003; 154:133–138.

44. Gayer G, Zandman-Goddard G, Raanani P, Hertz M, Apter S. Widespread abdominal venous thrombosis in paroxysmal nocturnal hemoglobinuria diagnosed on CT. Abdom Imaging 2001; 26:414–419.

45. Tedde R, Sechi LA, Marigliano A, Loriga V. Paroxysmal nocturnal hemoglobinuria with multiple venous thrombosis and acute renal insufficiency. Description of a case. Minerva Med 1989; 80:615–618.

46. Engelhardt TC, Kerstein MD. Pregnancy and mesenteric venous thrombosis. South Med J 1989; 82:1441–1443.

47. Dubina MV, Petrishchev NN, Anisimov VN. Microvascular endothelium dysfunction in rats bearing 1,2-dimethylhydrazine-induced colon tumors. Cancer Lett 1999; 144:125–129.

48. Cornu-Labat G, Kasirajan K, Simon R, Smith DJ, Herman ML, Rubin JR. Acute mesenteric vein thrombosis and pancreatitis. A rare association. Int J Pancreatol 1997; 21:249–251.

49. Crowe PM, Sagar G. Reversible superior mesenteric vein thrombosis in acute pancreatitis. The CT appearances. Clin Radiol 1995; 50:628–633.

50. Jensen K, Bradley EL, III. Mesenteric venous infarction in acute pancreatitis. Int J Pancreatol 1989; 5:213–219.

51. Sanghavi P, Paramesh A, Dwivedi A, Markova T, Phan T. Mesenteric arterial thrombosis as a complication of Crohn's disease. Dig Dis Sci 2001; 46:2344–2346.

52. Uthman SM, Harb A. Mesenteric venous thrombosis 11 years after splenectomy. J Med Liban 1971; 24:53–58.

53. Balz J, Minton JP. Mesenteric thrombosis following splenectomy. Ann Surg 1975; 181:126–128.

54. Germain MA, Soukhni N, Bouzard D. Mesenteric venous thrombosis complicating acute appendicitis. Ann Chir 2002; 127:381–384.

55. van Spronsen FJ, de Langen ZJ, van Elburg RM, Kimpen JL. Appendicitis in an eleven-year-old boy complicated by thrombosis of the portal and superior mesenteric veins. Pediatr Infect Dis J 1996; 15:910–912.

56. Davies M, Satyadas T, Akle CA. Spontaneous resolution of a superior mesenteric vein thrombosis after laparoscopic nissen fundoplication. Ann R Coll Surg Engl 2002; 84:177–180.

57. Millikan KW, Szczerba SM, Dominguez JM, McKenna R, Rorig JC. Superior mesenteric and portal vein thrombosis following laparoscopic-assisted right hemicolectomy. Report of a case. Dis Colon Rectum 1996; 39:1171–1175.

58. Fichera A, Cicchiello LA, Mendelson DS, Greenstein AJ, Heimann TM. Superior mesenteric vein thrombosis after colectomy for inflammatory bowel disease: a not uncommon cause of postoperative acute abdominal pain. Dis Colon Rectum 2003; 46:643–648.

59. Ashida H, Kotoura Y, Nishioka A, et al. Portal and mesenteric venous thrombosis as a complication of endoscopic sclerotherapy. Am J Gastroenterol 1989; 84:306–310.

60. Deboever G, Elegeert I, Defloor E. Portal and mesenteric venous thrombosis after endoscopic injection sclerotherapy. Am J Gastroenterol 1989; 84:1336–1337.

61. Horing E, Muller-Beissenhirtz W, Dipper S, von Gaisberg U. Portal hypertension due to thromboses of the portal, splenic and mesenteric veins in congenital protein c deficiency. Dtsch Med Wochenschr 1988; 113:1847–1849.

62. Amitrano L, Guardascione MA, Brancaccio V, et al. Risk factors and clinical presentation of portal vein thrombosis in patients with liver cirrhosis. J Hepatol 2004; 40:736–741.

63. Winslow ER, Brunt LM, Drebin JA, Soper NJ, Klingensmith ME. Portal vein thrombosis after splenectomy. Am J Surg 2002; 184:631–635; discussion 5–6.

64. Matsumoto T, Kuwabara N, Abe H, et al. Zahn infarct of the liver resulting from occlusive phlebitis in portal vein radicles. Am J Gastroenterol 1992; 87:365–368.

65. Dubina MV, Petrishchev NN, Anisimov VN. Microvascular endothelium dysfunction during growth of transplanted lymphosarcoma and glioma in rats. J Exp Clin Cancer Res 1999; 18:537–542.

66. Ibrarullah M, Wagholikar G, Srinivas M, Mishra A, Reddy DG, Prasadbabu TL. Acute mesenteric venous thrombosis complicating endoscopic variceal sclerotherapy with absolute alcohol. Indian J Gastroenterol 2003; 22:27–29.

67. Boley SJ, Kaleya RN, Brandt LJ. Mesenteric venous thrombosis. Surg Clin North Am 1992; 72:183–201.

68. Kumar S, Sarr MG, Kamath PS. Mesenteric venous thrombosis. N Engl J Med 2001; 345:1683–1688.

69. Kitchens CS. Evolution of our understanding of the pathophysiology of primary mesenteric venous thrombosis. Am J Surg 1992; 163:346–348.

70. Morasch MD, Ebaugh JL, Chiou AC, Matsumura JS, Pearce WH, Yao JS. Mesenteric venous thrombosis: a changing clinical entity. J Vasc Surg 2001; 34:680–684.

71. Archibald RB, Burnstein AV, Knackstedt VE, Tolman KG, Holbrook JH. Ischemic colitis in a young adult due to inferior mesenteric vein thrombosis. Endoscopy 1980; 12:140–143.

72. Roman RJ, Loeb PM. Massive colonic dilatation as initial presentation of mesenteric vein thrombosis. Dig Dis Sci 1987; 32:323–326.

73. Dagenais M, Langer B, Taylor BR, Greig PD. Experience with radical esophagogastric devascularization procedures (Sugiura) for variceal bleeding outside Japan. World J Surg 1994; 18:222–228.

74. Murray MJGM, Nowak LR, Cobb CF. Serum D(−)-lactate levels as an aid to diagnosing acute intestinal ischemia. Am J Surg 1994; 167:575–578.

75. Jonas JSS, Alebrahim-Dehkordy A. Behavior of the lactate level in occlusion and reperfusion of the right superior mesenteric artery. An animal experiment study. Langenbecks Arch Chir 1996; 381:1–6.

76. Lange H, Jackel R. Usefulness of plasma lactate concentration in the diagnosis of acute abdominal disease. Eur J Surg 1994; 160:381–384.

77. Lange H, Toivola A. Warning signals in acute abdominal disorders. Lactate is the best marker of mesenteric ischemia. Lakartidningen 1997; 94:1893–1896.

78. Ljungdahl M, Rasmussen I, Raab Y, Hillered L, Haglund U. Small intestinal mucosal pH and lactate production during experimental ischemia-reperfusion and fecal peritonitis in pigs. Shock 1997; 7:131–138.

79. Boverie JH, Counet D, Meunier P, Dondelinger RF. Small bowel enema and diagnosis of chronic nonischemic disturbance of superior mesenteric venous blood flow. Abdom Imaging 1993; 18:265–270.

80. Bradbury AW, Brittenden J, McBride K, Ruckley CV. Mesenteric ischemia: a multidisciplinary approach. Br J Surg 1995; 82:1446–1459.

81. Steinkamp HJ, Jochens R, Zendel W, et al. Color duplex sonography of liver transplantation. The vascular status. Rofo 1993; 159:222–228.

82. Bradbury MS, Kavanagh PV, Chen MY, Weber TM, Bechtold RE. Noninvasive assessment of portomesenteric venous thrombosis: current concepts and imaging strategies. J Comput Assist Tomogr 2002; 26:392–404.

83. Kreft B, Strunk H, Flacke S, et al. Detection of thrombosis in the portal venous system: comparison of contrast-enhanced MR angiography with intraarterial digital subtraction angiography. Radiology 2000; 216:86–92.

84. Cho YP, Jung SM, Han MS, et al. Role of diagnostic laparoscopy in managing acute mesenteric venous thrombosis. Surg Laparosc Endosc Percutan Tech 2003; 13:215–217.

85. Hassan HA, Raufman JP. Mesenteric venous thrombosis. South Med J 1999; 92:558–562.

86. Rhee RY, Gloviczki P. Mesenteric venous thrombosis. Surg Clin North Am 1997; 77:327–338.

87. Sehgal M, Haskal ZJ. Use of transjugular intrahepatic portosystemic shunts during lytic therapy of extensive portal splenic and mesenteric venous thrombosis: long-term follow-up. J Vasc Interv Radiol 2000; 11:61–65.

88. Brunaud L, Antunes L, Collinet-Adler S, et al. Acute mesenteric venous thrombosis: case for nonoperative management. J Vasc Surg 2001; 34:673–679.

89. Opitz T, Buchwald AB, Lorf T, Awuah D, Ramadori G, Nolte W. The transjugular intrahepatic portosystemic stent-shunt (TIPS) as rescue therapy for complete Budd-Chiari syndrome and portal vein thrombosis. Z Gastroenterol 2003; 41:413–418.

90. Bickelhaupt A, Jehle M, Eisele R. Thrombolytic therapy of antithrombin III-deficiency-induced mesenteric vein thrombosis in a newly operated patient. Vasa 1991; 20:78–81.

91. Antoch G, Taleb N, Hansen O, Stock W. Transarterial thrombolysis of portal and mesenteric vein thrombosis: a promising alternative to common therapy. Eur J Vasc Endovasc Surg 2001; 21:471–472.

92. Klempnauer J, Grothues F, Bektas H, Pichlmayr R. Results of portal thrombectomy and splanchnic thrombolysis for the surgical management of acute mesentericoportal thrombosis. Br J Surg 1997; 84:129–132.

93. Wang Y, Li J, He S. Early diagnosis and treatment of mesenteric venous thrombosis. Zhonghua Wai Ke Za Zhi 1997; 35:443–445.

94. Uenishi T, Hirohashi K, Haba T, et al. Portal thrombosis due to intrahepatic cholangiocarcinoma following successful treatment for hepatocellular carcinoma. Hepatogastroenterology 2003; 50:1140–1142.

95. Dorffel T, Wruck T, Ruckert RI, Romaniuk P, Dorffel Q, Wermke W. Vascular complications in acute pancreatitis assessed by color duplex ultrasonography. Pancreas 2000; 21:126–133.

96. Mortele KJ, Mergo PJ, Taylor HM, et al. Peripancreatic vascular abnormalities complicating acute pancreatitis: contrast-enhanced helical CT findings. Eur J Radiol 2004; 52:67–72.

97. Chang TN, Tang L, Keller K, Harrison MR, Farmer DL, Albanese CT. Pylephlebitis, portal-mesenteric thrombosis, and multiple liver abscesses owing to perforated appendicitis. J Pediatr Surg 2001; 36:E19.

98. Pitcher R, McKenzie C. Simultaneous ultrasound identification of acute appendicitis, septic thrombophlebitis of the portal vein and pyogenic liver abscess. S Afr Med J 2003; 93:426–428.

99. Chan SC, Chan FL, Chau FM, Mok FP. Portal thrombosis complicating appendicitis: ultrasound detection and hepatic computed tomography lobar attenuation alteration. J Comput Tomogr 1988; 12:208–210.

100. Verna EC, Larghi A, Faddoul SG, Stein JA, Worman HJ. Portal vein thrombosis associated with Fusobacterium nucleatum septicemia in a patient with ulcerative colitis. J Clin Gastroenterol 2004; 38:611–612.

101. Mijnhout GS, Klinkenberg EC, Lycklama G, Linskens R, Meuwissen SG. Sepsis and elevated liver enzymes in a patient with inflammatory bowel disease: think of portal vein thrombosis. Dig Liver Dis 2004; 36:296–300.

102. Perez-Cruet MJ, Grable E, Drapkin MS, Jablons DM, Cano G. Pylephlebitis associated with diverticulitis. South Med J 1993; 86:578–580.

103. Yonemitsu Y, Yanaga K, Matsumata T, Sugimachi K. Portal vein thrombosis due to antithrombin III deficiency. A case report. Angiology 1995; 46:1043–1047.

104. Janssen HL. Changing perspectives in portal vein thrombosis. Scand J Gastroenterol Suppl 2000;69–73.

105. Godeau B, Leroy-Matheron C, Gouault-Heilmann M, Schaeffer A. A case of portal vein thrombosis associated with protein S deficiency. J Hepatol 1993; 18:258.

106. Condat B, Pessione F, Helene Denninger M, Hillaire S. Recent portal or mesenteric venous thrombosis: increased recognition and frequent recanalization on anticoagulant therapy. Hepatology 2000; 32:466–470.

107. Denninger MH, Chait Y, Casadevall N, et al. Cause of portal or hepatic venous thrombosis in adults: the role of multiple concurrent factors. Hepatology 2000; 31:587–591.

108. Amitrano L, Brancaccio V, Guardascione MA, et al. Portal vein thrombosis after variceal endoscopic sclerotherapy in cirrhotic patients: role of genetic thrombophilia. Endoscopy 2002; 34:535–538.

109. Susani M, Asboth f, Feigl W. Portal vein thrombosis and portal vein sclerosis in liver cirrhosis. Vasa 1986; 15:392–396.

110. Karoui S, Sfar S, Kallel M, Boubaker J, Makni S, Filali A. Antiphospholipid syndrome revealed by portal vein thrombosis in a patient with celiac disease. Rev Med Interne 2004; 25:471–473.

111. Belli AM, Jennings CM, Nakielny RA. Splenic and portal venous thrombosis: a vascular complication of pancreatic disease demonstrated on computed tomography. Clin Radiol 1990; 41:13–16.

112. Araki T, Suda K, Sekikawa T, Ishii Y, Hihara T, Kachi K. Portal venous tumor thrombosis associated with gastric adenocarcinoma. Radiology 1990; 174:811–814.

113. Fujita F, Lyass S, Otsuka K, et al. Portal vein thrombosis following splenectomy: identification of risk factors. Am Surg 2003; 69:951–956.

114. Lonardo A, Grisendi A, Frazzoni M, Pulvirenti M, Della Casa G. Portal vein thrombosis (PVT) associated with oral contraceptive steroids (OCS). J Gastroenterol Hepatol 1994; 9:314.

115. Goodrich MA, James EM, Baldus WP, Lomboy CT, Harms RW. Portal vein thrombosis associated with pregnancy. A case report. J Reprod Med 1993; 38:969–972.

116. Beaufort P, Perney P, Coste F, Masbou J, Le Bricquir Y, Blanc F. Post-traumatic thrombosis of the portal vein. Presse Med 1996; 25:247–248.

117. Mathieu E, Fain O, Trinchet JC, Aurousseau MH, Sterin D, Thomas M. Portal vein thrombosis: a rare complication of Crohn disease. Rev Med Interne 1994; 15:589–592.

118. Cuffari C, Seidman E, DuBois J, Brochu P, Alvarez F. Acute intrahepatic portal vein thrombosis complicating cholangitis in biliary atresia. Eur J Pediatr 1997; 156:186–189.

119. Inoguchi H, Nakata K, Sugimachi K. Portal vein thrombosis complicated with disseminated intravascular coagulation due to acute cholecystitis. Hepatogastroenterology 2004; 51:661–663.

120. Bakthavatsalam R, Marsh CL, Perkins JD, Levy AE, Healey PJ, Kuhr CS. Rescue of acute portal vein thrombosis after liver transplantation using a cavoportal shunt at re-transplantation. Am J Transplant 2001; 1:284–287.

121. Settmacher U, Nussler NC, Glanemann M, et al. Venous complications after orthotopic liver transplantation. Clin Transplant 2000; 14:235–241.

122. Goldstein MJ, Salame E, Kapur S, et al. Analysis of failure in living donor liver transplantation: differential outcomes in children and adults. World J Surg 2003; 27:356–364.

123. Saing H, Fan ST, Tam PK, et al. Surgical complications and outcome of pediatric liver transplantation in Hong Kong. J Pediatr Surg 2002; 37:1673–1677.

124. Atweh N, Kavic SM, Dudrick SJ. Portal vein thrombosis after splenectomy. J Am Coll Surg 2001; 192:551–552.

125. Valla DC, Condat B. Portal vein thrombosis in adults: pathophysiology, pathogenesis and management. J Hepatol 2000; 32:865–871.

126. Cohen J, Edelman RR, Chopra S. Portal vein thrombosis: a review. Am J Med 1992; 92:173–182.

127. Ueno N, Sasaki A, Tomiyama T, Tano S, Kimura K. Color doppler ultrasonography in the diagnosis of cavernous transformation of the portal vein. J Clin Ultrasound 1997; 25:227–233.

128. Martinoli C, Cittadini G, Pastorino C, et al. Gradient echo MRI of portal vein thrombosis. J Comput Assist Tomogr 1992; 16:226–234.

129. Davis CP, Debatin JF, Fuchs WA. MRI venous angiography of the abdomen. Schweiz Med Wochenschr 1995; 125:639–648.

130. Takahashi S, Kim T, Murakami T, et al. Three-dimensional gadolinium-enhanced dynamic MRI of whole liver using spectrally selected enhanced fast gradient recall sequence. Nippon Igaku Hoshasen Gakkai Zasshi 1998; 58:99–101.

131. Sheen CL, Lamparelli H, Milne A, Green I, Ramage JK. Clinical features, diagnosis and outcome of acute portal vein thrombosis. QJM 2000; 93:531–534.

132. Vogl T, Hidajat N, Schroder RJ, Felix R. Recanalization of an extensive fresh portal vein thrombosis by transjugular intrahepatic portosystemic stent-shunt (TIPS). Rofo 1999; 171:163–165.

133. Hanig V, Stenzel G, Rossle M. Acute portal vein thrombosis in liver cirrhosis: successful recanalization with the use of a portosystemic shunt (TIPS). Rofo 1996; 165:403–405.

134. Honda M, Nishida H, Takashina T, et al. A case of alcoholic liver cirrhosis associated with portal vein thrombosis which was successfully treated by TIPS. Nippon Igaku Hoshasen Gakkai Zasshi 1993; 53:220–222.

135. Webster GJ, Burroughs AK, Riordan SM. Review article: portal vein thrombosis—new insights into etiology and management. Aliment Pharmacol Ther 2005; 21:1–9.

136. Condat B, Pessione F, Hillaire S, et al. Current outcome of portal vein thrombosis in adults: risk and benefit of anticoagulant therapy. Gastroenterology 2001; 120:490–497.

137. Aytekin C, Boyvat F, Kurt A, Yologlu Z, Coskun M. Catheter-directed thrombolysis with transjugular access in portal vein thrombosis secondary to pancreatitis. Eur J Radiol 2001; 39:80–82.

138. Kercher KW, Sing RF, Watson KW, Matthews BD, LeQuire MH, Heniford BT. Transhepatic thrombolysis in acute portal vein thrombosis after laparoscopic splenectomy. Surg Laparosc Endosc Percutan Tech 2002; 12:131–136.

139. Rossi C, Zambruni A, Ansaloni F, et al. Combined mechanical and pharmacologic thrombolysis for portal vein thrombosis in liver-graft recipients and in candidates for liver transplantation. Transplantation 2004; 78:938–940.

140. Sainz-Barriga M, Baccarani U, Risaliti A, et al. Successful minimally invasive management of late portal vein thrombosis after splenectomy due to splenic artery steal syndrome following liver transplantation: a case report. Transplant Proc 2004; 36:558–559.

141. Kaplan JL, Weintraub SL, Hunt JP, Gonzalez A, Lopera J, Brazzini A. Treatment of superior mesenteric and portal vein thrombosis with direct thrombolytic infusion via an operatively placed mesenteric catheter. Am Surg 2004; 70:600–604.

142. Uflacker R. Applications of percutaneous mechanical thrombectomy in transjugular intrahepatic portosystemic shunt and portal vein thrombosis. Tech Vasc Interv Radiol 2003; 6:59–69.

143. Stein M, Link DP. Symptomatic spleno-mesenteric-portal venous thrombosis: recanalization and reconstruction with endovascular stents. J Vasc Interv Radiol 1999; 10:363–371.

144. Cherukuri R, Haskal ZJ, Naji A, Shaked A. Percutaneous thrombolysis and stent placement for the treatment of portal vein thrombosis after liver transplantation: long-term follow-up. Transplantation 1998; 65:1124–1126.

145. Wolff M, Hirner A. Current state of portosystemic shunt surgery. Langenbecks Arch Surg 2003; 388:141–149.

146. Warren WD, Henderson JM, Millikan WJ, Galambos JT, Bryan FC. Management of variceal bleeding in patients with noncirrhotic portal vein thrombosis. Ann Surg 1988; 207:623–634.

147. Janssen HL. Role of coagulation in the natural history and treatment of portal vein thrombosis. J Gastroenterol Hepatol 2001; 16:595–596.

148. Plemmons RM, Dooley DP, Longfield RN. Septic thrombophlebitis of the portal vein (pylephlebitis): diagnosis and management in the modern era. Clin Infect Dis 1995; 21:1114–1120.

149. Alam H, Kim D, Provido H, Kirkpatrick J. Portal vein thrombosis in the adult: surgical implications in an era of dynamic imaging. Am Surg 1997; 63:681–684; discussion 4–5.

34

Superior Vena Caval Obstruction

Enrico Ascher and Anil Hingorani
Division of Vascular Surgery, Department of Surgery, Maimonides Medical Center,
Brooklyn, New York, U.S.A.

ETIOLOGY

The initial paper on superior vena caval (SVC) obstruction was reported in 1757 by William Hunter in a case caused by a syphilitic aortic aneurysm (1). Presently, the most common cause of this syndrome is malignancy (80–90% of presentations) (2). The most frequent reported malignancy causing this syndrome is bronchogenic cancer; however many other types of mediastinal neoplasms have also been cited to cause this syndrome including lymphomas, thymomas, teratomas, germ cell tumors, metastatic tumors etc.

Benign causes of this syndrome consist of mediastinal fibrosis (greater than 40% of the benign cases), graulomatous disease such as histoplasmosis and sarcoidosis, constrictive pericarditis, aneurysms of the aortic arch, prior radiation, retrostenal goiter, thrombophilia, dialysis access, Bechet's disease (3) and idiopathic thrombosis. The increased use of short- and long-term venous catheters and pacemakers make their usage a factor as well (4,5).

PRESENTATION

The most common presenting symptoms of SVC obstruction are fullness of the head or neck. These symptoms may become more severe when the patients bends over or lies flat in bed. Other patients may also present with dyspnea, othopnea, tongue swelling, nasal stuffiness, stridor or cough. Additionally, nausea, dizziness, and mental confusion, headache, visual disturbance or syncope may result from cerebral venous hypertension. In the worst case scenario, this can result in cerebral edema and cerebellar herniation.

Physical signs consist of head swelling, prominent chest wall and neck collateral vessels, facial cyanosis, proptosis, arm swelling, stridor, hoarseness, respiratory distress, conjunctival edema and ecchymosis. SVC syndrome can also result in laryngeal and airway edema.

The determinant factors in the severity of symptoms include duration, progression, extent of venous occlusive disease and the amount of collaterals that develop. The major collaterals that develop involve the azygos and hemiazygos veins, and these can be established only if obstruction occurs below the entrance of the azygos vein into the SVC. Lumbar veins subsequently drain into the inferior vena cava. The second pathway involves the internal mammary venous system, with its tributaries and communication with the inferior epigastric vein. The third and fourth collateral routes include the thoracoepigastric vein, with its connection to the saphenous vein, and the vertebral veins (6).

DIAGNOSIS

The initial work-up begins with a detailed history and physical examination. Chest X-ray and computed tomography with intravenous contrast are the mainstays of the diagnostic testing that is needed. Currently, magnetic resonance venography plays a limited role. Duplex scans can assess the patency of the internal jugular vein for an inflow vein. However, invasive procedures such as brochoscopy, mediasinoscopy, thorascopy, throrocotomy or median sternotomy may be needed to provide tissue diagnosis. If surgical reconstruction is planned, diagnostic venography via simultaneous injection of bilateral superficial arm veins is mandatory.

TREATMENT

The first SVC bypass was reported in 1951 (7). In 1974, Chiu et al. (8) helped to further progress this field when they first suggested autologous spiral vein grafts for replacement of larger veins. However, it was Doty et al. (9–11) who established this technique for reconstruction of the occluded SVC using autologous saphenous vein.

Initial conservative therapy consisting of head elevation, anticoagulation, oxygen, steroids and diuretics can at times relieve acute SVC syndrome. If this therapy is unsuccessful, the additional types of treatment are determined by evaluation of the underlying cause(s) of the SVC syndrome. In benign and malignant causes, thrombolytic therapy can also be used to help resolve acute thrombosis (12,13).

Additionally, in malignant SVC syndrome, if conservative therapy and radiation or chemotherapy fail to resolve the symptoms, some authors have suggested that good short-term results can be obtained with endovascular therapy (14–17). However, for malignant SVC syndrome following balloon angioplasty, stents are needed to avoid early restenosis and recurrence. A pressure gradient should be measured before and after the intervention to document the benefit of the intervention in addition to the documentation of resolution of the clinical symptoms.

Since many of these patients have a limited life span and the endovascular therapy is minimally invasive, the role of open surgery in this patient population has been limited to patients with a life expectancy of greater than one year (such as cases of lymphoma, thymoma, metastatic medullary or follicular carcinoma of the thyroid). In patients with residual carcinoma, some authors have suggested that using PTFE for the bypasses as this would be less likely to be compressed by recurrence (18).

It has been suggested that the type of therapy to be employed is affected by the anatomy of the lesion. Venographic classification of SVC syndrome has been divided into four types (19). Type I has a <90% stenosis of the SVC with patency and antegrade flow of the azygous-right atrium pathway. Type II has a >90% stenosis or occlusion of the SVC with patency and antegrade flow in the azygous-right atrial pathway. Type III has >90% stenosis or occlusion of the SVC with reversal of azygous blood flow. Type IV has occlusion of the SVC and one or more other caval tributary including the azygous systems. Some authors have suggested using endovascular therapy for type I and II lesions (20).

Open surgical bypass has been largely employed for benign disease. The types of conduits that have been used include: spiral vein graft, superficial femoral vein bypass, human allograft, PTFE and pericardial tube graft (21). When using a spiral vein graft, some authors, when dealing with fibrosing mediastinitis, have suggested external support with a PTFE graft to prevent extrinsic compression due to the recurrence (18).

To construct a spiral saphenous vein bypass graft (SSVG), the saphenous vein is harvested and opened longitudinally, and valve leaflets are excised under loop magnification. The opened vein is wrapped around a 32F or 36F polyethylene chest tube, and the edges are stapled or sutured with 7.0 continuous monofilament nonabsorbable suture, interrupting the suture line every three-quarter turn. To obtain adequate length as in those patients where the SSVG originates from the internal jugular vein, the saphenous vein from both legs often has to be harvested. The additional operating time required to prepare a 10 cm long spiral vein graft ranges been between 60 and 90 minutes. This is performed while a separate team performs the median sternotomy (22). If clamping of the vessels result in hemodynamic changes with an increase in the venous pressure greater than 30 mmHg, one may consider using a temporary venovenous shunt (21).

If the peripheral anastomosis is performed to the subclavian vein or more distally, an addition of a brachial artery arteriovenous fistula is suggested to maintain patency. If the peripheral anastamosis is performed to the internal jugular vein, a vein conduit for the bypass is needed as the relatively low flow in this system will not maintain patency. If the greater saphenous vein is not available, some authors have used the superficial femoral vein with good results (7,23–25). In general the patency of these bypasses has been better with vein as compared to PTFE. However, PTFE with a minimum diameter of 10 mm has been used with good results for the lesions 5–10 cm long (26). These bypasses and endovascular procedures only need to decompress one side even with bilateral innominate vein thrombosis, as collaterilization across the midline is adequate to decompress both sides with a single graft (27).

Post-operative heparin is started in 24–48 hours and then long-term coumadin is initiated. If a vein graft was used, then only three months of coumadin is needed. Life-long anticoagulation is used if PTFE was used for the bypass or if the underlying disorder is a hypercoaguable state (6).

With both endovascular and open procedures, long term patency can be maintained with surveillance (28). Gloviczki et al. (6) have suggested venography as a surveillance tool. Attempts at checking patency with contrast tomography and magnetic resonance venography does not seem to offer the needed resolution, and lesions can be missed. With these surveillance techniques, often patency can be extended with secondary endovascular procedures. Therefore, surveillance with venography every three months for one year is essential. After one year, venography is needed if symptoms recur (6).

Often the immediate results in terms of the resolution of the symptoms can be quite prompt and dramatic, and the patients can be some of the most grateful, which can make treating these patients a most rewarding experience.

KEY POINTS

- The superior vena cava obstruction is due to malignancy in 80–90% of cases.
- Patients usually present with head swelling, prominent chest wall and neck collateral vessels, facial cyanosis, proptosis, arm swelling, stridor, hoarseness,

respiratory distress, conjunctival edema and ecchymosis and sometimes with laryngeal and airway edema.

- Chest X-ray and computed tomography with intravenous contrast are the mainstays of the diagnostic testing that is needed.
- Conservative therapy consists of head elevation, anticoagulation, oxygen, steroids and diuretics.
- Good short-term results can be obtained with balloon angioplasty and stenting. This is usually done for patients with limited life span.
- Surgery with various types of grafts is performed in patients with benign disease.

ACKNOWLEDGMENT

Special thanks to Anne Ober for editorial assistance.

REFERENCES

1. Hunter W. The history of an aneurysm of the aorta with some remarks on aneurysms in gerneral. Med Obsinq 1757; 1:323–357.
2. Gloviczki P, Yao JST, eds. In: Handbook of Venous Disorders: Guidelines of the American Venous Forum., 2nd ed. London, England: Arnold Publishers, 2001:401–418.
3. Hanta I, Ucar G, Kuleci S, Ozbek S, Kocabas A. Superior vena cava syndrome: a rare clinical manifestation of Behcet's disease. Clin Rheumatol 2004.
4. Spittell PC, Vlietstra RE, Hayes DL, Higano ST. Venous obstruction due to permanent transvenous pacemaker electrodes: treatment with percutaneous transluminal balloon venoplasty. Pacing Clin Electrophysiol 1990; 13:271–274.
5. Schindler N, Vogelzang RL. Superior vena cava syndrome. Experience with endovascular stents and surgical therapy. Surg Clin North Am 1999; 79:683–694.
6. Alimi YS, Gloviczki P, Vrtiska TJ, et al. J Vasc Surg 1998; 27:287–299 pp. 300–301.
7. Klassen KP, Andrews NC, Curtis GH. Diagnosis and treatment of superior vena cava obstruction. Arch Surg 1951; 63:311–325.
8. Chiu CJ, Terzis J, Mac Rae ML. Replacement of superior vena cava with the spiral composite vein graft. Ann Thorac Surg 1974; 17:555–560.
9. Doty DB, Baker WH. Bypass of superior vena cava with spiral vein graft. Ann Thorac Surg 1976; 22:490–493.
10. Doty DB, Bypass of superior vena cava: six years' experience with spiral vein graft for obstruction of superior vena cava due to benign and malignant disease. J Thorac Cardiovasc Surg 1982; 83:326–338.
11. Doty DB. Composite spiral saphenous vein graft for occlusion of the superior vena cava. In: Bergan JJ, Yao JST, eds. Surgery of the veins. Orlando: Grune & Stratton, Inc., 1985:413–422.
12. Dayal R, Bernheim J, Clair DG, et al. Multimodal percutaneous intervention for critical venous occlusive disease. Ann Vasc Surg 2005.
13. Bornak A, Wicky S, Ris HB, Probst H, Milesi I, Corpataux JM. Endovascular treatment of stenoses in the superior vena cava syndrome caused by non-tumoral lesions. Eur Radiol 2003; 13:950–956.
14. Kee ST, Kinoshita L, Razavi MK, Nyman UR, Semba CP, Dake MD. Superior vena cava syndrome: treatment with catheter-directed thrombolysis and endovascular stent placement. Radiology 1998; 206:187–193.
15. Garcia Monaco R, Bertoni H, Pallota G, et al. Use of self-expanding vascular endoprostheses in superior vena cava syndrome. Eur J Cardiothorac Surg 2003; 24:208–211.

16. Thony F, Moro D, Witmeyer P, et al. Endovascular treatment of superior vena cava obstruction in patients with malignancies. Eur Radiol 1999; 9:965–971.

17. Young N, Yeghiaian-Alvandi R, Chin YS. Use of endovascular metal stents to alleviate malignant superior vena cava syndrome. Intern Med J 2003; 33:542–544.

18. Marshall WG, Kouchoukos NT. Management of recurrent superior vena caval syndrome with an externally supported femoral vein bypass graft. Ann Thorac Surg 1988; 46:239–241.

19. Stanford W, Doty DB. The role of venography and surgery in the management of patients with superior vena cava obstruction. Ann Thorac Surg 1986; 41:158–163.

20. Dondelinger RF, Trotteur, G. Expandable stents in the venous system. Abstracts of the International Symposium, Leuven, Belgium. 1996.

21. Seelig MH, Oldenburg WA, Klingler PJ, Odell JA. Superior vena cava syndrome caused by chronic hemodialysis catheters: autologous reconstruction with a pericardial tube graft. J Vasc Surg 1998; 28:556–560.

22. Kalra M, Gloviczki P, Andrews JC, et al. Open surgical and endovascular treatment of superior vena cava syndrome caused by nonmalignant disease. J Vasc Surg 2003; 38:215–223.

23. Hagino RT, Bengtson TD, Fosdick DA, Valentine RJ, Clagett GP. Venous reconstructions using the superficial femoral-popliteal vein. J Vasc Surg 1997; 26:829–837.

24. Marshall WGJ, Kouchoukos NT. Management of recurrent superior vena caval syndrome with an externally supported femoral vein bypass graft. Ann Thorac Surg 1988; 46:239–241.

25. Gladstone DJ, Pillai R, Paneth M, Lincoln JC. Relief of superior vena caval syndrome with autologous femoral vein used as a bypass graft. J Thorac Cardiovasc Surg 1985; 89:750–752.

26. Gloviczki P, Pairolero PC, Toomey BJ, et al. Reconstruction of large veins for nonmalignant venous occlusive disease. J Vasc Surg 1992; 16:750–761.

27. Dinkel HP, Mettke B, Schmid F, Baumgartner I, Triller J, Do DD. Endovascular treatment of malignant superior vena cava syndrome: is bilateral wallstent placement superior to unilateral placement? J Endovasc Ther 2003; 10:788–797.

28. Kalra M, Gloviczki P, Andrews JC, et al. Open surgical and endovascular treatment of superior vena cava syndrome caused by nonmalignant disease. J Vasc Surg 2003; 38:215–223.

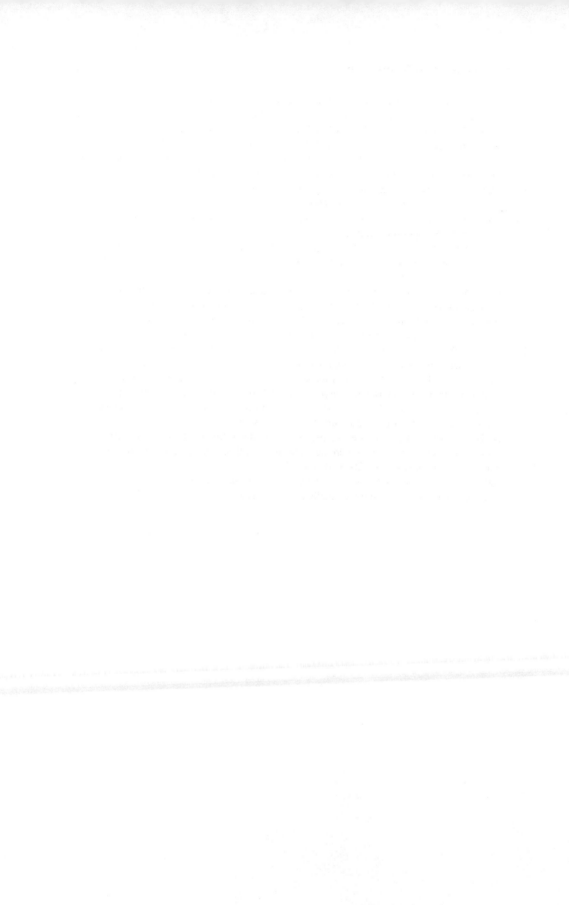

35
Congenital Venous Malformations: Venous Tumors

Sachiendra V. Amaragiri
Freeman Hospital, University of Newcastle upon Tyne, Newcastle upon Tyne, U.K.

Nicos Labropoulos
Vascular Laboratory, Division of Vascular Surgery, New Jersey Medical School, Newark, New Jersey, U.S.A.

CONGENITAL VENOUS MALFORMATIONS

When one considers that venous anatomical variations are common, it is surprising that congenital venous malformations are seen quite uncommonly in specialist venous clinics. There is a wide spectrum of congenital variation—absence of major veins, incomplete development, multiple vessels, dextra-position of vessels and hereditary diseases. Attempts are being made to map the genetic signatures for these venous malformations but no single chromosome or gene has yet been implicated. There is however evidence that some of the hereditary forms are associated with some chromosomal defects, but the findings have not been consistent. Awareness of these anomalies, such as double inferior vena cava, left side inferior vena cava, etc., have implications in surgical practice, especially for vascular surgeons and radiologists. Some of these such as venous aneurysm, agenesis, congenital and hereditary anomalies, etc., are associated with complications such as varicose veins, thrombosis, embolism, and the secondary effects of venous thrombosis—venous hypertension leading to chronic venous disease.

Venous Aneurysm

There are numerous published case reports of venous aneurysms but it a relatively rare disorder. The term venous aneurysm is synonymous with the terms phlebectasia, venous congenital cyst, venous ectasia and essential venous dilatation. It is an isolated abnormal fusiform or saccular dilatation of a vein. They are either primary, which is idiopathic (congenital), or secondary due to trauma.

   Venous aneurysm differs from varicose vein in that it is a solitary lesion that can affect any vein and there is no associated venous elongation as in a varicosity. It has no relation to sex and it can occur at any age and has been reported even in a child as young as 2 years (1).

Sites

Venous aneurysms can occur at any site. In the lower limbs, they have been reported in the popliteal vein, the femoral vein, the great saphenous vein, the small saphenous vein (2), foot veins and the superficial communicating veins of the legs. In the pelvis they have been reported in the external and internal iliac veins (3). In the neck they are commonly found in the internal jugular vein (4), the external jugular vein (5,6), anterior jugular vein (7), the facial vein and the parotid gland veins. In the upper limbs, they have been reported in the subclavian vein, the cephalic vein, the basilic vein, and the brachial vein. Intra-abdominally they have been reported in the superior vena cava (8), the inferior vena cava, the superior mesenteric vein, the portal vein (9), and the splenic vein and in the chest in the azygos venous system (10). About 60% of them are found in the deep venous system of the lower extremities and the remaining 40% are distributed in the rest of the venous system (11).

Pathology

The pathogenesis of these rare lesions is unknown. There is elastic tissue dysplasia and smooth muscle fiber fragmentation, both of which are replaced by fibrous tissue. The tunica media exhibits a reduced number of muscle fibers. Congenital focal defects of the elastic and muscle fibres have been proposed to contribute to the development of venous aneurysms (12).

Presentation

The most common presentations of venous aneurysm are pain (75%), swelling (67%) and a mass (42%) (11). However, there are region specific presentations and venous aneurysms in the lower limbs, and the pelvis can present with deep venous thrombosis. In a review of 117 patients with popliteal venous aneurysm by Sessa et al. 45% presented with pulmonary embolism, 26% with chronic venous disease (phlebitis, pain, and ulcer) and 26% with varicose veins (13). Most of the popliteal aneurysms were associated with varicose veins and were more common in females. Venous aneurysms of the neck veins present with swelling in almost all the published cases and are most often found in the internal jugular vein. The abdominal, pelvic and thoracic vein aneurysms are most often identified as incidental findings during routine diagnostic investigations for other diseases.

Complications

The most serious complication of venous aneurysm of the lower limb, abdominal and pelvic veins is pulmonary embolism. Cardiac arrest and death have been reported due to the thrombo-embolic events as complication of these aneurysms. Deep venous thrombosis and chronic venous disease (phlebitis, pain swelling, ulcers) are the most common complications. Paradoxical embolus via a patent foramen ovale has been reported leading to hemiplegia (14,15).

Nerve compression syndromes due to venous aneurysms have also been reported. They include radial nerve compression by cephalic vein aneurysm (16), tibial nerve compression by popliteal vein aneurysm (17), median nerve compression by brachial vein aneurysm (18), and brachial plexus compression by a subclavian vein aneurysm (19).

Investigations

Color duplex scan has been found to be accurate and sufficient in diagnosing limb venous aneurysms. It not only enables diagnosis but also provides valuable information on site,

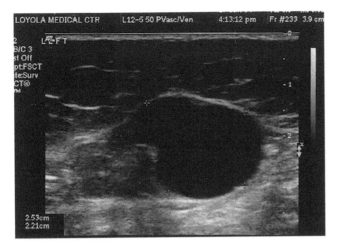

Figure 1 Ultrasound B-mode image of a great saphenous aneurysm. This was found in the lower thigh of a female patient who presented with local pain over the aneurysm. It measured 25×22 mm. The aneurysm was pushing the saphenous fascia and distorted the local anatomy in the saphenous canal. No varicose veins were found in either extremity. There was no thrombosis but only mild reflux exiting through a medial tributary. The diameter of the saphenous vein above and below the aneurysm measured 4.6 and 4.1 mm, respectively. The patient did not want any treatment, and she was scheduled to have follow-up once a year.

size, patency, the presence of thrombus, valve status and flow dynamics that are useful for managing these aneurysms (Fig. 1). Venographic methods have also been employed in a number of case studies in diagnosis and assessment of these aneurysms. However, not only is venography invasive but also does not give any information to the clinician about the haemodynamic status of the veins.

Other modalities such as contrast enhanced magnetic resonance imaging (MRI) and computed axial tomography (CAT) may need to be employed in certain circumstances and they have been found to be accurate in diagnosing venous aneurysms within the thorax and abdomen. However, CAT and MRI have been employed mostly when venous anomalies are identified incidentally during the diagnostic investigation of abdominal mass, some other disease or suspicious shadows on plain X-rays. In abdominal, pelvic and thoracic venous aneurysms, CT and MRI scans may perhaps be the most appropriate methods of investigations, given the limitations of other methods such as ultrasound, venogram, etc.

Treatment

Treatment of venous aneurysm is varied. The vast majority can be managed conservatively except deep venous aneurysms of the lower limbs. For popliteal vein aneurysm, surgery is the treatment of choice as they usually present with thrombosis and embolism which could be life threatening. The method of choice is tangential aneurysmectomy and lateral venorrhaphy. Other methods employed are resection with end-to-end anastomosis and resection with vein interposition graft (13). In a large retrospective study and review, surgery has mostly been the treatment of choice and this has been found to be effective in managing most such venous aneurysms (20,21).

Pelvic and abdominal vein aneurysms have usually been managed conservatively as well as surgically, but the vast majority of surgeons prefer surgery to conservative management because of the increased risk of thrombosis and embolism and rupture (21). Tangential excision and lateral venorrhapy or poly-tetra-fluoroethylene (PTFE) interposition graft have been employed in their surgical management.

Thoracic venous aneurysms can be managed conservatively. Most of the surgery is for rupture and increasing size, which are not common (21).

Neck vein aneurysms have been excised in most of the case reports. Most of these neck venous aneurysms have been found in the younger age group. Cosmetic appearance is the only indication for surgery and this is by surgical excision and direct suture (4,22,23). However the majority of these can be treated conservatively with routine follow up (24–26).

Blue Rubber Bleb Nevus Syndrome

Blue rubber bleb nevus syndrome (BRBNS) is a rare congenital venous disorder characterized by cutaneous and gastrointestinal venous malformation. It is associated with intestinal hemorrhage and iron deficiency anemia. It was first recognized by Gascoyen in 1860 and in 1958 Bean further described these lesions and coined the term BRBNS (27).

The cause of this syndrome is unknown. The majority of cases occur sporadically but Gallione et al. have studied two families with venous malformation syndrome and found a linkage to chromosome 9p (28). Vikkula et al. concluded that these families had an activating mutation in the tyrosine kinase (TIE2) receptor that participates in abnormal angiogenesis (29).

Cutaneous Lesions

In BRBNS, lesions are usually multiple and characteristically consist of deep-blue blebs which are soft and rubbery and are easily compressible.

They can be found anywhere over the body surface but the majority of them are located most commonly on the upper extremities and trunk. The size of the skin lesions varies from a few millimeters to 5 cm or more. They are usually covered with a layer of skin of varying thickness and in contrast to the gastrointestinal lesions they rarely bleed spontaneously.

Cutaneous lesions are of three types:

1. A large disfiguring lesion that may compress the surrounding tissues
2. A typical red to blue–violet nodule or macule covered with skin
3. An irregular macule or papule that may punctuate or merge with adjacent nevi

These cutaneous lesions are soft and are most often asymptomatic. The lesion can be emptied of blood on pressure. Excessive sweating has been described to occur from the overlying skin due to the close association of the nevi with sweat glands (30).

Gastrointestinal Lesions

These are again characteristically multiple and can occur anywhere from the mouth to the anus. The commonest occurrence of these lesions is in the small bowel. In the colon they have a predilection to the left side. The typical mucosal lesion is a nodule similar to the cutaneous lesion with a bluish tinge covered by a thin layer of mucosal cells. They may also appear as a bluish–red spot or polypoid lesions. They can bleed spontaneously and are a cause of gastrointestinal hemorrhage and iron deficiency anemia.

Presentations and Complications

The most common presentation in the skin is the obvious lesion, but in the gastrointestinal tract, anemia and frank bleeding are the presenting features. They constitute one of rare causes of bleeding in the gastrointestinal tract in infants, children and young adults (31–36). These lesions are also known to occur in the kidneys giving rise to hematuria in the brain leading to intracranial hemorrhage causing ataxia, dementia, focal neurological signs and symptoms (37) and in the vulva they can cause severe bleeding and distress (38). They have also been reported to cause consumptive coagulopathy (39), a cause of massive gastrointestinal bleeding (40), and endobronchial involvement leading to chronic cough (41).

Investigations

The skin lesions are obvious but the most common manifestation is anaemia and gastrointestinal bleeding and for this gastrointestinal endoscopy is the investigation of choice in the upper and lower gastrointestinal tract. In the small bowel, endoscopic techniques such as wireless capsule endoscopy and push enteroscopy have been employed in the investigation and wireless capsule endoscopy in particular has been found to be quite accurate in the diagnosis (42). In intracranial and intra-abdominal lesions other methods such as CAT and MRI angiography may be necessary for diagnosis. In certain circumstances technetium labeled red cells have been used to delineate the lesions at times of active bleeding (43).

Treatment

The cutaneous lesions do not usually cause any symptoms except occasional pain and discomfort. No reports of thrombosis in these lesions have been noted so far. They very rarely bleed spontaneously, however trauma to these lesions may cause profuse bleeding. Resuscitation with fluids, blood and blood products is the goal of treatment of gastrointestinal bleeding. Specific treatment of gastrointestinal bleeding due to BRBNS includes: sclerotherapy, rubber band ligation and argon beam laser coagulation of the lesions. In intractable cases bowel resection may have to be undertaken to control the bleeding. Multiendoscope (simultaneous use of laparoscope and gastrointestinal endoscope) assisted resection of these lesions in the gastrointestinal tract has also been undertaken with good results (44).

Congenital Angiodysplasias

These are congenital vascular anomalies encompassing three variations in presentation (45).

1. *Klippel–Trenaunay syndrome (KTS)*. This consists of a triad of varicosity, hemangioma and hypertrophy of soft tissues and bones.
2. *Parks-Weber syndrome*. This consists of hypertrophy of the lower limbs with hemodynamically active congenital arterio-venous fistulae, usually of an intra- and extraosseous location.
3. *Servelle-Martorell type*. This consists of hemangiomatosis usually of a venous (cavernous) type, affecting soft tissues as well as bones in association with skeletal hypoplasia. There is a retardation of bone growth by substitution and destruction of the epiphysial cartilages by the intraosseous hemangioma.

From a clinical perspective, this classification has little relevance because management of these in most cases are identical. Hence all these are clubbed and termed Klippel–Trenaunay–Weber syndrome or just Klippel–Trenaunay syndrome.

In 1988 the Hamburg Classification came into existence and is the most comprehensive classification and is based on clinical, anatomical and pathophysiological features of the disease. This classified all congenital vascular malformations into five groups based on the predominance of the anatomic component: arterial, venous, atreriovenous shunting, lymphatic, and combined (hemolymphatic). Each one of these is further classified into "Extratruncular form" and "Truncular form." The extratruncular form develops from the embryonic remnant because of the developmental arrest during the embryonic life. This embryonic remnant originates from the mesodermal cells and hence retains the capacity of organogenesis and to differentiate further at a later stage in life when subjected to various normal physiological stimuli. However the truncal form lacks this feature of differentiation as it is a growth defect which occurs at later stages of embryonic life and hence lacks the capacity to differentiate (46,47).

Klippel–Trenauny Syndrome

KTS was originally described in 1900 and is characterized by a constellation of three anomalies (1) soft tissue and bony hypertrophy of the extremity, (2) cutaneous vascular naevi of the affected extremity mainly of the port-wine stain type and (3) varicose veins and lymphatic anomalies. The other added features are clinically absent aterio-venous shunting and the presence of deep venous anomalies which include atresia, hypoplasia or aneurysmal dilatation of the deep veins, external compression by fibrous bands, valvular incompetence or agensis (48,49).

Etiology.   The etiology of KTS is still obscure. A number of theories have been hypothesized, some of them quite controversial. One of the suggested theories is that KTS is due to an embryogenic abnormality of the vascular system at the mesodermal level (45,50).

Much genetic research has been undertaken to understand the etiology of KTS, but so far it has remained elusive. A few cases have been thought to be due to an autosomal dominant gene with low penetrance. Berry reviewed 49 cases of KTS and found that all of them were sporadic and suggested that it was due to somatic mutation (51).

Angiogenic factors critical in the initiation and maintenance of vascular architecture have been studied. Two genetic defects of angiogenic factor VG5Q have been identified in patients with KTS, i.e., excessive expression and enhanced activity. The autocrine effect of VG5Q promotes uncontrolled vascular proliferation. Two mutations have been identified, one of these is chromosomal translocation (5:11) which increases the VG5Q transcription and the second mutation is E133K which enhances the angiogenic effect of VG5Q. In addition, the angiogenic factor TNFSF-12 also called TWEAK interacts with VG5Q to summate the angiogenic effect (52). However, none of these have been demonstrated consistently in KTS.

Clinical Features.   In addition to the venous malformation, KTS is not uncommonly associated with lymphatic malformations. In a study of 252 patients, 63% had the triad of varicose veins, limb hypertrophy and cutaneous vascular naevi, 37% had just two of the triad, however in 94% of patients with KTS, one of the triad was noted shortly after birth (53). None of the reports show any gender differences nor significant family history. Lower limbs are more often affected (88% to 95%), unilateral involvement occurs in 85% of cases, upper and lower limb involvement in 15% of cases, and all four extremity involvement is very rare (49,53,54).

Due to the venous congestion and the lymphedema, pain, heaviness and fatigability are some of the common presenting complaints.

Capillary Malformation.   This is the commonest of the triad of KTS and occurs in 62% (49). It presents as a port-wine patch which is red to purple in color, flat and has an irregular distribution. On the trunk it has a clear sharp border and does not cross the midline whereas in the extremities it has a patchy distribution. In addition to skin, the subcutaneous tissue, muscles, abdominal and thoracic cavities can be also involved (54). These capillary malformations, although they do not disappear, they may however fade significantly on aging. In addition they can bleed, develop skin atrophy, hyperhidrosis, infection etc (53,54).

Venous Anomalies.   The venous anomalies in KTS are mainly varicosities. Unlike common varicose veins these are extensive and large. They take an erratic course and begin in childhood. Trelat and Monod described the "vein of Servelle" which is a large dilated vein starting from a plexus of veins over the dorsum of the foot running laterally over the lower limbs before entering the deep system at sites such as the profunda vein, popliteal vein, superficial femoral or the iliac system via the gluteal veins. In 33% of cases it extends the whole length of the lower extremity terminating in the iliac vein system (55).

In a study involving 144 patients with KTS, it was observed that the lower limbs were the more commonly affected. In the 559 operations performed for KTS by Servelle, he has observed that the commonest veins affected in the lower limbs was the popliteal (54).

The other commonly described anomalies of the venous system in KTS are hypoplasia, agenesis, venous and valvular incompetence and aneurysmal dilation of the deep venous system. Other frequently occurring defects are fibrous bands and hypoplasia. Servelle in 448 operations for KTS has observed that in the popliteal veins, the lesions were compression and fenestration in 71%, peirvenous sheath in 15% and the remaining 14% accounts for hypoplesia and agensis. In 252 operations on the superficial femoral vein, compression and fenestration were observed in 54%, hypoplasia in 41% and perivenous sheath and agensis in the remaining 5%. Whereas in the 19 operations on iliac veins, hypoplesia accounts for 63% and agenesis for 37%. In the upper limbs, in 80 patients, the brachial and axillary veins were involved in the pathology, compression in 63%, hypoplasia in 22% and agenesis in 15% (48).

Limb Hypertrophy.   This usually manifests at a later age in life. Soft tissue, bone or both may be involved. Increase in limb length is due to involvement of bone whereas increase in the girth is due to the soft tissue involvement. In 144 patients, limb hypertrophy has been observed in 93%. Increase in the length was observed in 66% and increase in the girth in 69% (49).

Other Anomalies.   Anomalies of the lymphatic in KTS are the most common and can be disabling. The most common anomalies are aplasia, hypoplasia and a decrease in the number of lymph trunks and lymph nodes are noticed in 70% of patients. Cutaneous lymphatic vesicles, cutaneous lymphatic leakage can occur due to the associated lymphatic abnormalities.

Complications.   At least one episode of deep vein thrombosis and thrombophlebitis occurs in 17% of patients with KTS and venous thrombosis has a potential risk of throwing pulmonary emboli.

Bleeding from hemangioma can cause rectal, vaginal, vulvar or esophageal bleeding and hematuria due to pelvic vein involvement that accounts for 23% (49). Hematochezia is a common form of bleeding in KTS. The pathophysiology is the internal iliac vein normally drains the rectal, pudendal, vesicular and genital veins. In KTS, the lateral vein in the lower limbs and the sciatic vein form the posterior venous system. They unite in the thigh and divide to enter the superior and the inferior sciatic notch to join the internal iliac vein. The internal iliac vein in turn is overloaded by these veins and hence its normal draining tributaries become varicose with concomitant bleeding and hematochezia and hematuria (56).

Cavernous hemangiomas can enlarge rapidly, usually in the first year of life, producing high-output congestive heart failure or a consumptive coagulopathy (Kasabach–Merritt syndrome). This syndrome is marked by anemia, thrombocytopenia, prolonged prothrombin time (PT) and activated partial thromboplastin time (APTT), reduced levels fibrinogen and fibrin split products.

Investigation. Diagnosis of KTS is clinical. However, investigations are only needed to identify any surgically correctable lesions and, if surgery is indicated, to assess the feasibility and the extent of surgery because the majority of patients with this disorder are managed conservatively. Generally color duplex scanning is sufficient to map the venous anomaly. Venogram and contrast enhanced MRI scans may be needed in identifying the architecture, the defect and the extent of the lesions. Lymphangiogram and lymphoscinti-graphy may delineate the lymphatic defects and may help in managing the patients. Scanogram of the skeletal system and CT scans may be helpful in identifying the skeletal discrepancy and help in determining the timing of surgery (51,53).

Treatment. KTS is a life-long disease. To date there is no treatment available to completely cure the abnormality. Patients have to learn to live with the anomaly. There are a number of KTS support organizations that are helpful in bringing together patients and helping them to understand the disease, provide psychological support and disseminate information, and also keep them updated with ways of adjusting and managing their life styles.

Common presenting complaints in KTS are due to varicosities of the lower limbs and cosmetic appearance. The majority of the patients can be treated symptomatically with support stockings, elevation, rest and continued reinforcement to wear graduated compression stockings. The secondary effects of varicosities such as phlebitis, cellulitis and ulcers are treated with antibiotics and compression. Surgery has been undertaken in the past for KTS. Servelle has reported remediable causes for the venous congestion and varicosities in the lower limbs such as bands, perivenous sheath, hypoplasia and agenesis. He claims that resolving these anomalies can improve the venous circulation and varicosity (48). Treating varicosities with traditional varicose vein surgery—vein stripping, ligation, and multiple stab avulsions—is fraught with the risk of worsening the situation with development of new varicosities, difficulties of wound healing, bleeding, infection etc (57). Sclerosing agents (sodium tetradecyl sulphate, ethanolamine oleate) have been used with some success in obliterating the varicosities. In one study 44% of the venous malformation over the face disappeared and 28% decreased on foam sclerotherapy (58). In another study 1% polidocanol has been used and has shown promising results (59).

Capillary malformations usually diminish in size and appearance on aging. However, they present a common problem in the earlier years. Surgery should be withheld, as it is complicated with bleeding, non healing wounds, ulcers etc. With the advent of laser therapy many of these disfiguring appearances could be minimized. Ordinary pulse dye laser has not shown to be effective in improving the port wine stain (60). Flashlamp pump dye laser has found to be quite effective in treating port wine staining in childhood, (61,62) although it may darken and thicken the skin. A multilayer technique has been developed that seems to cause less skin damage (63). However the intelligent application of modern cosmetic products helps in masking these lesions to almost invisibility.

Hypertrophy and limb elongation are usually treated based on the degree of overgrowth. A discrepancy of less than 2 cm length can be adjusted by altering the soles of the shoes. Greater than 2 cm may need surgical correction (53). A number of methods have been employed. Servelle showed that ligating the deep veins of the opposite leg increased the limb length of that leg compensating for the over growth of the anomalous leg in 48 children (48). However, this is not the standard current practice. Limb length discrepancy is tailored to the needs of individual patient. Predicting the overgrowth is difficult in children and it is still debated as to when, how and where intervention should be undertaken. Current practice is to cause epiphyseal arrest by stapling of the epiphysis but this is not always effective. Epiphysiodesis described by Mullikne and Young is considered to be more reliable and permanent (64). However, prior to undertaking such surgery, scanogram and CAT may be useful in determining the best time for this procedure.

Lymphedema is usually managed with compression stockings, massage and surgery is rarely indicated. General skin care and prevention of trauma is important to prevent the complications of healing, ulcers, infection etc.

Gastrointestinal bleeding usually stops spontaneously. Esophageal varices may need sclerotherapy or rubber band ligation. Hemorrhoidal bleeds can be similarly managed. Occasionally in rectosigmoid bleeding, rectosigmoidectomy may have to be undertaken to control the bleeding (56).

VENOUS TUMORS

Venous tumors are one of the rarest neoplasms encountered in venous clinical practice. They are either benign or malignant, however most venous tumors are malignant. They arise from the tissues of the vessel wall and they include endothelioma from the endothelial lining of the tunica intima, fibrosarcoma from the connective tissue of all the three layers, and leiomyoma and leiomyosarcoma from the smooth muscles of the tunica media. Leiomyosarcoma is the most common among these rare neoplasms. Two cases of primary malignant lymphoma of the veins have also been reported (65,66).

Leiomyosarcoma

The commonest site of occurrence of these tumors is in the inferior vena cava and in the extremities the great saphenous vein (67). Their occurrence in the azygos vein (68) pulmonary veins (69), femoral vein, internal jugular vein (70), portal vein (71), renal vein (72), iliac veins (73), and ovarian vein (74) has also been reported. Potentially they can occur in any vein.

Leimyosarcoma of the inferior vena cava is the more common (60% overall); 80% of these occur in women and the majority of them have been detected in the elderly (75). The mean age of detection in two big reviews was between 50 and 60 years (76,77). In the extremities they occur more commonly in the great saphenous vein.

The distribution of primary IVC leiomyosarcoma is described in relation to the renal and hepatic veins: segment I infrarenal, segment II suprarenal, and segment III suprahepatic (78). The majority of them are intramural but intravenous extension of these tumors have also been reported (79).

Histology

The tumor consists of an elongated pinkish-white, lobulated, moderately circumscribed, and encapsulated fibrous mass. Histologically they consists of hyperchromatic, enlarged, solid spindle-cell lesion with elongated spindled irregular nuclei arranged in interwoven fascicles with small focal areas of necrosis. The smooth muscle cells are typical for leiomyoma with a whorled pattern without nuclear pleomorphism. Mitotic activity is no greater than 1 per 15 high-power fields. The tumor cells display desmin, vimentin, and smooth muscle cell actin but not S-100 protein (80,81).

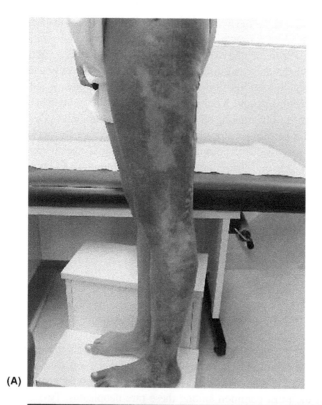

(A)

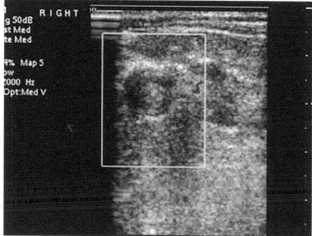

(B)

Figure 2 Klippel–Trenauny syndrome. (**A**) Young female patient with hypertrophy of the left lower extremity, staining of the skin, and varicose veins. The lateral thigh veins were enlarged and had reflux. The femoral vein was hypoplastic. (**B**) Thrombosis of the lateral vein in a young male. He also had bleeding in the intestine and for this reason an IVC filter was placed. (*See color insert.*)

Clinical Presentation

Clinically they are often asymptomatic and hence remain undetected for great periods. They may present as a palpable mass (40% to 80%), back pain (70%) or abdominal pain (60%). Suprarenal inferior vena caval involvment may present as renal failure however this is infrequent because of the rich collateral network retroperitonially via the left renal vein (75).

Although obstruction of the hepatic veins is uncommon, this has been reported in 36 patients. In these cases the clinical symptoms may present as an acute or chronic form of Budd-Chiari syndrome (82–85). These tumors can invade the right atrium and patients may present with acute heart right heart failure, with symptoms similar to pulmonary hypertension or pulmonary embolism.

These tumors are slow growing and there is usually adequate time for the development of venous collateral circulation and as a result clinical presentation with signs and symptoms of acute deep venous obstruction is rare. Lower limb swelling is more frequent if the iliac or femoro-popliteal veins are invaded. Primary tumors of the superficial leg veins usually present as a painless mobile mass, whereas those arising from deep veins can be fixed to the surrounding tissues (86,87).

Investigations

Ultrasound scan, contrast enhanced CAT, and MRI are usually sufficient in delineating these lesions. As they are retroperitoneal other surrounding structures such as ureter, aorta, bowel, biliary structures may be involved in the disease process hence intravenous urography, angiography, barium examination, etc. may also be useful in assessing their involvement. However, a definitive diagnosis can often only be made on histopathological examination of the resected specimen. Duplex scan may be useful in assessing the venous anatomy and hemodynamics.

Treatment

Resection of the neoplasm is the treatment of choice. After resection, the caval defect can be dealt with caval interruption, patch repair, or interposition graft using spiral saphenous vein or ePTFE prosthetic graft. Recently several studies have shown that reconstructing the inferior vena cave with prosthetic material is not only possible but also the graft patency maintained is good (88,89). Due to the close proximity of other important anatomical structures, nephrectomy, cholecystectomy, hepatectomy may have to be undertaken to free the margins. However vena caval reconstruction should be selective. If the pre operative investigations shows that the vena cava is occluded without secondary effects this could be safely treated with caval interruption, as there are usually enough venous collaterals to prevent secondary effects of interruption (75). Given the median survival of about three years, the longest survival has been recorded to be 13 and 17 years after resection (75,90).

Adjuvant treatment such as radiotherapy and chemotherapy can be instituted but they have not shown to be of much benefit.

Leiomyoma

Intravenous leiomyomatosis is an extremely rare, benign, well-differentiated tumor that can cause venous obstruction or cardiac irritability due to its propensity to extend into the inferior vena cava and to the right heart. The tumor is confined to the vascular channels (91). Although they are benign, they can recur. This disorder is more common in women who have had

Table 1 Venous Involvement in 144 Patients with KTS

Region involved	Percentage
Upper limbs in association with other organs	26
Upper limbs in isolation	18
Lower limbs in association with other organs	92
Lower limbs in isolation	73
Thorax	17
Pelvis and abdomen	14
Head and neck	5

Source: From Ref. 49.

Table 2 Lower Limb Veins Involvement in 559 Operations for KTS

Lower limb veins involved	Percentage
Popliteal vein	50
Femoral vein	16
Combined femoral and popliteal veins	29
Iliac vein	3
Inferior vena cava	1

Source: From Ref. 54.

previous hysterectomy (64%) for uterine leiomyomatosis. The mean age of the patient is 50 years (91,92). An interval range of six months to 20 years passed before presentation with the intravenous portion of the tumor and 76% of these women were postmenopausal. Presentation is usually related to signs of increased venous obstruction or decreased venous return to the heart. Recurrence rate is high and has poor outcome (Fig. 2, Tables 1, 2).

KEY POINTS

- Congenital venous malformations and tumors are uncommon.
- Ultrasound CT and MRI are usually adequate for diagnosis.
- There are many venous malformations and their treatment could be conservative, endovenous and surgical.
- Symptoms can improve after treatment but most of these diseases do not have a complete cure.
- There are benign and malignant venous tumors but the latter is most common.

REFERENCES

1. Sakallioglu AE, Yagmurlu A, Yagmurlu B, Gokcora HI. An asymmetric ballooning of the neck: jugular vein aneurysm. J Pediatr Surg 2002; 37:111–113.
2. Kim DH, Lescault EJ. Aneurysm of the small saphenous vein presenting as a popliteal mass: a case report. Am J Orthop 1999; 28:304–305.
3. Banno H, et al. External iliac venous aneurysm in a pregnant woman: a case report. J Vasc Surg 2004; 40:174–178.

4. Arnaudov D. Surgical treatment of congenital aneurysms of the internal jugular vein in children. Khirurgiia (Sofiia) 1972; 25:290–292.

5. Verbeeck N, Hammer F, Goffette P, Mathurin P. Saccular aneurysm of the external jugular vein, an unusual cause of neck swelling. J Belge Radiol 1997; 80:63–64.

6. Fishman G, DeRowe A, Singhal V. Congenital internal and external jugular venous aneurysms in a child. Br J Plast Surg 2004; 57:165–167.

7. Zorn WG, Zorn TT, Van Bellen B. Aneurysm of the anterior jugular vein. J Cardiovasc Surg (Torino) 1981; 22:546–549.

8. Modry DL, Hidvegi RS, LaFleche LR. Congenital saccular aneurysm of the superior vena cava. Ann Thorac Surg 1980; 29:258–262.

9. Kim EE, Romero J, Kim CG. Portal venous aneurysm demonstrated by magnetic resonance imaging. Clin Imaging 1998; 22:360–363.

10. Olbert F, Kobinia G, Russe OJ, Denck H. Aneurysmal dilatation of the bulb of the azygos vein. Radiological and clinical value. Wien Med Wochenschr Suppl 1980; 65:1–26.

11. Gillespie DL, et al. Presentation and management of venous aneurysms. J Vasc Surg 1997; 26:845–852.

12. Goto Y, Sakurada T, Nanjo H, Masuda H. Venous aneurysm of the cephalic vein: report of a case. Surg Today 1998; 28:964–966.

13. Sessa C, et al. Management of symptomatic and asymptomatic popliteal venous aneurysms: a retrospective analysis of 25 patients and review of the literature. J Vasc Surg 2000; 32:902–912.

14. Manthey J, Munderloh KH, Mautner JP, Kohl M, Frohlich G. Popliteal venous aneurysm with pulmonary and paradoxical embolization. Vasa 1994; 23:264–267.

15. Willinek WA, Strunk H, Born M, Remig J, Becher H, Schild H. Popliteal venous aneurysm with paradoxical embolization in a patient with patent foramen ovale. Circulation 2001; 104:E60–E61.

16. Kassabian E, Coppin T, Combes M, Julia P, Fabiani JN. Radial nerve compression by a large cephalic vein aneurysm: case report. J Vasc Surg 2003; 38:617–619.

17. Coffman SW, Leon SM, Gupta SK. Popliteal venous aneurysms: report of an unusual presentation and literature review. Ann Vasc Surg 2000; 14:286–290.

18. Marquardt G, Angles SM, Leheta FD, Seifert V. Median nerve compression caused by a venous aneurysm. Case report. J Neurosurg 2001; 94:624–626.

19. Gabriel EM, Friedman AH. Brachial plexus compression by venous aneurysms. Case illustration. J Neurosurg 1997; 86:311.

20. Aldridge SC, et al. Popliteal venous aneurysm: report of two cases and review of the world literature. J Vasc Surg 1993; 18:708–715.

21. Calligaro KD, et al. Venous aneurysms: surgical indications and review of the literature. Surgery 1995; 117:1–6.

22. Bosshardt TL, Honig MP. Congenital internal jugular venous aneurysm: diagnosis and treatment. Mil Med 1996; 161:246–247.

23. Gao Y, et al. Diagnosis and treatment of internal jugular phlebectasia (three cases report). Hua Xi Kou Qiang Yi Xue Za Zhi 1999; 17:352–354.

24. al Dousary S. Internal jugular phlebectasia. Int J Pediatr Otorhinolaryngol 1997; 38:273–280.

25. Calligaro KD, et al. Congenital aneurysm of the internal jugular vein in a pregnant woman. Cardiovasc Surg 1995; 3:63–64.

26. Lubianca-Neto JF, Mauri M, Prati C. Internal jugular phlebectasia in children. Am J Otolaryngol 1999; 20:415–418.

27. Atten MJ, Ahmed S, Attar BM, Richter H, III, Mehta B. Massive pelvic hemangioma in a patient with blue rubber bleb nevus syndrome. South Med J 2000; 93:1122–1125.

28. Gallione CJ, et al. A gene for familial venous malformations maps to chromosome 9p in a second large kindred. J Med Genet 1995; 32:197–199.

29. Vikkula M, et al. Vascular dysmorphogenesis caused by an activating mutation in the receptor tyrosine kinase TIE2. Cell 1996; 87:1181–1190.

30. Oksuzoglu BC, Oksuzoglu G, Cakir U, Bayir T, Esen M. Blue rubber bleb nevus syndrome. Am J Gastroenterol 1996; 91:780–782.

31. Tatar G, Ozyilkan E, Telatar H. Blue rubber bleb nevus syndrome: report of a case. Turk J Pediatr 1993; 35:131–134.

32. Goraya JS, Marwaha RK, Vatve M, Trehan A. Blue rubber bleb nevus syndrome: a cause for recurrent episodic severe anemia. Pediatr Hematol Oncol 1998; 15:261–264.

33. Boente MD, Cordisco MR, Frontini MD, Asial RA. Blue rubber bleb nevus (bean syndrome): evolution of four cases and clinical response to pharmacologic agents. Pediatr Dermatol 1999; 16:222–227.

34. Rodrigues D, et al. Blue rubber bleb nevus syndrome. Rev Hosp Clin Fac Med Sao Paulo 2000; 55:29–34.

35. Domini M, et al. Blue rubber bleb nevus syndrome and gastrointestinal haemorrhage: which treatment? Eur J Pediatr Surg 2002; 12:129–133.

36. Dobru D, Seuchea N, Dorin M, Careianu V. Blue rubber bleb nevus syndrome: case report and literature review. Rom J Gastroenterol 2004; 13:237–240.

37. Vig EK, Brodkin KI, Raugi GJ, Gladstone H. Blue rubber bleb nevus syndrome in a patient with ataxia and dementia. J Geriatr Psychiatry Neurol 2002; 15:7–11.

38. Busund B, Stray-Pedersen S, Iversen OH, Austad J. Blue rubber bleb nevus syndrome with manifestations in the vulva. Acta Obstet Gynecol Scand 1993; 72:310–313.

39. Apak H, et al. Blue rubber bleb nevus syndrome associated with consumption coagulopathy: treatment with interferon. Dermatology 2004; 208:345–348.

40. Rehman SU, et al. Blue rubber bleb nevus syndrome: associated with severe GI bleeding requiring one hundred blood transfusions. J Pak Med Assoc 2003; 53:570–573.

41. Gilbey LK, Girod CE. Blue rubber bleb nevus syndrome: endobronchial involvement presenting as chronic cough. Chest 2003; 124:760–763.

42. Fish L, Fireman Z, Kopelman Y, Sternberg A. Blue rubber bleb nevus syndrome: small-bowel lesions diagnosed by capsule endoscopy. Endoscopy 2004; 36:836.

43. Fernandes C, Silva A, Coelho A, Campos M, Pontes F. Blue rubber bleb naevus: case report and literature review. Eur J Gastroenterol Hepatol 1999; 11:455–457.

44. Watanabe Y, et al. Multiendoscope-assisted treatment for blue rubber bleb nevus syndrome. Surg Endosc 2000; 14:595.

45. Vollmar J, Vogt K. Angiodysplasia and the skeletal system. Chirurg 1976; 47:205–213.

46. Belov S. Classification of congenital vascular defects. Int Angiol 1990; 9:141–146.

47. Leu HJ. Pathomorphology of vascular malformations. Analysis of 310 cases. Int Angiol 1990; 9:147–154.

48. Servelle M. Klippel and Trenaunay's syndrome. 768 operated cases. Ann Surg 1985; 201:365–373.

49. Gloviczki P, et al. Klippel–Trenaunay syndrome: the risks and benefits of vascular interventions. Surgery 1991; 110:469–479.

50. Baskerville PA, Ackroyd JS, Browse NL. The etiology of the Klippel–Trenaunay syndrome. Ann Surg 1985; 202.624–627.

51. Berry SA, et al. Klippel–Trenaunay syndrome. Am J Med Genet 1998; 79:319–326.

52. Tian XL, et al. Identification of an angiogenic factor that when mutated causes susceptibility to Klippel–Trenaunay syndrome. Nature 2004; 427:640–645.

53. Jacob AG, et al. Klippel–Trenaunay syndrome: spectrum and management. Mayo Clin Proc 1998; 73:28–36.

54. Gloviczki P, et al. Surgical implications of Klippel–Trenaunay syndrome. Ann Surg 1983; 197:353–362.

55. Cohen MM, Jr. Klippel–Trenaunay syndrome. Am J Med Genet 2000; 93:171–175.

56. Servelle M, et al. Hematuria and rectal bleeding in the child with Klippel and Trenaunay syndrome. Ann Surg 1976; 183:418–428.

57. Lindenauer SM. The Klippel–Trenaunay syndrome: varicosity, hypertrophy and haemangioma with no arteriovenous fistula. Ann Surg 1965; 162:303–314.

58. Yamaki T, Nozaki M, Sasaki K. Color duplex-guided sclerotherapy for the treatment of venous malformations. Dermatol Surg 2000; 26:323–328.

59. Jain R, Bandhu S, Sawhney S, Mittal R. Sonographically guided percutaneous sclerosis using 1% polidocanol in the treatment of vascular malformations. J Clin Ultrasound 2002; 30:416–423.

60. Edstrom DW, Ros AM. The treatment of port-wine stains with the pulsed dye laser at 600 nm. Br J Dermatol 1997; 136:360–363.

61. Scherer K, Lorenz S, Wimmershoff M, Landthaler M, Hohenleutner U. Both the flashlamp-pumped dye laser and the long-pulsed tunable dye laser can improve results in port-wine stain therapy. Br J Dermatol 2001; 145:79–84.

62. Edstrom DW, Hedblad MA, Ros AM. Flashlamp pulsed dye laser and argon-pumped dye laser in the treatment of port-wine stains: a clinical and histological comparison. Br J Dermatol 2002; 146:285–289.

63. Bencini PL. The multilayer technique: a new and fast approach for flashlamp-pumped pulsed (FLPP) dye laser treatment of port-wine stains (preliminary reports). Dermatol Surg 1999; 25:786–789.

64. Mulliken JB, Glowacki J. Hemangiomas and vascular malformations in infants and children: a classification based on endothelial characteristics. Plast Reconstr Surg 1982; 69:412–422.

65. Nomori H, Nara S, Morinaga S, Soejima K. Primary malignant lymphoma of superior vena cava. Ann Thorac Surg 1998; 66:1423–1424.

66. Rulli F, et al. Primary malignant lymphoma of the saphenous vein. J Vasc Surg 2002; 35:168–171.

67. Humphrey M, Neff J, Lin F, Krishnan L. Leiomyosarcoma of the saphenous vein. A case report and review of the literature. J Bone Joint Surg Am 1987; 69:282–286.

68. Dasika U, Shariati N, Brown JM, III. Resection of a leiomyosarcoma of the azygos vein. Ann Thorac Surg 1998; 66:1405.

69. Gurbuz A, Yetkin U, Yilik L, Ozdemir T, Turk F. A case of leiomyosarcoma originating from pulmonary vein, occluding mitral inflow. Heart Lung 2003; 32:210–214.

70. Thomas MA. Leiomyosarcoma of veins. Cancer 1960; 13:96–101.

71. Celdran A, et al. Leiomyosarcoma of the portal venous system: a case report and review of literature. Surgery 2004; 135:455–456.

72. Hiratuka Y, Ikeda H, Sugaya Y, Tozuka K, Yamada S. A case of leiomyosarcoma of the renal vein. Nippon Hinyokika Gakkai Zasshi 2001; 92:38–41.

73. Taheri SA, Conner GW. Leiomyosarcoma of iliac veins. Surgery 1983; 94:516–520.

74. Iannelli A, et al. Leiomyosarcoma of the ovarian vein: report of a case. Int Surg 2003; 88:6–8.

75. Dzsinich C, et al. Primary venous leiomyosarcoma: a rare but lethal disease. J Vasc Surg 1992; 15:595–603.

76. Bailey RV, Stribling J, Weitzner S, Hardy JD. Leiomyosarcoma of the inferior vena cava: report of a case and review of the literature. Ann Surg 1976; 184:169–173.

77. Griffin AS, Sterchi JM. Primary leiomyosarcoma of the inferior vena cava: a case report and review of the literature. J Surg Oncol 1987; 34:53–60.

78. Bower TC, Stanson AW. Diagnosis and management of tumors of the inferior vena cava. In: Rutherford RB, ed. Vascular Surgery. Philadelphia. WB Saunders Company, 2000:2077–2092.

79. Okur N, Inal M, Akgul E, Binokay F. Case report: pedunculated leiomyosarcoma of the inferior vena cava. Tani Girisim Radyol 2003; 9:78–80.

80. Burke AP, Virmani R. Sarcomas of the great vessels. A clinicopathologic study. Cancer 1993; 71:1761–1773.

81. Mingoli A, et al. The effect of extend of caval resection in the treatment of inferior vena cava leiomyosarcoma. Anticancer Res 1997; 17:3877–3881.

82. Kracht M, et al. Acute Budd-Chiari syndrome secondary to leiomyosarcoma of the inferior vena cava. Ann Vasc Surg 1989; 3:268–272.

83. Justiniani FR, Cohen GH, Roen SA, Arribas I, Kushner DS. Budd-Chiari syndrome due to leiomyosarcoma of the inferior vena cava. Am J Dig Dis 1973; 18:337–346.

84. Taylor RW, Sylwestrowicz T, Kossakowska AE, Urbanski SJ, Minuk GY. Leiomyosarcoma of the inferior vena cava presenting as Budd-Chiari syndrome. Liver 1987; 7:201–205.

85. Satoh M, Katoh J, Onodera S. Leiomyosarcoma of the inferior vena cava causing Budd-Chiari syndrome—a case report. Angiology 1993; 44:673–676.

86. Basu SK, Scott TD, Wilmshurst CC, MacEachern AG, Clyne CA. Leiomyosarcomata of the popliteal vessels: rare primary tumours. Eur J Vasc Surg 1988; 2:423–425.

87. Berlin O, Stener B, Kindblom LG, Angervall L. Leiomyosarcomas of venous origin in the extremities. A correlated clinical, roentgenologic, and morphologic study with diagnostic and surgical implications. Cancer 1984; 54:2147–2159.

88. Bower TC, et al. Vena cava replacement for malignant disease: is there a role? Ann Vasc Surg 1993; 7:51–62.

89. Bower TC, et al. Replacement of the inferior vena cava for malignancy: an update. J Vasc Surg 2000; 31:270–281.

90. Kalsbeek HL. Leiomyosarcoma of the inferior vena cava. Arch Chir Neerl 1974; 26:35–40.

91. Harris LM, Karakousis CP. Intravenous leiomyomatosis with cardiac extension: tumor thrombectomy through an abdominal approach. J Vasc Surg 2000; 31:1046–1051.

92. Norris HJ, Parmley T. Mesenchymal tumors of the uterus V. Intravenous leiomyomatosis. A clinical and pathologic study of 14 cases. Cancer 1975; 36:2164–2178.

36
Popliteal Vein Entrapment

Seshadri Raju and Peter Neglén
*River Oaks Hospital and University of Mississippi Medical Center,
Jackson, Mississippi, U.S.A.*

Popliteal vein compression as an intra-operative finding was first reported by Rich and Hughes in 1967 (1). Sporadic case reports (2–13) and two large series (14,15) have appeared since. Popliteal vein compression is frequently seen on routine venography even in asymptomatic extremities. When ankle maneuvers are carried out, popliteal vein compression can be seen in 42% of ascending venograms (15) performed for a variety of unrelated indications. Leon et al. (16) have shown that positional compression of the popliteal vein with reduction in outflow fraction can be demonstrated in as many as 27% of limbs of normal healthy adults. In this regard the situation is not unlike thoracic outlet syndrome; anatomic vascular compression occurs ubiquitously but is clinically significant in only a small fraction. Diagnosis is frequently uncertain due to the lack of reliable specific testing. Under the circumstances, clinical approach should be one of caution: the diagnosis should be considered only when other more common causes of chronic venous insufficiency have been eliminated. Surgical decompression should be considered only when conservative measures have been adequately tried and failed.

INCIDENCE

As a pathologic entity, popliteal vein compression is estimated to have a prevalence of less than 4% of patients presenting with symptoms of chronic venous insufficiency (15). Contrary to expectations, the disease is not confined to the young; there appears to be no age or sex predilection.

CLINICAL FEATURES

Symptoms and signs are the same as in chronic venous insufficiency: swelling, pain and stasis skin changes including ulceration. Limb swelling extending above the knee joint probably rules out the condition as the primary pathology. Some patients may complain of increased limb pain on ambulation (venous claudication); patients with non–obstructive venous insufficiency generally report relief of pain on ambulation. Hyperpigmentation

483

may extend beyond the gaiter area to involve the middle and upper third of the calf as well. Isolated popliteal valve reflux, when symptomatic, should arouse suspicion of associated vein compression as the former by itself is seldom symptomatic.

VENOGRAPHY

Popliteal vein compression on ascending venography is not specific for the clinical syndrome but is very sensitive. For credible diagnosis, compression should be demonstrated on active plantar flexion; passive dorsiflexion may also reproduce the lesion in some. In one series of symptomatic patients (15) the venographic site of compression was high popliteal in 11%, midpopliteal in 39%, low popliteal in 18% and diffuse in 32%, thus suggesting varied compressive mechanisms; in 34%, the contralateral limb also showed venographic compression. Associated popliteal artery compression could be demonstrated by photoplethysmography in 57% of limbs in this series even though none had clinical features of arterial insufficiency. Demonstration of arterial compression does not signify functionally significant associated venous compression.

OTHER IMAGING TECHNIQUES

Duplex examination with ankle maneuvers can readily demonstrate popliteal vein compression without any inference to causality of symptoms (16). Magnetic resonance imaging (17,18) may display abnormal features of the gastrocnemius muscle that is frequently a part of the compressive mechanism, and it can also help rule out other causes of compression such as the Baker's cyst (7,12).

FUNCTIONAL TESTS

Increased postexercise pressure and reduced outflow fraction may be suggestive but these tests are neither sensitive nor specific (15). Similar comments apply to airplethysmography with regard to subnormal ejection fraction and increased residual volume (Fig. 1).

Dynamic popliteal vein pressure measurements (Fig. 2) with ankle exercise may be diagnostic and help document successful surgical lysis of the compressive elements (15).

PATHOLOGY

The most frequent external compressive mechanism is abnormalities in the origin of the medial head of the gastrocnemius muscle (Table 1). Other muscular anomalies including that of the lateral head of the gastrocnemius and soleal sling are relatively rare. In contrast to popliteal artery entrapment, anatomic course variations of the vein appear to be relatively uncommon. Migration of the medial head extending its origin from the medial femoral condyle to involve portions of the adjacent femoral shaft is a normal postnatal event in the development of the gastrocnemius muscle; excessive migration involving more of the femoral shaft appears to result in compression of the vein. The compressed segment becomes sclerosed and stenotic; both prestenotic and poststenotic dilatations may occur, occasionally large enough to be classified as aneurysms. A thick perivenous fascia fused to the gastrocnemius muscle fascia was noted in nearly half the cases and may play a significant part in the compressive mechanism. Traction on the perivenous sheath by the

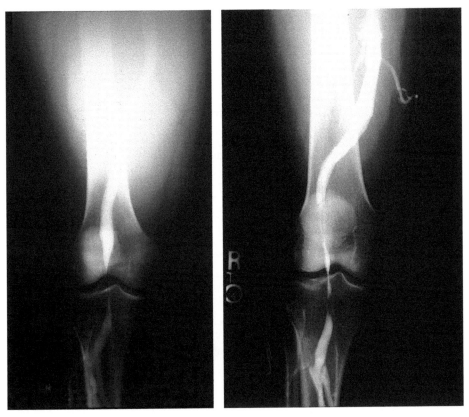

Figure 1 Popliteal vein compression with ankle maneuvers: mid popliteal (*left*), and diffuse (*right*). Compressive lesions at high and low popliteal locations (not shown) also occur.

adherent contracting muscle leading to stretching of the vein may explain the varied location of vein compression noted on venography. The entrapment mechanism is likely more complex than simple external compression by adjacent muscle; this is signified by the prolonged interval for normalization of the popliteal vein pressure after cessation of

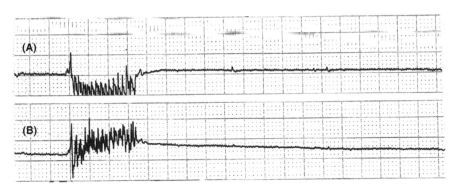

Figure 2 Simultaneous pressure tracings in the dorsal foot vein and popliteal vein with calf exercise. Note elevation in popliteal pressure and decrease in foot venous pressure after exercise. Popliteal pressure elevation persists for 100 seconds after cessation of exercise before slowly declining to baseline.

Table 1 Pathological Features in 30 Cases Undergoing Entrapment Release

	Number
Compressive entrapment mechanism	
Gastrocnemius medial head anomalous origin	18[a]
Additional "3rd" head of gastrocnemius	1
Gastrocnemius lateral head origin from medial condyle	5
Soleus sling	3
Thick perivenous fascia	13[b]
Abnormal course of vascular bundle lateral to the lateral head	2
Unknown	1
Pathological changes in the popliteal vein	
Sclerosis	13
Pre-stenotic dilatation	1
Post-stenotic dilatation	4[c]
Postthrombotic changes	2

[a] One case associated with atrophic lateral head.
[b] Associated with other entrapment mechanisms.
[c] Two saccular aneurysms.

active muscle contraction (Fig. 2). Popliteal vein entrapment may lead to thrombosis (19). There is speculation that entrapment may eventually lead to popliteal valve reflux (15) and perforator incompetence (20).

OPERATIVE LYSIS

The posterior approach (20) to the popliteal fossa is standard for release of the entrapment and to recognize anatomic course variations of the vessel; the authors have found the familiar medial approach (15) to be satisfactory as well; it also provides the necessary exposure. The medial head of the gastrocnemius is taken down and the vein is freed of any other restrictive elements. Iwai et al. (9) recommend actual resection of the medial head to reduce the chance of recurrence. The vein is cleared of its perivenous sheath and tributaries over a generous 10 cm length centred on the compressive point. Aneurysmal and stenotic segments should be resected and the vein repaired without any hint of tension using a saphenous graft If necessary, The popliteal valve should be repaired if reflexive, particularly when skin changes are present. Axillary vein transfer may be required if primary valve reconstruction is not possible (15). Perioperative antithrombotic prophylaxis including use of low molecular weight heparin, meticulous hemostasis, and closed drainage are necessary to achieve clean primary healing without local complications that may predispose to recurrence.

CLINICAL RESULTS

Excellent clinical results with relief of pain, swelling and stasis skin changes have been reported, particularly when the diagnosis was firmly established on the basis of dynamic popliteal vein pressure measurements.

KEY POINTS

- *Anatomic* popliteal vein compression with ankle maneuvers can be demonstrated frequently in patients with chronic venous insufficiency and even in many normal limbs. Anatomic compression alone, therefore, does not indicate clinical entrapment syndrome.
- *Clinical* popliteal vein entrapment is a rare entity that should be considered in the differential diagnosis only when the more common causes of chronic venous insufficiency have been ruled out or corrected.
- As yet, a widely accepted specific diagnostic test is lacking. Dynamic popliteal vein pressure measurement holds promise.
- When patients are carefully selected, entrapment release can be expected to yield good to excellent clinical results.
- Many aspects of the pathophysiology of the syndrome are obscure and remain to be fully understood.

REFERENCES

1. Rich NM, Hughes CW. Popliteal artery and vein entrapment. Am J Surg 1967; 113:696–698.
2. Edmondson HT, Crowe JA, Jr. Popliteal arterial and venous entrapment. Am Surg 1972; 38:657–659.
3. Connell J. Popliteal vein entrapment. Br J Surg 1978; 65:351.
4. Mastaglia FL, Venerys J, Stokes BA, Vaughan R. Compression of the tibial nerve by the tendinous arch of origin of the soleus muscle. Clin Exp Neurol 1981; 18:81–85.
5. Koplic S, Maskovic J, Radonic V. Musculotendinous pressure on the arteries of the knee observed in a patient with obstructive entrapment syndrome of the popliteal artery and vein. Acta Chir Iugosl 1982; 29:189–193.
6. Zelli GP, Mattei E. Unusual phlebopathy of the lower limbs. Considerations on a case of congenital compression (entrapment) of the popliteal vein. Ann Ital Chir 1982; 54:245–252.
7. Zygmunt S, Keller K, Lidgren L. Baker cyst causing nerve entrapment. Scand J Rheumatol 1982; 11:239–240.
8. van Berge Henegouwen DP, Salzmann P, Lindner F. Entrapment and cystic degeneration of the adventitia as a cause of occlusion of the popliteal artery. Chirurg 1986; 57:797–800.
9. Iwai T, Sato S, Yamada T, et al. Popliteal vein entrapment caused by the third head of the gastrocnemius muscle. Br J Surg 1987; 74:1006–1008.
10. Van Damme H, Dallnux JM, Dereume JP. Femoro-popliteal venous graft entrapment. J Cardiovasc Surg (Torino) 1988; 29:50–55.
11. Nelson MC, Teitelbaum GP, Matsumoto AH, Stull MA. Isolated popliteal vein entrapment. Cardiovasc Intervent Radiol 1989–1990; 12:301–303.
12. Rettori R, Boespflug O. Popliteal vein entrapment, popliteal cyst, desmoid tumor and fabella syndrome. J Mal Vasc 1990; 15:182–187.
13. Sieunarine K, Prendergast FJ, Paton R, Goodman MA, Ibach EG. Entrapment of popliteal artery and vein. Aust NZ J Surg 1990; 60:533–537.
14. di Marzo L, Cavallaro A, Sciacca V, Mingoli A, Tamburelli A. Surgical treatment of popliteal artery entrapment syndrome: a ten-year experience. Eur J Vasc Surg 1991; 5:59–64.
15. Raju S, Neglen P. Popliteal vein entrapment: a benign venographic feature or a pathologic entity? J Vasc Surg 2000; 31:631–641.
16. Leon M, Volteas N, Labropoulos N, et al. Popliteal vein entrapment in the normal population. Eur J Vasc Surg 1992; 6:623–627.
17. Fermand M, Houlle D, Cormier JM, Vitoux JF, Lignieres G. Popliteal vein entrapment shown by MR imaging. AJR Am J Roentgenol 1990; 155:424–425.

18. Di Cesare E, Marsili L, Marino G, et al. Stress MR imaging for evaluation of popliteal artery entrapment. J Magn Reson Imaging 1994; 4:617–622.
19. Gerkin TM, Beebe HG, Williams DM, Bloom JR, Wakefield TW. Popliteal vein entrapment presenting as deep venous thrombosis and chronic venous insufficiency. J Vasc Surg 1993; 18:760–766.
20. Di Marzo L, Cisternino S, Sapienza P, et al. Entrapment syndrome of the popliteal vein: results of the surgical treatment. Ann Ital Chir 1996; 67:515–519; discussion 519–520.

37

Management of Venous Trauma

Denis W. Harkin and Paul H. Blair
Regional Vascular Surgery Unit, Royal Victoria Hospital, Belfast, Northern Ireland

INTRODUCTION AND MAGNITUDE OF PROBLEM

A paucity of good quality evidence exists in the literature concerning the management of venous trauma. Most available information arises from retrospective case-control or cohort studies, and of course expert opinion. Considerable heterogeneity is seen within and between series in the population, clinical characteristics, associated factors, mechanism and extent of injury, anatomical distribution, operative management, and clinical outcome in these patients. This somewhat limits generalizations to other patient populations. Therefore, in this chapter we shall endeavor to present the best quality available information, qualified by our own experience with the management of civilian vascular trauma over 25 years of urban conflict in Northern Ireland, at the Royal Victoria Hospital (1).

Premature death and disability due to trauma has been highlighted as one of the major public health concerns in the developed world. As such the epidemiology of trauma has been well-characterized. It is the leading cause of death in adults under 40 years in the developed world, and more concerning trauma accounts for the greatest number of years of life lost. In recent years data quality has improved with the centralization of trauma services and the adoption by many regions of computerized registries. However, information on the incidence and etiology of venous trauma, or indeed any vessel trauma, with respect to the population as a whole, is still scarce. Epidemiological studies of vascular injuries are largely based on the clinical experience accumulated with military campaigns and civilian trauma (1–3). Overall the civilian incidence of vascular injuries is relatively low, estimated at 0.9 to 2.3 per 100,000 of the population (4). In military settings the incidence of vascular injury remains devastatingly high.

Ideally major vascular trauma should be dealt with in a facility that combines appropriate expertise, access to diagnostic modalities, and the full range of endovascular and open treatment options. The severely injured patient with multiple injuries requires a multidisciplinary approach in assessment, management, and rehabilitation from injury. Individualized management may include the coordinated activities of general, vascular, cardio-thoracic, plastic, and orthopaedic surgeons. Furthermore, in order to achieve restoration of optimal function many other allied heathcare professionals will be required, such as physiotherapists, occupational therapists, psychologists, nutritionists, and specialist nurses.

PATHOPHYSIOLOGY OF VENOUS TRAUMA

Vein trauma has often played a supporting role to arterial trauma, with respect to clinical importance in the setting of vascular trauma. However, as every practicing vascular surgeon knows, there is nothing more deadly than the progressive exsanguination seen with major venous injury. Historically there was a clear distinction between the mechanism of injury between military and civilian trauma. The former mainly arising from high velocity penetrating injury (bullets, missiles, shrapnel) the later mainly high velocity blunt trauma (road traffic accident) or low velocity penetrating injury (knife injuries). However, many large urban civilian centers now experience similar rates of "military style" injury to the battlefield, an experience which shall surely increase if modern trends continue in respect to gun crime and civilian terrorism.

Environment and Population

Over the last century military conflict involving modern weapons of war have taught us many important lessons in respect to the management of vascular trauma, albeit with considerable cost to limb and life. Much of our current practice in the management of vascular trauma owes origin to seminal studies arising from major conflict in World War II, the Korean War, the Vietnam War, and Bosnian War (5–8). The majority of these injuries were caused by high velocity penetrating injury from bullet, missile, or blast associated shrapnel. The injuries reported involve mainly the extremities, and this in part reflects the battlefield mortality with high velocity penetrating injuries to the neck or trunk. Venous injuries are rarely seen in isolation with high velocity penetrating trauma, but are often accompanied by injuries to arteries, nerves, bones, or soft-tissues. Many lessons have been learned with respect to the early stabilization, rapid transport, and operative exposures used with these casualties (9). However, one must be cautious in drawing conclusions in civilian practice based on military series, dealing as they do with a much higher proportion of penetrating and high velocity injury, often in a healthy young adult male population (3). Historically, the incidence of civilian vascular trauma roughly paralleled the increasing mechanization of society with accidents encountered with mans exposure to industry, agriculture and transport. Despite major public health initiatives to make road transport safer, road traffic accidents remain a leading cause of traumatic death in developed societies. Vascular injuries may arise from blunt trauma, deceleration injuries, and penetrating injuries. In the urban setting low velocity penetrating injury from knives or other weapons remain common. However, many large urban centers are now also facing the challenge of "battlefield" injuries in the urban setting, due to the proliferation of firearm crime and urban terrorism (10). Wide geographical variation does exist for instance in the developed world. Rates of firearm crime are much higher in urban centers in the United States of America when compared to Europe (4).

Mechanism of Vascular Injury

With respect to firearms related injuries, low velocity injuries are often defined as those caused by hand guns (muzzle velocity of up to 300 m/s) whereas high velocity injuries are defined as those caused by rifles and semi-automatic rifles (muzzle velocity > 900 m/s). It is also known that a bullet often may not follow a straight path through tissues, especially where kinetic energy is low (11,12). Indeed vascular injury may occur without apparent direct trauma to the vessel. Shockwave experiments have demonstrated significant damage to all layers of the vessel wall. This "percussion" effect may sufficiently displace and distort the vessel anatomy to produce thrombosis, embolism, and extravasation (12). High velocity weapons in particular dissipate a large amount of energy as the projectile passes through the tissues. This cavitational effect can cause tissue destruction well beyond the path of the missile (13).

Blunt vascular injury resulting from road traffic accidents, and to a lesser degree, falls from height and crush injury, may account for over 50% of all non-iatrogenic vascular injuries. A strong correlation has been noted between increasing severity of injury and incidence of associated vascular injury (14). As expected, increased dissipation of kinetic forces to the trauma victim generated during deceleration result in more severe injuries and poor outcome. Furthermore, blunt injury to vessels in the neck, thorax, and abdomen is often associated with severe brain, lung or abdominal visceral injury (15). Blunt trauma, if extreme, may simply crush and devitalize tissue exposed to such injury. More commonly the stretching effect on tissues of varying compliance leads to tearing of the inelastic intima with exposure of the thrombogenic media, which may become a nidus for embolism or for propagation of thrombus and thrombosis. Major skeletal trauma is often associated with specific vascular injury patterns. Blunt thoracic vascular injuries are more common in the presence of first rib or sternal fractures (16,17). Pelvic arterial and venous injuries are common in the presence of major pelvic fractures or dislocations (18). Extremity fractures and dislocations are often associated with vessel injury, most notably knee dislocation and popliteal injury (19). These skeletal injuries in part reflect the degree of force transmitted but also exemplify how bones can become secondary internal missiles in certain traumatic settings.

Currently iatrogenic vascular trauma is responsible for 5% to 75% of vascular injuries in civilian practice, an incidence that varies according to the type of vascular practice studied and the referral bias (20). With the increased trend for invasive monitoring and central venous catheterization there has been an inevitable increase in iatrogenic venous injuries. These may include thrombotic occlusion, perforation, or arterio-venous fistula. Retroperitoneal hematoma is the most frequent major mechanical complication of femoral venous catheterization, occurring in up to 1.3% of cases (21), whereas pneumothorax is the most frequent major complication of subclavian venous catheterization, occurring in 1.5 to 2.3% of cases (22). Reported rates of catheter related thrombosis range from 6.6 to 25% with femoral vein catheterization, and 10% to 50% with subclavian catheterization (23). There is little doubt that any current frequency estimates of iatrogenic venous trauma are a gross underestimate as many do not lend to major adverse events. A small proportion of these are iatrogenic operative injuries, but when they involve low-pressure high-flow venous systems in difficult anatomic locations, such as pelvic, retrohepatic caval, and portal venous regions, they can be especially treacherous (24). Several specific surgical procedure carry increased risk of inadvertent venous trauma. Hepatic and pancreaticobiliary procedures inevitably expose hepatic, portal and splanchnic veins to risk. Operations involving the lower lumbar spine are occasionally associated with vena caval injuries. Furthermore, as oncological surgery, particularly in the pelvis and retroperitoneum, continues to approach increasingly advanced tumours injuries to associated veins shall continue to increase. One special area worthy of mention are iatrogenic vascular injury associated with blind-insertion of laparoscopic insufflation devices, these injuries in the past caused several fatalities but with the advent of open-insertion techniques they are now essentially of historical interest only (25).

DIAGNOSIS OF VENOUS TRAUMA

The modern clinician can call on a vast array of complementary imaging modalities to confirm or refute any suspicion raised of major venous trauma. Perhaps reassuringly for those treating the trauma patient, clinical assessment by an experienced clinician with a high index of suspicion will identify the majority of clinically significant venous injuries. In the acute phase clinical signs relate to hemorrhage, occlusion, or acute venous hypertension. Hemorrhage in the setting of penetrating trauma may be apparent, particularly if an extremity is primarily involved. Blunt trauma, and particularly injury to the deep torso veins, may be much more subtle where it is often at least temporarily concealed by tamponade of this low-pressure system by surrounding tissues. In the chronic phase clinical signs relate to venous thrombo-embolism, stenosis, and chronic venous hypertension. Many deep venous occlusions are initially clinically inconspicuous due to an ample collateral circulation, but may later cause serious problems with distal venous hypertension. At present, the available diagnostic modalities are clinical examination, ultrasound (US), contrast venography, computed tomography (CT), and magnetic resonance (MR) imaging.

Clinical Examination

A thorough clinical examination from an experienced vascular surgeon is an obvious prerequisite to any more advanced diagnostic modality. This is particularly relevant in the unstable patient when rapid decisions about treatment paradigms must be made. The correct interpretation of clinical signs in the context of knowledge of the mechanism of injury can be enough to dictate immediate surgical care or order further confirmatory investigations. In arterial injury hard signs may be an obvious spur to invasive management, but with isolated venous injury the signs may be much more subtle. Clinical signs of vascular injury may be "soft" signs (history of bleeding, non-pulsatile hematoma) or "hard" signs (pulsatile hematoma, bruit, thrill, pulse deficit) (Table 1). With major venous injury in chest or abdomen signs of hemorrhage or hypotension will be frank. With penetrating injury, in particular if soft-tissue loss is extensive, venous bleeding may be profuse but often controlled with simple direct application of pressure and elevation. Blunt venous injury is often contained by local tissue tamponade and coagulum formation, and the only visible external signs may be hematoma and distal evidence of venous hypertension.

Venous Imaging (Ultrasound, Computed Tomography, Magnetic Resonance Imaging, Venography)

Duplex ultrasonography can provide a rapid mode of bedside assessment in the unstable trauma patient. Focused Assessment with Sonography for Trauma (FAST) has been

Table 1   The Clinical Manifestations of Vascular Injury

Hard signs	Soft signs
Pulsatile bleeding	Hematoma (small)
Expanding hematoma	History of hemorrhage at scene
Absent distal pulses	Unexplained hypotension
Cold, pale limb	Peripheral nerve deficit
Palpable thrill	
Audible bruit	

widely adopted by many trauma units worldwide and can identify free fluid (suggestive of hemorrhage) by rapid assessment of key area namely the peri-hepatic, peri-splenic, pelvis, and pericardium (26). In the setting of suspected cervical or extremity vascular injury it can also provide rapid confirmation of vessel integrity, blood-flow, bleeding, and associated solid organ pathology. However, it is operator dependant, site-specific, two-dimensional, and is of limited use in the thorax or indeed in the large gaseous abdomen.

Contrast-enhanced CT is becoming the examination of choice in major trauma, due in part to its widespread availability, speed, and three-dimensional capability. It gives information not only on the venous and arterial system but anatomical relations and associated injuries to other solid viscera.

MR imaging undoubtedly can provide superb images of venous anatomy and integrity. However, it has limitations perhaps most apparent in the emergency situation, in that it is not readily available in many units, the confined space makes it unsuitable for some trauma patients, and the data-acquisition and interpretation time can be long.

Contrast venography in the elective setting remains the gold standard for assessment of the venous system (27). The sensitivity of venography is almost 100%, and in theory it can identify venous pathology at any bodily site. The classical findings of acute venous thrombosis are a filling defect with surrounding contrast medium "tram-tracking," or abrupt vessel cut-off distant from a valve in the case of total occlusion. However, venography is invasive and has associated complications such as allergic reactions, nephrotoxicity, and phlebitis, and thus its use is limited to carefully selected patients. Increasingly, a variety of endoluminal venous therapies may be conducted to staunch hemorrhage (such as placement of a covered-stent or embolization), or to aid recanalization (such as clot aspiration, catheter-directed lysis, venoplasty, and venous stenting) (27).

MANAGEMENT PRINCIPLES FOR VENOUS TRAUMA

Once the diagnosis of acute venous trauma has been verified, the next step is adequate treatment. The objectives of any acute therapeutic regime are restoration of unimpeded venous return, prevention of recurrent occlusion, preservation of valve function, and prevention of thrombo-embolism. However, the importance of associated injury must be at the forefront of any treatment algorithm. Often the venous injury is only one of several life or limb threatening injuries and the vascular clinician, as part of a multidisciplinary healthcare, must address these injuries and management on the basis of clinical priority. In the setting of civilian trauma, and the practice in our unit, all patients are evaluated by the general surgery/trauma service upon arrival in the emergency department, and resuscitation carried out in accordance with the Advanced Trauma Life Support (ATLS) guidelines (28).

Resuscitation must be considered holistically in the unstable trauma patients remembering the priority is operative control of hemorrhage. Excessive fluid resuscitation in an attempt to normalize blood pressure in the absence of hemorrhage control will simply encourage clot dislodgement and re-bleeding (29). Furthermore, the dilution effect may well compound hypothermia and coagulopathy. Common practice in most centers now is to allow permissive-hypotension sufficient to maintain cerebral perfusion (30). Indeed in a conscious patient who is talking and orientated, blood pressure may be assumed adequate regardless of any measured value. In the unconscious patient a systolic pressure of 60–70 mmHg is adequate in most circumstances. If volume depletion from hemorrhage is the obvious cause of hypotension then fluid resuscitation should be the action of choice. Inappropriate use of inotropes to support the circulation in a hypovolaemic patient shall simply increase myocardial work and oxygen demand. Venous access should be secured with at least two large bore peripheral lines, and warmed fluids should be given as required through a rapid infusion system. Once hemorrhage control has been achieved vigorous resuscitation efforts should aim to restore adequate tissue perfusion and oxygen delivery. A combination of blood replacement, crystalloid, and clotting factors should help correct volume, acidosis, hypothermia, and coagulopathy.

Nonoperative Management of Venous Trauma

The management of minimal, non-occlusive, clinically asymptomatic venous injuries detected by imaging remains controversial. At all points the surgeon must give considered thought to nonoperative management to the hemodynamically stable patient as this policy undoubtedly saves lives. In a stable patient conservative management has been successfully employed for retroperitoneal blunt retroperitoneal and hepatic injuries (31). It is also advocated for pelvic fractures associated with venous injury (32), and can be selectively employed for cervico-thoracic injury (33). However, observation must be carried out in a high dependency environment and imaging modalities fully utilized to exclude serious associated injuries.

Surgical Management of Venous Trauma

Operative strategy considered by the surgeon in charge is crucial as patient positioning and exposure, particularly in polytrauma where several procedures are contemplated often with a multidisciplinary team of surgeons, can aid or hinder the success of the procedures. The procedure sequencing priority, to include any potential "bail-out" options, is best considered at this stage. In particular with vascular or orthopaedic injuries the operating table and patient position should be compatible with the use of on-table angiography. The full extent of the injury, including any possible missile tracts, as well as proximal vessel control access point must be prepared. Often other limbs shall be required for vein conduit harvest. Distal parities should be transparently draped to allow assessment of distal perfusion. Attention should also be given to the prevention of hypothermia and external warming, using warm air or fluid–mattress. Liberal exposure cannot be overemphasized in the setting of uncontrolled bleeding and the original incision may be extended or supplemented by a secondary incision. In general the approach follows standard exposure principles in the thorax, abdomen and extremities and is dictated by the suspected site of injury. In the unstable patient open packing with scheduled repeat operation for hemostasis is often lifesaving and allows correction of coagulopathy, hypothermia, and acidosis (34,35).

In general, vascular control is obtained initially by digital or sponge–stick compression. Balloon occlusion catheters are occasionally useful to assist with vascular control. With profuse venous bleeding associated with significant hypotension despite venous compression, temporary aortic cross-clamping may allow time for hemorrhage control. With hepatic or retrohepatic venous trauma the Pringle maneuver may staunch bleeding and give valuable time for exposure and control. Vessel exposure and control can be particularly difficult in "hostile" settings where anatomy has been distorted and tissue plains obscured by previous surgery, radiation therapy, cancer, or inflammation. Vessel related complications are more likely in the setting of dirty wounds, subsequent anastamotic dehiscence and vessel "blow-out" may result in fatal exsanguinations.

Therefore, we advocate meticulous vascular coverage in this situation using available means omental flap, muscle flap, or even bovine pericardium.

Temporary intraluminal shunts have revolutionized the management of both arterial and venous trauma care (36,37). A variety of commercial shunts are available, but even sterile heparinized polyethylene tubing or chest tubes will suffice for most vessel sizes encountered. These versatile conduits allow rapid restoration of vessel flow prior to any considered reconstruction. Restoration of arterial inflow arrests tissue hypoxia and prevents further ischaemic damage, while restoration of venous outflow reduces capillary bed pressure and allows controlled release of cellular metabolites. This allows time for a multi-disciplinary approach to these complex multisystem injuries, adequate wound toilet, debridement, orthopaedic manipulation and fixation. Shunts are also used as part of "damage control" surgery, once flow is restored and shunt securely fixed, definitive repair can be delayed by up to 24–48 hours to allow treatment of hypothermia, acidosis, and coagulopathy. Flow can be confirmed with a Doppler transducer.

Venous injuries may be treated by ligation, primary repair (lateral venorrhaphy or end-to-end anastimosis), or complex repair [vein patch, interposition autogenous vein graft or interposition ringed expandable poltetrafluoroethylene (PTFE) graft]. Venous thrombectomy may be necessary as an adjunct. We generally attempt lateral venorrhaphy for partial lacerations, and end-to-end anastimosis for complete lacerations without segmental loss. If venorrhaphy is not possible because of significant vessel narrowing, patch angioplasty with autologous vein or ePTFE graft should be considered. Short interposition graft, most often externally supported ePTFE, are used when multiple lacerations or significant segmental loss, prevent a tension-free anastimosis. In dirty wounds we would recommend the use of autologous vein, usually the contralateral long saphenous or occasionally superficial femoral vein. Size disparities can be overcome with the construction of composite vein grafts using a spiral or panelled graft technique, and although additional time is required for vein harvest with a team surgical approach, this does not usually significantly add to operative time. When using interposition PTFE grafts larger sizes are favored (average 8 mm).

If primary repair is not possible due to the extent of injury and ligation contraindicated due to vessel location, interposition grafting of the vein is required. Several factors influence the choice of conduit, namely: the calibre and length required; the wound contamination, the availability of suitable autologous tissue, the stability of the patient and time available. Although the most appropriate conduit would naturally be a suitably sized portion of autologous vein. In practice this is always compromised by concerns relating to potential size and length mismatches, unavailability of one or both saphenous veins, and the risk of anastamotic disruption with exposed vein grafts. The construction of panelled or spiral vein grafts overcome concerns regarding size mismatch, but although elegant they are time consuming and often inappropriate in the trauma setting. The stability of the patient, associated injuries, and the passage of time may all need to be factored into the surgical equation. In the critically ill patient with significant blood loss prosthetic grafting is a more expedious alternative. However, the use of prosthetic graft carries the risk of graft infection and poor long-term patency.

Endoluminal Management of Venous Trauma

One of the major advances in vascular therapy in the last decade has been the rapid proliferation of endoluminal vascular techniques and therapies. Although invasive venous catheterization itself has lead to an increase in iatrogenic venous injuries, so too have the endoluminal treatments evolved to deal with many of these complications. The endovascular management of hemodynamically stable patients with venous trauma is an appealing concept. In particular, lesions that occur at the base of skull or at infraclavicular or pelvic regions often pose far less difficulty when managed by endoluminal techniques than by traditional surgical exposure. Surgical access is made more challenging by hemorrhage and anatomical distortion in the trauma setting and potentially endoluminal therapy would reduce associated morbidity. Catheter-directed embolization is an adaptable technique, whether with coils or procoagulants, and is particularly useful in management of pelvic hemorrhage (38). More recently it has been used to treat traumatic injuries to larger veins (39). One area of interest is that of covered-stents to treat major venous hemorrhage. One such report describes how fenestrated stent-graft may be used to treat traumatic juxtahepatic vena cava injury (40). The management of these surgically challenging injuries by endoluminal means may also complement open surgical techniques (41). Although evidence is lacking regarding stent patency in trauma, if used in large veins stent patency is quite acceptable even in the treatment of malignant stenosis (42). However, little is known about the long-term patency of venous stents placed for trauma or the potential infective risks, and therefore treatments should be individualized and often combined with complementary open techniques.

Adjuvant Therapy

Medical therapy should include aspirin (75 mg daily), unless contraindicated, and prophylaxis of venous thromboembolism with subcutaneous heparin in all patients. Once postoperative coagulopathy and risk of bleeding have been controlled, it is our practice for all patients to receive 20 mg of subcutaneous low molecular weight heparin (LMWH) every 12 hours. There is little role for post-operative systemic therapeutic heparinization in these patients as more often than not this would be contraindicated by the risk of further hemorrhage from the vascular repair or associated injuries. Intermittent mechanical calf compression has shown promise in the prevention of symptomatic lower limb venous thrombosis in those in whom routine anticoagulant prophylaxis is contraindicated. Postoperatively, injured extremities are kept elevated, thrombo-embolic stocking are presecribed, or in the setting of significant lower limb venous obstruction wrapped with a compression bandage applied from the distal foot to the proximal thigh. Patients begin ambulation once their other injuries allow.

Complications

Major injury related complications include: repeated exploration because of bleeding; permanent organ failure, such as dialysis dependant renal failure or ventilatory-dependent respiratory failure; life-threatening complications from massive hemorrhage or transfusion therapy, such as disseminated intravascular coagulation, acute respiratory distress syndrome, venous thrombosis or pulmonary embolism.

EXTREMITY VENOUS TRAUMA

Epidemiology

It is fair to say that the majority of published literature on venous trauma relates to the lower limb. Rich, drawing on his experience with vascular trauma from the Vietnam War, reported that popliteal and femoral vein ligation was associated with high amputation rates, post-operative edema, and post-thrombotic syndrome (43,44). This was supported at that time by some elegant research studies supporting the role of venous preservation where possible (45,46). However, more recent reports from civilian practice showed no increase in amputation rates when vein ligation was performed, or vein repairs thrombosed (47,48). In one of the few papers where patency of venous reconstruction was quantified by venography in all cases, the thrombosis rate varied from 21% (local repair) to 59% (complex repair) (47). However, in the trauma setting the early use of intraluminal arterial and venous shunts restores vascular homeostasis allowing time for full assessment and vascular reconstruction. In our experience venous repair in the acute setting, even if subsequent patency is limited, reduces limb associated morbidity and amputation (1).

Investigation

Hemorrhage from major venous trauma may be free or contained depending on the injury and anatomical location. In extremity trauma a significant quantity of blood can be lost and concealed in the buttock or thigh, and should be considered in the setting of unexplained hypotension. The diagnosis of significant vascular injury is initially clinical, based on the mechanism of injury and any consequent symptoms or signs. Figure 1 demonstrates the rather inconspicuous external signs of hematoma despite subsequent angiographic evidence of significant blunt vascular injury to the groin resulting in an arteriovenous fistula. Hard signs of vascular injury necessitate immediate surgical intervention. With high velocity injuries, the possibility of fragmentation must be considered well beyond the site of penetration and appropriate pre-operative imaging sought. Duplex US is a useful non-invasive mode of assessing integrity of the peripheral venous system, and in recent year most vascular units and indeed emergency departments have equipped themselves with high-quality portable duplex US scanners. Contrast-enhanced CT, can give rapid assessment of vascular integrity in the injured extremity while also allowing assessment of other injuries to the head, chest, or abdomen. However, delays for imaging may be clinically unacceptable in the unstable patient who would be better served by direct transfer to the operating room.

Management

The priorities of vascular injury are the arrest of hemorrhage and the restoration of normal circulation. As with all traumatic injuries the clinical priority must be to maintain vital organ systems in the first instance namely, airway, breathing, and circulation. Soft-signs are most often best treated expectantly by watchful waiting unless significant associated injury to other structures artery, nerve, or muscle cannot be excluded. This policy should use clinical and radiological means to exclude serious associated injury and involve at least 24-hours of in-hospital observation.

Immediate hemorrhage control by application of direct pressure over the site of injury is the best first-aid measure that can be instituted with minimal resources, targeted dressings or even manual compression by a defined team member will usual control hemorrhage sufficiently for transportation to a definitive care setting. Control of the low-pressure venous system can be achieved in most instances by pressure and elevation. If hemorrhage is welling-up from a deep cavity, such as the tract of a deep knife or gunshot wound, surface control can be difficult and temporary control may be achieved by placing a large urinary catheter (or sengstaken tube) into the cavity, inflating the balloon, and applying traction. Blind attempts at clamping artery or vein in deep cavities without adequate exposure shall inevitably fail and can extensively damage the vessels and surrounding structures. The underlying principles of vascular control dictates that

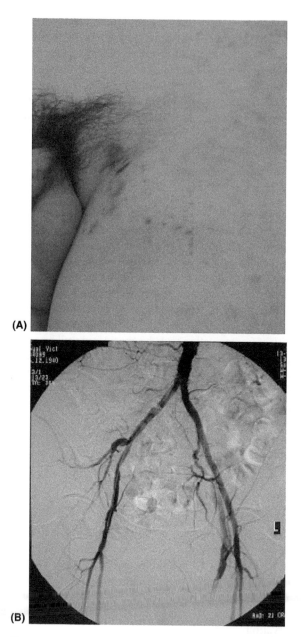

Figure 1 Hematoma in left groin. (**A**) This blunt crush injury to the left groin showed external signs of ecchymosis and hematoma. (**B**) Although apparently vascularly intact on examination, subsequent angiogram reveals a traumatic femoral arteriovenous fistula. (*See color insert.*)

proximal and distal control should be sought prior to exploration of the bleeding site. When isolated venous injury of an extremity warrants exploration, due to uncontrolled hemorrhage or mass effect, then control of arterial inflow may be necessary to reduce venous bleeding. In some settings it is a reasonable precaution to place a proximal pneumatic tourniquet; however, inflation times should be kept to a minimum if secondary ischaemic injury is to be avoided. While it may be tempting to explore a wound that is not actively bleeding, disruption of the local tamponade will rapidly reactivation bleeding

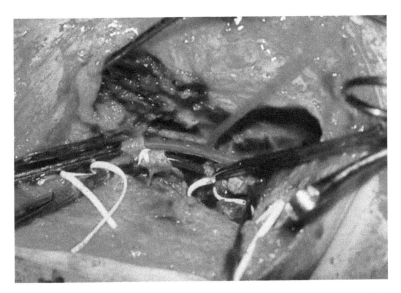

Figure 2 In complex limb trauma intraluminal shunting of both artery and vein is achieved with commercial vessel shunts. Intraluminal shunts rapidly restore blood flow to ischemic distal tissues and allow venous return to decompress the leg. (*See color insert.*)

obscuring anatomy. In general, large veins are easily controlled with elastic vessel slings, passed twice around the vessel to effect closure when tightened. While veins can be clamped care must be taken to use the minimum force necessary. Often digital or sponge stick pressure will be sufficient for local control.

Once the bleeding site is identified adequate segments of the involved vessel must be displayed proximal and distal to the site of injury. Traction injuries in particular can cause extensive intimal injury well beyond the site of external damage, with risk of subsequent thrombosis. Clot should be milked from the vein to restore uninterrupted flow. Figure 2 shows the use of intraluminal arterial and venous shunts to restore vascular homeostasis to an injured limb. Small, clean, transverse wound may undergo simple lateral suture if only part of the circumference is involved. A vein patch may be required to repair a larger defect in the vein wall where direct suture wound lead to vessel narrowing. If a longer segment is damaged, and despite full mobilization primary repair would result in tension, then interposition grafting must be considered. Ideally the most suitable graft would be autologous contralateral reversed long saphenous vein. In certain settings synthetic PTFE can be considered. Some surgeons advocate the construction of panel and spiral grafts from undersized veins, but these are time consuming in practice and unproven to improve patency or outcome. Simple ligation is of course always an option particularly in the hemodynamically unstable patient. Intra-operative venography is indicated if the location of the vessel injury is in doubt or to confirm the patency of the vessel repair. Direct distal introduction of a 18-gauge catheter through a small venotomy will allow the delivery of intravenous contrast which can be mapped with fluoroscopy and digital subtraction venograpy. Many surgeons elect to perform a prophylactic fasciotomy to prevent compartment syndrome particularly if there are major associated injuries (bone, soft tissue), crush injuries, concurrent arterial injury, or if presentation is delayed. Figure 3 demonstrates the typical findings at fasciotomy in a patient with penetrating arterial and venous trauma to the leg, grossly oedematous but viable muscle is seen. Although there is some associated morbidity with respect to the wounds, many of these can be incrementally closed at ward level using a "shoelace" or "pre-placed" suture technique, skin grafts are occasionally required. It also has a role in protecting fragile low-pressure low-flow venous reconstructions.

Damage Control. The basic principles of damage control surgery can be applied equally to arterial or venous trauma. These include ligation, packing, and shunting. Severely injured limbs for which attempted salvage would be futile can be identified using the Mangled Extremity Severity Score (MESS) (49) and require primary amputation not heroic efforts and subsequent mortality. In the unstable patient almost all veins, including the common femoral and even the inferior vena cava, can be ligated where necessary. However, lower limb edema will occur and may be severe in some. Where a significant risk of limb loss exists yet associated systemic injuries limit definitive repair an intraluminal shunt may be used in more commonly in arterial injury but also in major venous trauma, this will also help determine the viability of a severely threatened or dismembered limb. We would suggest that repair of major venous injuries in a stable patient is a reasonable undertaking: however, when venous repair would be complex or the patient is hemodynamically unstable, simple lateral suture or ligation is often appropriate.

Outcomes

Repair of major venous injuries in the lower extremities is felt to decrease the incidence of postoperative venous hypertension and associated chronic venous insufficiency, improve

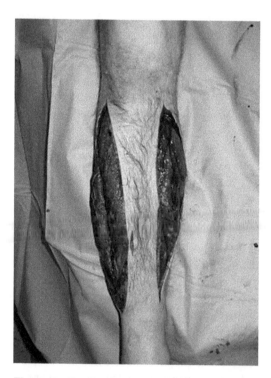

Figure 3 Fasciotomy. This leg suffered gun-shot injuries disrupting arteries and veins below knee; wound tract is included in medial and lateral incisions as part of a four-compartment fasciotomy. Edematous but viable muscle tissue is seen bulging through medial and lateral decompression wounds. (*See color insert.*)

arterial flow as well as patency, and improve limb salvage (1,50). Such complications are most notable with ligation of the popliteal vein (51). Early concerns about increased risks of thrombo-embolism with venous repair of major lower extremity veins have never been proven. Occlusion of the venous repair has been most studied in extremity injury. Meyer et al. (47), found that venous repairs with interposition vein grafting had a significantly higher rate of thrombosis than lateral repair. In contrast more recently, Pappas et al. (52), in a study including 27 primary repairs and 37 complex repairs (including 27 with interposition ringed PTFE) reported overall patency on follow-up venous imaging (Duplex or venography) was 73.8%, with no difference in patency between primary and complex repairs. Adjuncts believed to improve patency rates are subcutaneous infractionated heparin or LMWH, elevation, and graduated compression wrapping. Opponents of complex venous repairs state that most will thrombose, thus negating any potential benefits of the repair. However, recanalization after thrombosis of venous repairs is well documented, and even short-term patency may provide the necessary time to allow recruitment of collaterals. Inevitably chronic venous insufficiency will ensue in some patients, causing symptoms of limb pain, heaviness, edema, skin pigmentation, or ulceration.

NECK VENOUS TRAUMA

Epidemiology

Cervicothoracic vascular injuries are often combined in the literature, even less evidence exists in respect to isolated cervical venous injuries. Carotid artery injuries typically account for 10% of all vascular trauma although wide variation exists depending on the demographics of the reporting vascular practice (53). Associated venous injuries are believed to be grossly under-reported in the literature and isolated venous injury even less so.

Investigation

For the purposes of clinical assessment the neck is often divided into three zones, based on anatomical landmarks (Table 2). Using this system the likely vessels at risk of injury can be considered and management tailored accordingly. However, in a more recent prospective study to test the validity of physical examination in the detection of vascular injury in stable patients with gunshot wounds to the neck, physical examination alone had merely a sensitivity 57% and specificity 53%, positive predictive value 43%, and negative predictive value 67% (54). Therefore other imaging modalities should be used to complement clinical examination such as angiography ultrasonography, and contrast-enhanced CT scanning. Modern endovascular theaters provide the optimal balance between endovascular imaging quality and access to full operative capability, although a portable fluoroscopy unit can provide adequate visualization in most instances.

Management

The management of penetrating and indeed blunt neck trauma has changed in recent years from a position of mandatory exploration to one of selective non-surgical management in a monitored environment. Much of this shift has been influenced by the availability of a range of new diagnostic imaging and therapeutic modalities, including DSA, CT, and MRI. Furthermore, experience with urban trauma has allowed us to better predict clinically the likelihood of negative exploration. The previous policy of routine

Table 2 Anatomical Subdivision of the Neck with Respect to Penetrating Trauma

Region[a]	Anatomical landmarks	Vessels at risk
Zone I	The area of the base of the neck	Subclavian and innominate vessels, the common carotids and lower vertebral arteries and the jugular veins
Zone II	The mid-neck from clavicle to the inferior border of the mandible	Common carotid, carotid bifurcation, the vertebral arteries and the jugular veins
Zone III	Extending from the lower border of the mandible to the base of the skull	Branches of the external carotid artery, the internal carotid artery, vertebral artery and the internal jugular and facial veins

[a] The cervical region is divided into three zones.
Source: From Ref. 63.

exploration of all neck wounds deep to the platysma undoubtedly results in many unnecessary operations. With experience diagnostic adjuncts may be safely used to allow a safe policy of watchful waiting in many individuals provided on can exclude significant injuries to major structures such as the airway, major vessels, esophagus, spinal cord, and nerves.

As always priority lies with life saving measures, protecting airway, ensuring adequate oxygenation, and circulatory support. With respect to venous injury significant external hemorrhage can occur from neck wounds involving the great veins of the neck or their confluence in the upper thorax. In general carefully directed pressure to the point of hemorrhage is an adequate first-aid measure until definitive exploration is possible. Care must be taken to avoid airway compromise either from pressure or from the expanding hematoma. Associated injury to the larynx or trachea is common in penetrating injury, and with the progression of laryngeal edema and hemorrhage, the airway can be rapidly compromised. Prophylactic endotracheal intubation, often with the use of flexible larynoscopy, may avoid subsequent need for emergency cricothyroidotomy, or tracheostomy. Immediate airway compromise is suggested by respiratory distress with stridor, and abnormal see–saw motion of the chest. Low velocity midline injuries and any high velocity penetrating injury are particularly dangerous.

In the neck, especially in zones 2 and 3, hemorrhage can often be controlled externally initially, in zone 1 where injuries often extend into the chest, hemorrhage is often catastrophic. Any penetrating missile still in situ should be left undisturbed. Patients with uncontrollable hemorrhage, expanding hematomas, or shock, need emergency control of hemorrhage. This is best achieved in a fully equipped vascular operating theater. Operative approach is dictated by the site of suspected injury determined by a collation of the mechanism of injury, missile tract, and any preoperative imaging information from angiography (including venography) or CT scan. Where external pressure is insufficient or contraindicated for the control of bleeding a balloon catheter may be introduced into a penetrating wound tract and inflated, once under a degree of traction this should temporarily halt external bleeding. If vessels are visible rapid placement of an occlusive balloon embolectomy catheter may represent a lifesaving measure until definitive care is delivered. Careful inspection for associated injuries to the esophagus, larynx, or nerves should follow definitive vascular care. As in all trauma situations there is a place for damage limitation surgery. While lateral suture will preserve patency in all but the worst injuries, young adults will tolerate unilateral ligation of major neck vein well with minimal morbidity.

Outcomes

Outcomes in many respects are dictated by the degree of vessel related complications and associated injuries. Initial hemorrhage control is essential. Morbidity is generally low from neck venous injuries in the absence of concurrent arterial injury and associated neurological sequelae. Even with complete unilateral occlusion edema or congestion is rarely more than temporary due to the abundance of collateral channels in the head and neck. Although venous thrombo-embolism is a potential concern, especially with venous ligation, again the overall risk is low and this is rarely clinically apparent.

THORACIC VENOUS TRAUMA

Epidemiology

Perhaps the most catastrophic vascular sequelae of blunt or penetrating injuries occur within the chest. With a paucity of surrounding structures to provide tamponade a major venous injury within the chest can bleed catastrophically. Indeed many high velocity injuries shall result in exsanguinations or death before reaching the arena of hospital care. One large reported civilian experience of penetrating cervicomediastinal venous trauma involves 49 patients, with approximately equal numbers undergoing ligation and repair, reports an overall mortality of 16%, with no difference between ligation or repair. In this retrospective study involving mainly young adult males, the majority involving stab injuries, these impressive results appear to have been achieved by a simplistic surgical approach avoiding complex repairs entirely using lateral suture or ligation. However, with high velocity penetrating trauma, and in particular battlefield injuries, mortality is much higher and often occurs in the pre-hospital phase.

Investigation

Apart from hypotension there may be few clinical signs of major intra-thoracic hemorrhage. In the spontaneously breathing patient decreased air entry on one hemithorax may indicate hemothorax, although a late sign. In the ventilated patient again unequal air entry may be elicited or rising airway pressures and falling saturations may indicate a loss of lung capacity. The placement of a chest tube for hemothorax that drains a large rush of blood, or has significant ongoing losses may clinch the diagnosis of intrathoracic vascular injury and dictate immediate transfer for emergency thoracotomy. A chest radiograph is a standard adjunct to any patient with suspected blunt thoracic injury. Signs of major venous injury may include signs of mediastinal hemorrhage or frank hemothorax. Figure 4 demonstrates typical findings of hemothorax on chest radiograph, with subsequent CT scan revealing significant extravasation from a pulmonary vein injury. Although the plain chest radiograph has low sensitivity, when normal it has a 98% predictive value. In the presence of an abnormal mediastinum even in a stable patient further diagnostic imaging is mandatory. As CT technology has developed it has established itself as the best screening modality for major thoracic vascular injury. The sensitivity of modern CT scanners is reported at 97–100%, with a negative predictive value of 100% and specificity of 83–99%. As the newer multi-detector scanners become

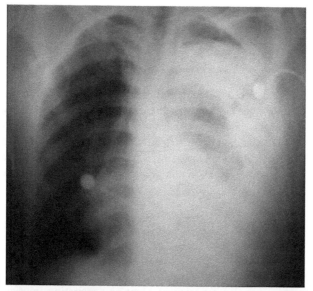

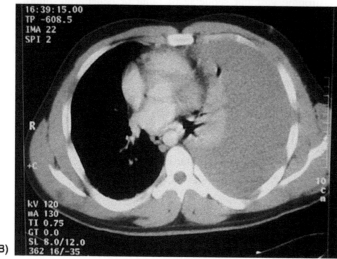

Figure 4 Typical appearances of a massive left hemothorax secondary to penetrating thoracic venous trauma. (A) Chest radiograph shows opacification of left hemithorax due to blood. (B) Contrast-enhanced computed tomography scan of chest confirms massive extravasation from large mediastinal vein (pulmonary vein).

more widespread, their increased resolution, bolus-tracking technology and improved processing software will allow more surgeons to rely solely on the CT scan to plan operative or endovascular repair.

Management

In high velocity blunt injuries sudden deceleration creates shearing and traction forces on major veins and arteries leading to laceration, rupture, or thrombosis. Penetrating injuries may range from small lacerations to complete transaction. Of those patients surviving to the hospital, care must be taken to limit secondary hemorrhage due to over aggressive fluid resuscitation. Cyclical resuscitation attempts, which only temporarily restore normotension to be followed by further rebleeding and hypotension, should alert the clinician to a major vascular injury and prompt urgent investigation and control or hemorrhage. Unfortunately in many rebleeding, iatrogenic hypothermia, and coagulopathy will supervene at which point all attempts at salvage are often futile. Once aortic injury is excluded the extent and stability of the venous injury may be assessed. Contained mediastinal venous injury is best observed in a high-dependancy environment, and shall seldom require delayed open surgical care. If uncontained hemorrhage is present urgent surgical intervention is indicated.

Outcomes

Although the mortality of these injuries is significant, in survivors most morbidity is related only to thoracic wound pain. Edema, of the upper limb is most common after subclavian vein injuries but is often a transient phenomenon. However, often even unilateral internal jugular vein ligation demonstrated no clinical evidence of venous hypertension.

ABDOMINAL VENOUS TRAUMA

Epidemiology

With respect to abdominal trauma most evidence relates to military conflict. During the Lebanese conflict one Israeli trauma center received between 1975 and 1989, 1860 patients with abdominal injuries, reporting that 107 patients (6%) had major abdominal vascular injuries involving 141 vessels (55). Of these injuries 113 (80%) affected the venous system: inferior vena cava (35%), common iliac vein (15.6%), internal iliac vein (15.6%), external iliac vein (9.2%), renal vein (2.1%), and hepatic vein (2.1%) (55). The low mortality rate of 36.5% may be explained in part by the young healthy adult population involved and the rapid transport with short injury to exploration times (mean 45 minutes, range 10 minutes to 5 hours) (55). However, mortality was significantly greater in certain subgroups, in particular vena caval injuries associated with liver fracture (78.5% mortality), vascular injury associated with pelvic fractures (57% mortality), and those with shock (55). Even low-velocity penetrating injury has the potential to cause massive venous bleeding, in Fig. 5, CT scan demonstrates significant intra-abdominal hemorrhage from a penetrating knife injury to the inferior mesenteric vein.

Retrohepatic and juxtahepatic venous trauma has a daunting mortality, which bares testimony to the difficulties inherent in their management. These injuries offer enormous challenges to the vascular surgeon due to the combination of fragmented liver tissue, avulsed or lacerated hepatic veins, and major inferior vena caval injury (56). Atriocaval shunting, balloon shunting, sequential vascular clamping, and perihepatic packing are all methods of treatment with which the surgeon must be familiar (57). Blunt trauma can cause devastating juxta-hepatic venous injury. Figure 6 shows blunt injury due to a motorcycle crash has caused a grade 5 liver injury, with disruption of the right renal vein and vena cava.

Abdominal and pelvic venous traumas similarly carry a very high mortality rate, ranging from 36% to 65% (55,58), particularly where the vena cava is involved. Although historically these injuries expected 100% mortality (59), this failure to enhance survival is despite significant improvements in transport, resuscitation, surgery, and intensive care. It is certainly true that because of the factors mentioned we now have the opportunity to treat

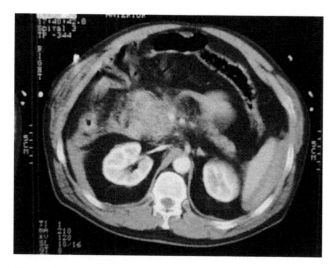

Figure 5 In penetrating trauma this patient sustained a laceration to the superior mesenteric vein and pancreas. Contrast-enhanced computed tomography scan shows extravasation of blood in the upper retrosperitoneum.

those patients who previously would have died in the pre-hospital phase. Death is generally associated with the location of injury and with factors such as hypotension and blood loss, which often herald shock.

Management

Rapid control of hemorrhage is essential and as such outcomes are improved where vessel access and control is more straightforward and simple repair is possible. Where possible,

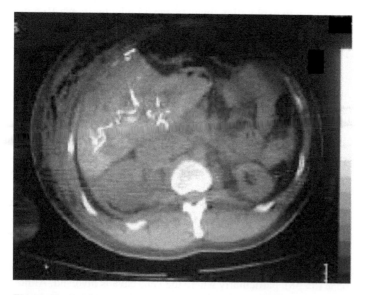

Figure 6 In blunt trauma this patient sustained a grade 5 liver injury and disruption of the vena cava. Contrast-enhanced computed tomography scan shows a large hematoma in the retrohepatic space in the region of the right kidney as a result of injury to the right renal vein and vena cava.

simple repair with venorrhaphy is recommended. When more complex repair, patch, or interposition graft is required, mortality is higher. Although infrarenal caval ligation can and should be carried out if required, suprarenal and juxtahepatic ligation is often fatal in the trauma setting (58). When dealing with the retrohepatic cava the authors have most experience with the direct approach with finger fracture technique (digitoclasia), as described by Patcher et al. (60,61), and direct repair or ligation of the inferior vena cava or hepatic veins. However, others have found benefits from the use of atriocaval shunting, as described by Burch et al. (62).

Outcomes

In one large series from civilian practice when comparing survivors with non survivors, factors relating to hemorrhagic shock strongly predict non survival (systolic blood pressure, hemoglobin, bicarbonate levels, volume of blood products, blood loss, temperature, and coagulation) (58). In this same study blunt trauma also carried a significantly higher mortality than penetrating trauma (80% compared to 44%), and the authors suggest this was related to the higher number of significant injuries in this group. In addition to physiological factors, the type and location of injury also influence mortality. As would be expected, a more extensive injury to the inferior vena cava, such as avulsion and lacerations larger than 5 cm, were associated with the highest mortality (50–67%) in one series (58). Whereas infrarenal location was associated with the lowest mortality rate (23%); both suprarenal and retrohepatic locations were associated with mortality rates of greater than 70% (58). The same is true of military series, were involvement of the inferior vena cava alone was associated with mortality rates of 31.8% compared to 78.6% when the inferior vena cava was involved in the retrohepatic position, often with major associated liver injury (55).

KEY POINTS

- Venous trauma is grossly under-reported but more commonly accompanies penetrating trauma.
- Iatrogenic venous injury is common, particularly in respect to central venous catherization, but often of limited clinical significance.
- Clinical examination alone by an experienced vascular surgeon has a high sensitivity and specificity for the detection of significant vascular trauma.
- In the unstable trauma patient contrast-enhanced CT scanning provides important information on vascular and soft tissue architecture.
- Priorities in management of venous trauma are arrest of hemorrhage, restoration of functional venous anatomy, and prevention of thrombotic complications.
- Nonoperative treatment of the stable patient with venous trauma undoubtedly saves lives.
- Endoluminal treatments, such as embolization and stenting, are gaining popularity in many centers.
- In extremity vascular trauma the insertion of intraluminal vascular shunts to vein and artery provides time for a thorough assessment and appropriate management.
- In an unstable patient with multiple-injuries control of venous bleeding is best achieved by lateral suture or ligation.
- Complex venous repairs when clinically indicated are best achieved with an autologous vein conduit.

REFERENCES

1. Barros D'Sa AA. Twenty five years of vascular trauma in Northern Ireland. BMJ 1995; 310:1–2.
2. Rich NM. Vascular trauma in Vietnam. J Cardiovasc Surg (Torino) 1970; 11:368–377.
3. Mattox KL, Feliciano DV, Burch J, Beall AC, Jr., Jordan GL, Jr., De Bakey ME. Five thousand seven hundred sixty cardiovascular injuries in 4459 patients. Epidemiologic evolution 1958 to 1987. Ann Surg 1989; 209:698–705.
4. Fingerhut A, Leppaniemi AK, Androulakis GA, et al. The European experience with vascular injuries. Surg Clin North Am 2002; 82:175–188.
5. Shumacker HB, Jr. The surgical volumes of the history of the United States Army Medical Department in World War II. Vascular surgery. Arch Surg 1960; 80:379–383.
6. HUGHES CW. Acute vascular trauma in Korean War casualties; an analysis of 180 cases. Surg Gynecol Obstet 1954; 99:91–100.
7. Chandler JG, Knapp RW. Early definitive treatment of vascular injuries in the Vietnam conflict. JAMA 1967; 202:960–966.
8. Lovric Z, Wertheimer B, Candrlic K, et al. War injuries of major extremity vessels. J Trauma 1994; 36:248–251.
9. Rich NM, Rhee P. An historical tour of vascular injury management: from its inception to the new millennium. Surg Clin North Am 2001; 81:1199–1215.
10. Barros D'Sa AA. Management of vascular injuries of civil strife. Injury 1982; 14:51–57.
11. Ordog GJ, Wasserberger J, Balasubramanium S. Wound ballistics: theory and practice. Ann Emerg Med 1984; 13:1113–1122.
12. Sykes LN, Jr., Champion HR, Fouty WJ. Dum-dums, hollow-points, and devastators: techniques designed to increase wounding potential of bullets. J Trauma 1988; 28:618–623.
13. Hirshberg A, Wall MJ, Jr., Allen MK, Mattox KL. Causes and patterns of missed injuries in trauma. Am J Surg 1994; 168:299–303.
14. Oller DW, Rutledge R, Clancy T, et al. Vascular injuries in a rural state: a review of 978 patients from a state trauma registry. J Trauma 1992; 32:740–745.
15. McIntyre WB, Ballard JL. Cervicothoracic vascular injuries. Semin Vasc Surg 1998; 11:232–242.
16. Mattox KL. Contemporary issues in thoracic aortic trauma. Semin Thorac Cardiovasc Surg 1991; 3:281–285.
17. Fisher RG, Oria RA, Mattox KL, Whigham CJ, Pickard LR. Conservative management of aortic lacerations due to blunt trauma. J Trauma 1990; 30:1562–1566.
18. Yelon JA, Scalea TM. Venous injuries of the lower extremities and pelvis: repair versus ligation. J Trauma 1992; 33:532–536.
19. Bishara RA, Pasch AR, Lim LT, et al. Improved results in the treatment of civilian vascular injuries associated with fractures and dislocations. J Vasc Surg 1986; 3:707–711.
20. Nehler MR, Taylor LM, Jr., Porter JM. Iatrogenic vascular trauma. Semin Vasc Surg 1998; 11:283–293.
21. Williams JF, Seneff MG, Friedman BC, et al. Use of femoral venous catheters in critically ill adults: prospective study. Crit Care Med 1991; 19:550–553.
22. Mansfield PF, Hohn DC, Fornage BD. Complications and failures of subclavian-vein catheterization. N Engl J Med 1994; 331:1735–1738.
23. Timsit JF, Farkas JC, Boyer JM, et al. Central vein catheter-related thrombosis in intensive care patients: incidence, risks factors, and relationship with catheter-related sepsis. Chest 1998; 114:207–213.
24. Oderich GS, Panneton JM, Hofer J, et al. Iatrogenic operative injuries of abdominal and pelvic veins: a potentially lethal complication. J Vasc Surg 2004; 39:931–936.
25. Nordestgaard AG, Bodily KC, Osborne RW, Jr., Buttorff JD. Major vascular injuries during laparoscopic procedures. Am J Surg 1995; 169:543–545.
26. Yeo A, Wong CY, Soo KC. Focused abdominal sonography for trauma (FAST). Ann Acad Med Singapore 1999; 28:805–809.

27. Haage P, Krings T, Schmitz-Rode T. Nontraumatic vascular emergencies: imaging and intervention in acute venous occlusion. Eur Radiol 2002; 12:2627–2643.

28. Bell RM, Krantz BE, Weigelt JA. ATLS: a foundation for trauma training. Ann Emerg Med 1999; 34:233–237.

29. Bickell WH, Wall MJ, Jr., Pepe PE, et al. Immediate versus delayed fluid resuscitation for hypotensive patients with penetrating torso injuries. N Engl J Med 1994; 331:1105–1109.

30. Martin RR, Bickell WH, Pepe PE, Burch JM, Mattox KL. Prospective evaluation of preoperative fluid resuscitation in hypotensive patients with penetrating truncal injury: a preliminary report. J Trauma 1992; 33:354–361.

31. Asensio JA, Roldan G, Petrone P, et al. Operative management and outcomes in 103 AAST-OIS grades IV and V complex hepatic injuries: trauma surgeons still need to operate, but angioembolization helps. J Trauma 2003; 54:647–653.

32. Heetveld MJ, Harris I, Schlaphoff G, Balogh Z, D'Amours SK, Sugrue M. Hemodynamically unstable pelvic fractures: recent care and new guidelines. World J Surg 2004; 28:904–909.

33. Nair R, Robbs JV, Muckart DJ. Management of penetrating cervicomediastinal venous trauma. Eur J Vasc Endovasc Surg 2000; 19:65–69.

34. Hirshberg A, Mattox KL. "Damage control" in trauma surgery. Br J Surg 1993; 80:1501–1502.

35. Hirshberg A, Wall MJ, Jr., Mattox KL. Planned reoperation for trauma: a two year experience with 124 consecutive patients. J Trauma 1994; 37:365–369.

36. Barros D'Sa AA. The rationale for arterial and venous shunting in the management of limb vascular injuries. Eur J Vasc Surg 1989; 3:471–474.

37. Barros D'Sa AA, Moorehead RJ. Combined arterial and venous intraluminal shunting in major trauma of the lower limb. Eur J Vasc Surg 1989; 3:577–581.

38. Maull KI, Sachatello CR. Current management of pelvic fractures: a combined surgical-angiographic approach to hemorrhage. South Med J 1976; 69:1285–1289.

39. Cooper SG. Complication of subclavian vein catheterization: treatment with coil embolization. J Vasc Interv Radiol 1999; 10:379.

40. Watarida S, Nishi T, Furukawa A, et al. Fenestrated stent-graft for traumatic juxtahepatic inferior vena cava injury. J Endovasc Ther 2002; 9:134–137.

41. Denton JR, Moore EE, Coldwell DM. Multimodality treatment for grade V hepatic injuries: perihepatic packing, arterial embolization, and venous stenting. J Trauma 1997; 42:964–967.

42. Smayra T, Otal P, Chabbert V, et al. Long-term results of endovascular stent placement in the superior caval venous system. Cardiovasc Intervent Radiol 2001; 24:388–394.

43. Rich NM, Hobson RW. Venous trauma: emphasis for repair is indicated. J Cardiovasc Surg (Torino) 1973;571–575.

44. Rich NM, Collins GJ, Jr., Andersen CA, McDonald PT, Ricotta JJ. Venous trauma: successful venous reconstruction remains an interesting challenge. Am J Surg 1977; 134:226–230.

45. Hobson RW, Howard EW, Wright CB, Collins GJ, Rich NM. Hemodynamics of canine femoral venous ligation: significance in combined arterial and venous injuries. Surgery 1973; 74:824–829.

46. Hobson RW, Yeager RA, Lynch TG, et al. Femoral venous trauma: techniques for surgical management and early results. Am J Surg 1983; 146:220–224.

47. Meyer J, Walsh J, Schuler J, et al. The early fate of venous repair after civilian vascular trauma. A clinical, hemodynamic, and venographic assessment. Ann Surg 1987; 206:458–464.

48. Timberlake GA, Kerstein MD. Venous injury: to repair or ligate, the dilemma revisited. Am Surg 1995; 61:139–145.

49. Johansen K, Daines M, Howey T, Helfet D, Hansen ST, Jr. Objective criteria accurately predict amputation following lower extremity trauma. J Trauma 1990; 30:568–572.

50. Rich NM, Leppaniemi A. Vascular trauma: a 40-year experience with extremity vascular emphasis. Scand J Surg 2002; 91:109–126.

51. Rich NM. Principles and indications for primary venous repair. Surgery 1982; 91:492–496.

52. Pappas PJ, Haser PB, Teehan EP, et al. Outcome of complex venous reconstructions in patients with trauma. J Vasc Surg 1997; 25:398–404.

53. Pearce WH, Whitehill TA. Carotid and vertebral arterial injuries. Surg Clin North Am 1988; 68:705–723.

54. Mohammed GS, Pillay WR, Barker P, Robbs JV. The role of clinical examination in excluding vascular injury in haemodynamically stable patients with gunshot wounds to the neck. A prospective study of 59 patients. Eur J Vasc Endovasc Surg 2004; 28:425–430.

55. Khoury G, Sfeir R, Khalifeh M, Khoury SJ, Nabbout G. Penetrating trauma to the abdominal vessels. Cardiovasc Surg 1996; 4:405–407.

56. Feliciano DV, Mattox KL, Jordan GL, Jr., Burch JM, Bitondo CG, Cruse PA. Management of 1000 consecutive cases of hepatic trauma (1979–1984). Ann Surg 1986; 204:438–445.

57. Phelan H, Hunt JP, Wang YZ. Retrohepatic vena cava and juxtahepatic venous injuries. South Med J 2001; 94:728–731.

58. Hansen CJ, Bernadas C, West MA, et al. Abdominal vena caval injuries: outcomes remain dismal. Surgery 2000; 128:572–578.

59. Graham JM, Mattox KL, Beall AC, Jr., Debakey ME. Traumatic injuries of the inferior vena cava. Arch Surg 1978; 113:413–418.

60. Pachter HL, Spencer FC, Hofstetter SR, Coppa GF. Experience with the finger fracture technique to achieve intra-hepatic hemostasis in 75 patients with severe injuries of the liver. Ann Surg 1983; 197:771–778.

61. Pachter HL, Spencer FC, Hofstetter SR, Liang HG, Coppa GF. Significant trends in the treatment of hepatic trauma. Experience with 411 injuries. Ann Surg 1992; 215:492–500.

62. Burch JM, Feliciano DV, Mattox KL, Edelman M. Injuries of the inferior vena cava. Am J Surg 1988; 156:548–552.

63. Monson DO, Saletta JD, Freeark RJ. Carotid vertebral trauma. J Trauma 1969; 9:987–999.

38

Lymphedema: Clinical Features and Investigation

Alok Tiwari and George Hamilton
University Department of Surgery, Royal Free Hospital, UCL and Royal Free Medical School, London, U.K.

INTRODUCTION

Lymphedema is the swelling of a body part due to an accumulation of lymphatic fluid caused by an abnormality in the lymphatic drainage (1). It is thought that 38%–100% of all circulating proteins leave the intravascular compartment every 24 hours (2). The lymphatic system is responsible for return to the vascular system of these extravascular molecules and colloids which are too large to re-enter directly (3). Lymphedema thus occurs when the lymphatics are unable to cope with this protein rich fluid that is filtered out of the vasculature but not reabsorbed. This happens because of three reasons: (1) increased fluid filtered out of vascular capillaries, (2) reduced reabsorption into distal capillaries and venules, and (3) failure of the lymphatics—i.e., lymphedema. Any of these (or a combination) leads to an accumulation of fluid in the interstitial tissues. The normal lymphatic system has some reserve to compensate for mild increases in fluid filtered or reduction in fluid reabsorption, therefore edema is not usually clinically recognizable until the normal interstitial volume has doubled (4). It is worth noting that lymphatic function declines with age (especially after the age of 65 years) and may account for the relatively late age at which some patients present (5).

Lymphedema is seen most commonly seen in the lower limbs. Arm lymphedema is usually a consequence of breast surgery and axillary lymph node dissection. This is made worse by radiotherapy. Treatments of arm lymphedema is undertaken generally by breast surgeons and breast physiotherapists and thus rarely referred to vascular surgeons. Lymphedema has also been described in the face, trunks and external genitalia.

It is estimated that 140 million people worldwide suffer from some form of lymphedema with filariasis accounting for 45 million of these cases, post-mastectomy lymphedema about 20 million cases, 20 million traumatic lymphedema, 0.5–2 million cases of primary lymphedema and the rest are thought to have damaged lymphatics but no clinical lymphedema (5).

511

ETIOLOGY OF LYMPHEDEMA

This is summarized in Table 2.

Primary Lymphedema

This is caused by a congenital abnormality or dysfunction in the lymphatic system. It can be classified according to either age of presentation or due to the primary pathology. Edgar V. Allen in 1934 wrote one of the key papers on this subject in classifying lymphedema based on his experience with 300 patients. According to the age of presentation it is classified into congenitum, praecox, and tarda (6,7):

1. *Congenitum*: This is lymphedema which is either detected at birth or in the first year of life. This comprised approximately 10% of patients. It may be either sporadic or familial. The familial form is known as Milroy's disease. This rare form is thought to result from an autosomal inheritance of a single gene.
2. *Praecox*: This is lymphedema presenting between the ages of one and 35 years. This is the most common form of lymphedema (approximately 71% of patients). In females this is more common around menarche. Meige disease is familial lymphedema praecox due to an inheritance of an autosomal recessive gene and usually presents at puberty.
3. *Tarda*: This is lymphedema presenting after the age of 35 years. This is the second most common form of primary lymphedema and comprises approximately 19% of patients.

Alternatively primary lymphedema can be classified according to the abnormality found in the lymphatics. Thus it may be aplastic, hypoplastic and hyperplastic. Wolfe and Kinmonth have suggested that aplasia might be an extreme form of hypoplasia and they believe that true aplasia is rare (7). These terms suggest an abnormality in the development of the lymphatic system. While this is true for congenital lymphedema, cases of later onset primary lymphedema might be due to an acquired abnormality. It is difficult to prove whether the abnormal lymphatics seen when these patients are investigated have existed in the same state since birth.

In a study of 372 patients with primary lymphedema, the most common form of primary lymphedema was proximal and distal hypoplasia followed by distal hypoplasia and then proximal hypoplasia with hyperplasia being the least common (7). Primary hypoplastic lymphedema is milder, often bilateral and symptoms are confined to below the knee. Not surprisingly proximal disease causes more severe symptoms with whole limb swelling. Patients with primary hyperplastic lymphedema have an increased number and size of lymphatics. It is unusual in that it has a male preponderance and is more often familial (8). An association with other congenital abnormalities (Table 1) is sometimes seen. The thoracic duct may be absent or abnormal in such patients (8).

Secondary Lymphedema

This is edema due to a reduction in lymph flow by an acquired cause. This can be through a physical disruption of the lymphatics as in trauma or surgery, through extrinsic compression of lymphatic vessels or through obstruction from within the lymphatic ducts (Table 2). The causes of this are:

Table 1 Congenital Syndromes Associated with Primary Lymphedema

Turner's syndrome
Noonan's syndrome[a]
Pes cavus
Distishiasis (double eyelashes)
Yellow nail syndrome
Ptosis
Hypoparathyroidism
Microcephaly
Arteriovenous malformations
Facial anomalies
Cholestasis

[a] An autosomal dominant inherited disorder with features similar to Turners syndrome.
Source: From Ref. 8.

Infection

This is the most common cause worldwide due to infection with the parasitic nematode *Wuscheria bancrofti* otherwise known as filariasis. Filariasis is transmitted in larval form by insect vectors with the adult form living in the peripheral lymphatic channel and nodes (9). It is mainly found in developing countries with very few cases in the western world except possibly in immigrants. Recurrent cellulitis typically due to streptococcus used to be an important factor for development of lymphedema in the Western population. However, because of the ready availability of antibiotics this is more important in affecting the limited lymphatics in patients already with lymphedema.

Malignancy

In the Western world this is the most common cause of secondary lymphedema. The common primary malignancies include prostate, gynecological and lymphoma or metastatic disease to the regional lymph nodes such as from melanoma. Even after radical lymph node excision for malignancy, lymphedema does not always ensue. When it does occur, it is often a late complication. The reasons for this late development are uncertain but gradual failure of distal lymphatics, which have to "pump" lymph at a greater pressure through damaged proximal ducts, has been postulated. The transected lymphatics will regenerate after node clearance procedures, but if combined with radiotherapy, the risk of lymphedema is higher as fibrous scarring reduces regrowth of ducts. Metastasis to the lymphatic is a common cause of lymphedema in patients but is usually difficult

Table 2 Causes of Lymphedema

Primary lymphedema
Secondary lymphedema
Filariasis
Recurrent cellulitis
Radiotherapy
Surgery
Lymph node excision/dissection
Arterial reconstruction
Venous surgery
Trauma

to treat. Radiotherapy for the treatment of malignancy causes damage to the lymphatics and this is also responsible for the development of lymphedema.

Trauma

Traumatic injury of the lymphatics due to fractures can lead to the development of lymphedema. It may also worsen the lymphatics in patients who may have mild lymphedema but have never had any symptoms before. These patients believe that their lymphedema was caused by the traumatic injury rather than worsened by the injury.

Venous Disease

It is unusual for surgery alone to cause lymphedema as lymphatics have excellent regenerative capabilities. Some series have shown significant lymphatic damage in over 60% of patients undergoing varicose vein surgery (10). Patients with venous disease have been shown to have impaired lymphatic drainage (11). Lymphedema is unusual after varicose vein surgery but patients should be examined preoperatively as vein stripping can significantly exacerbate mild lymphedema (10).

Peripheral Bypass Surgery

The incidence of peripheral edema following arterial reconstruction is 62–100% (12). The most common operation causing this is a femoro-popliteal bypass with occasional cases occurring after aorto-iliac and aorto-femoral bypass (12). The swelling becomes apparent after two to three days when the patient first starts to mobilize. This swelling if significant can itself lead to problems with mobilization and wound healing especially as the swelling may persist for up to six months. This type of edema is thought to mainly results from damage to the lymphatics resulting in impairment and interruption of lymphatic drainage secondary to the extensive surgical dissection in the thigh and popliteal region (12–15). Others have suggested that this could be due to deep vein thrombosis or because of increased filtration from capillaries of the legs following revascularization. If the swelling is significant (more than 4.5 cm) then it is thought to be more likely due to thrombosis of the tibial or popliteal veins (16). Some authors have tried to reduce the extensive dissection in bypass surgery by using smaller and separate incisions in the groin for dissecting the femoral artery and long saphenous vein but have not been universally successful (17,18).

Other Cause of Limb Swelling

General Causes

Generalized causes of lower limb swelling include congestive cardiac failure, hepatic failure, renal failure, hypoalbuminaemia and protein losing nephropathy i.e. nephrotic syndrome (19). These may be excluded by a full clinical examination and simple blood tests including full blood count, urea and electrolytes, liver function tests including albumin and urine microscopy especially looking for proteinuria. Other tests may include a chest radiograph and echocardiogram for congestive cardiac failure, abdominal ultrasound and biopsy of the organ to exclude liver and renal pathology. Other causes include drug treatment such as anti-hypertensives, certain hormones and antidepressants, hyperthyroidisms leading to pretibial myxedema and retroperitoneal fibrosis. Other rare causes may include neurofibromatosis, hemihypertrophy, macrodystrophia lipomatosa, reflex sympathetic dystrophy and multiple enchondromatosis (8).

Lipedema

Lipedema (lipomatosis of the leg) is thought to result from abnormal deposition of subcutaneous fat associated with edema. It can be easily mistaken for lymphedema unless there is awareness of this condition. In a review of 250 patients cases with lymphedema, Rudkin and Miller found that nine (3.6%) patients had lipedema. These patients present with swollen limbs which may have been present for many years. The clinical features of this condition are the early age of onset (around puberty in 60% of patients), exclusively or mostly found in females and a positive family history in some patients (20,21). These patients may also complain of pain, tenderness and easy bruising of their limbs (21). The clinical signs are elastic symmetrical enlargement of both the legs with sparing of the feet (20,21), so called "riding breech thighs" and "stove pipe legs" (22), hypothermia of the skin, a negative Stemmer sign and plantar positioning alterations (21,23). There is usually non-pitting swelling of the leg. Even though this is thought to be due to accumulation of fatty tissue, there is no real effect on the leg appearance with weight loss (Fig. 1) (21). In one series lymphoscintigraphy and photoplethysmography in these patients demonstrated very little impairment of venous and lymphatic function (21) while in another series it was found that lymphatic system was slow and that this was asymmetrical (23).

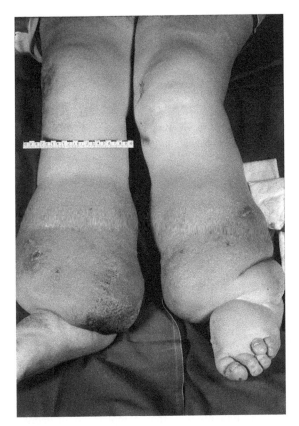

Figure 1 A typical patient with lower limb lymphedema showing all the characteristic features. (*See color insert.*)

Chronic Venous Disease

Deep venous thrombosis has already been discussed in a previous chapter. The resulting edema is usually pitting in nature and is usually much softer than in established lymphedema. Often there are underlying risk factors such as recent surgery or immobility, malignancy, a preceding long haul flight or thrombophilia. The diagnosis is confirmed with duplex scanning or venography. Treatment is with anticoagulation.

One of the long-term sequela of deep venous thrombosis is the post-phlebitic syndrome. On clinical grounds alone, this may be more difficult to differentiate from lymphedema and further investigation as outlined later in this article may be required. Other venous causes of swollen limbs are Klippel–Trenaunay–Weber syndrome and arterio-venous fistulae. In the former the features are limb hypertrophy, varicose veins and port wine stains while in the latter there may be thrills, hemangiomas and large varicose veins.

Baker's Cyst

These popliteal cysts cause lower limb swelling and acute leg pain especially if they have ruptured. Treatment is mostly conservative because of their recurrent and generally benign clinical course. If the cyst is very large and symptomatic aspiration, which may need to be repeated, is commonly used. Infrequently surgical excision is required.

Artifact

This occurs when there is prolonged immobility of the limb such as in patients with neurological disorders. It is also seen in some patients with psychiatric disorders who fake lower limb paralysis or as part of Munchausen's syndrome where the patients used a tourniquet on their limb to cause lower limb swelling.

Cyclical Edema

In cyclical edema the mechanism is thought to be due to increased microvascular permeability (24). The edema can affect the face, breast, abdomen and legs with symptoms worse at the end of the day.

Idiopathic Edema

In one series of patients investigated for limb swelling, 28.3% of patients were diagnosed with idiopathic edema (25).

Rheumatoid Arthritis

In children lower limb swelling has been seen in association with arthritis but the exact reason for this is unknown (26).

Clinical Features of Lymphedema

Symptoms

The most common symptom of lymphedema is a swelling of the limb. The patient may complain of shoes not fitting or a heaviness/swollen foot at the end of the day or in hot weather. The swelling is progressive and patients may thus complain about decreased activity because of the heavy legs (27). Some patients with bilateral lymphedema may not realize that their legs are abnormal until they seek treatment for other symptoms such as cellulite where the first diagnosis of lymphedema might be made. The swelling is usually painless unless there has been an infection. Symptoms may vary throughout the menstrual cycle (28).

Lymphedema is found in both sexes though women are investigated for this disease more often than men (25). Two-thirds of the cases have unilateral lymphedema (25). The distal part of the leg is affected initially with proximal extension and the feet are not spared. In patients with complete absence of lymphatics, the history is of long-term swelling while those with impaired lymphatics have shorter histories (29).

The sign of lymphedema is a swollen limb initially with pitting edema. In advance disease process fibrosis in the subcutaneous tissues causes the classical non-pitting signs (27). A typical patients limb is shown in Figure 1. The distribution is asymmetrical and patients have a positive Stemmer sign (impossibility to pinch with fingers the skin of the second toe) (21). Stemmer sign is positive in approximately 80% of patients though negative Stemmer's do not exclude lymphedema. Early in the disease process the edema can spread proximally (or distally) but this is uncommon after the first year and extremely unlikely after the first five years. Radial enlargement, however, is usually progressive if treatment is not instituted. With time skin changes are seen over the affected area, the skin becomes thicker (hyperkeratosis) and rougher (papillomatosis) and skin turgor is increased (27,30).

The skin can break down in severe cases with lymph exuding through any skin breaks. This compromises healing and leads to an increased risk of infection. Recurrent infections, cellulitis and lymphangitis are common. This unfortunately can lead to a further deterioration in lymphatic drainage ending in a vicious cycle of infection and worsening edema.

Lymphangiosarcoma (now classified as an angiosarcoma) is a rare late complication of lymphedema (also known as Stewart-Treves syndrome). This is most commonly seen in the lymphedematous arms of patients following radical mastectomy but has also been described in patients with Milroy's disease and in patients with secondary lymphedema (31,32). It appears to be an earlier complication (average 10 years) in patients with arm lymphedema than in patients with congenital lymphedema (average 38 years) (33). The prognosis for this disease is poor with only 10% surviving five years from diagnosis. Treatment is with a combination of radiotherapy and surgery.

Assessment of Limb Swelling

General Clinical Examination

It is important to examine both legs for the distribution of the swelling, presence or absence of pitting edema, any associated skin changes as well as a generalized examination to exclude typical medical causes such as congestive cardiac failure. The urine should also be analyzed to exclude any protein nephropathy. In a review of non-invasive assessment of the lymphedematous limb, Stanton et al. have looked at the non-invasive assessment of the lymphedematous limb and explained that the opposite leg may be useful as a comparison (34). However it may be confounded by the fact that the disease may itself affect the opposite leg or the unaffected leg may normally have been larger than the diseased leg.

Limb Girth

A normal tape measure will assess the swelling relative to the contralateral leg but this is not a reliable technique. It is used to measure the limb girth at various points. It is important to note that many points need to be measured as baseline and then to look at whether treatment is having any effect. If too few points are used then it may difficult to know whether the reduction in limb girth is because fluid has left the limb or has just been redistributed (35).

Limb Volume

This is probably the most common method for assessing lymphedema. This can be achieved by the following methods:

Surface Volume.   A tape measure is used as above to measure circumference at various points and the leg volume then calculated using geometric formulae (35). For obvious reasons volume of hands and feet are difficult to measure but otherwise this is a simple and inexpensive test with surprising accuracy.

Water Displacement Volumetry.   This technique, though not commonly used, gives a measurement of the limb volume and is a more accurate measurement than calculating the leg volume using circumferential measurement with tape measures (36). It also allows measurement of the volume of hand and feet.

Optoelectronic Volumetry.   This measures limb volume using light beams and a computer software to calculate the limb volume. It is good for follow-up because the machine can record and store limb shape and contour. It is simple and easy to use but is expensive and the machinery is large. Two commercial devices have been used for measuring leg volume using computers. The Perometer™ has been used in patients with postmastectomy lymphedema, and compared to the tape measure technique, found to be a highly reproducible technique (37). Kim et al. have used the Volometer™ to assess limb volume and to investigate venous dynamics in patients with lymphedema (38).

Tissue Tonicity

In lymphedema the tissue tonicity (degree of tissue resistance to mechanical compression) is either higher or lower compared to the non-edematous leg (39). This is more useful in assessing response to treatment. There is debate whether this is a good measure as differing authors have shown that tissue tonicity may go up or down even with successful treatment of lymphedema.

Bioelectrical Impedance

This method has been used successfully for evaluation of swelling in post-mastectomy patients but has not yet been evaluated for leg edema (40). More research in this technique is awaited.

Edema Tester

Cesarone et al. have described a technique for testing edema by the use of plastic plates with either protrusions or holes (41). This is applied over a swollen area for fixed period (one to three minutes) and pressure (50 mmHg) and then the marks left by the device are measured. This test allowed the differentiation between primary and chronic lymphedema in 13 patients. It has been recommended by the author for this to be used as a screening tool to allow only patients with positive results to be further investigated.

Radiology

Invasive Investigation

Lymphangiogram. This technique involves the direct cannulation of the lymphatics in the foot usually in the subcutaneous web spaces. This requires a skin incision in a patient with an edematous leg and thus the propensity towards infection, local inflammation and fibrosis. It is also painful and time consuming, with an increased risk of hypersensitivity reaction and emboli and subsequently this technique has largely been abandoned (42). However, it is still useful if operative intervention; i.e., bypass procedure is to be undertaken as the lymphatics anatomy is properly visualized including the site of the obstruction (43). It may also be undertaken if the results of the lymphoscintigram are perceived to be incorrect (43).

Lymphoscintigram. This is the gold standard for assessing lymphatic function at this present time. This technique was first introduced in 1953. It utilizes a radioactive labeled protein which is usually [99]Technetium-labeled colloid including antimony sulphur and albumin. Non-ionic contrast agents have also been used with reportedly less side effects (42). This is injected in to the web space of the feet and pictures taken at various time intervals. It allows measurement of lymphatic function, lymph movement and lymph drainage function and is also useful in looking at the response to treatment (3,9). Lymphoscintigram may be sufficient if any bypass procedure is intended but some patients may also require a contrast lymphogram to fully elucidate the lymphatic anatomy (43,44).

Lymphoscintigram when used to measure lymph flow can be further improved by taking an oral dose of heptaminol adenosine phosphate which can increase lymphatic flow (45). The amount of time that the lymphatics are visualized is important. If lymphatics are not imaged within the first hour the diagnosis may be missed (46). In some patients the one hour image may show normal lymphatics while only delayed films (two–24 hours postinjection) may show the true abnormality (47,48). In one series 32% of patients would have had a normal lymphoscintigram if only the one-hour film had been considered.

Other techniques to improve the sensitivity of this test detection include condensed image processing, which involves condensing images from multiple images into a single image. This allows improved detection of abnormality that are not readily apparent on standard analysis (49). Using a modified Kleinhans score (a semiquantitative score) using the following criteria: transport kinetics, distribution pattern, time to visualization of regional nodes, transport kinetics and time to appearance of lymph nodes and vessels with higher the numbers the higher the abnormality of the lymphatics (25). Time activity curves are also better at diagnosis than standard film scintigrams (50).

The sensitivity of the this test is 73–97% and specificity is 94–100% (25,46,51,52). Lymphoscintigram alone can exclude lymphedema as a cause of limb swelling in approximately one-third of patients (25,53). Lymphoscintigram will also differentiate between lymphedema and edema of venous origin (47). In patients with venous leg ulcers, lymphoscintigram shows there is a significantly lower lymph drainage as well lower drainage in the nonulcerated leg compared to controls (3). It is also lower in patients with varicose veins and especially if deep vein incompetence was present (3). This suggests chronic venous insufficiency is also associated with lymphatic insufficiency. In post-thrombotic disease there is reduction of the subfascial lymphatic flow while the epifascial flow remains normal, while in lymphedema both epifascial and subfascial lymphatics remains abnormal (54). Therefore, both epifascial and subfascial compartments must be evaluated to differentiate between postthrombotic and lymphedema (24,54). In lipedema, lymphoscintigraphy will confirm that peripheral lymphatics are essentially normal though there may be slowness of the lymphatic (21,23). The lymphoscintigram pictures are often asymmetrical in lipedema though the disease is bilateral with the disease process affecting mainly the lower third of the leg (23). Lymphoscintigram also shows impairment of lymphatic drainage or lymphatic disruption following arterial reconstruction (13–15). Typical lymphoscintigrams are shown in Figure 2.

Noninvasive Investigation

All these investigation may not only be used for confirming the diagnosis but all are useful in monitoring response to treatment.

Ultrasound. Very few studies on the use of ultrasound exist in diagnosing lymphedema. The ultrasound features of lymphedema are minimal increase in the thickness of the dermis (55), increase in the subcutaneous layer of between 46–79% (38,55) with hyperechogenic dermis and hypoechogenic subcutaneous layer (55). It allows an assessment of soft tissue changes but does not give information about the truncal anatomy of the lymphatics (55). It can also rule out other soft tissue causes for the limb swelling but will obviously be limited by operator experience.

Duplex Ultrasound. In patients with lymphedema there is gradual impedance of venous return which then aggravates the edema and thus duplex may be an useful investigation in patients with lower limbs swelling (38). Others have however not found any association between chronic edema and increased venous reflux (56). A combination of a duplex scan and lymphoscintigram may find a cause of limb swelling in up to 82% of patients in whom clinical examination could not elicit the cause of the swelling (29). The main role of the duplex examination would be to rule out superficial and deep venous reflux as a possible cause of the swelling and depending on the experience of the radiographer other causes of lower limb swelling including Baker's cyst may be found. It is worth noting that diagnosing and then treating varicose veins in patients with lymphedema can aggravate leg swelling.

Computed Tomography. The common computed tomography (CT) findings in lymphedema are calf skin thickening (57–59), thickening of the subcutaneous compartment (57–59), increased fat density (57,59) and thickening of the perimuscular aponeurosis (59). A typical honeycomb appearance is seen in 83% of patients (58). CT scan can be used not only to confirm the diagnosis but also to monitor the effect of treatment (59). When a CT scan is being dome the pelvis may be scanned at the same time which can show the primary lesion in patients with malignancy (57). CT can also differentiate lymphedema as a cause of swelling compared to patients with chronic venous disease, ruptured Baker's cyst and lipedema. In chronic venous disease there is enlargement of the subcutaneous compartment and skin thickening but the honeycomb appearance is not seen (58) while in lipedema there is enlargement of the subcutaneous compartment with normal skin thickness and subfascial compartment (58). CT scans in patients with deep venous thrombosis showed an increase in the subcutaneous layer with signs of lymphedema as well as showing increase in the cross sectional muscle area with presence of enlarged superficial veins (57). However, if calf swelling is not present following a deep vein thrombosis there will be no change in the muscle area and so becomes an unreliable investigation. All the studies have been undertaken in a small number of patients. Overall CT is a reasonable investigation for the swollen limb and to look for any causes of lymphedema by scanning the pelvis at the same time.

Magnetic Resonance Imaging. The typical magnetic resonance imaging (MRI) features of lymphedema are circumferential edema, increased volume of subcutaneous tissue and honeycomb pattern above the fascia between muscle and subcutis and marked

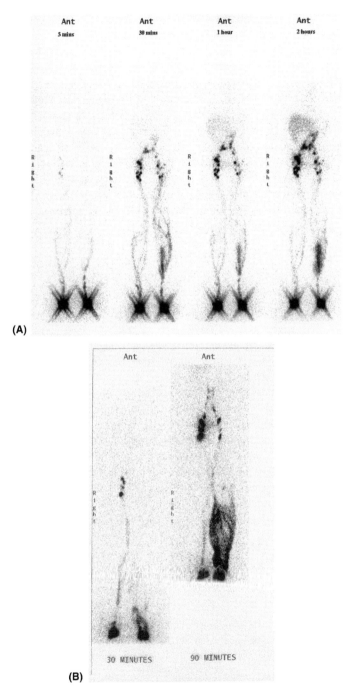

Figure 2 (**A**) Typical lymphoscintigram showing the time sequence in demonstrating left leg lymphatic blockage and recanalization. (**B**) This lymphoscintigram demonstrates left leg lymphatic obstruction and channeling through dermal lymphatics.

thickening of the dermis (60–62). It is however generally difficult to differentiate primary and secondary lymphedema using MRI (63). MRI has been used to investigate the lower limb following peripheral bypass procedure and to see whether it can differentiate between differing causes of leg edema (60). This showed that following bypass the edema is located around the entire circumference and restricted to the subcutaneous tissue and increase in the leg volume of 26% (8–45%) (60) while in chronic lymphedema there is an increase in leg volume of 40% (27–120%). The distribution of the edema in the various compartments was, however, similar. In DVT there is edema of the leg muscles particularly in the posterior compartments with increase in the leg volume of 23% (60). MRI will also show the typical features of angiosarcoma when evaluating the swollen limb (32). Some of the radiologcal features described above will have been seen in other causes of limb swelling (61). MRI has been used to differentiate between lymphedema, lipedema and phlebedema (61). The feature of lipedema is an enlarged subcutaneous layer while in phlebedema it was increased fluid in both muscular and subcutaneous layer.

KEY POINTS

- Lymphedema is an accumulation of lymphatic fluid caused by an abnormality of lymphatic drainage.
- It is a differential diagnosis of lower limb swelling, other causes commonly being chronic venous disease, medical causes such as congestive and renal failure, lipedema and idiopathic.
- Lymphedema is either primary or secondary. Secondary causes are malignancy, trauma, infection (commonly filariasis) and peripheral bypass surgery.
- Diagnosis is made by clinical examination and radiological investigation. Common clinical features are edema (initially pitting before becoming non-pitting), positive Stemmer's sign, hyperkeratosis and papillomatosis.
- Gold standard for confirming the diagnosis is a lymphoscintigraphy. However other noninvasive investigation such as computed tomography, magnetic resonance imaging, and ultrasound of the limb are useful in confirming the diagnosis. The latter investigation do not give any information on the actual lymphatic abnormality.

REFERENCES

1. Tiwari A, Cheng KS, Button M, Myint F, Hamilton G. Differential diagnosis, investigation, and current treatment of lower limb lymphedema. Arch Surg 2003; 138:152–161.
2. Browse NL, Stewart G. Lymphedema: pathophysiology and classification. J Cardiovasc Surg (Torino) 1985; 26:91–106.
3. Mortimer PS. Evaluation of lymphatic function: abnormal lymph drainage in venous disease. Int Angiol 1995; 14:32–35.
4. Mortimer PS. Implications of the lymphatic system in CVI-associated edema. Angiology 2000; 51:3–7.
5. Piller NB, Morgan RG, Casley-Smith JR. A double-blind, cross-over trial of O-(beta-hydroxyethyl)-rutosides (benzo-pyrones) in the treatment of lymphedema of the arms and legs. Br J Plast Surg 1988; 41:20–27.
6. Allen EV. Lymphedema of the extremities: classification, etiology and differential diagnosis. Arch Intern Med 1934; 54:606–624.

7. Wolfe JH, Kinmonth JB. The prognosis of primary lymphedema of the lower limbs. Arch Surg 1981; 116:1157–1160.
8. Wright NB, Carty HM. The swollen leg and primary lymphedema. Arch Dis Child 1994; 71:44–49.
9. Williams WH, Witte CL, Witte MH, McNeill GC. Radionuclide lymphangioscintigraphy in the evaluation of peripheral lymphedema. Clin Nucl Med 2000; 25:451–464.
10. Foldi M, Idiazabal G. The role of operative management of varicose veins in patients with lymphedema and/or lipedema of the legs. Lymphology 2000; 33:167–171.
11. Bull RH, Gane JN, Evans JE, Joseph AE, Mortimer PS. Abnormal lymph drainage in patients with chronic venous leg ulcers. J Am Acad Dermatol 1993; 28:585–590.
12. Eickhoff JH, Engell HC. Local regulation of blood flow and the occurrence of edema after arterial reconstruction of the lower limbs. Ann Surg 1982; 195:474–478.
13. Esato K, et al. 99mTc-HSA lymphoscintigraphy and leg edema following arterial reconstruction. J Cardiovasc Surg (Torino) 1991; 32:741–746.
14. Suga K, et al. Lymphoscintigraphic assessment of leg oedema following arterial reconstruction using a load produced by standing. Nucl Med Commun 1991; 12:907–917.
15. Howarth DM. Increased lymphoscintigraphic flow pattern in the lower extremity under evaluation for lymphedema. Mayo Clin Proc 1997; 72:423–429.
16. Hamer JD. Investigation of edema of the lower limb following sucessful femoropopliteal by-role of phlebography in demonstrating venous thrombosis. Br J Surg 1972; 59:979–982.
17. Porter JM, Lindell TD, Lakin PC. Leg edema following femoropopliteal autogenous vein bypass. Arch Surg 1972; 105:883–888.
18. Haaverstad R, Johnsen H, Saether OD, Myhre HO. Lymph drainage and the development of post-reconstructive leg edema is not influenced by the type of inguinal incision. A prospective randomised study in patients undergoing femoropopliteal bypass surgery. Eur J Vasc Endovasc Surg 1995; 10:316–322.
19. Young JR. The swollen leg. Clinical significance and differential diagnosis. Cardiol Clin 1991; 9:443–456.
20. Rudkin GH, Miller TA. Lipedema: a clinical entity distinct from lymphedema. Plast Reconstr Surg 1994; 94:841–847.
21. Harwood CA, Bull RH, Evans J, Mortimer PS. Lymphatic and venous function in lipedema. Br J Dermatol 1996; 134:1–6.
22. Loughlin V. Massive obesity simulating lymphedema. N Engl J Med 1993; 328:1496.
23. Bilancini S, Lucchi M, Tucci S, Eleuteri P. Functional lymphatic alterations in patients suffering from lipedema. Angiology 1995; 46:333–339.
24. Brautigam P, et al. Analysis of lymphatic drainage in various forms of leg edema using two compartment lymphoscintigraphy. Lymphology 1998; 31:43–55.
25. Cambria RA, Gloviczki P, Naessens JM, Wahner HW. Noninvasive evaluation of the lymphatic system with lymphoscintigraphy: a prospective, semiquantitative analysis in 386 extremities. J Vasc Surg 1993; 18:773–782.
26. Bardare M, Falcini F, Hertzberger-ten Cate R, Savolainen A, Cimaz R. Idiopathic limb edema in children with chronic arthritis: a multicenter report of 12 cases. J Rheumatol 1997; 24:384–388.
27. Lewis JM, Wald ER. Lymphedema praecox. J Pediatr 1984; 104:641–648.
28. Schirger A. Lymphedema. Cardiovasc Clin 1983; 13:293–305.
29. Wheatley DC, Wastie ML, Whitaker SC, Perkins AC, Hopkinson BR. Lymphoscintigraphy and colour Doppler sonography in the assessment of leg edema of unknown cause. Br J Radiol 1996; 69:1117–1124.
30. Mortimer PS. Swollen lower limb-2: lymphedema. BMJ 2000; 320:1527–1529.
31. Brostrom LA, Nilsonne U, Kronberg M, Soderberg G. Lymphangiosarcoma in chronic hereditary edema (Milroy's disease). Ann Chir Gynaecol 1989; 78:320–323.
32. Nakazono T, et al. Angiosarcoma associated with chronic lymphedema (Stewart–Treves syndrome) of the leg: MR imaging. Skeletal Radiol 2000; 29:413–416.

33. Chen KT, Gilbert EF. Angiosarcoma complicating generalized lymphangiectasia. Arch Pathol Lab Med 1979; 103:86–88.
34. Stanton AW, Badger C, Sitzia J. Non-invasive assessment of the lymphedematous limb. Lymphology 2000; 33:122–135.
35. Sitzia J, Stanton AW, Badger C. A review of outcome indicators in the treatment of chronic limb edema. Clin Rehabil 1997; 11:181–191.
36. Casley-Smith JR. Measuring and representing peripheral edema and its alterations. Lymphology 1994; 27:56–70.
37. Stanton AW, Northfield JW, Holroyd B, Mortimer PS, Levick JR. Validation of an optoelectronic limb volumeter (Perometer). Lymphology 1997; 30:77–97.
38. Kim DI, Huh S, Hwang JH, Kim YI, Lee BB. Venous dynamics in leg lymphedema. Lymphology 1999; 32:11–14.
39. Liu NF, Olszewski W. Use of tonometry to assess lower extremity lymphedema. Lymphology 1992; 25:155–158.
40. Ward LC. Regarding Edema and leg volume: methods of assessment. Angiology 2000; 51:615–616.
41. Cesarone MR, et al. The edema tester in the evaluation of swollen limbs in venous and lymphatic disease. Panminerva Med 1999; 41:10–14.
42. Weissleder H, Weissleder R. Interstitial lymphangiography: initial clinical experience with a dimeric nonionic contrast agent. Radiology 1989; 170:371–374.
43. Burnand KG, et al. Value of isotope lymphography in the diagnosis of lymphedema of the leg. Br J Surg 2002; 89:74–78.
44. Vaqueiro M, et al. Lymphoscintigraphy in lymphedema: an aid to microsurgery. J Nucl Med 1986; 27:1125–1130.
45. Thibaut G, Durand A, Follignoni P, Bertrand A. Measurement of lymphatic flow variation by noninvasive method cases of lymphedema. Angiology 1992; 43:567–571.
46. Ter SE, Alavi A, Kim CK, Merli G. Lymphoscintigraphy. A reliable test for the diagnosis of lymphedema. Clin Nucl Med 1993; 18:646–654.
47. Proby CM, Gane JN, Joseph AE, Mortimer PS. Investigation of the swollen limb with isotope lymphography. Br J Dermatol 1990; 123:29–37.
48. Larcos G, Foster DR. Interpretation of lymphoscintigrams in suspected lymphedema: contribution of delayed images. Nucl Med Commun 1995; 16:683–686.
49. Baulieu F, et al. The potential usefulness of condensed image processing of sequential lymphoscintigrams in patients with lymphedema. Lymphology 1990; 23:15–22.
50. Rijke AM, Croft BY, Johnson RA, de Jongste AB, Camps JA. Lymphoscintigraphy and lymphedema of the lower extremities. J Nucl Med 1990; 31:990–998.
51. Gloviczki P, et al. Noninvasive evaluation of the swollen extremity: experiences with 190 lymphoscintigraphic examinations. J Vasc Surg 1989; 9:603–689.
52. Stewart G, Gaunt JI, Croft DN, Browse NL. Isotope lymphography: a new method of investigating the role of the lymphatics in chronic limb edema. Br J Surg 1985; 72:906–909.
53. Nawaz MK, Hamad MM, Abdel-Dayem HM, Sadek S, Eklof BG. Lymphoscintigraphy in lymphedema of the lower limbs using 99mTc HSA. Angiology 1992; 43:147–154.
54. Brautigam P, Vanscheidt W, Foldi E, Krause T, Moser E. The importance of the subfascial lymphatics in the diagnosis of lower limb edema: investigations with semiquantitative lymphoscintigraphy. Angiology 1993; 44:464–470.
55. Doldi SB, et al. Ultrasonography of extremity lymphedema. Lymphology 1992; 25:129–133.
56. Valentin LI, Valentin WH. Comparative study of different venous reflux duplex quantitation parameters. Angiology 1999; 50:721–728.
57. Vaughan BF. CT of swollen legs. Clin Radiol 1990; 41:24–30.
58. Hadjis NS, Carr DH, Banks L, Pflug JJ. The role of CT in the diagnosis of primary lymphedema of the lower limb. AJR Am J Roentgenol 1985; 144:361–364.
59. Marotel M, et al. Transaxial computer tomography of lower extremity lymphedema. Lymphology 1998; 31:180–185.

60. Haaverstad R, Nilsen G, Myhre HO, Saether OD, Rinck PA. The use of MRI in the investigation of leg edema. Eur J Vasc Surg 1992; 6:124–129.
61. Werner GT, Scheck R, Kaiserling E. Magnetic resonance imaging of peripheral lymphedema. Lymphology 1998; 31:34–36.
62. Duewell S, et al. Swollen lower extremity: role of MR imaging. Radiology 1992; 184:227–231.
63. Idy-Peretti I, et al. Lymphedematous skin and subcutis: in vivo high resolution magnetic resonance imaging evaluation. J Invest Dermatol 1998; 110:782–787.

39

Lymphedema: The Role of Conservative Medical and Surgical Treatments

Alok Tiwari and George Hamilton
University Department of Surgery, Royal Free Hospital, UCL and Royal Free Medical School, London, U.K.

INTRODUCTION

In the previous chapter we have discussed the clinical features and diagnosis of arm and leg lymphedema. In this chapter we will discuss the medical and surgical treatment of this condition.

AIM OF TREATMENT

Lymphedema is a chronic disease with no cure. Therefore the main aim of treating patients with lymphedema is to prevent the progression of disease and to get symptomatic control. This is achieved by a combination of mechanical reduction and maintenance of limb size and preventing skin infection. Treatment will thus depend upon the symptoms and the severity of the condition. The mainstay of treating lymphedema is by conservative means with surgery reserved for a small proportion of patients (1).

CONSERVATIVE TREATMENT

Compression Stockings

Most patients who are seen in clinic and either have suspicion of lymphedema or have had the diagnosis confirmed will be offered compression stockings. Compression stocking can reduce leg volume, circumference and pain even at low pressures (2). However in lymphedema higher compression pressures are needed than for the treatment of chronic venous disease. Yashura et al. looked at the use of simple stocking in both primary and secondary lymphedema. They showed that after a median follow-up of five years (1.5–28 years) 92% of patients with primary lymphedema and 98% of patients with secondary lymphedema showed either an improvement or no difference following the use of simple compression hosiery. There were some patients whose lymphedema did get worse even after wearing compression stockings. The compression pressure of the stockings in this study was 40–60 mmHg.

Multilayer bandaging is another form of compression, which has been shown to be effective in both upper and lower limb lymphedema. This form of compression consists of an inner layer of tubular stockinette followed by foam and padding to protect the joint flexures and to even out the contours of the limb so that the pressure is evenly distributed. An outer layer of short-stretch extensible bandages provides compression where a minimum of two bandages is required. In a randomized trial of using multilayer bandaging followed by compression versus hosiery alone in patients with both upper and lower limb lymphedema, there was a 32.6% reduction in limb volume in the former group compared to 19.6% for the latter group. These were results in 78 patients after a follow up of 24 weeks (3). In lipedema no difference is made by compression stockings (4).

Another form of compression and massage comes from pneumatic pumps (5–7). These pump allow the development of high pressure up to 150 mmHg. They work in a sequential inflation/deflation way to allow the lymphatic fluid to flow into the systemic circulation (8). The treatment cycle per day can last up to 8 hours. Patients may sometimes need to be treated initially as inpatients especially if they are due to undergo surgery. Post treatment patients should continue to wear compression stocking else there is a high-risk of recurrence. These pump can reduce the limb girth measurements by 37–68.6% (7–9). When Klien et al. used a Wright® Linear pump for 8 hours a day for two days in 74 patients, they showed that in 90% of the patients limb circumference was reduced significantly in this short time (6). There was a greater effect in men though why this should be so was difficult to explain. After this procedure the patients wore compression stockings in the day and used the pump at night. In one study using external pump compression a significant number of patients developed genital edema (10). The pumps may not be suitable for use in patients with co-existing renal failure or congestive heart failure. Patients should ideally also be free of metastasis in the limb to prevent the risk of spreading the malignancy (6).

Complex (Combined) Physical Therapy

This is a combination of the various methods to achieve and maintain the reduction in limb size. It should to be the mainstay for the treatment of lymphedema. This was described by Foldis in the 1970s in Germany and has increasingly become popular in the last 20 years (11). The largest experience with this technique is thus from this group where they have regularly demonstrated limb reduction of 50% in more 2500 patients annually (12). Therefore the aim of all centers has been to reproduce the results from Germany. In the United States where this is known as complex decongestive physiotherapy this was evaluated in 291 patients (13). Treatment consisted of manual lymphatic massage, multilayered compression bandaging and skin care. This 90-minutes treatment was conducted every day taking between 4 to 25 days to complete. After this patients were put into compression stocking with some still requiring weekly massage therapy. This led to a 59.1% reduction in upper limb and 67.7% reduction in lower limb girth. 82–84% of the patients maintained this reduction in the limb girth as well as reducing the frequency of cellulitis. Casley-Smith et al. looked at this treatment in Australia in 78 patients with arm and 128 patients with leg lymphedema (14). One of the authors (Judith R. Casley-Smith), learned the technique of complex physical therapy from Germany and then taught their own physiotherapist. They showed an overall reduction in limb edema of 60% in the upper limb and 50% for the lower limbs. The summary of their complex physical therapy is summarized in Figure 1. In another large study from the United States, Boris et al. demonstrated 63.8% reduction in arm and 62.7% reduction in leg volume after three years of follow-up (9). Their treatment lasted two to four hours a day and was administered for 30 days.

The general principle of complex physical therapy involves the division of the trunk and limb into lymphotomes by lymphatic watersheds (14). These lymphotomes drain the superficial body region into the deeper lymphatic pathways and collecting lymphatics. When a lymphotomes is blocked then collaterals, which cross these lymphotomes, are used to carry the lymph to allow drainage. Thus the lymphatic massage encourages the use of these collaterals to improve lymphatic flow. The physiotherapy involved in this is discussed in Table 1. Because of the specialized nature of this massage it is performed by trained physiotherapy. It is the specialized nature of his treatment and the time and expense required which prevents many patients having access to this treatment.

Franzeck et al. measured the pressure in cutaneous lymph capillaries in 12 patients with lower limb lymphedema to look at the effect of complex physical therapy (15). When the patients had undergone manual lymph drainage and compression bandaging the microlymphatic hypertension was reduced to 5.9 mmHg from 12.8 mmHg. This pressure continued to drop when a combination of compression bandaging and ergotherapy (involving active circular and bicycle riding movements of the feet with the trunk in a supine position and legs elevated) was carried on for three months. Following the initial stages of complex physical therapy it is important for these patients to continue to wear their compression garments to prevent any relapse (9).

The effect of physical treatment has also been studied histologically (16). High-pressure compression (70–100 mmHg) produces focal lymphatic damage, initially affecting the endothelial lining of the lymphatics followed by alteration of the lymphatic pools or collectors. Edema is reduced because the fluid in lymphedema is translocated from the interstitium into the lymphatic lumens by means of open junctions and by artificial connections formed from damage in the lymphatic wall. Skin induration is decreased from the loosening of the subcutaneous tissue, formation of large tissue channels and the release of lipid droplets that enter the lymphatics. Some patients with leg edema may benefit from raised leg exercise but this has not shown any benefit when the cause of the leg swelling is due to lymphedema (17).

Table 1 Summary of the Treatment Stages of Complex Physical Therapy

1. Skin care to cure any existing infection and to prevent any further infection from destroying any further lymphatics and to improve skin condition. This involves the use of antibiotics and antifungals as well as educating the patients on the signs and prompt treatment of infection.
2. Lymphatic massage, which lasts about one hour a day, five to six days a week and last for four weeks. The massage starts from the trunk and the normal areas and then moves distally towards the feet or the hands. The massage is light and the lymph is moved toward an already cleared area and encouraging crossing watersheds. After the massage the patients will wear compression garments with pressure of 40-60 mmHg. Eventually greater pressure massage is used to increase collateral lymphatic flow or to soften fibrotic areas.
3. Compression garments are worn after and indefinitely once the massage is finished.
4. Special exercises to supplement the massage are continued indefinitely and some of this has been eluded to in the treatment section above.

Source: Adapted from Ref. 14.

Heat Therapy

This can be achieved by hot water immersion (18), microwave (19) and electromagnetic irradiation (20). Microwave heat therapy treatment lasts for about one hour per day for up to 40 days. Chang et al. used heat therapy in combination with hosiery to reduce limb circumference and tonometry by 5.5% and 10.8% respectively (19). When this was combined with benzopyrones there was further improvement in leg volume and tonometry. This is supported by another group using both microwave (at a frequency of 2450 MHz for 45 minutes each day for a total for 15 days as a single course and repeated for three courses) and hot water immersion (at 44°C for the same amount of time) (18). This method of treatment had no complication during or after treatment.

The mechanism of action of thermal treatment is not fully known. One group suggested that heat by means of electromagnetic radiation produced its effect by increasing the venous return rather than by lymphatic flow (20). Histologically, the skin in lymphedema after heat treatment shows a near resolution of perivascular cellular infiltration, disappearance of the so-called lymph lakes and dilatation of blood capillaries (18). This decrease in the dermal inflammatory process associated with alteration of extracellular matrix may explain the reduction of lymphedema seen after heat treatment.

MEDICAL TREATMENT

Benzopyrones

Benzopyrones are thought to work by increasing the number of macrophages thus enhancing proteolysis resulting in removal of protein and thereby edema (21). In addition, the stimulus it provides for inflammatory and fibrotic process is removed and its presence as a good culture medium for bacterial growth is also eliminated.

Numerous studies exist where benzopyrones have been useful in treating both lymphedema and elephantiasis. In a study of 31 patients with post–mastectomy lymphedema and 21 with leg lymphedema, coumarin (5,6-benzopyrone) given at 400 mg daily for six months was shown to significantly reduce the edema fluid, arm circumference, to increase the softness of the limb and to decrease the elevated skin temperature (22). There were markedly fewer attacks of secondary infection as well as improvement in the symptoms, such as reduction in the bursting pain and feeling of hardness, tightness, heaviness and swelling associated with increased mobility. Side effects (nausea and diarrhea) were seen in only seven patients, which had disappeared by one month of treatment. These findings were supported by another group who showed that benzopyrones reduce limb volume by 20% compared to placebo (23).

In a review of four trials on lymphedema and elephantiasis due to numerous causes including filariasis and elephantiasis, benzopyrones alone provided adequate reduction in the symptoms and signs as well as a decrease in the number of secondary infection, (24). However, its effect was slower when compared to physical therapy and also slower in cases of elephantiasis. The reported advantages of benzopyrones included low toxicity, oral or topical application and with no need for compression therapy, which is particularly helpful for patients who do not tolerate high-pressure treatment (25). The combination of benzopyrones, whether in a topical or oral preparation and CPT is significantly better than CPT alone (26). Benzopyrones are however not licensed in many countries including the United Kingdom, Australia and France because of reports of hepatotoxcity in a small number of patients (27). They may still be being used in other parts of the world because of lack of any other effective treatment such as combined physical therapy.

Micronized Purified Flavonoid Fraction (MPFF)

This is a phlebotropic drug which has been used in the treatment of chronic venous insufficiency, idiopathic cyclic edema and post–mastectomy lymphedema (28). It exerts its action by reducing the capillary permeability and inflammatory component typical of this condition (28). However, to our knowledge no trials of this drug are available at present to look at its efficacy for lower limb lymphedema.

SURGICAL TREATMENT

Only a small number of patients are thought to be suitable for surgery. These are because of unsuitable lymphatic anatomy, the good results obtained with conservative treatment and only if the morbidity cause by the lymphedema leads to problems with lifestyle. Because of the variable results and the small number of patients treated surgically these procedure are generally undertaken in specialized units. There are two types of surgical options: procedures to reduce the limb girth and procedures to improve the lymphatic drainage. Another option is to undertake prophylactic surgery to prevent lymphedema and this is discussed briefly at the end of the chapter.

LIMB REDUCTION PROCEDURES

Before any operative procedures are undertaken, all the patients should undergo lymphangiogram and lymphoscintigram to elucidate the anatomy and to assess if the patients are suitable for bypass. The patients need to be admitted one to two weeks before the procedure for intensive physiotherapy to reduce the limb swelling to allow the operative procedure to proceed with less perioperative fluid loss.

Liposuction

Liposuction has been mainly used in the treatment of arm lymphedema where it has shown very promising results. There is very little published work on the use of this technique in lower limb lymphedema. However there are reports of its use and its effectiveness when used during a bypass procedure or a secondary procedure after a lymphatic bypass (29). Further work is needed to identify this treatment in the management of lower limb lymphedema.

Charles Procedure

Sir Richard Charles described the treatment of scrotal lymphedema by excision of tissue and skin grafting. However erroneously he is credited with the surgical treatment of lower limb lymphedema. This involves the excision of skin, subcutaneous tissue and deep fascia followed by skin grafting (Fig. 1). The skin graft is either taken from the already excised tissues or harvested from a nonaffected area. This technique had shown a reduction in improvement in mobility as well as reduction in cellulitis. However it has numerous complication including the skin graft not taking and subsequent poor cosmetic results. The patients should wear stockings following this procedure as with any of the surgical procedure to reduce the risk of lymphedema.

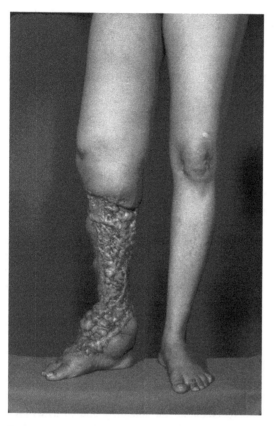

Figure 1   Keloid scarring in skin grafts following a Charles procedure; this intervention effectively reduces bulk but gives poor cosmetic results. (*See color insert.*)

Homan Procedure

This procedure involves raising of skin flaps from the subcutaneous fat followed by excision of tissue down to the deep fascia. The skin flaps are then resutured. It is normal practice to do the debulking procedure in two stages. Initially the medial aspect of the leg or thigh is undertaken because more tissue is removed from this area followed by a lateral reduction a few months later (30). A modification of this method is the Thompson procedure where the skin flap is sutured to the deep fascia to try and increase lymphatic collaterals. However this is no longer routinely undertaken because of complications including scarring and sinuses. Servelle described another technique where the whole limb undergoes a two stage reduction similar to the Homan procedure. This is thought to reduce the chances of recurrence and has been claimed to give good results (31). All of these procedures should only be undertaken if the skin is in good condition.

BYPASS PROCEDURES

Enteromesenteric Bridge Bypass

This procedure was developed by Kinmonth. This involves the mobilization of the ileum and its mesentery which is then isolated from the rest of the small bowel. The resected ileum with its mesentery is then opened up, the mucosa is excised and this is then sutured over bivalved lymph nodes. This is undertaken in patients who have proximal obstruction and has shown moderate long-term results (32).

Lymphovenous Bypass

In this procedure the lymph nodes are anastomosed to veins in either end to end or end to side anastomosis. In a number of studies this procedure has been shown to reduce limb swelling and reduce the incidence of cellulitis (33–35). The procedure is time consuming taking typically four to six hours. There is also the risk of failure of anastomosis which occurs more often in patients with long standing lymphedema. It has also been shown that end-to-end anastomosis are likely to thrombose because of blood reflux into the lymphatic vessel (36). The series by Campisi et al. using end-to-side lymphovenous anastomosis showed marked edema regression in 40% of patients, moderate in 38% of patients, mild in 17% of patients and no improvement in 5% of patients (36).

Lymphatic-Venous-Lymphatic Bypass

This is done in patients who have co-existing venous disease of the legs precluding direct lymphovenous bypass. In this procedure autogenous venous valve grafts are taken from the ipsilateral long or short saphenous veins and used as an interposition graft between lymphatics above and below the obstruction. In a series of 59 patients, Campisi et al. showed significant reduction of edema in 40 of these patients after a five year follow up (37).

Adipo-Lymphatico-Venous Transfer

This procedure was developed because of concerns that microlymphaticovenous anastomosis may have poor patency rates especially in the long-term. This utilizes the long saphenous vein along with 3–6 cm cuff of adipose tissue from the unaffected limb to be transferred on its axis to the contralateral side and anastomosed to the saphenous vein. There is therefore no lymphatic anastomosis. It is thought that the transferred lymphatic tissue will remain viable and result in spontaneous lymphatic drainage. In a preliminary study on five patients there was reduction in the limb swelling after a two to five years follow up (38).

Autotransplantation of the Greater Omentum

This has been developed for use in patients who have hypoplastic lymphedema or long standing secondary lymphedema. This utilizes a free autograft of the omentum which is then anastomosed to the femoral artery followed by lymph nodal-venous anastomosis between the lymph node of the greater omentum and a tributary of the long saphenous vein. In a series of 19 patients there was a more than 50% reduction in limb swelling in 14 of the patients (39). Complications included partial necrosis of the omental transplant and wound infection.

PROPHYLACTIC SURGERY

Two types of prophylactic surgery have been undertaken, lymphovenous anastomosis and omentoplasty. In the first group, 30 patients had a lymphovenous anastomosis done following a ilio-inguinal dissection for metastatic disease. They found that the incidence of lymphedema was only 30% compared to 75% who did not have prophylactic surgery as well as reducing hospital stay (40). Complications included lymphocoele, skin necrosis and wound infection. In the second study patients undergoing retroperitonral dissection for cervical cancer had a pedicled omentoplasty done. There was a reduction in the number of patients with lymphedema compared to the untreated group (41). No complications were reported from this procedure.

SUMMARY

We would emphasize that many different surgical procedures have been performed on small numbers of patients with indifferent short and generally poor long-term results. However the lymphovenous bypass in some centers, particularly in Egypt, has shown good results. In respect to U.K. practice there is an important role for reduction procedures in the most severe cases but the lack of evidence for the other surgical approaches mitigates against their use.

KEY POINTS

- The treatment of lymphedema involves a multidisciplinary approach. The aim of treatment is to control the symptoms and prevent progression of the disease.
- The mainstay of treatment is complex physical (decongestive) therapy. This involves a cycle of massage, wearing of compression stockings, and education to prevent infection and reduce swelling.
- There is no effective licensed drug treatment available in the U.K. for lymphedema. Benzopyrones, which were effective, have been discontinued because of hepatotoxicity.
- Surgery is of benefit to a small number of selected patients. These patients should undergo extensive investigation including lymphangiogram and lymphoscintigram before surgery can be considered.
- Two surgical options exist: debulking and bypass. Debulking involves either excision of skin, subcutaneous tissue and deep fascia followed by skin grafting (Charles procedure) or formation of skin flap, and then excision of subcutaneous tissue (Homan procedure). The former gives at best mediocre cosmetic results while the latter can only be undertaken if skin condition is good.
- The main form of bypass surgery is end-to-end lymphvenous anastomosis or lymphatic-venous-lymphatic bypass. The enteromesenteric bridge bypass is suitable only in a very selective group of patients. Good results have been obtained for the bypass procedure but these are mainly from a few centers.
- Promising early results are available for prophylactic surgery but the role of this modality still needs to be defined.

REFERENCES

1. Tiwari A, Myint F, Hamilton G. Management of lower limb lymphedema. In: Beard J, Murray S, eds. Pathways in Vascular Surgery. Shropshire, UK: TFM Publishing, 2002:106–108.
2. Pierson S, Pierson D, Swallow R, Johnson G, Jr. Efficacy of graded elastic compression in the lower leg. JAMA 1983; 249:242–243.

3. Badger CM, Peacock JL, Mortimer PS. A randomized, controlled, parallel-group clinical trial comparing multilayer bandaging followed by hosiery versus hosiery alone in the treatment of patients with lymphedema of the limb. Cancer 2000; 88:2832–2837.
4. Rudkin GH, Miller TA. Lipedema: a clinical entity distinct from lymphedema. Plast Reconstr Surg 1994; 94:841–847.
5. Zelikovski A, Manoach M, Giler S, Urca I. Lympha-press—A new pneumatic device for the treatment of lymphedema of the limbs. Lymphology 1980; 13:68–73.
6. Klein MJ, Alexander MA, Wright JM, Redmond CK, LeGasse AA. Treatment of adult lower extremity lymphedema with the Wright linear pump: statistical analysis of a clinical trial. Arch Phys Med Rehabil 1988; 69:202–206.
7. Richmand DM, O'Donnell TF, Jr., Zelikovski A. Sequential pneumatic compression for lymphedema. A controlled trial. Arch Surg 1985; 120:1116–1119.
8. Yamazaki Z, Idezuki Y, Nemoto T, Togawa T. Clinical experiences using pneumatic massage therapy for edematous limbs over the last 10 years. Angiology 1988; 39:154–163.
9. Boris M, Weindorf S, Lasinkski S. Persistence of lymphedema reduction after noninvasive complex lymphedema therapy. Oncol (Huntingt) 1997; 11:99–109.
10. Boris M, Weindorf S, Lasinski BB. The risk of genital edema after external pump compression for lower limb lymphedema. Lymphology 1998; 31:15–20.
11. Foldi E, Foldi M, Weissleder H. Conservative treatment of lymphedema of the limbs. Angiology 1985; 36:171–180.
12. Foldi M. Treatment of lymphedema. Lymphology 1994; 27:1–5.
13. Dicken SC, Lerner R, Klose G, Cosimi AB. Effective treatment of lymphedema of the extremities. Arch Surg 1998; 133:452–458.
14. Casley-Smith JR. Modern treatment of lymphedema. I. Complex physical therapy: the first 200 Australian limbs. Australas J Dermatol 1992; 33:61–68.
15. Franzeck UK, Spiegel I, Fischer M, et al. Combined physical therapy for lymphedema evaluated by fluorescence microlymphography and lymph capillary pressure measurements. J Vasc Res 1997; 34:306–311.
16. Eliska O, Eliskova M. Are peripheral lymphatics damaged by high pressure manual massage? Lymphology 1995; 28:21–30.
17. Ciocon JO, Galindo-Ciocon D, Galindo DJ. Raised leg exercises for leg edema in the elderly. Angiology 1995; 46:19–25.
18. Liu NF, Olszewski W. The influence of local hyperthermia on lymphedema and lymphedematous skin of the human leg. Lymphology 1993; 26:28–37.
19. Chang TS, Han LY, Gan JL, Huang WY. Microwave: an alternative to electric heating in the treatment of peripheral lymphedema. Lymphology 1989; 22:20–24.
20. van der Veen P, Kempenaers F, Vermijlen S, et al. Electromagnetic diathermia: a lymphoscintigraphic and light reflection rheographic study of leg lymphatic and venous dynamics in healthy subjects. Lymphology 2000; 33:12–18.
21. Casley-Smith JR. The pathophysiology of lymphedema and the action of benzo-pyrones in reducing it. Lymphology 1988; 21:190–194.
22. Casley-Smith JR, Morgan RG, Piller NB. Treatment of lymphedema of the arms and legs with 5,6-benzo-[alpha]- pyrone. N Engl J Med 1993; 329:1158–1163.
23. Chang TS, Gan JL, Fu KD, Huang WY. The use of 5,6 benzo-[alpha]-pyrone (coumarin) and heating by microwaves in the treatment of chronic lymphedema of the legs. Lymphology 1996; 29:106–111.
24. Casley-Smith JR. Modern treatment of lymphedema. II. The benzopyrones. Australas J Dermatol 1992; 33:69–74.
25. Piller NB, Morgan RG, Casley-Smith JR. A double-blind, cross-over trial of O-(beta-hydroxyethyl)-rutosides (benzo-pyrones) in the treatment of lymphedema of the arms and legs. Br J Plast Surg 1988; 41:20–27.
26. Casley-Smith JR. Treatment of lymphedema by complex physical therapy, with and without oral and topical benzopyrones: what should therapists and patients expect. Lymphology 1996; 29:76–82.

27. Tiwari A, Cheng KS, Button M, Myint F, Hamilton G. Differential diagnosis, investigation, and current treatment of lower limb lymphedema. Arch Surg 2003; 138:152–161.

28. Olszewski W. Clinical efficacy of micronized purified flavonoid fraction (MPFF) in edema. Angiology 2000; 51:25–29.

29. O'Brien BM, Khazanchi RK, Kumar PA, Dvir E, Pederson WC. Liposuction in the treatment of lymphedema; a preliminary report. Br J Plast Surg 1989; 42:530–533.

30. Miller TA, Wyatt LE, Rudkin GH. Staged skin and subcutaneous excision for lymphedema: a favorable report of long-term results. Plast Reconstr Surg 1998; 102:1486–1498.

31. Servelle M. Surgical treatment of lymphedema: a report on 652 cases. Surgery 1987; 101:485–495.

32. Hurst PA, Stewart G, Kinmonth JB, Browse NL. Long term results of the enteromesenteric bridge operation in the treatment of primary lymphedema. Br J Surg 1998; 72:272–274.

33. Gong-Kang H, Ru-Qi H, Zong-Zhao L, et al. Microlymphaticovenous anastomosis for treating lymphedema of the extremities and external genitalia. J Microsurg 1981; 3:32–39.

34. Ipsen T, Pless J, Frederiksen PB. Experience with microlymphaticovenous anastomoses for congenital and acquired lymphedema. Scand J Plast Reconstr Surg Hand Surg 1988; 22:233–236.

35. Huang GK, Hu RQ, Liu ZZ, et al. Microlymphaticovenous anastomosis in the treatment of lower limb obstructive lymphedema: analysis of 91 cases. Plast Reconstr Surg 1985; 76:671–685.

36. Campisi C, Boccardo F, Alitta P, Tacchella M. Derivative lymphatic microsurgery: indications, techniques, and results. Microsurgery 1995; 16:463–468.

37. Campisi C, Boccardo F, Tacchella M. Reconstructive microsurgery of lymph vessels: the personal method of lymphatic-venous-lymphatic (LVL) interpositioned grafted shunt. Microsurgery 1995; 16:161–166.

38. Tanaka Y, Tajima S, Imai K, et al. Experience of a new surgical procedure for the treatment of unilateral obstructive lymphedema of the lower extremity: adipo-lymphatico venous transfer. Microsurgery 1996; 17:209–216.

39. Egorov YS, Abalmasov KG, Ivanov VV, et al. Autotransplantation of the greater omentum in the treatment of chronic lymphedema. Lymphology 1994; 27:137–143.

40. Orefice S, Conti AR, Grassi M, Salvadori B. The use of lympho-venous anastomoses to prevent complications from ilio-inguinal dissection. Tumori 1988; 74:347–351.

41. Logmans A, Kruyt RH, de Bruin HG, et al. Lymphedema and lymphocysts following lymphadenectomy may be prevented by omentoplasty: a pilot study. Gynecol Oncol 1999; 75:323–327.

40

Surgical Management of Chylous Ascites and Chylothorax

Ian Nichol

Department of Vascular Surgery, The James Cook University Hospital, Middlesbrough, U.K.

CHYLOUS ASCITES

Following disruption or obstruction of the abdominal lymphatic channels lymphatic fluid may accumulate within the peritoneal or thoracic compartments, termed chylous ascites and chylo-thorax respectively. Chylous ascites is the extravasation of milky or creamy peritoneal fluid that is rich in triglycerides as a result of the presence of lymphatic fluid in the abdominal cavity. Asellio in 1622 described the lymphatics in a dog and observed a white milky fluid having transected a mesenteric lymphatic. In 1647 Pecquet described the thoracic duct and its connection to the bowel lymphatics. The first reports of chylothorax and chyloperitoneum are attributed to Bartholin in 1651 and Morton in 1694 respectively (1). Press reported an incidence of one case of chyloperitoneum per 20,000 admissions over a 20 years period (2). The incidence is however increasing due to increasing retroperitoneal and thoracic surgery and increasing survival of patients with malignant disease. During the later years of Press' study there was an incidence of one per 12,000.

Anatomy of the Lymphatics

The lymphatic system provides a means by which fluids and protein can return to the vascular circulation and is composed of numerous channels containing one-way valves that drain the interstitial spaces of tissues. The lymphatics also play an essential role on transporting debris and bacteria to the lymph nodes where phagocytosis can occur (1). Gastrointestinal lymphatics transport absorbed water and lipids in the form of chylomicrons to the circulation. Lymphatics in the abdominal cavity are located in the omentum, the diaphragm and the small intestinal wall. The first lymphatic vessels are saccular structures originating from interconnecting endothelial tubes. These lymphatics lie adjacent to capillaries and can be seen in the seromuscular layer of the small intestine. Abdominal lymphatic vessels converge to form the cisterna chyli which classically lies on the anterior aspect of the first or second lumber vertebrae on the right side of the aorta.

Usually the cisterna chyli is formed by the ascending vertical lumbar lymphatic trunks merging posterior and medial to the aorta behind the left crus of the diaphragm. The cisterna chyli represents the termination of the retroperitoneal lymphatics and the beginning of the thoracic duct that emerges from the superior end. The cisterna chyli may be absent in 50% of subjects and may then be replaced by a retroperitoneal plexus that then merges with the thoracic duct. The thoracic duct passes through the aortic hiatus entering the right posterior mediastinum, where it crosses to the left at the level of the fifth lumbar vertebrae and enters the venous system at the confluence of the left internal jugular and subclavian veins (3). The daily volume of lymph ranges between 1500 and 2400 ml, this can be altered by diet as starving reduces while long chain triglycerides increase flow (4).

Physiological Mechanisms of Chylous Ascites

The underlying pathophysiological mechanisms of chylous ascites are related to disruption of the lymphatic system which may occur due to either traumatic injury or benign or malignant obstruction. There are three described mechanisms for the development of chylous ascites (5,6):

1. Lymph node fibrosis due to malignant change can obstruct lymph flow from the gut into the cisterna chyli and lead to extravasation of lymph from dilated subserosal and mesenteric lymphatics into the peritoneal cavity. Chronic obstruction can lead to thickening of the basement membrane due to collagen deposition which can impair gut absorption and a resulting protein losing enteropathy with diarrhea, malabsorption and malnutrition.
2. Exudation of lymph through the walls of retroperitoneal megalymphatics may occur with or without a visible fistula into the peritoneal cavity may occur as a result of congenital lymphangiectasia or thoracic duct obstruction.
3. Thoracic duct obstruction may result in dilated retroperitoneal lymphatics and cause direct chyle leakage through a lymphoperitoneal fistula.

Chylous ascites may also result from increased lymph production as consequence of increased caval or hepatic venous pressures as occurs in patients with heart failure of various aetiologies (7). Cirrhosis also increases lymph production (8). A high fat diet enhances intestinal lymph flow and protein flux. Thoracic duct lymph flow averages 1 ml/kg/h but may increase to 200 ml/kg/hr after a fatty meal (9). This leads to an average of 70 g of fat and 50 g of protein passing down the thoracic duct daily. Conversely fasting and low fat elemental diets reduce lymphatic flow. Medium and short chain triglycerides can be absorbed directly in the portal circulation, whereas long chain fatty acids are incorporated into chylomicrons and absorbed into the lymphatic circulation (10). Obstruction of lymphatic flow results in intestinal edema and exudation of lymph into the peritoneal cavity with significant protein and fat loss (6).

Etiology

Chylous ascites may result from numerous aetiologies including congenital lymphatic defects, infective causes, liver cirrhosis, malignancy, abdominal trauma and iatrogenic injury (Table 1) (3). In the developed world malignancy and cirrhosis account for two-thirds of all cases of chylous ascites (2). In the developing world however infections such as filariasis and tuberculosis account for the majority of cases (11,12). Determination of the cause of a patient's chylous ascites is extremely important in planning the management of these patients. Malignant lymphoma accounts for 85% of all cases in the developed

Table 1 Etiology of Chylous Ascites

	Primary lymphatic hypoplasia
Congenital	Yellow nail syndrome
	Klippel–Trenaunay syndrome
	Primary lymphatic hyperplasia
Neoplastic	Lymphoma
	Lymphangiomyomatosis
	Carcinoid tumors
Cirrhosis	
Infections	Tuberculosis
	Filariasis
Inflammatory	Radiation
	Pancreatitis
Postoperative	Abdominal aortic aneurysm repair
	Retroperitoneal node dissection
Trauma	Blunt abdominal trauma
	Battered-child syndrome
Cardiac	Dilated cardiomyopathy
	Right heart failure

world (13). Congenital lymphatic abnormalities are more frequently observed in children. Primary lymphatic hypoplasia presents with lower limb lymphedema, chylothorax, chylous ascites or a combination of these (10,14). Turners and yellow nail syndrome are associated, indeed 80% of Turners syndrome patients suffer some degree of lymphoedema. The yellow nail syndrome consists of lower limb lymphedema resulting from hypoplastic lymphatics associated with a yellow nail dystrophy (15). The Klippel–Trenaunay syndrome is an autosomal dominant disorder characterized by venous and lymphatic hypoplastic malformations that result in lower limb lymphedema and tissue hypertrophy and often chylous ascites (16). Primary lymphatic hyperplasia can cause chylous ascites and consists of two forms. In bilateral hyperplasia the lymphatics are not severely dilated and contain valves whereas in lymphangiectasia they are very dilated and lack valves. Abdominal radiotherapy causes fibrosis that may result in lymphatic obstruction in the small bowel and mesentery and consequent lymph extravasation (17). Typically this occurs 12 months after radiotherapy (18,19). Pancreatitis can rarely cause chylous ascites by compression of retroperitoneal lymphatics and direct damage by the inflamed pancreas producing enzymes (20). By increasing hepatic venous pressure constrictive pericarditis can cause chylous ascites by increasing lymph production and decreasing drainage (21). Other causes include retroperitoneal fibrosis, sarcoidosis, retractile mesenteritis and Whipple's disease. Tumors cause chylous ascites by obstruction and invasion of lymphatic channels (1). Lymphoma is the most common cause. Others include breast, pancreatic, colon, renal, testicular, ovarian, prostate, lymphangiomyomatosis and carcinoid tumors. Chylous ascites can occur early after one week from surgical disruption of the lymphatic vessels or after several weeks to months due to adhesions or extrinsic compression. Divided lymphatic vessels remain patent for several days in contrast to blood vessels that thrombose rapidly (22). It takes several weeks for a divided lymphatic to reconstitute. The surgical procedures that may result in chylous ascites are retroperitoneal lymphnode dissection, abdominal aortic aneurysm repair, inferior vena cava resection and peritoneal dialysis catheter insertion. Aneurysm repair is the most common cause (80%) of all postoperative cases of chylous ascites due to surgical injury to retroperitoneal lymphatics or the cisterna chyli (23). It is, however, still a rare complication accounting for less than 1% of all complications post-aneurysm repair (24). Repair of ruptured aneurysm and inflammatory aneurysm may increase the risk of developing chylous ascites post-operatively (23). Blunt abdominal trauma resulting in intestinal or mesenteric injury may also produce chylous ascites (1,25,26). In children the so called Battered-Child syndrome is responsible for 10% of pediatric cases of chylous ascites. Chylous ascites is present in 0.5–1% of patients with cirrhosis and ascites and be the result of hepatocellular carcimoma, shunt surgery or thoracic duct injury from sclerotherapy (27–29). In cirrhosis chylous ascites results from rupture of serosal lymphatics due to the excessive lymph production caused by cirrhosis.

Symptoms and Signs of Chylous Ascites

Chylous ascites presents as progressive painless abdominal distension that occurs over a period of weeks to months depending on the etiology. Patients may complain of weight gain and dyspnoea due to diaphragmatic splinting. Other non-specific symptoms may be abdominal pain, weight loss, diarrhea, steatorrhea, edema, nausea, anorexia, fevers and night sweats (1,2,5). Children may present with vomiting and scrotal edema due to a patent processus vaginalis (1). Examination may reveal ascites, pleural effusions, lymphadeno-pathy, lymphedema, and signs of weight loss and malnutrition. The features of liver disease may be present if cirrhosis is the cause. Uncommonly the presentation is with acute abdominal pain due to acute chylous peritonitis. The pain is very severe and on examination signs of peritonism may be present (30). Usually this is diagnosed as being due to appendicitis, cholecystitis or a perforated viscus. The correct diagnosis is usually only established at laparotomy. Peritoneal chyle is non-irritating and therefore should not cause pain unless infection is present. Pain may also result from stretching of the retroperitoneum or mesenteric serosa (20). Morbidity and mortality associated with chylous ascites are primarily related to the underlying pathology. Those cases associated with malignancy have a poor outcome. High output fistulas are associated with haemodynamics instability, renal impairment, and malnutrition. There is an increased risk of infection due to reduced humoral and cellular immunity due to the loss of the large number of lymphocytes in chyle. When the daily chyle output exceeds 1 l the loss of 20–30 g/day protein and 5–30 g/day of fat occurs (31). Should this loss continue for more than a few days the total parenteral nutrition is unable to compensate for the protein loss in addition to basal energy requirements.

Investigation of Chylous Ascites

Abdominal paracentesis is fundamental to the diagnosis of chylous ascites as chyle is the only body fluid with a fat content greater than plasma (1). Chyle has the appearance of a cloudy milky fluid which separates into a creamy layer on standing, in contrast to the straw coloured fluid of normal ascites due to cirrhosis. The protein level is half that of plasma; however, the electrolyte composition is similar to plasma (1). An ascitic fluid triglyceride concentration greater than 200 mg/dl is diagnostic although some authors suggest a level of greater than 110 mg/dl as a threshold for diagnosis (2,32). The triglycerides ascites/serum ratio >1 and cholesterol ascites/serum ration <1 has been advocated (33). Importantly these parameters may not be accurate in cirrhotic patients due to dilution from transudative ascites. In addition the chemical composition of chyle varies greatly between individuals and protein and fat content vary with diet. In patients in whom the triglyceride level is equivocal (50–100 mg/dl) then lipoprotein analysis can be useful which reveals predominantly chylomicrons. It is important to distinguish chylous ascites from pseudochylous ascites in which the turbid milk-like appearance is due to cell degeneration bacterial peritonitis or malignancy. Analysis in these cases reveals a low triglyceride content. Ascitic fluid should be analysed for cell count, culture, Gram stain, protein concentration, albumin, glucose, lactate dehydrogenase, amylase, carcinoembryonic antigen (CEA) and cytology (34). A CEA level greater than 10 ng/ml suggests malignancy despite a negative cytology result (35). In rare cases if carcinoid is suspected urine 5HIAA should be measured and ascitic fluid hyaluronic acid in suspected mesothelioma (1).

Computed tomography (CT) can distinguish between chyle, which has a low attenuation, and acute hemorrhage. CT is also useful in identifying intra-abdominal pathology that may be responsible for the ascites such as lymph nodes and tumors. Hibbeln described CT findings pathognomonic of chylous ascites (36). The formation of a fluid-fluid level in the supine patient was observed with the non-dependent fluid layer having a density consistent with fat. This is analogous to the separation of oil and vinegar in salad dressing (37). The finding of intra- and extra-peritoneal collections in trauma patients may indicate rupture of the cisterna chyli. Lymphoscintigraphy involves the injection of technetium Tc^{99m}-labeled colloid and dextran into the toe web spaces. This allows a functional assessment of the lymphatic system and can demonstrate leakage of chyle from disrupted lymphatics (38–40). Intraperitoneal radioisotope injection to identify the site of leakage has also been described to identify the source of post-operative chylothorax. The advantages of lymphoscintigraphy over lymphangiography are that it is non-invasive, has no contraindications and can be repeated. Pedal lymphangiography is considered the gold standard in defining the exact sites of lymphatic obstruction and extravasation in cases of chylous ascites facilitating repair or identifying the lymph node hyperplasia that results from chylous ascites. Serious side effects of the contrast agent have been reported in 1.2% of procedures with over half of these being pulmonary oil emboli. Exacerbation of chylous ascites is reported in 4% of patients (41).

Treatment of Chylous Ascites

The aims of the management of chylous ascites are to maintain nutrition, decrease chyle formation and correct the underlying problem. Aalami reported a review of 156 cases with 67% being successfully managed with conservative techniques with the remainder managed surgically (1). A study from the Mayo Clinic treated patient with post-radiation chylous ascites with diuretics alone and reported success in 86% of cases (19). Nine of 18 patients with post retroperitoneal lymph node dissection chylous ascites were managed successfully with a low-fat, high protein, medium chain triglyceride diet and diuretics (42). Dietary manipulation has also been described in patient with protein losing enteropathy due to primary intestinal lymphangiectasia. Dietary intervention is the mainstay of non-operative management and aims to reduce lymphatic flow in the major lymphatic vessels and facilitate closure of any disrupted lymphatics (43,44). Closure usually takes one or two weeks and compensation for chyle output during this period is achieved by giving fluid, protein and electrolytes. Dietary restriction of long chain triglycerides avoids the conversion of these into monoglycerides and free fatty acids that are transported as chylomicrons to the intestinal lymphatics. Patients who fail to respond to these methods should be fasted and total parenteral nutrition (TPN) initiated as fasting further reduces lymph production (45). TPN has the advantage that it addresses the nutritional deficits and electrolyte imbalances induced by prolonged chylous ascites. Octreotide, somatostatin and etilefrine have been used to treat post-operative lymphatic leaks and yellow nail syndrome with some success (46,47). The exact mechanisms of actions are unknown but it has been proposed that they act on receptors in the walls of intestinal lymphatic vessels and reduce lymphatic flow (46,48). Patients with underlying malignant disease respond poorly to these conservative methods.

Palliative paracentesis to relieve abdominal distension and dyspnea may be necessary and should be repeated as required. Replacement of intravascular volume with albumin is not necessary unless the patient has underlying cirrhosis. In some patients repeated paracentesis may lead to resolution of the ascites. Repeated paracentesis has the draw-back of introducing infection and peritonitis. Press reported serious complications in seven of 21 patients (2). Repeated paracentesis may also rapidly lead to cachexia due to large losses of protein, fluid and fat. Autogenous reinfusion of chylous ascites has been used but has a significant risk of coagulopathy, sepsis, fat embolism and sudden death (49). Embolisation of a leaking lymphatics has been described by Cope by percutaneous transabdominal catheterization of the cisterna chyli and retroperitoneal lymphatic vessels in post-operative patients. Successful embolization was performed in four of five patients (50).

Peritoneovenous shunts have been used in patients with chylous ascites refractory to medical therapy in poor surgical candidates, in patients with permanent unresponsive disorders and in traumatic and post-operative cases. The initial success with LeVeen or Denver shunts were reported as 75–90%, however, their use is associated with several complications (51,52). Chyle has a high viscosity and therefore the patency has been disappointing with 100% eventual occlusion within three to six months as reported by Browse (5). Sepsis, fever, disseminated intravascular coagulopathy, hypokalaemia, pulmonary edema and air embolism are other complications of shunts (2,53). An advantage over repeated paracentesis is that shunts do not cause nutritional depletion as the chyle is recirculated.

Surgical exploration is reserved for patients with chylous ascites of benign etiology that has been unresponsive to less invasive treatment modalities. Laparotomy for acute chylous peritonitis is essential. The timing of post-operative re-exploration for post-operative chylous ascites is controversial. Early re-exploration may allow identification of the lymphatic fistula which can then be repaired or ligated with immediate control of the leak (54). Identification can be assisted by giving a high fat meal pre-operatively or injecting lipophilic dye intraoperatively. If the leak cannot be identified then suturing of retroaortic tissue may resolve the leak, or fibrin glue may be used to seal the ruptured lymphatic (54,55). Early surgical intervention avoids the metabolic consequences of a protracted lymphatic leak with it ensuing complications. The hazards, however, of operating on malnourished and immunocompromised patients who may not have recovered from their previous operation are high. There is an added risk of graft infection for those patients who are post-aneurysm repair. Browse reported treating 45 patients with chylous ascites (5). Medical treatment failed in 66% and they were treated with either shunts or surgery. Complete resolution was obtained in 33%. Twelve patients underwent closure of a fistula at laparotomy and of these 58% were cured. Laparoscopy is being increasingly used for identifying and treating post-operative lymphatic fistulae (56).

Prognosis of Chylous Ascites

The prognosis depends on the underlying etiology of the chylous ascites. As most patients have underlying malignancy or congenital disorders the prognosis is usually poor. Post-operative chylous ascites, however, has a much better prognosis, an analysis by Pabst of patients with chylous ascites post-aortic surgery reported resolution in 90% overall including those who underwent intervention (54). Of the 27 patients, however, three died as a result of the chylous ascites, giving a mortality of 11%.

CHYLOTHORAX

Etiology

Chylothorax is defined as the accumulation of chyle in the pleural space due to obstruction or disruption of the thoracic duct or a major tributary as it passes through the thoracic cavity. The diagnosis is made by thoracocentesis and the fluid obtained subject to the same diagnostic criteria as those used to diagnose chylous ascites, that is high triglyceride levels and chylomicrons. Should the effusion be large then patients can suffer severe respiratory embarrassment. The loss of chyle leads to metabolic disturbances, malnutrition and immunodeficiency. Chylothorax may be the result of lymphangiectasia with or without thoracic duct obstruction or from chylous ascites moving through the diaphragm. The etiology may be due to malignancy, trauma, post-operative radiotherapy and rare lymphatic disorders such as lymphangioleimyomatosis (57).

Investigations

Lymphangiography is used to define the site of chyle leak or obstruction with penetrating trauma, spontaneous chylothorax and lymphangiomatous malformation (58). It is often difficult to identify the site of leak in patients who suffer a non-traumatic chylothorax and lymphoscintigraphy has been reported as an alternative in these patients (59). Lymphoscintigraphy allows a functional assessment of lymphatic transport and regional lymph nodes. It is fast, safe and non-traumatic. It has been reported as successful in identifying lymphatic obstruction and in the follow-up of patients following treatment (60).

Management

Conservative treatment follows lines similar to those described for the treatment of chylous ascites with dietary manipulation and drainage of the effusion. Repeated or continuous drainage of the effusion may be necessary to prevent respiratory embarrassment. Somatostatin has been used as an adjunct to reduce chyle flow and improve fistulae closure (61). Patients with chylothorax become lymphopenic due to loss of T- and B-lymphocytes in the chyle (62). This results in decreased immunity and septic complications particularly in children. The mainstay of treatment of acute infections is appropriate antibiotics. The loss of B-lymphocytes leads to a reduction in humoral immunity. There are reports of the use of prophylactic intravenous immunoglobulins reducing septic complications by enhancing humoral immunity in children with chylothorax (63). If fluid losses exceed 1.5 L/day for more than five days in an adult or 100 ml/day in a child then conservative treatment should be deemed to have been unsuccessful (64). Patients who fail conservative management require intervention. Ligation of the thoracic duct in cases of thoracic duct injury may be performed safely due to the extensive collaterals and has a 90% success rate. The flow of lymph is channeled to these collateral vessels and new lymphatic vessels will be formed in two to three weeks (62). This may be performed by using either thoracotomy or using video-assisted thoracoscopic surgery (VATS) (65). Patients with lymphoma related chylothorax refractory to conservative techniques have been managed with thoracoscopic chemical pleurodesis with talc or open pleurectomy (66). Adult respiratory distress syndrome (ARDS) is an unusual complication of talc pleurodesis (67). Tetracycline and bleomycin have also been used to achieve pleurodesis (68). After a fatty meal thoracotomy or VATS is performed and the lymphatics oversewn or clipped and then pleurodesis performed. A series of eight patients treated by the Mayo Clinic reported good early results with these interventional procedures (69). Browse reported that from a series of 22 patients parietal pleurectomy was the most successful procedure when no distinct leak could be identified (5). Thoracic duct to azygous vein anastomosis has also been reported with good early results, however Browse reported that all the shunts were occluded by one year follow-up (5). Pleuroperitoneal shunting has been found to be safe and effective in the management children with persistent chylothorax (70). Shunting usually fails in patients with simultaneous chylous ascites and in these patients the diaphragmatic defect must be identified and closed with either glue or a clip. Cope has described percutaneous embolisation of the thoracic duct to treat primary and secondary chylothorax with some success. Intra-operative injury during thoracic surgery is a common cause of chylothorax and it has been suggested that should thoracic duct injury be suspected during open surgery then the duct should be ligated as a prophylactic procedure (71). There are some reports of using fibrin glue either placed directly on the leak site or via a chest tube after thoracic surgery (72,73).

Prognosis

The prognosis of patients with chylothorax depends on the etiology. The mortality rate of adults with non-traumatic chylothorax was 76% after a mean follow-up of 22 months (74). Thoracic duct injury and resulting chylothorax following chest surgery or major neck dissections, untreated, has a mortality is 50% and therefore early treatment is imperative.

KEY POINTS

Chylous Ascites

- Chylous ascites have many causes but the most common are malignancy and chronic liver disease.
- Ascites may also occur postoperatively with aneurysm repair the most common operation involved.
- The aims of the management of chylous ascites are to maintain nutrition, decrease chyle formation and correct the underlying problem.
- The majority can be managed successfully with a low-fat, high protein, medium chain triglyceride diet.
- Surgical exploration is reserved for patients who fail to respond to conservative treatment.
- The prognosis depends on the underlying etiology, with postoperative chylous ascites having a better prognosis and cases related to malignancy a worse prognosis.

Chylothorax

- Chylothorax also has many causes but malignancy, congenital abnormalities and traumatic or postsurgical are the most common.
- Lymphangiography is used to define the site of chyle leak or obstruction.
- Initially treatment should be conservative with dietary manipulation and drainage of the effusion.
- Repeated or continuous drainage of the effusion may be necessary to prevent respiratory embarrassment in some patients.

- If fluid loss exceeds 1.5 liters/day for more than 5 days in an adult or 100 ml/day in a child then conservative treatment should be deemed to be unsuccessful.
- If conservative treament fails, ligation of the thoracic duct is done in cases of thoracic duct injury.
- Patients with lymphoma-related chylothorax refractory to conservative techniques have been managed with thoracoscopic chemical pleurodesis.
- The prognosis of patients with chylothorax depends on the etiology. The mortality rate of adults with non-traumatic chylothorax was 76% after 22 months.

REFERENCES

1. Aalami OO, Allen DB, Organ CH. Chylous ascites: A collective review. Surgery 2000; 128:761–778.
2. Press O, Press N, Kaufman S. Evaluation and management of chylous ascites. Ann Intern Med 1982; 96:258–264.
3. Cardenas A, Chopra S. Chylous ascites. Am J Gastroenterol 2002; 97:1896–1899.
4. McKenna M, Chu JW, Kahkonen DM. Disturbances in lipid metabolism associated with chylothorax and its management. Henry Ford Hosp J 1991; 39:45–51.
5. Browse N, Wilson N, Russo F, Al-Hassan H, Allen DR. Aetiology and treatment of chylous ascites. Br J Surg 1992; 79:1145–1150.
6. Kinmonth J. Disorders of the circulation of Chyle. J Cardiovasc Surg (Torino) 1976; 17:329–339.
7. Hurler MK, Emiliani VJ, Corner GM, et al. Dilated cardiomyopathy associated with chylous ascites. Am J Gastroenterol 1989; 84:1567–1569.
8. Cheng WS, Gough IR, Ward M, et al. Chylous ascites in cirrhosis: A case report and review of the literature. J Gastroenterol Hepatol 1989; 4:95–99.
9. Meinke AH, Estes NC, Ernst CB. Chylous ascites following abdominal aortic aneurysm repair. Ann Surg 1979; 190:631–633.
10. Lesser G, Bruno M, Enselberg K. Chylous ascites: newer insights and many remaining enigmas. Arch Intern Med 1970; 125:1073–1077.
11. Jhittay P, Wolverston R, Wilson A. Acute chylous peritonitis with associated intestinal tuberculosis. J Paediatr Surg 1986; 21:75–76.
12. Patel KC. Filariasis, chyluria and chylous effusion. J Assoc Physicians India 1983; 31:801–803.
13. Oosterbosch L. Chylothorax and chylous ascites due to malignant lymphoma. Acta Clin Belg 1995, 50:20 24.
14. Unger S, Chandler J. Chylous ascites in infants and children. Surgery 1983; 93:455–461.
15. Duhra P, Quingley B, Marsh M. Chylous ascites, intestinal lymphangiectatsia and the "yellow nail" syndrome. Gut 1985; 26:1266–1269.
16. Cohen MM. Klippel-Trenaunay syndrome. Am J Med Genet 2000; 93:171–175.
17. Fox U, Lucani G. Disorders of the intestinal mesenteric lymphatic system. Lymphology 1993; 26:261–266.
18. Keung Y, Whitehead R. Chemotherapy treatment of chyloperitoneum and peritoneal carcinomatosis due to cervical cancer-review of literature. Gynaecol Oncol 1996; 61:448–450.
19. Lentz S, Schray M, Wilson T. Chylous ascites after whole body irradiation for gynaecologic malignancy. Radiat Oncol Biol Phys 1990; 19:435–438.
20. Goldfarb J. Chylous effusions secondary to pancreatic case report and review of the literature. Am J Gastroenterol 1984; 79:133–135.
21. Guneri S, Nazli C, Kinay O, et al. Chylous ascites due to constrictive pericarditis. Int J Card Imaging 2000; 16:49–54.
22. DeBartolo T, Etzkorn J. Conservative management of chylous ascites after abdominal aortic aneurysm repair: case report. Mo Mod 1976; 73:611–613.

23. Coombe J, Buniet JM, Douge C, et al. Chylothorax and chylous ascites following surgery of an inflammatory aortic aneurysm. Case report and review of the literature. J Mal Vasc 1992; 17:151.

24. Halloul Z, Meyer F, Berger T, et al. Chylous ascites, a rare complication of aortic surgery. Vasa 1995; 24:377.

25. Maurer C, Wildi S, Muller MF, et al. Blunt abdominal trauma causing chyloperitoneum. J Trauma 1997; 43:696–697.

26. Bal A, Gormley C, Gordon D, Ellis CM. Chylous ascites: A manifestation of blunt abdominal trauma in an infant. J Pediatr Surg 1998; 33:650–652.

27. Rector WG. Spontaneous chylous ascites of cirrhosis. J Clin Gastroenterol 1984; 6:369–372.

28. Sultan S, Pauwels A, Poupon R, Levy VG. Chylous ascites in cirrhosis. Retrospective study of 20 cases. Gastroenterol Clin Biol 1990; 14:842–847.

29. Vargas-Tank L, Estay R, Ovalle L, et al. Esophageal sclerotherapy and chylous ascites. Gatsrointest Endosc 1994; 40:396.

30. Rosser B, Poterucha J, McKusick M, Kamath P. Thoracic duct-cutaneous fistula in a patient with cirrhosis of liver: successful treatment with a trans-jugular intrahepatic portosystemic shunt. Mayo Clin Proc 1996; 71:793–796.

31. Machleder HI, Paulus H. Clinical and immunological alterations observed in patients undergoing long-term thoracic duct drainage. Surgery 1978; 84:157–165.

32. Runyon BA, Hoefs JC, Morgan TR. Ascitic fluid analysis in malignancy related ascites. Hepatology 1988; 8:1104–1109.

33. Staats BA, Ellefson RD, Budhan LL, et al. The lipoprotein profile of chylous and nonchylous pleural effusions. Mayo Clin Proc 1980; 50:700–704.

34. Runyon BA. Care of patients with ascites. N Engl J Med 1994; 330:337–342.

35. Lowenstein MS, Rittgers RA, Feinerman AE, et al. CEA assay of ascites and detection of malignancy. Ann Intern Med 1978; 88:635–638.

36. Hibbeln JF, Wehmueller MD, Wilbur AC. Abdom Imaging 1995; 20:138.

37. Arsura E. Chylous ascites associated with tuberculosis in a patient with AIDS. Clin Inf Dis 1994; 19:973.

38. Baulieu F, Baulieu JL, Mesny J, et al. Visualisation of the thoracic duct by Lymphoscintigraphy. Eur J Nucl Med 1987; 13:264.

39. Gregg DC, Wells RG, Sty JR. Lymphoscintigraphy. Chylous ascites and lymphocele demonstration. Clin Nucl Med 1988; 13:300.

40. Cope C. Diagnosis and treatment of postoperative chyle leakage via percutaneous transabdominal catheterisation of the cisterna chyli: a preliminary study. J Vasc Interv Radiol 1998; 9:727–734.

41. Nubie M. lymphoedema and chylo-ascites: an unusual complication of lymphography. Neth J Med 1977; 20:18–22.

42. Baniel J, Foster RS, Rowland R, Management of Chylous ascites after retroperitoneal lymph node dissection for testicular cancer. J Urol 1993; 150:1422–1424.

43. Weinstein LD, Scanlon GT, Hersh T. Chylous ascites. Management with medium-chain triglycerides and exacerbation by lymphangiography. Am J Dis 1969; 14:500–509.

44. Ohri SK, Patel T, Desa LA, Spencer J. The management of postoperative chylous ascites. A case report and literature review. J Clin Gastroenterol 1990; 12:693–697.

45. Ablan CJ, Littoy FN, Freeark RJ. Postoperative chylous ascites: Diagnosis and treatment. A series report and literature review. Arch Surg 1990; 125:270–273.

46. Widjaja A, Gratz KF, Ockenaga J, et al. Octreotide for therapy of chylous ascites in yellow nail syndrome. Gastroenterology 1999; 116:1017–1018.

47. Rimensberger PC, Muller-schenker B, Kalangos A, et al. Treatment of persistent post-operative chylothorax with somatostatin. Ann Thorac Surg 1998; 66:253.

48. Shapiro AM, Bain VG, Sigalet DL, Kneteman NM. Rapid resolution of chylous ascites after liver transplantation using somatostatin analog and total parenteral nutrition. Transplantation 1996; 61:1410–1411.

49. Vasko J, Trapper R. The surgical significance of chylous ascites. Arch Surg 1967; 95:355–368.

50. Cope C. Diagnosis and treatment of postoperative chyle leakage via percutaneous transabdominal catheterisation of the cisterna chyli: a preliminary study. J Vasc Interv Radiol 1998; 9:727–734.

51. Varga J, Palmer RC, Koff RS. Chylous ascites in adults. South Med J 1985; 78:1244–1247.

52. LeVeen HH, Wapnick S, Grosberg S, et al. Further experience with peritoneo-venous shunt for ascites. Ann Surg 1976; 184:574–581.

53. Sanger R, Wilmshurst CC, Clyne CA. Chylous ascites following aneurysm surgery. Eur J Vasc Surg 1991; 5:689.

54. Pabst T, McIntyre KE, Schilling JD. Management of chyloperitoneum after abdominal aortic surgery. Am J Surg 1993; 166:194–198.

55. Carones S, Caprossi M, Di Paola S, et al. Postoperative chylous ascites: its etiology and treatment. G Chir 1996; 17:586.

56. Inadomi JM, Kapur S, Kinkhabwala M, et al. The laparoscopic evaluation of ascites. Gastrointest Endosc Clin N Am 2001; 11:79.

57. Romero S. Nontraumatic chylothorax. Curr Opin Pulm Med 2000; 6:287–291.

58. Schulman B, Fataar S, Dalrymple R, Rad FF, Tidbury I. The lymphographic anatomy of chylothorax. Br J Radiol 1977; 51:420–427.

59. Pui MH, Yueh TC. Lymphoscintigrapghy in chyluria, chyloperitoneum and chylothorax. J Nucl Med 1998; 39:1292–1296.

60. Ngan H, Fok M, Wong J. The role of lymphangiography in chylothorax following thoracic surgery. Br J Radiol 1988; 61:1032–1036.

61. Ullibari JI, Sanz Y, Fuentes C, et al. Reduction of lymphorrhagia from ruptured thoracic duct by somatostatin. Lancet 1990; ii:258.

62. Paes ML, Powell H. Chylothorax: an update. Br J Hosp Med 1994; 51:482–490.

63. Mohan H, Paes ML, Haynes S. Use of intravenous immunoglobulins as an adjunct in the conservative management of chylothorax. Paediatr Anaesthesia 1999; 9:89–92.

64. Selle JG, Snyder WH, Schreiber JT. Chylothorax: indications for surgery. Ann Surg 1973; 177:245–249.

65. Janssen JP, Joosten HJM, Postmus PE. Thoracoscopic treatment of postoperative chylothorax after coronary bypass surgery. Thorax 1994; 49:1273.

66. O'Callaghan AM, Mead GM. Chylothorax in lymphoma: mechanisms and management. Ann Oncol 1995; 6:603–607.

67. Mares DC, Mathur PNM. Medical Thoracoscopic talc pleurodesis for chylothorax due to lymphoma. Chest 1998; 114:731–735.

68. Aoki M, Kato F, Saito H, Mimatsu K, Iwata H. Successful treatment of chylothorax by bleomycin for Gorham's disease. Clin Orthop 1996; 330:193–197.

69. Noel AA, Gloviczki P, Bender CE, Whitley D, Stanson AW, Deschamps C. Treatment of symptomatic primary chylous disorders. J Vasc Surg 2001; 34:785–791.

70. Engum GA, Rescoria FJ, West KW, Scherer T, Grosfeld JL. The use of pleuroperitoneal shunts in the management of persistent chylothorax in infants. J Pediatr Surg 1999; 34:286–290.

71. Cerfolio RJ, Allen MS, Deschamps C, et al. Postoperative chylothorax. J Thorac Cardiovasc Surg. 1996; 112:1361–1366.

72. Shirai T, Amano J, Takabe K. Thoracoscopic diagnosis and treatment of chylothorax after pneumonectomy. Ann Thorac Surg 1991; 52:306–307.

73. Akaogi E, Mitsui K, Sohara Y, et al. Treatment of postoperative chylothorax with intrapleural fibrin glue. Ann Thorac Surg 1989; 48:116–118.

74. Romero S, Martin C, Hernandez L, et al. Chylothorax in cirrhosis of the liver: analysis of its frequency and clinical characteristics. Chest 1998; 114:154–159.

Index

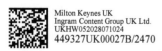

9 780367 390853